WORST PILLS BEST PILLS II

The Older Adult's Guide to Avoiding Drug-Induced Death or Illness

119 Pills You Should Not Use
245 Safer Alternatives

Sidney M. Wolfe, M.D.
Rose-Ellen Hope, R.Ph
Public Citizen
Health Research Group

The authors of *Worst Pills Best Pills*, first edition, in addition to Dr. Sidney Wolfe, were Lisa Fugate, Elizabeth P. Hulstrand and Laurie E. Kamimoto.

To Our Parents and Grandparents

ISBN # 0-937188-52-2

Preface

by **Paul D. Stolley, M.D.**
Professor and Chairman
Department of Epidemiology and Preventive Medicine
University of Maryland
School of Medicine

For older Americans, nothing less than the closest attention to their health problems is adequate. Although many older adults can benefit from drugs which lower blood pressure, reduce the pain and discomfort of angina or arthritis, or treat other common ailments, they are extraordinarily sensitive to adverse effects of medicines, such as drug-induced parkinsonism, confusion, decreased coordination, falls and hip fractures, and mental deterioration. Thus, the best medicine may be no medicine.

But if a drug is needed, the choice should be made by the active and informed participation of the patient with a sympathetic and unhurried physician. Furthermore, the continual monitoring of the patient is necessary after drug treatment is initiated: is the desired therapeutic effect occurring? are there adverse effects? when should the drug be stopped? is there the possibility of an undesirable drug interaction because of other drugs the patient is taking?

The well-informed consumer should ask these and other questions before and after drugs are prescribed. *Worst Pills Best Pills II* spells out the questions you should ask and explains the risks and benefits of the 364 most commonly used drugs for older adults in an easily understandable and interesting manner. The book is printed in a large format and with larger than usual type so that it can be readily used by older persons.

This second edition updates the important work in the first edition in two ways. By reviewing new studies on the 287 drugs in the first edition, it updates information on their safety and adds new information on their interactions with other drugs. In addition, many new drugs, not included in the first edition either because they were not on the market in 1988 or their sales were not yet large enough, are now included in *Worst Pills Best Pills II*. Whereas a small number of them are important drugs, most are either duplicative of existing drugs or have little advantage over those already available. Fifteen of the drugs newly listed as "Do Not Use" add to the 104 listed as "Do Not Use" in the first edition for a total of 119 "Do Not Use" drugs.

Most doctors want their patients to know about the drugs they prescribe and will, if asked, explain and put on the patient's **drug worksheet** the reasons why they have prescribed the drug and what they hope its use will accomplish. This book, and the **drug worksheet** that comes with it, will help guide discussions between patients and doctors, promote safer drug prescribing, and also provide invaluable material for patients to learn on their own. The Public Citizen's Health Research Group and its outside medical experts have once again provided essential information, information which is not available anywhere else, about the most commonly used medicines. As a result, both practicing doctors and patients will benefit from owning and using this volume.

Our medical drugs can provide us with symptomatic relief, comfort, and sometimes cure, but only if they are used with caution and prudence. *Worst Pills Best Pills II* will help older patients, their families, and their doctors reduce the amount of drug-induced disease and increase the likelihood of benefiting from appropriate drug therapy.

Acknowledgements

Worst Pills Best Pills II is the result of the talent, time, labor, and dedication of many people, including past and present members of the staff of Public Citizen's Health Research Group as well as many others outside the group.

The Authors
◆ Sidney M. Wolfe, M.D., Director, Public Citizen's Health Research Group
◆ Rose-Ellen Hope, pharmacist, Veneta, Oregon

The Editorial and Production Staff
Thank you to:
◆ *Phyllis M. McCarthy* for her exceptional organizational skills, limitless know-how, attention to important details, preparation of the manuscript, proof-reading, editing suggestions and her profound caring for those who will use and benefit from this book.

Five other people deserve special thanks. The book would not have been finished without them:
◆ *Alana Bame*, Consumer Specialist, Public Citizen's Health Research Group and *Durrie McKnew*, former Consumer Specialist, Public Citizen's Health Research Group, for editing, proofreading, fact checking and helping out in 100 other ways.
◆ *Lauren Marshall*, Production Manager, Public Citizen, for designing the report, typesetting the report and giving numerous suggestions for improving it.
◆ And, *Dr. Syed Rizwanuddin Ahmad* and *Dr. Ida Hellander*, S.R.A. for research on the newly added drugs.

Other staff helped in numerous ways during the editing and production of the book. They include from the Health Research Group Paul Roney, Benita Adler and Dana Hull. From Public Citizen, they include Linda Beaver, Bess Bezirgan, and Susan Peloquin. And freelancer Kathy Cashel.

Cover design by Joseph Freda.

Overview

When you have read even the first chapters of the book you will know that drug-induced illness is the leading cause of preventable disease in older people, but first, you might have some questions.

Question: **What do the following people have in common?**

❑ **a 58-year-old man who just developed parkinsonism**

❑ **a 68-year-old woman with a hip fracture**

❑ **a 63-year-old woman whose daughter says her memory and ability to think clearly are slipping**

❑ **a 62-year-old man with recent onset of extreme dizziness and occasional fainting when he first gets up**

❑ **a 52-year-old woman who suddenly died while having some dental work done**

Answer: The main thing these five people have in common is that they are all tragic victims of serious but entirely preventable adverse reactions to prescription drugs. In each case, the drug was too dangerous to be used at all or was misprescribed. (See Chapter 2, *Adverse Drug Reactions*, p. 9.)

Question: **I am sure that once in a while prescription drugs, whether prescribed properly or not, can cause adverse drug reactions. But these five cases are unusual, aren't they?**

Answer: Unfortunately, they are all too common. Each year there are approximately *61,000 older adults with drug-induced parkinsonism, 32,000 with hip fractures including 1,500 deaths attributable to drug-induced falls, 16,000 injurious car crashes caused by adverse drug reactions, 163,000 with drug-induced or drug-worsened memory loss, 659,000 who have to be hospitalized because of adverse drug reactions, including 41,000 hospitalizations — 3,300 deaths — from ulcers caused by nonsteroidal anti-inflammatory drugs, usually for arthritis, and hundreds of thousands with drug-induced dizziness or fainting. Over half (50.5%) of the Food and Drug Administration adverse reaction reports of deaths and 39% of hospitalizations related to adverse drug reactions are in older adults. All told, 9.6 million older adults suffer an adverse drug reaction each year.*

Other drug reactions can also lead to death. Older drugs such as *digoxin* (see p. 134), a heart medicine, cause 28,000 cases of life-threatening or fatal adverse reactions a year in hospitals alone, often because the prescribed dose is too high or the drug is given to people who do not need to be taking the drug in the first place. Newer drugs such as the powerful sedative/tranquilizer *Versed* can also be extremely dangerous. Used for so-called conscious sedation during oral surgery or during diagnostic procedures such as gastroscopy, this drug has also caused dozens of preventable deaths. Most were in older people.

Question: **But why are so many people getting adverse drug reactions and how can they be prevented?**

Answer: There are a number of reasons why older adults suffer more and more serious adverse drug reactions than younger people. In Chapter 2, *Adverse Drug Reactions*, p. 9, we discuss nine reasons including physical differences and differences and deficiencies in doctors' prescribing habits.

Recent studies have found that:

❑ 70% of doctors treating Medicare patients flunked an exam concerning their knowledge of prescribing to older adults.

❑ Between 40% and 50% of drugs prescribed for older adults outside the hospital were overused.

❑ Among older patients being given three or more prescriptions upon leaving the hospital, 88% of them had prescriptions with one or more problems, 22% had prescription errors which were potentially serious or life-threatening. The types of these frequent, often-serious prescribing mistakes included:

❑ 59% of patients were prescribed a less-than-optimal drug or one not effective for their disease;

❑ 28% of patients were given doses which were too high;

❑ 48% of patients were given drugs with one or more harmful interactions with other drugs.

But, according to the World Health Organization:

"quite often, the history and clinical examination of patients with side effects reveal that no valid indication (purpose) for the drug has been present."[1]

One of the most succinct explanations for why there is what is clearly an epidemic of drug overuse and preventable damage to older adults is by British geriatric drug expert, Dr. George Carruthers:

"Unfortunately, for a variety of reasons, medications are often used to treat the physical, psychological, social, and economic problems associated with aging, even when there is scientific evidence that drugs are the least appropriate way of managing some of these problems. Rather than having the quality of life improved, the elderly patient may actually suffer adverse effects of drug intervention which was initiated, presumably, with the best intentions. Overuse of medications in the elderly may result."

Dr. Carruthers attributes this serious problem to ignorance on the part of the doctor, differences between younger and older people, and ignorance of the "limitations" of drug therapy. Patients too often see doctors as "drug givers" and themselves as "drug receivers," also because of their own ignorance of nondrug alternatives to many of these problems.

Finally, he discusses the *"illness-medication spiral,"* in which adverse reactions to drugs already being used may be incorrectly interpreted as a new "illness," leading to the prescription of yet another drug, instead of stopping or reducing the dose of the one actually causing the "illness."[2] (See the case of Larry, with drug-induced parkinsonism, in Chapter 2, *Adverse Drug Reactions*, p. 9, for a classic example of this.)

Question: **Are you and the World Health Organization saying that if older people used fewer drugs, more selectively, most adverse reactions would be prevented?**
Answer: Yes, without a doubt that is exactly what we are saying. Most older people are using too many drugs, often for problems which are better treated with nondrug therapy. (See sections on sleeping pills and tranquilizers, p. 198, diabetes, p. 516, and hypertension, p. 62.)

Question: **Just how many drugs do older adults take?**
Answer: Although **older adults (60 and older) make up one-sixth of the population, they use almost 40% of the prescription drugs, an average of 15.4 prescriptions filled a year.** Thirty seven percent of older adults are using five or more different prescription drugs and 19% are using seven or more. Older Americans fill 650 million prescriptions a year. (See Chapter 1, *Are Older Adults Prescribed Too Many Drugs*, page 1, for more information on drug use.)

Question: **If I am not 60 or over, do I really need to worry about these problems?**
Answer: You certainly do, for two reasons. The first reason why this book is also important to people under 60 has to do with the fact that serious problems with prescription drugs do not suddenly start at age 60. Beginning in our 30s, the ability of the liver to metabolize drugs and even more importantly, of the kidney to clear drugs out of the body, and the output of the heart begin to decrease. Since most people in their 30s or 40s are not given many prescription drugs, these changes alone do not usually lead to a large number of drug-induced medical problems. **Many of the**

adverse reactions discussed in this book, however, can occur in anyone at any age. They just occur more often in older adults.

But as people enter their 50s, the amount of prescription drug use starts increasing significantly, and the odds of getting an adverse drug reaction also increase. **The risk of an adverse drug reaction is about 33% higher in people aged 50 to 59 than it is in people aged 40 to 49.**[3] It becomes two to three times higher as people get even older.[4]

For most of the categories of problems which can be caused by drugs, such as depression, sexual dysfunction, memory loss, hallucinations, insomnia, parkinsonism, constipation and many others, the lists of highly prescribed drugs can cause these problems in people of any age. Only for the categories of drug-induced injurious automobile crashes and hip fractures do the drug lists apply only to people 60 and older.

If you do not learn how to reduce (or keep the number low, if not at 0) the number of prescription drugs you are taking when you are in your 30s, 40s or 50s, you will be in great danger of becoming another over-medicated person at unnecessary risk of adverse drug reactions.

The second reason for concern, even though you may be less than 60 years old, is that all people under 60 have parents, grandparents, brothers, sisters, or friends who are over 60 and who could use some of your help in better coping with the onslaught of drugs and other treatments that most doctors are inclined to give out. (See Chapter 4, *Action To Stop the Drug-Induced Disease Epidemic in Older Adults*, p. 670, for specific ways you can help others with the information in this book.)

Question: **How many of the drugs in this book should not be used by older adults?**
Answer: 119 of the 364 most commonly prescribed drugs for older adults — one out of every three drugs — should not, according to published studies and/or Public Citizen's Health Research Group and its

medical consultants, be used by older adults because safer alternative drugs are available. (See Chapter 3, p. 55, for the 119 drugs which we say "Do Not Use" and their safer alternatives.)

This list of "Do Not Use" drugs includes widely used sleeping pills and tranquilizers such as Valium, Dalmane, Halcion, Restoril, Ativan, and Xanax, and antidepressants such as Elavil; painkillers or arthritis drugs such as Darvocet or Darvon, Indocin, and Feldene; heart drugs such as Persantine, Lopid, Aldomet, Dyrenium, and Catapres; gastrointestinal drugs such as Bentyl, Donnatal, Librax, Lomotil, and Tigan; and the widely used diabetes drug, Diabinese.

These 22 "Do Not Use" drugs alone account for more than 80 million prescriptions filled a year by older adults, at a cost of well in excess of one billion dollars a year.

When you look at the 119 "Do Not Use" drugs you will find 97 other drugs in addition to these 22. "Do Not Use" drugs account for approximately one out of every four prescriptions filled by older adults. In three of the major categories of drugs prescribed for older adults, a large proportion are categorized as "Do Not Use" by our medical experts. They include:

❑ 18 of 36, or 50%, of the mind drugs (tranquilizers, sleeping pills, etc.);
❑ 24 of 73, or 33%, of the heart/blood pressure drugs;
❑ 17 of 50, or 34%, of the gastrointestinal drugs.

Even for the 113 drugs which we categorize as "Limited Use" or the other drugs discussed in the book, the number of serious, life-threatening adverse reactions can be significantly reduced even more by using lower doses and avoiding the harmful interactions with other drugs or foods which we list.

Question: **What percentage of the drugs used by older adults are not necessary, too dangerous or are prescribed at a dose that is too high?**
Answer: A conservative estimate is that two-thirds of the prescriptions filled by

older adults — more than 429 million prescriptions a year — fall into one of these three categories.

That is, the drug is:

❏ not needed at all because the problem of the older patient is not one for which a drug is the proper solution.

❏ unnecessarily dangerous wherein a less dangerous drug would give the same benefit with lower risk.

❏ the right drug but the dose is unnecessarily high, again causing extra risks without extra benefits.

Question: **What can be done by older adults and their children and families about this serious epidemic of preventable drug-induced illness?**

Answer: The solution to this problem, a difficult one, will have to involve you, if you are the older adult, your parents, if they are the older adults, your doctor(s), and your pharmacist.

Awareness of the extraordinary variety of "illnesses," often written off to old age, which can be drug-induced is a good place to start. For example, all of the following medical problems have been found, in a significant number of instances, to occur as adverse drug reactions. The number of different drugs listed by name in the tables in Chapter 2 that can cause each type of adverse reaction is included:

❏ 86 drugs which can cause depression

❏ 105 drugs which can cause hallucinations or psychoses

❏ 119 drugs which can cause sexual dysfunction

❏ 65 drugs which can cause dementia

❏ 46 drugs which can cause falls and hip fractures

❏ 22 drugs which can cause injurious auto accidents

❏ 18 drugs which can cause insomnia

❏ 88 drugs which can cause constipation

❏ 29 drugs which can cause parkinsonism

This list does not include those kinds of adverse reactions which are more difficult for patients or their friends to detect, such as early evidence of liver or lung damage, nor does it contain every drug, no matter how few prescriptions there are, which can cause the adverse effects listed here.

The further specific details of how to significantly reduce the risks of drug-induced death and injury are discussed in Chapter 4, including *10 Rules for Safer Drug Use.*

The first step is to take an inventory of all the drugs you or your parents have used in the last month, including over-the-counter and prescription drugs. The most accurate way to do this is **to put all the drugs you are using in a brown bag** and, the next time you or your parents go to the doctor, bring all of these along and **get the doctor to help you fill out the drug worksheet** (p. 674). For each drug you or your parents are using you will need to list the doses, how often the drug is taken and for how long, the medical conditions for which the doctor says each drug is being used, the adverse effects you are having from any of these drugs and other information shown on the drug worksheet. Then you, your parents and the doctor can begin the process of reducing the number of drugs being taken by eliminating the ones which are not absolutely necessary or which are unnecessarily dangerous. At the same time, the drugs which are thought to be necessary can be reduced, if possible, to further decrease the risk of adverse drug reactions.

Question: **When I finally get down to the smallest number of drugs I really need to be taking and the lowest dose of each, is there any way that I can further cut down on the $1200 a year I am now spending on prescription drugs?**

Answer: As is discussed in much more detail in Chapter 5, *Saving Money By Buying Generic Drugs* (p. 678), each year a larger percentage of the drugs most commonly used by older adults are available in usually much less expensive generic form as the brand name version comes off patent. In this chapter, we also discuss and rebut the myths that brand name companies are using to frighten doctors and patients from using these much less expensive drugs.

In addition, many times more expensive, but no safer or effective drugs, are prescribed because they are promoted more to doctors.

A typical older adult might have arthritis and high blood pressure and get prescribed Feldene for the arthritis and Calan SR for the high blood pressure. At costs of $1,008 per year for the Feldene and about $190 a year for Calan SR, the total would be $1,198. But Feldene is a "Do Not Use" drug and the preferred *Worst Pills Best Pills II* alternatives for arthritis, either generic enteric-coated aspirin or ibuprofen, cost about $130 a year. Similarly, Calan SR costs about $190 a year but the first choice drug for hypertension, generic hydrochlorothiazide, can be obtained for only $12 a year. Thus, the yearly drug bill for this typical person would be $142 a year instead of $1,198, or less than one-ninth as much.

On the page with specific information on all drugs (except those in the "Do Not Use" category) the availability of a generic version of the drug is listed at the top.

One last thought: When we hear the phrase **Drug Abuse** these days, the first thing that comes to mind is heroin, cocaine, smack, crack or whatever drug is currently in the headlines. But what about drug abuse in older people? Well, older people do not use **those** kinds of drugs. **That** problem mainly has to do with younger people. But that is taking the narrow view that drug abuse means the drug-abusing person "chooses" to take drugs such as heroin, cocaine, etc. If instead, we broaden the definition of drug abuse to include victims of the choices of others — such as patients of doctors — then **the greatest epidemic of drug abuse in American society is among our older people.** Like other epidemics, it is preventable. This book will help you start that process.

Table Of Contents

Medical Advisors

The following physicians, with expertise in various medical subspecialties, gave generously of their time to read and make helpful suggestions about the drugs that fell into their area of expertise. The categories of drugs they reviewed for the first edition of *Worst Pills Best Pills* are listed in parentheses.

Murray Altose, M.D., Chief of Pulmonary Diseases, Cleveland Metropolitan General Hospital and Professor of Medicine, Case Western Reserve University, School of Medicine, Cleveland, Ohio. (Asthma Drugs)

James Butt, M.D., Acting Chief, Gastroenterology, Veterans Administration Hospital, Columbia, Missouri, and Professor of Medicine, University of Missouri School of Medicine. (Gastrointestinal Drugs)

* *Frank Calia, M.D.*, Chief of Infectious Diseases, University of Maryland and Chief of Medicine, Baltimore Veterans Administration Hospital. (Infectious Disease Drugs)

* *Charles Gerson, M.D.*, physician in private practice of gastroenterology, New York City, and attending physician, Mount Sinai School of Medicine, New York. (Gastrointestinal Drugs)

* *Phillip Gorden, M.D.*, Director, National Institute of Diabetes, Digestive Diseases and Kidney Diseases, National Institutes of Health, Bethesda, Maryland. (Diabetes Drugs)

William Havener, M.D., Chairman of Ophthalmology, The Ohio State University, Columbus, Ohio.

David Jacobs, M.D., physician in private practice of internal medicine, Washington D.C., and attending physician, George Washington University Medical Center. (Nutritional Supplements)

* *Sol Katz, M.D.*, Professor of Medicine, Georgetown University School of Medicine, Washington, D.C. (Asthma Drugs)

Elroy Kursh, M.D., Professor of Urology, Case Western Reserve University, School of Medicine, Cleveland, Ohio. (Urology Drugs)

* *Eric Larson, M.D.*, Professor of Medicine, University of Washington School of Medicine, Seattle, Washington, and author of key studies in which a significant proportion of cases of mental impairment and falls/hip fractures in older adults were found to be attributable to the use of prescription drugs. (All "Do Not Use" Drugs)

Michael Newman, M.D., physician in private practice of internal medicine, Washington, D.C., and attending physician, George Washington University Medical Center. (All Drugs)

George Paulson, M.D., Chairman of Neurology, The Ohio State University, Columbus, Ohio. (Neurological Drugs)

* *Paul Plotz, M.D.*, National Institute of Arthritis, National Institutes of Health, Bethesda, Maryland. (Arthritis Drugs)

Jerry Pomerantz, M.D., Department of Dermatology, Case Western Reserve University, School of Medicine and Cleveland Skin Pathology, Cleveland, Ohio. (Reviewed Retin-A and Rogaine for *Worst Pills Best Pills II*)

* *Linda Rabinowitz-Dagi, M.D.*, private practice, ophthalmology, Atlanta, Georgia and Faculty, Emory University School of Medicine. (Eye Drugs)

* *Louis Rakita, M.D.*, Chief of Cardiology, Cleveland Metropolitan General Hospital and Professor of Medicine, Case Western Reserve University, School of Medicine, Cleveland, Ohio. (Cardiovascular Drugs)

* *Fredric Solomon, M.D.*, Director, Division of Mental Health and Behavioral Medicine of the Institute of Medicine of the National Academy of Sciences, Washington D.C., and Study Director of the Institute of Medicine study *Sleeping Pills, Insomnia, and Medical Practice.* (Sleeping Pills and Minor Tranquilizers)

E. Fuller Torrey, M.D., practicing psychiatrist; author of *Surviving Schizophrenia*; former director of schizophrenic wards, St. Elizabeth's Hospital, Washington, D.C.; and staff member, Public Citizen's Health Research Group. (Antipsychotic Drugs and Antidepressants)

* *Maurice Victor, M.D.*, Distinguished Scholar, Veterans Administration, V.A. Hospital, White River Junction, Vermont; Professor Emeritus, Neurology, Case Western Reserve University, School of Medicine, Cleveland, Ohio; and co-author, *Principles of Neurology*. (Neurological Drugs)

---

* These reviewers also reviewed newly-added drugs for *Worst Pills Best Pills II.*

How This Book Was Compiled

Which Drugs Are Included in the Book?

The decision as to which drugs were to be included in the book was based in part on data from the National Disease and Therapeutic Index (NDTI), published by IMS, Plymouth Landing, Pennsylvania. The survey upon which the NDTI data is based includes the prescribing practices of a large, representative sample of U.S. physicians, determining which drugs they prescribe, how frequently they prescribe each one and for what medical indication, the age of the patients, whether the drugs are used in the hospital or out, the dosage form, and other information. We did not include in the book any drug if more than 50% of its use was in the hospital, such as a number of antibiotics, drugs for general anesthesia, and other drugs. We also did not include most drugs used primarily for the treatment of cancer.

After excluding the drug categories listed above, based on the number of prescriptions written for each, we ranked all the drugs and listed for the book those which were prescribed most often for people 60 and older. We added several drugs that have only recently come on the market but which we thought will shortly have usage that would place them among the most often prescribed drugs. The antibiotics azithromycin and clarithromycin are examples of such newer drugs. The total number of drugs listed in the book is 364; the names appear in the Index and the Table of Contents. The generic names are in lower-case letters, and the brand names are in capital letters.

What Information Goes Into the Discussions of Specific Drugs?

In addition to information that is referenced, much of the other information comes from the *Physicians' Desk Reference* and the *USP DI* (the United States Pharmacopeia Dispensing Information).

On What Basis Is a Drug Listed as "Do Not Use"?

For each of the 119 drugs listed as "Do Not Use" for older adults, at least one or more of the following reasons was used as the basis for the decision:

1. Published references explicitly stating not to use the drug in older adults.
2. Lack of evidence of effectiveness of the drug in the opinion of Public Citizen's Health Research Group and its consultants.* This was most commonly seen in combination drugs in which at least one ingredient has not been proven to be effective or the second ingredient has not been proven to significantly add to the effectiveness of the first. Therefore the drug is more dangerous than an alternative without the unproven ingredient because it has increased risks posed by the extra ingredient without any increased benefit.
3. Fixed-combination drugs that do not, in the opinion of Public Citizen's Health Research Group and its consultants,* meet the World Health Organization's criteria for justifying their use in older adults: " Use fixed combinations of drugs only when they are logical and well studied and they either aid compliance or improve tolerance or efficacy. **Few fixed combinations meet this standard.**"
4. Single-ingredient drugs that, in the opinion of Public Citizen's Health Research Group and its consultants,* are not as safe for older adults as the alternative drug or other treatment that is always listed on the page to the right of the "Do Not Use" designation.

On What Basis is a Drug Listed as "Limited Use"?

Drugs were designated for "Limited Use" on the basis of one or more of the following criteria:

1. Published studies stating that the drug should only be used as a second-line drug if another drug does not work.
2. Published studies showing that the drug is more dangerous than another, preferable drug but not so much so that it merits being listed as "Do Not Use."
3. Published evidence that the drug, although effective and safe enough for the treatment of certain conditions, is widely used in older adults for inappropriate and therefore unnecessarily unsafe purposes. The widespread use of antipsychotic drugs for treating older adults who are not psychotic (see p. 208) is an example of this serious problem.
4. Combination drugs that should be reserved for second-choice use. Examples are many combination high blood pressure drugs which are required to carry a warning label. The label states that, because it is a fixed-combination drug, the drug is not indicated for initial treatment of high blood pressure.

---

* *All drugs were initially reviewed by Public Citizen's Health Research Group staff to decide which ones should be listed as "Do Not Use." Subsequently, all drugs were also reviewed by a specialist in internal medicine, and, depending on their therapeutic category, most drugs were also reviewed by at least one specialist in areas including cardiology, gastroenterology, neurology, ophthalmology, and psychiatry. Finally, all of the "Do Not Use" drugs were reviewed by an internist specializing in geriatric medicine. Each drug met either criterion 1 or 2 listed above for "Do Not Use" and/or was thought by Public Citizen's Health Research Group staff and at least two or more of the above consultants to merit a "Do Not Use" designation for older adults. (The names and affiliations of these consultants are listed on p. xiv.)*

Notes for How This Book Was Compiled

1. *Drugs for the Elderly*. World Health Organization, Copenhagen, Denmark, 1985.

2. Carruthers SG. Clinical Pharmacology of Aging. In *Fundamantals of Geriatric Medicine*. New York: Raven Press, 1983.

3. Vestal RE, ed. *Drug Treatment in the Elderly*. Sydney, Australia: ADIS Health Science Press, 1984. Calculation of 33% increase in risk of adverse reaction (age 50-59 vs 40-49) is based on an average of all three studies listed on page 32.

4. Avorn JL, Lamy PP, Vestal RE. Prescibing for the elderly safely. *Patient Care*, June 30, 1982.

Index

You can use this index to look up any drug included in Chapter 3 of this book by either its generic name (lower-case letters) or its brand name (CAPITAL LETTERS). This index lists not only the limited number of brand names that are included in Chapter 3, but also additional brand names for the same drugs. If your brand name drug is listed below with a "see [generic name]" note after it, check the page number that is listed and look for that generic name. The information on that page will be applicable to your drug, even if the brand name you use is not listed there.

> People should seek physician consultation before deciding to make any change in their prescription drugs based on information in this book.

B

E

Q

R

U

CHAPTER 1

Are Older Adults Prescribed Too Many Drugs?

There are 42.3 million older adults, that is, people 60 and over, living in the United States.[1] **In 1991, older Americans filled 650 million prescriptions for drugs at retail drugstores, for an average of 15.4 prescriptions per person.**[2] **Thus, although people 60 and over make up just 16.7%, one-sixth, of the population, they use 38.5%, of the prescription drugs**[3] **at an annual cost of well over $14.3 billion. All other Americans got an average of only 4.9 prescriptions per year, less than one-third as many as older adults.**[4]

Another way of looking at the problem of too many drugs for older adults is to ask how many different drugs an average person takes in a year, since some of the 15.4 prescriptions per person are refills. A survey of older adults, this time people 65 and over, found that **61% of people 65-84 years old dwelling in the community (not in nursing homes or the hospital) got three or more different prescription drugs in a year, 37% got five or more, and 19% got seven or more different drugs.**[5] (In nursing homes, an even larger proportion of people were given an extraordinary number of drugs, with 34% of 65- to 84-year-old residents getting seven or more different prescription drugs in a year.)[6]

Yet another way of measuring the extent of prescription drug use by older adults is to find out what percentage are using different categories of drugs. The same study mentioned above found that:

❑ 65% of people 65 to 84 (who were not in nursing homes or hospitals) took a cardiovascular drug (for heart disease, high blood pressure, or other heart/blood vessel diseases) and 33% used a psychotropic drug (tranquilizer, sleeping pill, or antidepressant);

❑ 24% used a gastrointestinal drug (for ulcers, constipation, colitis, etc.).[7]

An even larger proportion of older adults in nursing homes were being given drugs in each of these therapeutic categories, especially the mind-altering drugs which were used by 61% of 65 to 84-year-olds.

Although older adults do have more chronic diseases than those who are younger and therefore may need more drugs than younger people, **there is mounting evidence that many of our older citizens are getting prescription drugs which are entirely unnecessary (the wrong diagnosis has been made or nondrug therapy would work), they are getting a more dangerous drug when a much less dangerous one would work (a Worst Pill, instead of a safer pill), or a lower dose of the same drug would give the same benefits with lower risks.**

A very serious problem concerning the use of drugs by older adults is that many of the "illnesses" for which they seek and are given drug treatment are problems which are, in fact, adverse drug reactions to drugs already being used which were not recognized by either patient or doctor as such.

In Chapter 2, *Adverse Drug Reactions*, p. 9, we list common adverse drug reactions which might be mistaken for diseases in older people. These "diseases," in this case drug-induced, include memory loss, confusion, depression, parkinsonism, falls and hip fractures, constipation, and urinary incontinence. We list, for each kind of adverse reaction, the drugs that have been shown to cause it.

A recent review of 19 studies measuring the appropriateness of medication use on the elderly — looking at the prescribing patterns of doctors for older adults outside of the hospital — found "that 40% to 50% of the medications studied were overused in outpatients." The categories of drugs included psychotropic drugs (tranquilizers, etc.), gastrointestinal drugs and antibiotics.[8]

The three categories of drugs that are most often overprescribed and misprescribed for older adults are mind-affecting drugs (tranquilizers, sleeping pills, and antipsychotic drugs), cardiovascular drugs, and gastrointestinal drugs.

To get an even better, more specific idea of the use of prescription drugs in older adults, we can look at the use and misuse of specific drugs within these three major categories.

Which Mind-Affecting Drugs Are Overprescribed?

This category of drugs, probably the one which older (and many younger) adults are most victimized by, includes minor tranquilizers, sleeping pills, antipsychotic drugs, and antidepressant drugs. These drugs are behind only heart drugs and painkillers, and are thus the third most frequently prescribed category of drugs for older adults. All together, **we list and discuss 36 of these drugs in this book. Eighteen (50%) of the drugs whose "purpose" it is to affect the mind are listed in this book as "Do Not Use" because of safety problems.** (See chapters on tranquilizers and sleeping pills, p. 198, antipsychotics, p. 208, antidepressants, p. 215.)

For example, the three most dangerously overused kinds of drugs within the larger

---

Older Adults, 60 and Older, Make Up One-Sixth of the Population But Are Prescribed:
Well over —
❑ **One-third of the minor tranquilizers**
❑ **One-third of the major tranquilizers (antipsychotics)**
❑ **One-half of the Sleeping Pills**
❑ **One-third of the Antidepressants**

---

category of psychotropic (mind-affecting) drugs are so-called *minor tranquilizers* such as **VALIUM, LIBRIUM, XANAX, and TRANXENE,** *sleeping pills* such as **DALMANE, HALCION, RESTORIL,** and the less-used *barbiturates,* and *antipsychotic* drugs, sometimes called *major tranquilizers.*

Minor Tranquilizers

As mentioned above, older adults (60 and over) make up one-sixth of the population but, for minor tranquilizers, they are given well over one-third of the prescriptions,[9] often for much longer periods of time than are safe or effective. As discussed in the section on tranquilizers, p. 198, **1.5 million older adults are being given minor tranquilizers daily for one year or more even though there is no evidence that they are effective for more than several months.**

Sleeping Pills

There is even more massive overprescribing of sleeping pills for older adults, wherein people 60 and over, again, one-sixth of the population, are prescribed over 50% of the sleeping pills used in the United States[10], **with more than a half million older people (see sleeping pills, p. 198) using these pills daily for one month or longer even though there is no evidence that they are effective for that long.**[11,12]

Antipsychotic Drugs (Major Tranquilizers)

The third category of widely overprescribed mind-affecting drugs for older people is the *antipsychotic drugs,* sometimes called *major tranquilizers.* These drugs are a major culprit in drug-induced Parkinson's disease and other serious adverse drug reactions even though the incidence of schizophrenia, the main disease for which these drugs are properly prescribed, is actually lower in people over 60 than in younger people.[13]

However, as with sleeping pills and the minor tranquilizers, a disproportionate fraction of these drugs is unleashed on older adults. **Again remembering that people 60 and over make up one-sixth of the population, more than one-third (37%) of these powerful antipsychotic drugs are prescribed for people 60 and over.** As discussed in the section on antipsychotic drugs, (p. 208) about 80% of the prescriptions in older adults for these powerful drugs are unjustified.

Which Heart, Blood Vessel, Cholesterol-lowering and Blood Pressure Drugs Are Overprescribed?

The largest category of drugs prescribed for older adults by far, 73 out of the 364 drugs in the book, are drugs for treating heart disease, high blood pressure, and diseases of blood vessels.

24 of the 73 drugs, or 32.9%, are listed in this book as "Do Not Use," mainly because of the unnecessary risks they pose.

Although high blood pressure is more common in older adults than in younger people, there is evidence that even the category of drugs used to treat this disease may be overprescribed.

In 1986, older adults filled 140 million prescriptions for antihypertensive drugs, including diuretics (water pills). This means that for every adult 60 and older, there was an average of 3.5 prescriptions for these antihypertensive drugs filled in 1986. One study found that 41% of patients 50 and older who were carefully taken off of their high blood pressure medications did not need them, having normal blood pressure 11 months after the drug was stopped.[14]

This suggests that a large proportion of older adults are being put on or kept on antihypertensive drugs who would do very well off them, gladly forgoing the adverse effects and the unnecessary expense.

> ❏ 65% of all high blood pressure drugs in the United States are used by older adults, who make up one-sixth of the population.

Another example of a dangerously misprescribed drug for older adults within the family of *high blood pressure drugs* are those containing *reserpine* (commonly prescribed examples include **SER-AP-ES**, **DIUPRES**, and **HYDROPRES**), a chemical which has caused many cases of drug-induced depression, sometimes leading to suicides. **All of these drugs are listed as "Do Not Use."**

> ❏ 69% of the reserpine-containing high blood pressure drugs used in the United States are used by older adults, who make up one-sixth of the population.

Drugs that are supposed to dilate blood vessels in the legs or head (to compensate for narrowed, hardened arteries) such as **PAVABID**, **VASODILAN**, and **CYCLOSPASMOL**, but which are not effective and present risks to older adults without any benefits are another class of drugs which victimize older adults.

> ❏ 84% of the blood vessel dilating drugs used in the United States are used by older adults, who make up one-sixth of the population.

Digoxin, used to treat heart failure and arrythmias, is another drug that is often overprescribed for older adults.[15] One recent study of people using digoxin outside the hospital found that four out of ten people were getting no benefit from the drug.[16] Because of digoxin's toxic effects, taking the drug when it has no benefit is not only wasteful but also dangerous. As many as one out of five digoxin users develops signs of toxic effects,[17] and much of this could be prevented if the people who did not need digoxin were taken off the drug. Evidence shows that **the majority (between 50 and 80%) of long-term digoxin users can stop using the drug** successfully, **under close supervision by a doctor, with no harmful results.**[18]

But as of now, there is an extraordinary amount of digoxin prescribed for older adults. In 1986, older adults filled 22 million prescriptions for digoxin, meaning that for every 100 older adults, there were 56 digoxin prescriptions filled that year.

> ❑ 86% of digoxin in the United States is used by older adults, who make up just one-sixth of the population.

Which Gastrointestinal Drugs Are Overprescribed?

In discussing the treatment of gastrointestinal problems in older patients and the tendency of doctors to overmedicate, the following points were made by two gastroenterologists:

"A knowledge of the patient's life situation and health concerns often allows the therapist [doctor] to use frequent visits, prescribed physical or social activities, detailed diet instructions, and the use of innocuous medications (vitamins, antiflatulents [we disagree about the antiflatulents, see page 359, Mylicon]) to overcome boredom and preoccupation with an unoptimistic future. Often patients are treated with substantial amounts of cathartics (laxatives), antispasmodics, when a more appropriate course would be to address diet, preoccupation with a daily bowel movement, and a monotonous daily existence.

"Modern treatment of gastrointestinal conditions usually favors four or six small meals daily, increases [in] the fiber content of the diet for all conditions . . . . Most gaseous conditions are controlled more effectively by deliberately chewing food (to lessen air swallowing) . . . ." [19]

In addition to the changes in eating and living habits that can "treat" many gastrointestinal complaints without resorting to drugs, many of these complaints can also be caused by the use of other drugs. In Chapter 2, *Adverse Drug Reactions*, we list,

by brand name and generic name, the large number of drugs used for a variety of different medical conditions which can cause loss of appetite, nausea, vomiting, abdominal pain, constipation or diarrhea (see p. 40).

> ❑ But again, as of now, although older adults make up just one-sixth of the population, 43% of all gastrointestinal drugs used in the United States were used by people 60 and older.

Looking at this problem another way, 31 drugs for treating gastrointestinal problems are listed in this book. (Many more such drugs, like antacids and laxatives, are purchased over-the-counter.) 12 of these drugs (38.7% of all these drugs), are listed in this book as "Do Not Use," largely because of the unnecessary risks they present.

Among the most dangerously overprescribed gastrointestinal drugs are those used for treating nausea or, in certain cases, for "heartburn," that is, the reflux of food from the stomach into the esophagus. These drugs include **REGLAN, TIGAN, PHENERGAN, COMPAZINE,** and **ANTIVERT.** They are often used before much safer and more conservative measures have been tried (see discussion of these drugs and alternatives in Chapter 3, p. 55). The first four of these can cause many adverse effects, such as drug-induced parkinsonism, similar to those seen with the antipsychotic drugs. Together, prescriptions filled for older adults for these five drugs accounted for about one-half of all use of these drugs.

Another category of misused gastrointestinal drugs, as referred to above, include the so-called antispasmodic drugs, sometimes combined with a tranquilizer such as **LIBRIUM.** Widely used examples, all of which we say **"Do Not Use,"** include **BENTYL, LOMOTIL, LIBRAX,** and **DONNATAL.** These four drugs alone account for more than 4 million prescriptions filled in 1986 by older adults and they subject patients to a variety of unnecessary risks.

Which Other Kinds of Drugs Are Overprescribed?

Two other categories that contain large numbers of drugs which we list as "Do Not Use" in this book are cold, cough, allergy, and asthma medicines, and painkillers. The 21 "Do Not Use" cough, cold, allergy, and asthma drugs account for about one-fifth of all prescriptions for this class of drugs filled by older adults.

In the category of painkillers and anti-inflammatory drugs there are 49 drugs listed, making this class of drugs second only to the heart/blood pressure drugs in how often they are prescribed. We list 17 of these drugs (35% of all these drugs) as "Do Not Use."

In summary, the answer to the question, "Are Older Adults Prescribed Too Many Drugs?" is yes.

Why Is There So Much Overprescribing and Misprescribing In Older Adults?

Although it is easy to blame older patients and allege that they just want to take more drugs, the overwhelming share of the blame must be placed on the drug industry and physicians. The drug industry is responsible for inadequately testing drugs in older adults and then heavily marketing them to doctors, often employing false and misleading advertising campaigns. Too many physicians, too often believing that their accepted role is to end a patient's visit by writing a prescription, fall easy prey to the industry's drug-pushing strategies, especially because of the doctors' often-appalling lack of information about the special problems of prescribing drugs for older adults.

The Role of The Drug Companies

A recently published study examined the extent to which older adults — major users of arthritis drugs — were actually tested during the studies which determined whether the drugs would or would not be approved.[20] Of those 83 randomized arthritis drug clinical trials which were analyzed, there were a total of 9,664 patients studied. Considering that about 33% of prescriptions for arthritis drugs are written for people 65 or older[21] and that older adults are particularly susceptible to serious life-threatening adverse effects of these drugs, such as gastrointestinal bleeding, the findings of this study were very disturbing. Of the 9,664 patients in the 83 studies, only 207 patients (2.1%) could be identified as being 65 or over. Thus, despite 33% of the prescriptions for arthritis drugs being written for those 65 or older, only 2.1% — or 1/15 as much representation — of these older adults occurred in the pre-marketing studies as occurs in the post-approval treatment use of the drugs.

Drug companies' failure to provide geriatric information in the labels of drugs most commonly prescribed to older adults was documented by the Food and Drug Administration. In a survey of 425 of the drugs most often used by the elderly, only 212 — less than one-half — had geriatric information.[22]

The lack of adequate testing and label information from the companies combines with the grossly inadequate amount of training that doctors get about prescribing for older adults to result in dangerous misprescribing and overprescribing.

The Role of Physicians

One study of physicians who treat Medicare patients found that 70% of the doctors who took an examination concerning their knowledge of prescribing for older adults failed to pass the test. The majority of physicians who were contacted for participation in the study refused to take the test, often giving as their reason that they had a "lack of interest in the subject." The authors concluded that "many of these physicians [who failed the exam] had . . . not made good use of the best information on prescribing for the elderly." [23]

It is clear that both the drug companies and physicians have a major responsibility for creating and perpetuating the largely preventable epidemic of drug-induced death and disease in older people caused by misprescribing of drugs.

In Chapter 2, *Adverse Drug Reactions*, we discuss the toll taken as a result of this misprescribing.

Notes for Chapter 1

1. *Statistical Abstract of the United States* 1992, Data for 1991.

2. From 1990 *National Disease and Therapeutic Index* (IMS, Plymouth Landing, Pa.), 38.5% of prescriptions written were for people 60 and older. We estimate this to be about the same in 1991. Using the methods of the Food and Drug Administration in its annual report, *Drug Utilization in the United States*, 1985, the % of prescriptions written for people 60 and older is applied to the actual number of prescriptions filled in the same year. In 1991, according to data from the *National Prescription Audit* (IMS, Plymouth Landing, Pa.), there were a total of 1.69 billion prescriptions filled in U.S. retail drug stores. Since 38.5% of these were written for people 60 and over, 38.5% of this total is 650 million prescriptions. Dividing this by the 42.34 million Americans 60 and older gives an average of 15.4 prescriptions filled per person in 1991.

3. Total U.S. population in 1991 was 252.685 million and the number of people 60 and older was 42.336 million (42.336/252.685=16.75%). *Statistical Abstract of the United States*, op. cit.

4. FDC Reports. *The Pink Sheet*, January 25, 1993. The average cost for a prescription was $22.44 in 1991.

5. Ray WA. Prescribing patterns of drugs for the elderly. In *Pharmaceuticals for the Elderly*. Washington: Pharmaceutical Manufacturers Association, 1986:35.

6. Ibid.

7. Ibid.

8. Brook RH, Kamberg CJ, Mayer-Oakes A, Beers MH, Raube K, Steiner A. Appropriateness of acute medical care for the elderly. *Health Policy* 1991; 14:225-42.

9. *National Disease and Therapeutic Index*, I.M.S. Inc., Ambler, Pa., 1985.

10. *Drug Utilization in the U.S.* 1985. Department of Health and Human Services, Food and Drug Administration, December 1986.

11. *Sleeping Pills, Insomnia, and Medical Practice*. Institute of Medicine, National Academy of Sciences, 1979.

12. Solomon F, White C, Arron D, Mendelson W. Sleeping pills, insomnia and medical practice. *New England Journal of Medicine* 1979; 300:803-8.

13. National Institute of Mental Health, Epidemiological Catchment Area Data from 1981-1982.

14. Hansen AG, Jensen H, Langesen LP, Peterson A. Withdrawal of antihypertensive drugs in the elderly. *Acta Medical Scandinavia* 1982; 676:178-85.

15. Carlson KJ. An analysis of physicians' reasons for prescribing long-term digitalis therapy in outpatients. *Journal of Chronic Diseases* 1985; 38:733-9.

16. Lee DC, et al. Heart failure in outpatients: A randomized trial of digoxin versus placebo. *New England Journal of Medicine* 1982; 306:699-705.

17. AMA Department of Drugs. *AMA Drug Evaluations.* 6th ed. Chicago: American Medical Association, 1984:423.

18. Fleg J. Lakatta E. How useful is digitalis in patients with congestive heart failure and sinus rhythm? *International Journal of Cardiology* 1984; 6:295-305.

19.Vestal RE, ed. *Drug Treatment in the Elderly.* Sydney, Australia: ADIS Health Science Press, 1984:246-7.

20. Rochon PA, Fortin PR, Dear KBG, Minaker KL, Chalmers TC. Reporting of age data in clinical trials of arthritis. *Archives of Internal Medicine* 1993; 153:243-8.

21. *National Disease and Therapeutic Index,* 1985, op. cit.

22. Medicare Drug Utilization Review. Office of the Inspector General, Health and Human Services, April, 1989, p. 9.

23. Ferry ME, Lamy P, Becker L. Physicians' knowledge of prescribing for the elderly. *Journal of the American Geriatrics Society* 1985; 33: 616-25.

CHAPTER 2

Adverse Drug Reactions:
How Serious Is the Problem
and Why Do They Occur?

Although some adverse drug reactions are not very serious, others cause the death, hospitalization, or serious injury of hundreds of thousands of older persons in the United States each year. Most of the time, these dangerous events could and should have been avoided. Even the less drastic reactions, such as change in mood, loss of appetite, or nausea, may seriously diminish the quality of life.

Data from the Food and Drug Administration (FDA) has put the magnitude of this problem of adverse drug reactions in older adults into sharp focus:

Older adults, with those 60 and older comprising just 16.7% or one-sixth of the population, make up a dangerously disproportionate share of deaths and hospitalizations from adverse drug reactions. **Over half (50.5%) of FDA reports of deaths from adverse drug reactions and 39% of hospitalizations from adverse drug reactions were in older adults — those 60 and over.**[1] The fact that much of this toll is a consequence of the dangerous amount of misprescribing of drugs to these increasingly vulnerable people is no longer in dispute.

In addition to these often serious adverse reactions occurring in older adults, many also occur in younger people.

Although the decisionmaking process of dividing all 364 drugs in this book into "Do Not Use," "Limited Use," and all others was based on the idea of the patient being 60 or older, the odds of suffering an adverse drug reaction really begin to increase by age 50. Many physical changes important to the way the body can handle drugs actually

begin when people are in their 30s but the increased prescribing of drugs for most people does not begin then. But as people enter their 50s, the amount of prescription drug use starts increasing significantly and the odds of getting an adverse drug reaction also increase. **The risk of an adverse drug reaction is about 33% higher in people aged 50 to 59 than it is in people aged 40 to 49.**[2]

The World Health Organization, discussing the problem of adverse drug reactions in the elderly, has stated,

"Quite often, the history and clinical examination of patients with side effects reveal that no valid indication [purpose] for the drug has been present. . . . Adverse reactions can to a large extent be avoided in the elderly by choosing safe and effective drugs and applying sound therapeutic principles in prescribing, such as starting with a small dose, observing the patient frequently, and avoiding excessive polypharmacy [the use of multiple drugs at the same time]."[3]

In other words, according to the World Health Organization, patients who suffer adverse drug reactions are very often victims of drugs which there was no valid reason for them to take.

A recent, carefully-controlled study examined the details of prescriptions of people with three or more prescriptions to treat chronic illnesses who were being discharged from a community hospital.[4]

The results of this study are quite disturbing both in what they say about the doctors' prescribing practices and the evidence as to the potential damage that could be done to older adults as a result of these practices. Of the 236 people intensively studied:

❏ 88% of the people had one or more prescribing problems with the prescriptions they were given. 22% of these patients had at least one potentially serious, life-threatening problem which could have occurred as a result of the prescriptions which had been written.

When the specific problems with the prescriptions were examined, the results were as follows:

❏ 59% of the patients had been given one or more prescriptions in which the drug was an inappropriate choice of therapy because it was either "less than optimal medication given the patient's diagnosis" or there was no established indication for the drug;

❏ 28% of the patients were given too high a dose of the drug, an "overdose;"

❏ 48% of the patients were given drugs with one or more harmful drug interactions;

❏ 20% of the patients were given drugs which unnecessarily duplicated the therapeutic effect of another drug they were taking.

The good news from this study, however, was that a consultant pharmacist, involved in the care of more than 50% of these patients, was able to reduce the risks by making recommendations to the prescribing physicians.

Another serious problem exists because doctors and patients do not realize that **practically any symptom in older adults can be caused or worsened by drugs.**[5] Also some doctors and patients assume that what are actually adverse drug reactions are simply signs of aging. As a result, many serious adverse reactions are entirely overlooked or not recognized until they have caused significant harm.

Later in this chapter we will list the most common drug-induced adverse effects along with the drugs which can cause them. In the box below are some of the changes

which, although they are frequently caused by drugs, are the kinds of problems that you or many doctors would first attribute simply to **"growing old," instead of to your drug.**

Mental Adverse Drug Reactions: depression, hallucinations, confusion, delirium, memory loss, impaired thinking

Nervous System Adverse Drug Reactions: parkinsonism, involuntary movements of the face, arms, legs (tardive dyskinesia), sexual dysfunction

Dizziness on Standing, Falls Sometimes Resulting in Hip Fractures, Automobile Accidents Resulting in Injury

Gastrointestinal Adverse Drug Effects: loss of appetite, constipation

Urinary Problems: difficulty urinating, leaking of urine

The drugs responsible for the most serious adverse reactions in older adults are tranquilizers, sleeping pills and other mind affecting drugs; cardiovascular drugs such as high blood pressure drugs, digoxin, and drugs for abnormal heart rhythms;[6] and drugs for treating intestinal problems.

How Extensive Is The Problem of Adverse Drug Reactions?

The following are national estimates based on well-conducted studies in the United States:

❏ *In 1990, an estimated 659,000 older American adults (60 and older) were hospitalized because of adverse reactions* to drugs they were taking before their hospitalization.[7]

❏ Each year, in hospitals alone, there are *28,000 cases of life-threatening heart toxicity from adverse reactions to digoxin*, the most commonly used form of digitalis in older adults.[8] Since as many as 40% or more of these people are using this drug unnecessarily (see discussion of this on p. 134), much of this injury is preventable.

❑ *41,000 older adults are hospitalized — 3,300 of whom die —each year from ulcers caused by NSAIDs* (non-steroidal anti-inflammatory drugs, usually for treatment of arthritis).[9]

❑ *Each year, more than 9.6 million adverse drug reactions occur in older Americans.* The referenced study found that 37% of these adverse reactions were not reported to the doctor, presumably because patients did not realize they were due to the drug. This is not too surprising since most doctors admitted that they did not explain possible side effects to their patients.[10]

❑ **At least 16,000 injurious auto crashes each year in older drivers are attributable to psychoactive drug use** (specifically benzodiazepines and tricyclic antidepressants.[11]

❑ *32,000 older adults a year suffer from hip fractures — contributing to more than 1,500 deaths — attributable to drug-induced falling.*[12] In one study, the main categories of drugs responsible for the falls leading to hip fractures were sleeping pills and minor tranquilizers (30%), antipsychotic drugs (52%), and antidepressants (17%). All of these categories of drugs are often being prescribed unnecessarily, especially in older adults. (See section on minor tranquilizers and sleeping pills, antipsychotic drugs, and antidepressants, p. 198.) Since in-hospital death rates for hip fractures in older adults is 4.9%,[13] multiplying this times the 32,000 hip fractures a year in older adults attributable to drug-induced falling results in 1,568 older adults who die each year from these adverse drug reactions which cause hip fractures.

❑ *163,000 older Americans suffer from serious mental impairment (memory loss, dementia) either caused or worsened by drugs.*[14] In a study in the state of Washington, in 46% of the patients with drug-induced mental impairment, the impairment was caused by minor tranquilizers or sleeping pills; in 14%, by high blood pressure drugs; and in 11%, by antipsychotic drugs.

❑ *2 million older Americans are addicted or at risk of addiction to minor tranquilizers or sleeping pills because of using them daily for at least one year,* even though there is no acceptable evidence that the tranquilizers are effective for more than four months and the sleeping pills for more than 30 days.[15]

❑ *73,000 older adults have developed drug-induced tardive dyskinesia, the most serious, common, and often irreversible adverse reaction to antipsychotic drugs.* Tardive dyskinesia is characterized by involuntary movements of the lips, tongue, and sometimes the fingers, toes, and trunk. Since most of the older people taking these drugs were not actually psychotic, they have a serious side effect from antipsychotic drugs prescribed without justification.[16]

❑ *61,000 older adults have developed drug-induced parkinsonism due to the prescribing of antipsychotic drugs such as Haldol, Thorazine, Mellaril, Stelazine, and Prolixin.* There are also other parkinsonism-inducing drugs such as Reglan, Compazine, and Phenergan, prescribed for gastrointestinal problems.[17] As mentioned above, most (about 80%) of older adults receiving antipsychotic drugs do not have schizophrenia or other conditions which justify the use of such powerful drugs.

Patient Examples

Sarah's 80-year-old Father's Confusion and Hallucinations Induced By His Ulcer Drugs

Sarah wrote us about her father saying that she had to repeatedly nag his doctor about the possible role of her dad's ulcer drugs in causing confusion and hallucinations before the doctor listened. Her father had been tried on three different ulcer drugs — Tagamet, Zantac, and Pepcid — each of which had caused these adverse reactions. When the doctor finally switched Sarah's father to an antacid, Maalox, his mind completely cleared and he was his old self, no longer confused or hallucinating.

58-year-old Man Develops Parkinsonism from Antipsychotic Drug Being Used to Treat His "Irritable Bowel" Problem

Larry, an otherwise healthy 58-year-old man with diarrhea believed to be due to "irritable bowel syndrome," was given Stelazine, a powerful antipsychotic tranquilizer to "calm down" his intestinal tract. Stelazine is not even approved for treating such medical problems. Six months after starting Stelazine, Larry developed severe parkinsonism and was started on L-dopa, a drug for treating Parkinson's disease. The Stelazine was continued because the doctor presumably did not realize the parkinsonism was drug-induced. For seven years, Larry took both drugs. Then a neurologist specializing in Parkinson's disease saw Larry, recognized the real cause of his problem, stopped the Stelazine, and slowly withdrew the L-dopa over a six-month period. Larry's severe, disabling parkinsonism cleared completely.

As mentioned above, 61,000 older adults develop drug-induced parkinsonism each year. At least 80% of them, like Larry, should never have been put on the drugs causing the parkinsonism in the first place. Also, as in Larry's situation, a large proportion of these people have doctors who think that their parkinsonism developed spontaneously.

The doctors not only fail to suspect that it is caused by a drug such as Stelazine, or other antipsychotic drugs, Reglan, Compazine, or Phenergan, but they add a second drug to treat the disease which has been caused by the first drug.

The same neurologist who "cured" Larry of his drug-induced parkinsonism saw, in just three years, 38 other patients with drug-induced parkinsonism and 28 with drug-induced tardive dyskinesia.

None of these people were psychotic, the one justification for antipsychotic medications. Rather, the most common reasons for using the

parkinsonism-inducing drugs were chronic anxiety and gastrointestinal complaints. The most frequent culprit (in 19 of these 39 patients) was Reglan (metoclopramide), usually prescribed for heartburn or for nausea and vomiting. Doctors often prescribe Reglan before trying other more conservative and safer methods. (See alternative treatment of nausea and vomiting, p. 343). Other drugs which brought on parkinsonism included Compazine, Haldol and Thorazine.[18]

79-year-old Woman Has Reversible Mental Impairment

Sally, the mother-in-law of a physician, was noted by her son-in-law, who had not seen her for several months, to have suffered severe impairment of her otherwise sharp mind. She was acting confused and, for the first time in her life, was unable to balance her checkbook. When questioned by her son-in-law, she was able to remember that her problem had started around the time she was put on a tranquilizer, Ativan. After this link was discovered, the drug was slowly discontinued and all of the mental impairment which had begun when the drug was started disappeared.

64-year-old Man Has Auto Accident After One Dose of Tranquilizer

Ben, the 64-year-old uncle of a physician, was scheduled to have a biopsy done at a local hospital at 8:00 in the morning. So that he would be relaxed for the biopsy, four days before it was to be done the doctor gave him a free sample of a tranquilizer, Xanax, to take an hour or so before the procedure. He was not told that he should not use drugs like this if he was going to drive and, while driving to the hospital for the biopsy, Ben blacked out. The car went over a fence, sustained $6,000 worth of damage, but fortunately Ben was unhurt. (See **Drugs That Can Cause Injurious Auto Accidents**, p. 36.)

63-year-old Gets Into "Drug-Illness" Cycle

Nancy, a healthy 63-year-old woman,

complained about difficulty going to sleep. Instead of taking a careful history and finding out that she had recently started drinking several cups of coffee at dinner, her doctor prescribed a sleeping pill. A subsequent referral was also made to a psychiatrist because of depression (possibly partly induced by the sleeping pill), and an antidepressant drug was also prescribed. If this patient also takes an antihistamine-containing drug for a cold (not an effective treatment), she will be using three drugs, all of which have powerful sedative effects, which could make her so groggy that standing would be difficult; falling would be easy.

60-year-old Woman Given "Overdose" of Propranolol

Elsie, a 60-year-old woman who worked as an assistant at a senior citizens' center, was started on propranolol to treat her high blood pressure. Unfortunately, her doctor did not realize that the dose of this sometimes useful drug (see p. 124) must be reduced in older adults, and she was started on 80 milligrams twice a day. Two days after she started taking the drug, she began feeling very weak, so much so that by the third day, she went to a hospital emergency room, where her pulse rate was found to be 36 beats per minute. This dangerously low rate fully explained her weakness. The drug was stopped and Elsie's heart rate returned to normal. She was later started on a low dose of a different drug and had no adverse effects.

Nine Reasons Why Older Adults Are More Likely Than Younger Adults To Get Adverse Drug Reactions (Unless They Are Given Fewer Drugs and Smaller Doses)

Many of the studies and much of the information concerning the epidemic of drug-induced disease focuses on people 60 and over. As we have mentioned previously, some of the changes which eventually lead to more adverse reactions in older

adults (in combination with increased drug use), really begin to occur in the mid-30s. In connection with the idea that drug-induced disease begins getting more common before age 60, it is interesting to notice that a number of studies comparing the way "older" people clear drugs out of the body in comparison to younger people, the definition of older is above 50, younger being below 50.[19]

1. *Smaller Bodies and Different Body Composition.* Older adults generally weigh less and have a smaller amount of water and a larger proportion of fat than younger adults. Body weight increases from age 40 to 60, mainly due to increased fat, then decreases from 60 to 70 with even sharper declines from 70 on. Therefore, the amount of a drug per pound of body weight or per pound of body water will often be much higher in an older adult than it would be if the same amount of the drug were given to a younger person. In addition, drugs which concentrate in fat tissue may stay in the body longer because there is more fat for them to accumulate in.

2. *Decreased Ability of the Liver to Process Drugs.* Because the liver does not work as well in older adults, they are less able than younger people to process certain drugs so that they can be excreted from the body. This has important consequences for a large proportion of the drugs used to treat heart conditions and high blood pressure, as well as many other drugs processed by the liver. The ability to get rid of drugs such as Valium, Librium and many others is affected by this decrease in liver function.

3. *Decreased Ability of the Kidneys to Clear Drugs Out of the Body.* As people grow older, the ability of their kidneys to clear many drugs out of the body decreases steadily from age 35-40 on. By age 65, the filtering ability of the kidneys has already decreased by 30%. This process keeps getting worse with age, along with other aspects of kidney function. This affects a large number of drugs.

4. *Increased Sensitivity To Many Drugs.*
The problems of decreased body size, altered body composition (more fat, less water), and decreased liver and kidney function cause many drugs to accumulate in older people's bodies at dangerously higher levels and for longer times than in younger people. These age-related problems are further worsened by the fact that even at "normal" blood levels of many drugs, older adults have an increased sensitivity to their effects, often resulting in harm. This is seen most clearly with drugs that act on the central nervous system such as many **sleeping pills, alcohol, tranquilizers, strong pain-killers such as morphine or pentazocine (Talwin), and most of the drugs which have "anticholinergic" effects. This latter group includes antidepressants, antipsychotic drugs, antihistamines, drugs which are used to calm the intestinal tract (for treating ulcers or some kinds of colitis) such as Donnatal, atropine, and Librax, anti-parkinsonians, and other drugs such as Norpace.**

For all of the drugs in the above-mentioned groups which are listed in this book, we include an "anticholinergic" warning box as follows:

Warning: Special Mental and Physical Adverse Effects
Older adults are especially sensitive to the harmful anticholinergic effects of (name of drug class). These drugs should not be used unless absolutely necessary.
Mental Effects: confusion, delirium, short-term memory problems, disorientation, and impaired attention.
Physical Effects: dry mouth, constipation, difficulty urinating (especially for a man with an enlarged prostate), blurred vision, decreased sweating with increased body temperature, sexual dysfunction, and worsening of glaucoma.

Yet another example of the marked increase in the sensitivity of older adults to drugs has to do with stimulant drugs which are in the same family as amphetamines or "speed." Despite the dangers of these drugs for anyone, especially older adults, they are widely promoted and prescribed. In 1986, for example, older adults filled well over 2 million prescriptions for such drugs including Ornade, Tavist-D, Entex LA, Novafed-A, and Actifed. All of these contain amphetamine-like drugs such as PPA (phenylpropanolamine) or pseudoephedrine. All of these drugs that are discussed in the book, most of which are listed as "Do Not Use," contain the following warning:

Warning
(name of drug) can cause or worsen high blood pressure. It is especially dangerous for people who have high blood pressure, heart disease, diabetes, or thyroid disease. People over 60 are more likely than younger people to experience effects on the heart and blood pressure, restlessness, nervousness, and confusion.

---

5. *Decreased Blood-Pressure-Maintaining Ability.* Because older adults are less able to compensate for some of the effects of drugs, there is yet another reason why they are more vulnerable to adverse effects of drugs and more sensitive to the intended effects. The most widespread example of older adults' decreased ability to compensate is seen when they get out of bed and/or suddenly rise from a seated position. As you rise, your blood pressure normally falls, decreasing the blood flow to your head, resulting in less blood flow to the brain. Younger peoples' bodies can compensate for this: receptors in the neck, sensing that the blood pressure is tending to fall as the person rises, tighten up the blood vessels in other parts of the body keeping the overall blood pressure high enough. In older adults, these receptors do not work as well. Often, upon standing, older adults feels giddy, light-headed, and dizzy. They may even faint because the blood pressure in the head fell too rapidly.

The ability to maintain a proper blood pressure is further weakened when you use any of a very long list of drugs, **the most common examples being high blood pressure drugs. Other categories of drugs which cause an exaggerated blood pressure drop include sleeping pills, tranquilizers, antidepressants, antipsychotic drugs, antihistamines, drugs for heart pain (angina), and antiarrhythmics.** (See p. 32 for a full list of drugs which can cause this difficulty.)

This problem of so-called postural hypotension — the sudden fall in blood pressure on standing, brought about by a combination of aging and drugs — can be catastrophic, and the falls which often result can end in hip fractures, a leading cause of death in older adults, or other serious injuries.

6. *Decreased Temperature Compensation.* Younger adults are more easily able than older people to withstand very high or very low temperatures. They sweat and dilate (widen) blood vessels to get rid of excess heat when it is hot, and constrict (narrow) blood vessels to conserve heat when it is cold. Older adult's bodies are less able to do this. As in the case of blood pressure compensation, this "normal" temperature-regulating problem of older adults can be significantly worsened by any of a large number of prescription and over-the-counter drugs, resulting in fatal or life-threatening changes in body temperature. **Many older adults' deaths during heat waves or prolonged cold spells, can be attributed to drugs which interfere with temperature regulation.**

Most of these people did not know they were at increased risk. All drugs in this book which contain a warning about anticholinergic effects can have this harmful effect on withstanding heat waves.

7. *More Diseases Which Affect The Response to Drugs.* Older adults are much more likely than younger adults to have at least one disease — such as liver or kidney damage (not just the decreased function of older age), poor circulation, and other chronic conditions — which alter their response to drugs. Little is known about the influence of multiple diseases on drug effects in the elderly.

One well-understood example, however, is the effect of heart failure on the way people can handle drugs. When the heart is not able to pump as much blood as it used to, the change which occurs in heart failure, there is also a decrease in the flow of blood to the kidneys. For the same reasons discussed in point #3, the reduced flow of blood to the kidneys harms the kidneys' ability to get rid of drugs from the blood and dump them in the urine.

8. *More Drugs and, Therefore, More Adverse Drug Reactions and Interactions.* Since older adults use significantly more prescription drugs than younger people, they have greatly increased odds of an adverse drug reaction caused by the dangerous interaction between two drugs. Often, older adults may be taking one or more over-the-counter drugs in addition to their prescription drugs. This further increases the likelihood of adverse drug interactions. One of the more common kinds of adverse drugs interactions is the ability of some drugs to cause a second drug to accumulate to dangerous levels in the body. At the end of the discussion of each drug in this book (see p. 55), except the 119 which we say "Do Not Use," there is a list of other drugs which can cause serious adverse interactions.

*Partial List Of Drug Interactions Of
Great Potential Harm To Patients -
Some Of Which Are Life-Threatening*
(see individual drugs for complete
lists of interactions)

Mevacor	with	Lopid
Seldane	with	erythromycin
Aldactone	with	potassium
Prozac	with	Desyrel
Butazolidin	with	Orinase
insulin	with	Inderal
Tegretol	with	erythromycin
Tagamet	with	Dilantin
Nardil	with	Larodopa
Inderal	with	Tagamet
Demerol	with	Nardil
Calan	with	Duraquin
Theo-Dur	with	Tagamet
Coumadin	with	Tagamet
Lanoxin	with	Calan

9. *Inadequate Testing of Drugs In Older
Adults Before Approval*. Although older
adults use a disproportionate share of
prescription drugs, few of these drugs
are adequately tested in older adults
before being approved by the Food and
Drug Administration (FDA). (See Chapter 1, *The Role of the Drug Companies*.)

Dr. Peter Lamy of the University of
Maryland, School of Pharmacy, has
stated that "We test drugs in young
people for 3 months; we give them to old
people for 15 years." The FDA is slowly
remedying this serious problem by
requiring that the people on whom a
drug is tested be representative of those
who will use the drug if it is approved.
Nonetheless, most drugs on the market
today, which are heavily used by older
adults, were not adequately tested in this
age group.

In summary, there are significant
differences between younger and older
patients, often not realized by doctors or
patients. By increasing the awareness of
everyone to these differences, there will be
far fewer drugs prescribed to older adults
and those which will still be prescribed will
be given at lower doses in most instances.

Which Adverse Effects Can Be Caused by Which Drugs?

The following charts are to be used by
patients who have any of a variety of medical problems (or by doctors) to find out
which drugs, especially ones they are using
or are considering using, can cause these
adverse reactions. The lists are compiled
from a variety of sources.[20,21,22]

Although these adverse effects occur
most commonly in older adults, most of
them have also been documented in
younger people, although not as often in
many instances.

Summary Of The Most Common Drugs Causing the Most Detectable Problems

Adverse Drug Reaction	(# Drugs)	Examples of Brand Names
Depression	(86)	Ser-Ap-Es, Valium, Dalmane, Xanax, Catapres, Moduretic, Inderal, Aldomet, Advil, Naprosyn, Tagamet, Talwin, Zantac, Pepcid, Axid, Norpace
Psychoses/Hallucinations	(105)	Lanoxin, Procan, Aldomet, Catapres, Inderal, Elavil, Valium, Actifed, Halcion, Benadryl, Hismanal, Seldane, Tagamet
Confusion/Delirium	(120)	Compazine, Mellaril, Elavil, Asendin, Luminal, Valium, Xanax, Benadryl, Sinemet, Catapres, Tagamet, Zantac, DiaBeta, Diabinese, Dymelor
Dementia	(65)	Mellaril, Valium, Xanax, Restoril, Aldomet, Ser-Ap-Es, Regroton, Inderal, Tagamet, Zantac, Maxzide
Insomnia	(18)	Sudafed, Inderal, Lasix, Mevacor, Habitrol, Theo-Dur, Nicotrol, Synthroid
Parkinsonism	(29)	Haldol, Mellaril, Thorazine, Elavil, Asendin, Aldomet, Ser-Ap-Es, Regroton, Compazine
Tardive Dyskinesia	(14)	Compazine, Haldol, Mellaril, Thorazine, Asendin, BuSpar, Wellbutrin
Dizziness on Standing	(108)	Nitro-Bid, Isordil, Lasix, Aldomet, Ser-Ap-Es, Calan, Cardizem, Catapres, Minipress, Procardia, Inderal, Tenormin, Valium, Xanax, Asendin, Elavil, Compazine, Haldol
Falls/Hip Fracture	(46)	Valium, Xanax, Restoril, Luminal, Nembutal, Elavil, Sinequan, Haldol, Compazine, Navane, Isordil, Dalmane
Injurious Auto Accidents	(22)	Valium, Xanax, Ativan, Elavil, Tofranil, Asendin, Norpramin, Pamelor, Sinequan
Sexual Dysfunction	(119)	TransdermScop, Axid, Pepcid, Tagamet, Zantac, Calan, Norpace, Tegretol, Lopid, Blocadron, Lopressor
Loss of Appetite, Nausea, Vomiting	(44)	Kaochlor, Lanoxin, Advil, Feldene, Demerol, E-Mycin, Sumycin, Feosol, Somophyllin, Bronkodyl

Summary Of The Most Common Drugs Causing the Most Detectable Problems, continued

Adverse Drug Reaction	(# Drugs)	Examples of Brand Names
Abdominal Pain, Ulcers, GI Bleeding	(37)	Advil, Motrin, Feldene, Indocin, Anaprox, Somophyllin, Bronkodyl, Cortone, Decadron
Constipation	(88)	Dilaudid, Talwin, Tylenol 3, Tylox, Benadryl, Cogentin, Urised, Maalox, Inderal, Alagel, Tums
Diarrhea	(35)	Aldomet, Ser-Ap-Es, Maalox, Milk of Magnesia, Dulcolax, Doxidan, Peri-Colace, Sumycin, Cleocin
Lung Toxicity	(63)	Tegretol, Inderal, Visken, Prinivil, Vasotec, Feldene
Blocked Urination	(53)	Sinequan, Asendin, Elavil, Compazine, Haldol, Antivert, Bentyl, Benadryl, Actifed, Tavist, Artane, Cogentin
Urine Leakage	(63)	Lasix, Esidrix, Zaroxolyn, Inderal, Tenormin, Minipress, Valium, Restoril, Xanax, Eskalith

Drugs That Affect the Mind
Drugs That Can Cause Depression

Drug Class	Brand Name	Generic Name
Antibiotics and other Anti-infective Agents	Flagyl	metronidazole
	INH	isoniazid
	Seromycin	cycloserine
	Trecator-SC	ethionamide
Corticosteroids, systemic	Acthar, Cortrophin-Zinc	corticotropin (ACTH)
	Aristocort, Kenacort	triamcinolone
	Celestone	betamethasone
	Cortef	hydrocortisone
	Cortone	cortisone
	Decadron, Hexadrol	dexamethasone
	Deltasone	prednisone
	Deproped, Medrol	methylprednisolone

	Prelone, Cortalone	prednisolone

Eye Drugs	Betagan	levobunolol

Gastrointestinal Drugs	Tagamet	cimetidine
	Zantac	ranitidine

Heart and Blood Vessel Drugs		
Antiarrhythmics	Norpace	disopyramide
	Procan SR	procainamide
High Blood Pressure Drugs (Beta-blockers)	Blocadren	timolol
	Corgard	nadolol
	Inderal	propranolol
	Inderide	propranolol/hydrochlorothiazide
	Lopressor	metoprolol
	Sectral	acebutolol
	Tenoretic	atenolol/chlorthalidone
	Tenormin	atenolol
	Trandate	labetalol
	Visken	pindolol
High Blood Pressure Drugs (Diuretics)	Diupres	chlorothiazide/reserpine
	Enduronyl	deserpidine/methyclothiazide
	Hydropres	reserpine/hydrochlorothiazide
	Regroton, Demi-Regroton	reserpine/chlorthalidone
	Salutensin	reserpine/hydroflumethiazide
	Ser-Ap-Es	reserpine/hydralazine/ hydrochlorothiazide
High Blood Pressure Drugs (Other)	Aldomet	methyldopa
	Catapres	clonidine
	Hytrin	terazosin
	Minipress	prazosin
	Serpasil, Sandril	reserpine
	Tenex	guanfacine

Mind Affecting Drugs		
Antidepressants	Wellbutrin	bupropion
Barbiturates	Butalan, Butisol	butabarbital
	Luminal	phenobarbital
	Nembutal	pentobarbital
	Seconal	secobarbital
Tranquilizers or Sleeping Pills	Ativan	lorazepam
	BuSpar	buspirone
	Centrax	prazepam

	Dalmane	flurazepam
	Halcion	triazolam
	Librium	chlordiazepoxide
	Limbitrol	chlordiazepoxide/amitriptyline
	Noludar	methyprylon
	Restoril	temazepam
	Serax	oxazepam
	Tranxene	clorazepate
	Valium	diazepam
	Xanax	alprazolam

Neurological Drugs

Anticonvulsants	Dilantin	phenytoin
	Klonopin	clonazepam
	Luminal	phenobarbital
	Mysoline	primidone
	Zarontin	ethosuximide
Antiparkinsonians	Dopar	levodopa
	Eldepryl	selegine, deprenyl
	Parlodel	bromocriptine
	Sinemet	carbidopa/levodopa

Painkillers/Narcotics

	Advil, Motrin, Nuprin, Rufen	ibuprofen
	Anaprox, Naprosyn	naproxen
	Ansaid, Ocufen	flurbiprofen
	Azolid, Butazolidin	phenylbutazone
	Clinoril	sulindac
	Dolobid	diflunisal
	Feldene	piroxicam
	Indocin	indomethacin
	Lodine	etodolac
	Meclomen	meclofenamate
	Nalfon	fenoprofen
	Orudis	ketoprofen
	Talwin	pentazocine
	Talwin-NX	pentazocine/naloxone
	Tolectin	tolmetin
	Voltaren	diclofenac

Other Drugs

		amphetamines (during withdrawal)
	Ampaque	metrizamide
	Antabuse	disulfiram

Drugs That Can Cause Psychoses, Such As Hallucinations

Drug Class	Brand Name	Generic Name
Antibiotics and Other Anti-infective Agents	Ambilhar	niridazole
	Aralen	chloroquine
	Atabrine	quinacrine
	DDS	dapsone
	Fungizone	amphotericin B
	INH	isoniazid
	Mintezol	thiabendazole
	NegGram	nalidixic acid
	Podofin	podophyllum
	Seromycin	cycloserine
	Symmetrel	amantadine
	Trecator-SC	ethionamide
	Wycillin	penicillin G procaine
	Zovirax	acyclovir
Corticosteroids, systemic	Acthar, Cortrophin-Zinc	corticotropin (ACTH)
	Aristocort, Kenacort	triamcinolone
	Celestone	betamethasone
	Cortef	hydrocortisone
	Cortone	cortisone
	Decadron, Hexadrol	dexamethasone
	Deltasone	prednisone
	Deproped, Medrol	methylprednisolone
	Prelone, Cortalone	prednisolone
Cold, Cough, Allergy and Asthma Drugs Antihistamines	Actifed, Actidil	triprolidine
	Atarax, Vistaril	hydroxyzine
	Benadryl, Benylin	diphenhydramine
	Chlor-Trimeton, Deconamine, Naldecon, Novafed A, Ornade	chlorpheniramine
	Dimetane, Dimetapp	brompheniramine
	Hismanal	astemizole

	Periactin	cyproheptadine
	Seldane	terfenadine
	Tavist, Tavist-1	clemastine
	Trinalin, Optimine	azatadine
Asthma Drugs	Maxair	pirbuterol
	Proventil, Ventolin	albuterol
Nasal Decongestants	Afrin, Dristan Long Lasting, Nostrilla, Sinex Long-Lasting	oxymetazoline
	Ephed II	ephedrine
	Neo-Synephrine	phenylephrine
	Sudafed	pseudoephedrine

Eye Drugs	Betagan	levobunolol

Gastrointestinal Drugs	Tagamet	cimetidine

Heart and Blood Vessel Drugs

Antianginal Drugs		digitalis
	Lanoxin	digoxin
Antiarrhythmics	Mexitil	mexiletine
	Pronestyl, Procan SR	procainamide
	Tonocard	tocainamide
	Xylocaine	lidocaine
High Blood Pressure Drugs	Aldomet	methyldopa
	Catapres	clonidine
	Hytrin	terazosin
	Inderal	propranolol
	Minipress	prazosin
	Tenex	guanfacine
	Trandate	labetalol

Mind-Affecting Drugs

Antidepressants	Adapin, Sinequan	doxepin
	Asendin	amoxapine
	Aventyl	nortriptyline
	Desyrel	trazodone
	Elavil	amitriptyline
	Limbitrol	chlordiazepoxide/amitriptyline
	Ludiomil	maprotiline
	Norpramin	desipramine
	Tofranil	imipramine
	Triavil, Etrafon	perphenazine/amitriptyline
	Wellbutrin	bupropion

Tranquilizers or Sleeping Pills	BuSpar	buspirone
	Halcion	triazolam
	Noludar	methyprylon
	Placidyl	ethchlorvynol
	Valium	diazepam

Neurological Drugs

Anticonvulsants	Dilantin	phenytoin
	Klonopin	clonazepam
	Mysoline	primidone
	Tegretol	carbamazepine
	Zarontin	ethosuximide
Antiparkinsonians	Dopar	levodopa
	Eldepryl	selegiline, deprenyl
	Parlodel	bromocriptine
	Sinemet	carbidopa/levodopa

Painkillers/Narcotics

	Arthropan*	choline salicylate*
	Ascriptin, Ascriptin A/D*	buffered aspirin*
	Aspirin, Easprin, Ecotrin, Empirin*	aspirin*
	Darvon	propoxyphene
	Disalcid*	salsalate*
	Doan's Pills*	magnesium salicylate*
	Indocin	indomethacin
	Ketalar	ketamine
	Orudis	ketoprofen
	Roxanol, MS Contin	morphine
	Talwin	pentazocine
	Talwin-NX	pentazocine/naloxone
	Trilisate*	choline and magnesium salicylates*

Other Drugs

		amphetamines
		atropine
		barbiturates
		cocaine
	Amicar	aminocaproic acid
	Amipaque	metrizamide
	Antabuse	disulfiram
	Lioresal	baclofen
	Nardil	phenelzine
	Oncovin	vincristine
	Ritalin	methylphenidate

* Salicylates can cause psychoses when they are used in high doses.

| | Sansert | methysergide |
| | Synthroid | thyroid hormone |

Drugs That Can Cause Sudden Onset of Confusion Or Delirium

Drug Class	Brand Name	Generic Name
Antibiotics and other Anti-infective Agents	Cipro	ciprofloxacin
	Floxin	ofloxacin
	Noroxin	norfloxacin
	Symmetrel	amantadine
	Urised	atropine/hyoscyamine/ methenamine/methylene blue/phenyl salicylate/ benzoic acid
Corticosteroids, systemic	Acthar, Cortrophin-Zinc	corticotropin (ACTH)
	Aristocort, Kenacort	triamcinolone
	Celestone	betamethasone
	Cortone	cortisone
	Cortef	hydrocortisone
	Decadron, Hexadrol	dexamethasone
	Deltasone	prednisone
	Deproped, Medrol	methylprednisolone
	Prelone, Cortalone	prednisolone
Cold, Cough, Allergy and Asthma Drugs Antihistamines	Actifed, Actidil	triprolidine
	Atarax, Vistaril	hydroxyzine
	Benadryl, Benylin	diphenhydramine
	Chlor-Trimeton, Deconamine, Naldecon, Novafed A, Ornade	chlorpheniramine
	Dimetane, Dimetapp	brompheniramine
	Hismanal	astemizole
	Periactin	cyproheptadine
	Seldane	terfenadine

	Tavist, Tavist-1	clemastine
	Trinalin, Optimine	azatadine

Diabetes Drugs	DiaBeta	glyburide
	Diabinese	chlorpropamide
	Dymelor	acetohexamide
	Glucotrol	glipizide
	Humulin Iletin, Insulatard, Mixtard, Novolin, Velosulin	insulin (beef, pork, human)
	Orinase	tolbutamide
	Tolinase	tolazamide

Gastrointestinal Drugs		atropine
	Antivert, Bonine	meclizine
	Axid	nizatidine
	Bentyl	dicyclomine
	Compazine	prochlorperazine
	Ditropan	oxybutynin
	Donnatal	phenobarbital/hyoscyamine/ atropine/scopolamine
	Librax	chlordiazepoxide/clidinium
	Lomotil	diphenoxylate/atropine
	Pepcid	famotidine
	Phenergan	promethazine
	Tagamet	cimetidine
	Tigan	trimethobenzamide
	Zantac	ranitidine

Heart and Blood Vessel Drugs	Catapres	clonidine
	Lanoxin	digoxin
	Norpace	disopyramide
	Tenex	guanfacine

Mind-Affecting Drugs Antidepressants	Adapin, Sinequan	doxepin
	Asendin	amoxapine
	Aventyl	nortriptyline
	Desyrel	trazodone
	Elavil	amitriptyline
	Eskalith	lithium
	Limbitrol	chlordiazepoxide/amitriptyline
	Ludiomil	maprotiline
	Norpramin	desipramine
	Prozac	fluoxetine
	Tofranil	imipramine

	Triavil, Etrafon	perphenazine/amitriptyline
Antipsychotics	Wellbutrin	bupropion
	Compazine	prochlorperazine
	Haldol	haloperidol
	Mellaril	thioridazine
	Navane	thiothixene
	Prolixin	fluphenazine
	Reglan	metoclopramide
	Stelazine	trifluoperazine
	Thorazine	chlorpromazine
	Triavil, Etrafon	perphenazine/amitriptyline
Barbiturates	Butalan	butabarbital
	Luminal, Solfoton	phenobarbital
	Nembutal	pentobarbital
Tranquilizers or Sleeping Pills	Atarax, Vistaril	hydroxyzine
	Ativan	lorazepam
	BuSpar	buspirone
	Centrax	prazepam
	Dalmane	flurazepam
	Doriden	glutethimide
	Halcion	triazolam
	Librium	chlordiazepoxide
	Miltown, Equanil	meprobamate
	Noctec	chloral hydrate
	Noludar	methyprylon
	Restoril	temazepam
	Serax	oxazepam
	Tranxene	clorazepate
	Valium	diazepam
	Xanax	alprazolam

Neurological Drugs

Anticonvulsants	Dilantin	phenytoin
	Klonopin	clonazepam
Antiparkinsonians	Artane, Trihexane	trihexyphenidyl
	Cogentin	benztropine
	Dopar	levodopa
	Parlodel	bromocriptine
	Sinemet	carbidopa/levodopa

Painkillers/Narcotics

	Advil, Motrin, Nuprin, Rufen	ibuprofen

Anaprox, Naprosyn	naproxen
Ansaid, Ocufen	flurbiprofen
Arthropan*	choline salicylate*
Ascriptin, Ascriptin A/D*	buffered aspirin*
Aspirin, Easprin,* Ecotrin,* Empirin*	aspirin*
Azolid, Butazolidin	phenylbutazone
Clinoril	sulindac
Disalcid*	salsalate*
Doan's Pills*	magnesium salicylate*
Dolobid	diflunisal
Feldene	piroxicam
Indocin	indomethacin
Lodine	etodolac
Meclomen	meclofenamate
Nalfon	fenoprofen
Orudis	ketoprofen
Talwin	pentazocine
Talwin-NX	pentazocine/naloxone
Tolectin	tolmetin
Trilisate*	choline and magnesium salicylates*
Voltaren	diclofenac

Drugs That Can Cause Or Worsen Dementia (Mental Impairment—Forgetfulness, Slow Thinking, Inability To Care For One's Self, Confusion)

Unlike the drugs listed on p. 24 that cause sudden confusion and/or delirium, these drugs cause mental impairment which is much slower and more subtle in onset.[23] **The categories of drugs with the biggest risk for mental impairment are the sleeping pills and so-called minor tranquilizers.**

Drug Class	Brand Name	Generic Name
Gastrointestinal Drugs	Axid	nizatidine
	Pepcid	famotidine
	Tagamet	cimetidine
	Zantac	ranitidine
Heart and Blood Vessel Drugs High Blood Pressure Drugs (Beta-blockers)	Blocadren	timolol

Salicylates can cause psychoses when they are used in high doses.

	Corgard	nadolol
	Inderal	propranolol
	Inderide	propranolol/hydrochlorothiazide
	Lopressor	metoprolol
	Tenoretic	atenolol/chlorthalidone
	Tenormin	atenolol
	Trandate	labetalol
	Visken	pindolol
High Blood Pressure Drugs (Diuretics)	Aldactazide	spironolactone/ hydrochlorothiazide
	Aldoril	methyldopa/ hydrochlorothiazide
	Apresazide	hydralazine/hydrochlorothiazide
	Combipres	clonidine/chlorthalidone
	Diupres	chlorothiazide/reserpine
	Diuril	chlorothiazide
	Dyazide, Maxzide	triamterene/hydrochlorothiazide
	Enduron	methyclothiazide
	Enduronyl	deserpidine/methyclothiazide
	Esidrix, HydroDIURIL	hydrochlorothiazide
	Hydropres	reserpine/hydrochlorothiazide
	Hygroton	chlorthalidone
	Inderide	propranolol/hydrochlorothiazide
	Lozol	indapamide
	Metahydrin	trichlormethiazide
	Moduretic	amiloride/hydrochlorothiazide
	Regroton, Demi-Regroton	reserpine/chlorthalidone
	Salutensin	reserpine/hydroflumethiazide
	Ser-Ap-Es	reserpine/hydralazine/ hydrochlorothiazide
	Tenoretic	atenolol/chlorthalidone
	Zaroxolyn, Diulo	metolazone
High Blood Pressure Drugs (Other)	Aldomet	methyldopa
	Serpasil, Sandril	reserpine

Mind-Affecting Drugs

Antidepressants	Prozac	fluoxetine
Antipsychotics	Compazine	prochlorperazine
	Haldol	haloperidol
	Mellaril	thioridazine
	Navane	thiothixene
	Prolixin	fluphenazine

	Stelazine	trifluoperazine
	Thorazine	chlorpromazine
	Triavil, Etrafon	perphenazine/amitriptyline
Barbiturates	Butalan	butabarbital
	Luminal, Solfoton	phenobarbital
	Nembutal	pentobarbital
Tranquilizers or Sleeping Pills	Atarax, Vistaril	hydroxyzine
	Ativan	lorazepam
	BuSpar	buspirone
	Centrax	prazepam
	Dalmane	flurazepam
	Doriden	glutethimide
	Halcion	triazolam
	Librium	chlordiazepoxide
	Miltown, Equanil	meprobamate
	Noctec	chloral hydrate
	Noludar	methyprylon
	Restoril	temazepam
	Serax	oxazepam
	Tranxene	clorazepate
	Valium	diazepam
	Xanax	alprazolam
Neurological Drugs Anticonvulsants	Klonopin	clonazepam

Drugs That Can Cause Insomnia

Drug Class	Brand Name	Generic Name
Antibiotics and other Anti-infective Agents	Symmetrel	amantadine
Cold, Cough, Allergy, and Asthmas Drugs	Sudafed	pseudoephedrine
	Elixophyllin, Theo-Dur	theophylline
Gastrointestinal Drugs	Tagamet	cimetidine
Heart and Blood Vessel Drugs	Aldomet	methyldopa
	HydroDIURIL	hydrochlorothiazide
	Inderal	propranolol
	Lasix	furosemide
	Mevacor	lovastatin
	Quinidex	quinidine

Mind-Affecting Drugs
  Tranquilizers or Sleeping Pills
  (Note: these drugs may
  cause rebound insomnia)

	Dalmane	flurazepam
	Halcion	triazolam

Neurological Drugs

	Dilantin	phenytoin
	Larodopa	levodopa

Other Drugs

		alcohol
		caffeine
	Habitrol,	nicotine
	Nicorette,	
	Nicoderm,	
	Nicotrol,	
	Prostep	
	Synthroid	l-thyroxine, thyroid

Drugs That Can Cause Abnormal, Involuntary Movements: Parkinsonism or Tardive Dyskinesia

Drug-induced Parkinsonism

The following drugs can cause a tremor often indistinguishable from Parkinson's disease. If signs of the disease develop after beginning to use one of these drugs, a trial off the drug will often result in the disappearance of the parkinsonism. Unfortunately, doctors often do not recognize the drug-induced nature of this problem, and instead of discontinuing the drug that caused the problem, they add another drug to treat the parkinsonism.

Drug Class	**Brand Name**	**Generic Name**
Heart and Blood Vessel Drugs		
High Blood Pressure Drugs (Diuretics)		
	Diupres	chlorothiazide/reserpine
	Enduronyl	deserpidine/methyclothiazide
	Hydropres	reserpine/hydrochlorothiazide
	Regroton, Demi-Regroton	reserpine/chlorthalidone
	Salutensin	reserpine/hydroflumethiazide
	Ser-Ap-Es	reserpine/hydralazine/ hydrochlorothiazide
High Blood Pressure Drugs (Other)		
	Aldomet	methyldopa
	Serpasil, Sandril	reserpine
Mind-Affecting Drugs		
Antidepressants		
	Adapin, Sinequan	doxepin
	Asendin	amoxapine
	Aventyl	nortriptyline
	Desyrel	trazodone

	Elavil	amitriptyline
	Limbitrol	chlordiazepoxide/amitriptyline
	Ludiomil	maprotiline
	Norpramin	desipramine
	Prozac	fluoxetine
	Tofranil	imipramine
	Triavil, Etrafon	perphenazine/amitriptyline
	Wellbutrin	bupropion
Antipsychotics	Compazine	prochlorperazine
	Haldol	haloperidol
	Mellaril	thioridazine
	Navane	thiothixene
	Prolixin	fluphenazine
	Stelazine	trifluoperazine
	Thorazine	chlorpromazine
	Triavil, Etrafon	perphenazine/amitriptyline
Tranquilizers	BuSpar	buspirone

Drug-induced Tardive Dyskinesia

Tardive dyskinesia is the most common and serious adverse effect of antipsychotic drugs and is often irreversible. It is characterized by involuntary movements of the lips, tongue, and sometimes the fingers, toes, and trunk. It may occur in as many as 40% of people over the age of 60 taking antipsychotic drugs. **Tardive dyskinesia is more common and more severe in older adults, and antipsychotic drugs are quite often prescribed unnecessarily in this age group.** (See discussion of this in *Antipsychotic Drugs*, p.211.)

Drug Class	Brand Name	Generic Name
Mind-Affecting Drugs		
Antidepressants	Asendin	amoxapine
	Prozac	fluoxetine
	Wellbutrin	bupropion
Antipsychotics	Compazine	prochlorperazine
	Haldol	haloperidol
	Mellaril	thioridazine
	Navane	thiothixene
	Phenergan	promethazine
	Prolixin	fluphenazine
	Stelazine	trifluoperazine
	Thorazine	chlorpromazine
	Triavil, Etrafon	perphenazine/amitriptyline
Tranquilizers	BuSpar	buspirone
Neurological Drugs	Eldepryl	selegiline, deprenyl

Drugs That Can Disturb Balance
Drugs That Can Cause Dizziness On Standing (Postural Hypotension)

Drug Class	Brand Name	Generic Name
Antibiotics and other Anti-infective Agents	Cipro	ciprofloxacin
	Vermox	mebendazole
Cold, Cough, Allergy and Asthma Drugs Antihistamines	Actified, Actidil	triprolidine
	Atarax, Vistaril	hydroxyzine
	Benadryl, Benylin	diphenhydramine
	Chlor-Trimeton, Deconamine, Naldecon, Novafed A, Ornade	chlorpheniramine
	Dimetane, Dimetapp	brompheniramine
	Hismanal	astemizole
	Periactin	cyproheptadine
	Seldane	terfenadine
	Tavist, Tavist-1	clemastine
	Trinalin, Optimine	azatadine
Eye Drugs	Betagan	levobunolol
	Neptazane	methazolamide
Heart and Blood Vessel Drugs Antianginal Drugs	Isordil	isosorbide dinitrate
	Nitro-Bid, Nitrodisc	nitroglycerin
High Blood Pressure Drugs (Beta-blockers)	Blocadren	timolol
	Corgard	nadolol
	Inderal	propranolol
	Inderide	propranolol/hydrochlorothiazide
	Lopressor	metoprolol
	Sectral	acebutolol
	Tenoretic	atenolol/chlorthalidone
	Tenormin	atenolol
	Trandate	labetalol
	Visken	pindolol
High Blood Pressure Drugs (Diuretics)	Aldactazide	spironolactone/

		hydrochlorothiazide
Aldoril	methyldopa/	
		hydrochlorothiazide
Apresazide	hydralazine/hydrochlorothiazide	
Bumex	bumetanide	
Combipres	clonidine/chlorthalidone	
Diupres	chlorothiazide/reserpine	
Diuril	chlorothiazide	
Dyazide,	triamterene/hydrochlorothiazide	
Maxzide		
Enduron	methyclothiazide	
Enduronyl	deserpidine/methyclothiazide	
Esidrix,	hydrochlorothiazide	
HydroDIURIL		
Hydropres	reserpine/hydrochlorothiazide	
Hygroton	chlorthalidone	
Inderide	propranolol/hydrochlorothiazide	
Lasix	furosemide	
Lozol	indapamide	
Metahydrin	trichlormethiazide	
Moduretic	amiloride/hydrochlorothiazide	
Regroton,	reserpine/chlorthalidone	
Demi-Regroton		
Salutensin	reserpine/hydroflumethiazide	
Ser-Ap-Es	reserpine/hydralazine/	
	hydrochlorothiazide	
Tenoretic	atenolol/chlorthalidone	
Zaroxolyn,	metolazone	
Diulo		

High Blood Pressure Drugs (Other)

Adalat,	nifedipine
Procardia	
Aldactone	spironolactone
Aldomet	methyldopa
Apresoline	hydralazine
Calan,	verapamil
Isoptin, Verelan	
Capoten	captopril
Cardene	nicardipine
Cardizem	diltiazem
Catapres	clonidine
Dynacirc	isradipine
Hytrin	terazosin
Ismelin	guanethidine
Minipress	prazosin
Prinivil,	lisinopril
Zestril	
Procardia	nifedipine

Serpasil Sandril	reserpine
Tenex	guanfacine
Vasotec	enalapril
Wytensin	guanabenz

Mind-Affecting Drugs

Antidepressants

Adapin, Sinequan	doxepin
Asendin	amoxapine
Aventyl	nortriptyline
Desyrel	trazodone
Elavil	amitriptyline
Limbitrol	chlordiazepoxide/amitriptyline
Ludiomil	maprotiline
Norpramin	desipramine
Prozac	fluoxetine
Tofranil	imipramine
Triavil, Etrafon	perphenazine/amitriptyline

Antipsychotics

Compazine	prochlorperazine
Haldol	haloperidol
Mellaril	thioridazine
Navane	thiothixene
Prolixin	fluphenazine
Stelazine	trifluoperazine
Thorazine	chlorpromazine
Triavil, Etrafon	perphenazine/amitriptyline

Tranquilizers or Sleeping Pills

Atarax, Vistaril	hydroxyzine
Ativan	lorazepam
Centrax	prazepam
Dalmane	flurazepam
Doriden	glutethimide
Halcion	triazolam
Librium	chlordiazepoxide
Miltown, Equanil	meprobamate
Noctec	chloral hydrate
Noludar	methyprylon
Placidyl	ethchlorvynol
Restoril	temazepam
Serax	oxazepam
Tranxene	clorazepate
Valium	diazepam
Xanax	alprazolam

Neurological Drugs

Anticonvulsants	Klonopin	clonazepam
Antiparkinsonians	Dopar	levodopa
	Eldepryl	selegiline, deprenyl
	Parlodel	bromocriptine
	Sinemet	carbidopa/levodopa

Drugs That Can Cause Falls/Hip Fractures

A recent study found that a significant proportion of hip fractures in older adults could be attributed to the use of four classes of drugs: sleeping pills, tranquilizers, antipsychotics, and antidepressant drugs. The following are examples of such drugs as well as others that have been associated with falls which could also increase the risk of hip fractures. In addition to these drugs, all of the drugs that are listed above as causing dizziness on standing can also cause falls.

Drug Class	Brand Name	Generic Name
Heart and Blood Vessel Drugs		
Antianginal Drugs	Isordil	isosorbide dinitrate
	Nitro-Bid, Nitrodisc	nitroglycerin
Mind-Affecting Drugs		
Antidepressants	Adapin, Sinequan	doxepin
	Asendin	amoxapine
	Aventyl	nortriptyline
	Desyrel	trazodone
	Elavil	amitriptyline
	Limbitrol	chlordiazepoxide/amitriptyline
	Ludiomil	maprotiline
	Norpramin	desipramine
	Prozac	fluoxetine
	Tofranil	imipramine
	Triavil, Etrafon	perphenazine/amitriptyline
	Wellbutrin	bupropion
Antipsychotics	Compazine	prochlorperazine
	Haldol	haloperidol
	Mellaril	thioridazine
	Navane	thiothixene
	Prolixin	fluphenazine
	Stelazine	trifluoperazine
	Thorazine	chlorpromazine
	Triavil, Etrafon	perphenazine/amitriptyline
Barbiturates	Butalan	butabarbital
	Luminal, Solfoton	phenobarbital
	Nembutal	pentobarbital

Tranquilizers or Sleeping Pills	Atarax, Vistaril	hydroxyzine
	Ativan	lorazepam
	BuSpar	buspirone
	Centrax	prazepam
	Dalmane	flurazepam
	Doriden	glutethimide
	Halcion	triazolam
	Librium	chlordiazepoxide
	Miltown, Equanil	meprobamate
	Noctec	chloral hydrate
	Noludar	methyprylon
	Placidyl	ethachlorvynol
	Restoril	temazepam
	Serax	oxazepam
	Tranxene	clorazepate
	Valium	diazepam
	Xanax	alprazolam
Neurological Drugs	Dilantin	phenytoin
	Klonopin	clonazepam
	Luminol	phenobarbital
	Tegretol	carbamazepine

Drugs That Can Cause Injurious Automobile Accidents

Drug Class	Brand Name	Generic Name
Mind-Affecting Drugs		
Antidepressants	Adapin	doxepin
	Anafranil	clomipramine
	Asendin	amoxapine
	Aventyl, Pamelor	nortriptyline
	Elavil, Endep	amitriptyline
	Etrafon, Triavil	amitriptyline/perphenazine
	Limbitrol	amitriptyline/chlordiazepoxide
	Ludiomil	maprotiline
	Norpramin	desipramine
	Pamelor	nortriptyline
	Sinequan	doxepin
	Surmontil	trimipramine
	Tofranil	imipramine
	Vivactil	protriptyline
Tranquilizers and Sleeping Pills	Ativan	lorazepam
	Centrax	prazepam
	Librium	chlordiazepoxide

	Paxipam	halazepam
	Serax	oxazepam
	Tranxene	clorazepate
	Valium	diazepam
	Xanax	alprazolam

Drugs That Can Cause Sexual Dysfunction

Drug Class	Brand Name	Generic Name
Antibiotics and Other Anti-Infective Agents	Nizoral	ketoconazole
	Tegison	etretinate
Anticholinergics	Banthine	methanetheline
	Bentyl	dicyclomine
	Cantil	mepenzolate
	Darbid	isopropamide
	Ditropan	oxybutynin
	Isopto Homatropine	homatropine
	Pamine	methscopolamine
	Pathlilon	tridihexethyl
	Probanthine	propantheline
	Quarzan	clidinium
	Robinul	glycopyrrolate
	Tral	hexocyclium
	TransdermScop	scopolamine
	Valpin	anisotropine
Cancer Drugs	Intron A	interferon alfa
	Lupron	leuprolide
	Folex, Mexate	methotrexate
	Nolvadex	tamoxifen
	Suprefact	buserelin
Eye Drugs	Diamox	acetazolamide
Gastrointestinal Drugs	Axid	nizatidine
	Azulfidine	sulfasalazine
	Pepcid	famotidine
	Prilosec	omeprazole
	Reglan	metoclopramide
	Tagamet	cimetidine
	Zantac	ranitidine
Heart and Blood Vessel Drugs Antianginal Drugs	Adalat, Procardia	nifedipine
	Calan, Verelan	verapamil
	Lanoxin	digoxin

Antiarrhythmics	Cordarone	amiodarone
	Mexitil	mexiletine
	Norpace	disopyramide
	Wytensin	guanabenz
Blood Vessel Dilators	Cerespan	papaverine
Cholesterol-lowering Drugs	Atromid-S	clofibrate
	Lopid	gemfibrozil
High Blood Pressure Drugs (Beta-blockers)	Blocadren	timolol
	Inderal	propranolol
	Lopressor	metoprolol
	Normodyne, Trandate	labetalol
	Tenormin	atenolol
High Blood Pressure Drugs (Diuretics)	Daranide	dichlorphenamide
	HydroDIURIL	hydrochlorothiazide
	Hygroton	chlorthalidone
	Lozol	indapamide
	Neptazane	methazolamide
High Blood Pressure Drugs (Other)	Aldactone	spironolactone
	Aldomet	methyldopa
	Apresoline	hydralazine
	Catapres	clonidine
	Demser	metyrosine
	Eutonyl	pargyline
	Hylorel	guanadrel
	Inversine	mecamylamine
	Ismelin	guanethidine
	Midamor	amiloride
	Minipress	prazosin
	Serpasil	reserpine
	Tenex	guanfacine

Mind-Affecting Drugs

Antidepressants	Asendin	amoxapine
	Aventyl	nortriptyline
	Desyrel	trazodone
	Elavil	amitriptyline
	Ludiomil	maprotiline
	Marplan	isocarboxazid
	Nardil	phenelzine
	Norpramin, Pertofrane	desipramine
	Parnate	trancylpromine
	Prozac	fluoxetine
	Sinequan	doxepin
	Tofranil	imipramine

	Vivactil	protiptyline
	Zoloft	sertraline
Antipsychotics	Clozaril	clozapine
	Eskalith	lithium
	Haldol	haloperidol
	Mellaril	thioridazine
	Moban	molidone
	Navane	thiothixene
	Orap	pimozide
	Prolixin	fluphenazine
	Serentil	mesoridazine
	Stelazine	trifluoperazine
	Taractan	chlorprothixene
	Thorazine	chlorpromazine
	Trilafon	perphenazine
Barbiturates	Nembutal	pentobarbital
Tranquilizers	BuSpar	buspirone
	Valium	diazepam
	Xanax	alprazolam

Neurological Drugs

Anticonvulsants	Dilantin	phenytoin
	Tegretol	carbamazepine
	Zarontin	ethosuximide
Antiparkinsonians	Dopar, Larodopa	levodopa
	Parlodel	bromocriptine
	Permax	pergolide

Painkillers/Narcotics

	Dolophine	methadone
	Indocin	indomethacin
	Naprosyn	naproxen
	Trexan	naltrexone

Other Drugs

		alcohol
		cocaine
	Antabuse	disulfuram
	Danocrine	danazol
	DepoTestosterone	testosterone
	Dexedrine	amphetamines
	Diprivan	propofol
	Fastin	phentermine
	Intralipid	fat emulsion
	Lioresal	baclofen
	Mazanor, Sanorex	mazindol
	Plegine	phendimetrazine
	Pondimin	fenfluramine
	Preludin	phenmetrazine
	Synarel	nafarelin

| | Tenuate, Tepanil | diethylpropion |

Drugs That Can Affect the Gastrointestinal (G.I.) Tract
Drugs That Can Cause Loss of Appetite, Nausea, or Vomiting

Drug Class	Brand Name	Generic Name
Antibiotics and Other Anti-infective Agents	Achromycin, Sumycin	tetracycline
	Diflucan	fluconazole
	Floxin	ofloxacin
	Ilotycin, E-Mycin	erythromycin
	Metronidazole	flagyl
	Noroxin	norfloxacin
Cancer Drugs	many anticancer drugs (not listed in this book)	
Cold, Cough, Allergy and Asthma Drugs	Amoline, Somophyllin	aminophylline
	Bronkodyl, Sustaire	theophylline
	Choledyl	oxtriphylline
Heart and Blood Vessel Drugs	Kaochlor, Kaon-Cl, K-Lor	potassium chloride
	Lanoxin	digoxin
	Mevacor	lovastatin
	Questran, Cholybar	cholestyramine
Mind-Affecting Drugs	BuSpar	buspirone
	Prozac	fluoxetine
	Wellbutrin	bupropion
Neurological Drugs	Dopar	levodopa
	Eldepryl	selegiline, deprenyl
	Sinemet	carbidopa/levodopa
Painkillers/Narcotics		codeine
	Advil, Motrin, Nuprin, Rufen	ibuprofen
	Anaprox, Naprosyn	naproxen
	Ansaid, Ocufen	flurbiprofen
	Azolid, Butazolidin	phenylbutazone

	Clinoril	sulindac
	Demerol	meperidine
	Dolobid	diflunisal
	Feldene	piroxicam
	Imuran	azathioprine
	Indocin	indomethacin
	Lodine	etodolac
	Meclomen	meclofenamate
	Nalfon	fenoprofen
	Orudis	ketoprofen
	Roxanol, MS Contin	morphine
	Talwin	pentazocine
	Talwin-NX	pentazocine/naloxone
	Tolectin	tolmetin
	Voltaren	diclofenac
Other Drugs	Estraderm	estradiol
	Feosol, Slow Fe	ferrous sulfate
	Feostat	ferrous fumarate
	Fergan, Simron	ferrous gluconate
	Premarin, Ogen, Estrace, DES	estrogen

Drugs That Can Cause Abdominal Pain, Ulcers, or Gastrointestinal Bleeding

Although all of these drugs can cause abdominal pain, bleeding, and ulcers, **piroxicam (Feldene), indomethacin (Indocin), and phenylbutazone (Butazolidin) are more dangerous than the others and should not be used by older adults.**

Drug Class	Brand Name	Generic Name
Antibiotics and Other Anti-infective Agents		
	Diflucan	fluconazole
Corticosteriods, systemic	Acthar, Cortrophin-Zinc	corticotropin (ACTH)
	Aristocort, Kenacort	triamcinolone
	Celestone	betamethasone
	Cortef	hydrocortisone
	Cortone	cortisone
	Decadron, Hexadrol	dexamethasone
	Deltasone	prednisone
	Deproped, Medrol	methylprednisolone
	Prelone, Cortalone	prednisolone

Cold, Cough, Allergy and Asthma Drugs	Amoline, Somophyllin	aminophylline
	Bronkodyl, Sustaire	theophylline
	Choledyl	oxtriphylline
Mind-Affecting Drugs	BuSpar	buspirone
	Wellbutrin	bupropion
Neurological Drugs	Eldepryl	selegiline, deprenyl
Painkillers/Narcotics	Advil, Motrin, Nuprin, Rufen	ibuprofen
	Anaprox, Naprosyn	naproxen
	Ansaid, Ocufen	flurbiprofen
	Arthropan	choline salicylate
	Ascriptin, Ascriptin A/D	buffered aspirin
	Aspirin, Easprin, Ecotrin, Empirin	aspirin
	Azolid, Butazolidin	phenylbutazone
	Clinoril	sulindac
	Disalcid	salsalate
	Doan's Pills	magnesium salicylate
	Dolobid	diflunisal
	Feldene	piroxicam
	Indocin	indomethacin
	Lodine	etodolac
	Meclomen	meclofenamate
	Nalfon	fenoprofen
	Orudis	ketoprofen
	Tolectin	tolmetin
	Trilisate	choline and magnesium salicylates
	Voltaren	diclofenac

Drugs That Can Cause Constipation

Drug Class	Brand Name	Generic Name
Antibiotics and Anti-infective Agents	Ditropan	oxybutynin

	Urised	atropine/hyoscyamine/ methenamine/methylene blue/phenyl salicylate/ benzoic acid

Cold, Cough, Allergy and Asthma Drugs
Antihistamines

	Actifed, Actidil	triprolidine
	Atarax, Vistaril	hydroxyzine
	Benadryl, Benylin	diphenhydramine
	Chlor-Trimeton, Deconamine, Naldecon, Novafed A, Ornade	chlorpheniramine
	Dimetane, Dimetapp	brompheniramine
	Hismanal	astemizole
	Periactin	cyproheptadine
	Seldane	terfenadine
	Tavist, Tavist-1	clemastine
	Trinalin, Optimine	azatadine

Eye Drugs   Betagan   levobunolol

Gastrointestinal Drugs

		atropine
	Alagel, Amphojel	aluminum hydroxide
	Antivert, Bonine	meclizine
	Bentyl	dicyclomine
	Compazine	prochlorperazine
	Dialose Plus,* Peri-Colace*	docusate/casanthranol*
	Donnatal	phenobarbital/hyoscyamine/ atropine/scopolamine
	Doxidan*	danthron/docusate*
	Dulcolax*	bisacodyl*
	Gaviscon	aluminum hydroxide/ magnesium trisilicate

prolonged use

Librax	chlordiazepoxide/clidinium
Lomotil	diphenoxylate/atropine
Maalox, Maalox-TC	aluminum and magnesium hydroxide
Mylanta, Mylanta II	aluminum and magnesium hydroxide/simethicone
Phenergan	promethazine
Reglan	metoclopramide
Tigan	trimethobenzamide
Tums, Alka-Mints	calcium carbonate

Heart and Blood Vessel Drugs

Antiarrhythmics	Mexitil	mexiletine
	Norpace	disopyramide
Cholesterol-lowering drugs	Mevacor	lovastatin
	Questran, Cholybar	cholestyramine
High Blood Pressure Drugs (Beta-blockers)	Blocadren	timolol
	Corgard	nadolol
	Inderal	propranolol
	Inderide	propranolol/hydrochlorothiazide
	Lopressor	metoprolol
	Sectral	acebutolol
	Tenoretic	atenolol/chlorthalidone
	Tenormin	atenolol
	Trandate	labetalol
	Visken	pindolol
High Blood Pressure Drugs (Other)	Adalat, Procardia	nifedipine
	Calan, Isoptin, Verelan	verapamil
	Cardene	nicardipine
	Dynacirc	isradipine

Mind-Affecting Drugs

Antidepressants	Adapin, Sinequan	doxepin
	Asendin	amoxapine
	Aventyl	nortriptyline
	Desyrel	trazodone
	Elavil	amitriptyline
	Limbitrol	chlordiazepoxide/amitriptyline
	Ludiomil	maprotiline
	Norpramin	desipramine

	Tofranil	imipramine
	Triavil	perphenazine/amitriptyline
	Wellbutrin	bupropion
Antipsychotics	Compazine	prochlorperazine
	Haldol	haloperidol
	Mellaril	thioridazine
	Navane	thiothixene
	Prolixin	fluphenazine
	Reglan	metoclopramide
	Stelazine	trifluoperazine
	Thorazine	chlorpromazine
	Triavil, Etrafon	perphenazine/amitriptyline
Tranquilizers and Sleeping Pills	BuSpar	buspirone
	Doriden	glutethimide

Neurological Drugs

Anticonvulsants	Klonopin	clonazepam
Antiparkinsonians	Artane, Trihexane	trihexyphenidyl
	Cogentin	benztropine

Painkillers/Narcotics		
	Bancap HC, Vicodin	hydrocodone/acetaminophen
	Darvocet-N, Wygesic	propoxyphene/acetaminophen
	Darvon, Darvon-N	propoxyphene
	Darvon Compound	propoxyphene/aspirin/caffeine
	Demerol	meperidine
	Dilaudid	hydromorphone
	Empirin with Codeine	aspirin/codeine
	Percodan, Percodan-Demi	oxycodone/aspirin
	Roxanol, M S Contin	morphine
	Synalgos-DC	dihydrocodeine/aspirin/caffeine
	Talwin	pentazocine
	Talwin-NX	pentazocine/naloxone
	Tylenol 3	acetaminophen/codeine
	Tylox, Percocet 5	oxycodone/acetaminophen

Drugs That Can Cause Diarrhea

Drug Class	Brand Name	Generic Name
Antibiotics and Other Anti-infective Agents	Achromycin, Sumycin	tetracycline

	Biaxin	clarithromycin
	Ceftin	cefuroxime
	Cipro	ciprofloxacin
	Cleocin	clindamycin
	Floxin	ofloxacin
	Ilosone	erythromycin estolate
	Lincocin	lincomycin
	Noroxin	norfloxacin
	Omnipen, Polycillin	ampicillin
	Suprax	cefixime
	Vermox	mebendazole
	Zithromax	azithromycin
Gastrointestinal Drugs	Cytotec	misoprostol
	Dialose Plus, Peri-Colace	docusate/casanthranol
	Doxidan	danthron/docusate
	Dulcolax	bisacodyl
	Maalox, Maalox-TC	aluminum and magnesium hydroxide
	Milk of Magnesia	magnesium hydroxide
	Mylanta, Mylanta II	aluminum/magnesium hydroxide/simethicone

Heart and Blood Vessel Drugs

Antianginal Drugs	Lanoxin	digoxin
Antiarrhythmics	Mexitil	mexiletine
High Blood Pressure Drugs (Diuretics)		
	Diupres	chlorothiazide/reserpine
	Enduronyl	deserpidine/methyclothiazide
	Hydropres	reserpine/hydrochlorothiazide
	Regroton, Demi-Regroton	reserpine/chlorthalidone
	Salutensin	reserpine/hydroflumethiazide
	Ser-Ap-Es	reserpine/hydralazine/ hydrochlorothiazide
High Blood Pressure Drugs (Other)	Aldomet	methyldopa
	Ismelin	guanethidine
	Serpasil, Sandril	reserpine

Mind-Affecting Drugs	BuSpar	buspirone
	Wellbutrin	bupropion

Painkillers/Narcotics	Imuran	azathioprine

Other Drugs	Habitrol, Nicorette, Nicoderm, Nicotrol, Prostep	nicotine

Drugs That Can Cause Lung Toxicity

Drug Class	Brand Name	Generic Name
Antibiotics and Other Anti-infective Agents	Blenoxane	bleomycin
	Daraclor	pyrimethamine-chloroquine
	Fansidar	pyrimethamine-sulfadoxine
	Furadantin	nitrofurantoin
	Maloprim	pyrimethamine-dapsone
	Mutamycin	mitomycin
Cancer Drugs	Alkeran	mephalan
	BiCNU	carmustine
	CeeNu	lomustine
	Cytosar-U	cytarabine
	Cytoxan	cyclophosphamide
	Eldisine	vindesine
	Folex	methotrexate
	Leukeran	chlorambucil
	Matulane	probarbazine
	Myleran	busulfan
	Proleukin	interleukin-2
	Semustine	methyl-CCNU
	Velban	vinblastine
Cold, Cough, Allergy and Asthma Drugs	Brethine	terbutaline
Eye Drugs	Pilocar	pilocarpine
Gastrointestinal Drugs	Azulfidine	sulfasalazine
Heart and Blood Vessel Drugs Antiarrhythmics	Cordarone	amiodarone
	Rythmol	propafenone
	Tonocard	tocainide
	Xylocaine	lidocaine
High Blood Pressure Drugs (Beta-blockers)	Blocadren	timolol
	Inderal	propranolol
	Visken	pindolol
High Blood Pressure Drugs (Diuretics)	Esidrix, HydroDIURIL	hydrochlorothiazide
High Blood Pressure Drugs (Other)	Capoten	captopril
	Heparin antagonist	protamine

	Prinivil, Zestril	lisinopril
	Vasotec	enalapril
Mind-Affecting Drugs	Placidyl	ethchlorvynol

Neurological Drugs		
Anticonvulsants	Dilantin	phenytoin
Antiparkinsonians	Parlodel	bromocriptine
	Tegretol	carbamazepine

Painkillers/Narcotics		
	Butazolidin	phenylbutazone
	Clinoril	sulindac
	Cuprimine, Depen	penicillamine
	Darvon	propoxyphene
	Dolophine	methadone
	Ecotrin	aspirin
	Feldene	piroxicam
	Imuran	azathioprine
	Indocin	indomethacin
	Motrin	ibuprofen
	Myochrysine	gold sodium thiomalate
	Naprosyn	naproxen
	Narcan	naloxone
	Sansert	methysergide
	Solganal	aurothioglucose
	Voltaren	diclofenac

Other Drugs		
		cocaine
		tryptophan
	Dantrium	dantrolene
	Metubine	tubocurarine
	Norcuron	vecuronium
	Pavulon	pancuronium
	Suxamethonium	succinylcholine
	Tracrium	atracurium
	Yutopar	ritodrine

Drugs That Affect the Urinary Tract
Drugs That Can Block Urination

All of the following drugs can cause urinary retention, the inability to urinate or difficulty in urinating, particularly in men with enlarged prostate glands.

Drug Class	**Brand Name**	**Generic Name**
Antibiotics and Other Anti-Infective Agents	Ditropan	oxybutynin
	Urised	atropine/hyoscyamine/ methenamine/methylene blue/ phenyl salicylate/ benzoic acid

Cold, Cough, Allergy and Asthma Drugs	Actified, Actidil	triprolidine
	Atarax, Vistaril	hydroxyzine
	Atrovent	ipratropium
	Benadryl, Benylin	diphenhydramine
	Chlor-Trimeton, Deconamine, Naldecon, Novafed A, Ornade	chlorpheniramine
	Dimetane, Dimetapp	brompheniramine
	Hismanal	astemizole
	Periactin	cyproheptadine
	Seldane	terfenadine
	Tavist, Tavist-1	clemastine
	Trinalin, Optimine	azatadine

Eye Drugs	Neptazane	methazolamide

Gastrointestinal Drugs		atropine
	Antivert, Bonine	meclizine
	Bentyl	dicyclomine
	Compazine	prochlorperazine
	Donnatal	phenobarbital/hyoscyamine/ atropine/scopolamine
	Librax	chlordiazepoxide/clidinium
	Lomotil	diphenoxylate/atropine
	Phenergan	promethazine
	Reglan	metoclopramide
	Tigan	trimethobenzamide

Heart and Blood Vessel Drugs		
Antiarrhythmics	Norpace	disopyramide
High Blood Pressure Drugs	Adalat, Procardia	nifedipine
	Cardene	nicardipine
	Dynacirc	isradipine

Mind-Affecting Drugs		
Antidepressants	Adapin, Sinequan	doxepin
	Asendin	amoxapine
	Aventyl	nortriptyline
	Desyrel	trazodone

	Elavil	amitriptyline
	Limbitrol	chlordiazepoxide/amitriptyline
	Ludiomil	maprotiline
	Norpramin	desipramine
	Prozac	fluoxetine
	Tofranil	imipramine
	Triavil, Etrafon	perphenazine/amitriptyline
Antipsychotics	Wellbutrin	bupropion
	Compazine	prochlorperazine
	Haldol	haloperidol
	Mellaril	thioridazine
	Navane	thiothixene
	Prolixin	fluphenazine
	Reglan	metoclopramide
	Stelazine	trifluoperazine
	Thorazine	chlorpromazine
	Triavil, Etrafon	perphenazine/amitriptyline
Tranquilizers	BuSpar	buspirone
Neurological Drugs	Artane, Trihexane	trihexyphenidyl
	Cogentin	benztropine
	Eldepryl	selegiline, deprenyl

Drugs That Can Cause Loss of Bladder Control (Incontinence)

All of the drugs listed above that may block urination can, when the bladder gets too full, cause "overflow" leakage. In addition, the following drugs can also cause urine to leak:

Drug Class	Brand Name	Generic Name
Antibiotics and Other Anti-infective Agents	Urised	atropine/ hyoscyamine/ methenamine/methylene blue/phenyl salicylate/ benzoic acid
Eye Drugs	Betagan	levobunolol
Gastrointestinal Drugs	Cytotec	misoprostol
Heart and Blood Vessel Drugs High Blood Pressure Drugs (Beta-blockers)	Blocadren	timolol
	Corgard	nadolol
	Inderal	propranolol
	Inderide	propranolol/hydrochlorothiazide
	Lopressor	metoprolol
	Sectral	acebutolol
	Tenoretic	atenolol/chlorthalidone
	Tenormin	atenolol

| | Trandate | labetalol |
| | Visken | pindolol |

High Blood Pressure Drugs (Diuretics)

	Aldactazide	spironolactone/hydrochlorothiazide
	Aldoril	methyldopa/hydrochlorothiazide
	Apresazide	hydralazine/hydrochlorothiazide
	Bumex	bumetanide
	Combipres	clonidine/chlorthalidone
	Diupres	chlorothiazide/reserpine
	Diuril	chlorothiazide
	Dyazide, Maxzide	triamterene/hydrochlorothiazide
	Enduron	methyclothiazide
	Enduronyl	deserpidine/methyclothiazide
	Esidrix, HydroDIURIL	hydrochlorothiazide
	Hydropres	reserpine/hydrochlorothiazide
	Hygroton	chlorthalidone
	Inderide	propranolol/hydrochlorothiazide
	Lasix	furosemide
	Lozol	indapamide
	Metahydrin	trichlormethiazide
	Moduretic	amiloride/hydrochlorothiazide
	Regroton, Demi-Regroton	reserpine/chlorthalidone
	Salutensin	reserpine/hydroflumethiazide
	Ser-Ap-Es	reserpine/hydralazine/hydrochlorothiazide
	Tenoretic	atenolol/chlorthalidone
	Zaroxolyn, Diulo	metolazone

High Blood Pressure Drugs (Other)

	Adalat, Procardia	nifedipine
	Aldactone	spironolactone
	Cardene	nicardipine
	Dynacirc	isradipine
	Hytrin	terazosin
	Minipress	prazosin

Mind-Affecting Drugs

Antidepressants

	Eskalith	lithium
	Prozac	fluoxetine
	Wellbutrin	bupropion

Tranquilizers or Sleeping Pills

| | Atarax, | hydroxyzine |

	Vistaril	
	Ativan	lorazepam
	BuSpar	buspirone
	Centrax	prazepam
	Dalmane	flurazepam
	Doriden	glutethamide
	Halcion	triazolam
	Librium	chlordiazepoxide
	Miltown, Equanil	meprobamate
	Noctec	chloral hydrate
	Noludar	methyprylon
	Placidyl	ethchlorvynol
	Restoril	temazepam
	Serax	oxazepam
	Tranxene	clorazepate
	Valium	diazepam
	Xanax	alprazolam
Neurological Drugs	Klonopin	clonazepam

Notes for Chapter 2

1. *Second Annual Adverse Drug/Biologic Reaction Report: 1986*. Food and Drug Administration, 1987.

2. Vestal RE, ed. *Drug Treatment in the Elderly*. Sydney, Australia: ADIS Health Science Press, 1984. Calculation on 33% increase in risk of adverse reaction (age 50-59 vs 40-49) is based on an average of all three studies listed on page 32.

3. *Drugs for the Elderly*. Denmark: World Health Organization, 1985.

4. Lipton HL, Bero LA, Bird JA, McPhee SJ. The impact of clinical pharmacists' consultations on physicians' geriatric drug prescribing. *Medical Care* 1992; 30:646-58.

5. Vestal, op. cit.

6. Ouslander JG. Drug therapy in the elderly. *Annals of Internal Medicine* 1981; 95:711-22.

7. The 659,000 hospitalizations of older adults due to adverse drug reactions is calculated in the following way: The rate of hospitalization (discharges per 1,000 people) for different age groups in 1985 is taken from the *National Center for Health Statistics Advanced Data*, September 24, 1987; 140:4 (327.1 per 1,000 for those 65 and older, an estimated 178 per 1,000 people for those 60-64). The population in these age groups is from *Statistical Abstracts of the United States*, 1992, reporting on 1990 population data. There were 31.22 million people 65 and older and 10.618 million people 60-64. This calculates to 12.1 million hospitalizations of people 60 and older in 1990 and approximately one-half of these hospitalizations were to the medical services of hospitals so that one half of the 12.1 million admissions or 6.05 million admissions were to medical (as opposed to surgical) or other services.   Most of the studies are based on patients admitted to the medical services of these hospitals, which make up approximately 50% of the total admissions of older adults. There have been several recent studies looking specifically at what proportion of hospital admissions for older adults are due to adverse drug reactions. Earlier studies had looked at people of all ages

and the percentages were therefore lower, most of these studies finding that adverse drug reactions accounted for from 3% to 6% of hospitalizations. The more recent studies were reviewed and the percentage of hospitalizations in older adults accounted for by adverse drug reactions ranged from 10% to 17%, with the largest study finding 10.5%. The weighted average of these studies was 10.9% so this figure will be used to compute the number of older adults hospitalized each year because of an adverse drug reaction. (The most recent study, from Denmark, reported that for 11.2% of older adults hospitalized, an adverse drug reaction was a "dominant or contributing cause of the admission"). Multiplying the 10.9% weighted average by the 6.05 million admissions to American hospitals of older adults (60 and older), there are 659,000 older adults hospitalized each year because of adverse drug reactions.

8. Using the same basis for estimating the number of admissions to medical wards of hospitals as used in reference #7 (above) of 6.05 million in 1990, and the estimate that 22.4% of medical admissions are using digoxin and that 2.06% of these get life-threatening heart toxicity from digoxin (both are from Miller RR, Greenblatt DJ. *Drug Effects in Hospitalized Patients.* John Wiley and Sons, New York. 1976), this amounts to 6.05 million times 22.4% times 2.06% or 27,917 older adults in hospitals who suffer from life-threatening heart toxicity from digoxin. This estimate understates the magnitude of the problem because the proportion of patients in the Miller/Greenblatt book using digoxin and experiencing life-threatening heart toxicity is based on all patients of all ages, whereas the rate of digoxin use and therefore the rate of life-threatening reactions is higher in older adults. The estimate is also lower because it does not include cases of digoxin toxicity which occur in surgical patients.

9. Ray WA, Griffin MR, Shorr RI. Adverse drug reactions and the elderly. *Health Affairs* Fall 1990:114-22.

10. Of the 42.34 million Americans 60 and older (*Statistical Abstracts of the United States* 1992, 1991 population data) approximately 90% are taking one or more medications for a total of 37.83 million older people. According to a recent study of verified adverse drug reactions (German PS, Klein LE. Adverse Drug Experience Among the Elderly. In *Pharmaceuticals for the Elderly.* Pharmaceutical Manufacturers Association, November 1986), 25.4% of the elderly patients 60 and older had at least one adverse drug reaction during the six month interval that the study encompassed. 25.4% of 37.83 million people is 9.61 million adverse reactions in six months. The number of adverse reactions in a year would certainly be higher. The actual number of adverse reactions is also much higher since this calculation assumes all patients were being seen outside of the hospital or nursing home. Because the use of drugs in nursing homes and hospitals is much higher than in clinics, the number of adverse reactions is also higher.

11. Ray WA, Fought RL, Decker, MD. Psychoactive drugs and the risk of injurious motor vehicle crashes in elderly drivers. *American Journal of Epidemiology* 1992; 136:873-83.

12. Ray WA, Griffin MR, Schaffner W, Baugh DK, Menton J. Psychotropic drug use and the risk of hip fracture. *New England Journal of Medicine* 1987; 316:363-9. The estimate of 32,000 hip fractures in older adults is based on projecting the findings of this study of drug-induced hip fractures in older Michigan Medicaid patients to the entire country.

13. Myers AP, Robinson EG, Van Natta ML, Michelson JD, Collins K, Baker SP. Hip fractures among the elderly: factors associated with in-hospital mortality. *American Journal of Epidemiology* 1991; 134:1128-37.

14. Larson EB, Kukull WA, Buchner D, Reifler BV. Adverse drug reactions associated with global cognitive impairment in elderly persons. *Annals of Internal Medicine* 1987; 107:169-73. This estimate is based on projecting the findings of the Larson study on the 1.43 million Americans 65 and older who have dementia. See discussion on sleeping pills and tranquilizers (p. 198) for more details about this serious problem.

15. See discussion on sleeping pills and tranquilizers, (p. 198), for more details on this estimate.

16. See discussion on antipsychotic drugs (p. 208) for more details about drug-induced tardive dyskinesia and misprescribing of antipsychotic drugs.

17. The estimate of 61,000 older adults suffering from drug-induced parkinsonism is derived as follows: As described in detail in the chapter on antipsychotic drugs (see p. 208), there are an estimated 750,000 people 65 and older in nursing homes or living in the community who are regularly (for three or four months or longer) being prescribed antipsychotic drugs. According to a survey in 1981 of 5,000 patients being treated with antipsychotic drugs, 13.2% had parkinsonism (see reference 66 in the Mind Drugs Section). Another study by the same researchers found that 62% became better (no longer had parkinsonism) within 30 days of discontinuing the drug. Thus, at least 62% of the 13.2% of patients getting antipsychotic drugs or 7.92% of all patients getting these drugs suffer from drug-induced parkinsonism. 7.92% of 750,000 patients getting these drugs for at least several months equals 61,380 patients with drug-induced parkinsonism. This is a very conservative estimate because it does not include either those patients using antipsychotic drugs for less than 3 to 4 months (an additional 1.16 million people) who are also at risk for drug-induced parkinsonism (because 90% of the cases occur within 72 days after beginning the drug) or those who get drug-induced parkinsonism from the related drugs Reglan (metoclopramide), Compazine (prochlorperazine) and Phenergan (promethazine) usually prescribed for nausea.

18. Grimes JD. Drug-induced parkinsonism and tardive dyskinesia in non-psychiatric patients. *Canadian Medical Association Journal* 1982; 126:468.

19. Vestal, op. cit., p. 364.

20. *Drugs for the Elderly*, op. cit.

21. *The Medical Letter on Drugs and Therapeutics*. New York: The Medical Letter Inc., 1986; 28:81-86

22. Davies DM, Ed. *Textbook of Adverse Drug Reactions*. Oxford University Press, 1977, New York. Other sources included the *Physicians' Desk Reference* and outside consultants.

23. Larson, op. cit. Although this study found specific drugs in certain therapeutic classes to cause an increased risk of mental impairment, we list all of the drugs in that class here, since for benzodiazepines, beta-blockers and major tranquilizers (antipsychotic drugs), for example, there is no reason to believe that the whole class would not have this adverse effect.

CHAPTER 3

The 364 Drugs Most Used by Older Adults

Guide to the Drug Listings

This page, showing the format of our description of each drug, will help you understand our listings for each of the 364 drugs in this chapter. If a drug listing lacks any of the sections described below, it means there is no relevant information.

DO NOT USE

We recommend that these drugs not be used and we suggest an alternative treatment. Listings for these drugs do not include information on Before You Use This Drug, When You Use This Drug, How To Use This Drug, Interactions With Other Drugs, Adverse Effects, or Periodic Tests.

LIMITED USE

We believe that these drugs offer limited benefit or benefit only certain people or conditions.

Generic Name

This is the chemical name of the active ingredient(s).

BRAND NAME (Manufacturer)

These are the brand names used by the manufacturers. The names are those of the most frequently prescribed drugs. In most cases, no more than five brand names appear because of space limitations. Check the Index (p. xviii) for more names if you do not see the brand name of your drug.

Generic: Tells if a generic product is available that is sold under the chemical name of the drug.
Family: This is the class of similar drugs.

The text section describes the drug's actions and effects, in older adults in particular, and the conditions for which the drug is prescribed. It explains how and why the drug should or should not be used.

Before You Use This Drug

❏ Presents information that your doctor should know before you start to use the drug, such as your past and present health conditions and prescription and non-prescription drugs that you use.

When You Use This Drug

◆ Presents information that will ensure your safety and maximum benefit while using the drug.

How To Use This Drug

◆ Tells you what to do about a missed dose and how to take the drug.

Interactions With Other Drugs

Alphabetically lists the names of the drugs that may interact most harmfully with the drug profiled if they are used at the same time. The generic drugs are in lower-case letters and the brand names are in CAPITAL LETTERS. Make sure you know the generic name of your drugs since most but not necessarily all brand names are listed.

Adverse Effects

❑ Presents the unwanted side effects that may occur while you use the drug (and sometimes after you stop). There are two categories of adverse effects: 1) those that require immediate medical attention, including signs of overdose for many drugs, and 2) other signs that do not require immediate attention, but you should let your doctor know if they persist.

Periodic Tests

❑ Names the medical tests that should or might need to be done during the time that you use this drug, such as complete blood count, complete urine test, electrocardiogram (EKG), or eye pressure exam. You should ask your doctor which of these tests you need.

People should seek physician consultation before deciding to make any changes in their prescription drugs based on the information in this book.

Heart, Blood Pressure, Blood Vessel And Cholesterol-lowering Drugs

Drugs for High Blood Pressure

Diuretics (fluid pills)

Other Drugs for High Blood Pressure

Drugs for Heart Failure or for Angina

Drugs for Abnormal Heart Rhythm

Cholesterol-lowering Drugs

Other Cardiovascular Drugs

High Blood Pressure

High blood pressure, or hypertension, is a major contributing factor to the development of strokes, heart attacks, kidney disease, and circulation disorders. The importance of high blood pressure, especially in older adults, has not always been appreciated. For a long time, an increase in blood pressure with age was considered helpful in maintaining blood flow as hardening of the arteries occurred. Studies have shown, however, that this increase in blood pressure can cause damage to organs and lead to a stroke or heart attack.

When your blood pressure is taken, you are given two numbers, which represent the systolic pressure and the diastolic pressure — 140/60 (mm Hg — millimeters of mercury, under pressure), for example. Systolic pressure, the upper number (140), reflects the pressure in the arteries as the heart contracts and pumps blood. As the arteries harden with age (arteriosclerosis), the systolic pressure increases. Diastolic pressure, the lower number (60), reflects the pressure in the arteries as the heart relaxes and fills with blood.

Either your systolic or your diastolic pressure can be elevated. Elevations of either one or both of these pressures can increase significantly your chance of having a stroke or heart attack.

What Is "Normal" Blood Pressure For Older Adults?

There is no single level of pressure that separates "normal" from "abnormal." This surprises most people who ask what is a good pressure. The age of the person is a determining factor, as older people are able to tolerate higher blood pressure with fewer adverse effects than younger people.

It is a common misconception that a blood pressure over 140/90 is too high for older adults. (This misconception is often supported by the media, such as a *Washington Post* article

on high blood pressure which stated that 64% of all people from age 65 to 74 had high blood pressure, defined as being over 140/90.)[1] Although 140/90 may be a high blood pressure for younger adults, it is not too high for adults over 60 years of age. The current blood pressure guidelines for older people are listed below.

Are Many Older Adults Being Given Antihypertensive Drugs Unnecessarily? One study found that 41% of patients 50 and older who were carefully taken off of their high blood pressure medications did not need them, having normal blood pressure 11 months after the drug was stopped.[2]

When Is Treatment Necessary?

Two things should be taken into account when considering whether your high blood pressure should be treated. One is the benefits of the treatment for your blood pressure, which vary depending on how high it is. The other consideration is the risks or the side effects of the treatment, which will vary depending on what is being considered.

Several studies have shown that the treatment of an elevated diastolic pressure does decrease your chance of having a stroke or heart attack. However, if only your systolic pressure is elevated, which often occurs in older adults, it is controversial as to what benefits are gained by treatment. Doctors generally agree that systolic blood pressure readings above a certain level are dangerous enough so that they require treatment. Treatment of systolic blood pressure below these levels is more controversial. The following guidelines for treating high blood pressure apply to people over 60 years of age.

People's blood pressure can be higher when measured at the doctor's office than when measured at home; feeling nervous probably contributes to the higher reading.

Ask your doctor about the various methods available for home monitoring of blood pressure, so you can see if it is lower at home. This result could mean that you actually do not have high blood pressure and do not have to be treated.

Nondrug Treatment of High Blood Pressure

Lowering high blood pressure should begin with methods that do not use drugs. Using one or more of these methods can often help reduce your blood pressure to the point where you do not need medication. Even if your high blood pressure does eventually require drugs, you should adhere to as many of the following recommendations as you can. A study of nutritional therapy showed that over one-third of people who previously needed drug treatment for high blood pressure had their blood pressure adequately controlled with nutritional therapy alone.[5] In addition, these methods are safer than using medication, since they have no adverse side effects. Trying them will often make other beneficial contributions to your health.

1. *Lose weight*: One in five adults in the United States is at least 20% above "desirable" weight. Many people in this category who lose weight can reduce their blood pressure by 15%.
2. *Reduce your salt intake*: Changing your diet by not using your salt shaker and reducing your intake of processed and salty foods is a good first step.
3. *Restrict alcohol*: Cutting alcohol intake to at most, one drink a day, also can reduce blood pressure.

Guidelines for Treating High Blood Pressure in Older Adults

Diastolic Blood Pressure[3]

Under 90 mm Hg	Does not have to be treated.
90-99 mm Hg	Mildly elevated blood pressure; it does not have to be treated with drugs, but nondrug measures can be started. Your blood pressure should be taken a few times during the next 6 months, to check that it has not increased.
100 mm Hg and over	Elevated blood pressure; it should be treated using nondrug measures first. If this is not effective, then drug treatment should be used. People over the age of 80 should discuss with their doctor whether their diastolic blood pressure is elevated enough to require treatment, as the cutoff level for treatment is debatable.

Systolic Blood Pressure[4]

140-160 mm Hg	Does not have to be treated. People over 60 have a higher systolic pressure than younger people. Although 140-160 mm Hg might be considered a high level in a younger person, it does not have to be treated in an older person.
160-180 mm Hg	Mildly elevated blood pressure; there is no one "best" type of treatment. Certainly, nondrug measures should be used; however, you may wish to discuss with your doctor whether a drug is necessary.
180 mm Hg and over	Most authorities agree that a systolic blood pressure of this level should be treated, beginning with nondrug measures and using drugs if necessary.

For older adults, the systolic pressure should not be reduced below the 140-160 mm Hg range with drugs. If you use a drug to control high blood pressure and this occurs, you should discuss with your doctor the need for decreasing the amount you take.

4. *Exercise: Mild* aerobic exercise such as walking 15 or 20 minutes a day at a comfortable pace will have a beneficial effect on heart and blood pressure.
5. *Decrease your fat intake*: Decreasing the amount of animal fat has a beneficial effect on blood pressure. Furthermore, a high-fat diet is a risk factor for heart disease independent of high blood pressure. Decreasing the amount of fat in your diet will therefore help reduce your overall risk of developing heart disease.
6. *Increase the fiber in your diet*: Diets with a high fiber content can lower blood pressure.[6] A recent study showed a drop of 10 mm Hg in systolic pressure and 5 mm Hg of diastolic pressure in people who took fiber supplements for 2 months, without any other dietary changes.[7] Fiber can be increased by eating more fruits, vegetables, and whole grains.
7. *Biofeedback*: Numerous studies have shown the value, in selected patients, of biofeedback as a way of reducing or eliminating the need for antihypertensive drugs.
8. *Other methods*: Increasing your potassium and calcium intake has been shown to have a beneficial effect on blood pressure, although this is somewhat controversial. If this is done through dietary means, however, it can have other health benefits and can be recommended as an overall healthy step.[8] (See p. 67 for foods that contain potassium and p. 559 for foods that contain calcium.)

Drug Treatment of High Blood Pressure

Most of the time, high blood pressure can be controlled with just one drug. Most specialists recommend beginning with a mild water pill (diuretic) at a low dose. The safest and best studied of the diuretics is hydrochlorothiazide (see p. 117), starting out at a low dose of 12.5 to 25 milligrams per day or even every other day. In general, the rule for treating high blood pressure, like so many other drug treatments for older adults is "start low and go slow." **According to experts in prescribing for older adults, for mild hypertension (or heart failure) start with half the standard starting dose and increase gradually.**

If a second drug is needed, beta-blockers are sometimes used, although they are not as effective in older adults as they are in younger adults. Because of this, beta-blockers should never be used as the first drug in treating high blood pressure in older adults. Calcium channel blockers are other effective drugs to use as a second agent. It is rarely necessary to take more than two drugs to treat high blood pressure. If you are taking more than two, a reassessment is indicated. Hydralazine (see p. 78), however, is a good agent to use if a third drug is required.

Common Adverse Effects of High Blood Pressure Drugs

The decision to use drugs to treat high blood pressure should be based on a consideration of both the benefits and the risks of the treatment. Therefore it is very important that you report any side effects of the drugs to your doctor, so that your situation can be reassessed. These are some of the possible side effects of the various antihypertensive drugs:[9]

❏ Depression — especially with beta-blockers, reserpine, methyldopa, and clonidine (see *Chapter 2, Drugs That Can Cause Depression*, p. 18).
❏ Sedation and fatigue — especially with beta-blockers, reserpine, methyldopa, and clonidine.
❏ Impotence and sexual dysfunction — especially with beta-blockers, methyldopa, and many other heart drugs (see *Chapter 2, Drugs That Can Cause Sexual Dysfunction*, p. 37).
❏ Dizziness (from a drop in blood pressure after standing up, which can result in accidental falls and broken bones)—seen with all high blood pressure drugs to some degree, and especially with guanethidine, prazosin, and methyldopa.

Older adults are more prone to this side effect because the internal blood pressure regulation system works more slowly (see *Chapter 2, Drugs That Can Cause Dizziness on Standing,* p. 32).

❑ Loss of appetite and nausea — especially with hydrochlorothiazide, digoxin and potassium supplements (see *Chapter 2, Drugs That Can Cause Loss of Appetite, Nausea or Vomiting,* p. 40).

These and other side effects can occur with any medication for high blood pressure. Those listed occur most often. If you experience any effects, or just feel worse in general, tell your doctor. It is often better to tolerate a slightly higher blood pressure with no side effects from medication, than to have a lower blood pressure along with serious side effects from medication that will adversely affect your life.

For example, let's consider the steps in devising a treatment for a 75-year-old woman whose baseline blood pressure is 200/90 mm Hg:

1. She is first treated with 12.5 milligrams of hydrochlorothiazide. This results in a blood pressure of 170/90, and she feels quite well.
2. Her doctor attempts to lower her blood pressure further by adding another drug, propranolol, to her treatment. This results in a blood pressure of 160/90, but she "feels awful" and complains of fatigue and confusion.
3. Her doctor might consider discontinuing the propranolol and using another drug. A better idea might be to accept a blood pressure of 170/90 on hydrochlorothiazide alone or to lower it further with nondrug therapy.

Stopping Drug Treatment

Historically, patients have been taught that hypertension means treatment for life, although countless thousands of patients have abandoned their treatment without their doctors' knowledge or consent. For some patients, this may be a dangerous idea but for many others, the treatment may no longer be needed. Two large studies in Australia and Britain have shown that one-half to one-third of patients with mild hypertension for whom treatment was stopped had normal blood pressures a year or more later.[10]

In a recent editorial in the *British Medical Journal,* it was stated that

"Treatment of hypertension is part of preventive medicine and like all preventive strategies, its progress should be regularly reviewed by whoever initiates it. Many problems could be avoided by not starting antihypertensive treatment until after prolonged observation. . . . Patients should no longer be told that treatment is necessarily for life: the possibility of reducing or stopping treatment should be mentioned at the outset."[11]

This view is shared by American experts in hypertension who have stated that "Once blood pressure has been normal for a year or more, a cautious decrease in antihypertensive dosage and renewed attention to non-pharmacologic treatment may be worth trying."[12]

Drugs Used For High Blood Pressure
Recommended Drugs
First drug to use: a diuretic such as hydrochlorothiazide (Esidrix, HydroDIURIL, or a generic)

Drug to add: a beta-blocker such as propranolol (Inderal), a calcium-channel blocker — nifedipine (Procardia) or an ACE inhibitor such as captopril (Capoten)

Another drug to add: hydralazine (Apresoline)

Potassium Supplementation: Diet Is the First Choice

Who Needs Nondietary Potassium Supplementation?

Very few people actually need to take a potassium supplement or a potassium-sparing diuretic (amiloride, spironolactone, triamterene). If, however, you take digoxin, have severe liver disease, or take large doses of diuretics (water pills) for heart disease, eating a potassium-rich diet may not be sufficient to replace the potassium that you are losing. If you fall into one of these categories, it is very important that your doctor precisely monitors and regulates the amount of potassium in your bloodstream. A potassium supplement or a potassium-sparing diuretic may be necessary. Read about the methods of increasing potassium discussed below and consult with your doctor about which will be best for you.

Who Does Not Need It?

Most people taking thiazide diuretics (hydrochlorothiazide, metolazone, for example) for high blood pressure (hypertension) do not need potassium-sparing diuretics[13] or potassium supplements. This is especially true if people are started on a low dose (12.5 milligrams of hydrochlorothiazide for treatment of mild hypertension). Supplementing the diet with potassium-rich foods or beverages (see below) is sufficient to prevent low levels of potassium.[14]

Mild potassium deficiency (between 3.0 and 3.5 millimoles potassium per liter of blood) can occur during diuretic therapy, but it usually has no symptoms and requires no treatment other than eating foods that are high in potassium. Most people do not get severe potassium deficiency (less than 3.0 millimoles per liter) from treatment with diuretics. Comparisons of people eating a potassium-rich diet, people taking potassium supplements, and people taking potassium-sparing drugs have shown that (1) diet is the safest method of replacing potassium and (2) potassium supplement drugs and potassium-sparing drugs return potassium levels to normal in only 50% of the users. Therefore, if you have mild potassium deficiency, eat a few bananas before risking the side effects of potassium supplements or potassium-sparing drugs. Ask your doctor what your potassium levels were before and after you started diuretic treatment. You probably do not need a nondietary potassium supplement or potassium-sparing drug.

Three Ways to Increase Your Potassium Levels

The safest and least expensive way is to increase the amount of potassium-rich food in your *daily* diet. This will provide sufficient potassium replacement for the overwhelming majority of people taking diuretics (people who also take digoxin or who have liver disease may be exceptions).

Restricting sodium (salt) intake also helps to maintain potassium levels while lowering sodium levels. In fact, salt substitutes containing potassium chloride may be an additional source of potassium intake.[15] Consult your doctor before using salt substitutes, however, if you are already taking potassium supplements or potassium-sparing diuretics. A dosage adjustment may be necessary to prevent too much potassium in the body, a potentially fatal condition.

Potassium supplement drugs are a second method for replacing potassium, but these can cause serious adverse reactions. Potassium is an irritant to the mucous membranes that line the mouth, throat, stomach, and intestines. If not properly dissolved and dispersed in the digestive tract, potassium can come in contact with these membranes and cause bleeding, ulcers, and perforations. Use of potassium supplements, because of serious potential side effects, should be restricted to people who are eating plenty of potassium-rich foods, yet still have a low level of potassium in their blood (less than 3.0 millimoles per liter).[16]

There are several kinds of potassium supplements:

❑ *Liquids*: Liquid supplements are safer than tablets[17] because, when taken in a dilute form over a 5 to 10 minute period, potassium is effectively dispersed in the digestive tract. They cause less stomach and intestinal irritation and ulceration. Packaged as a liquid, powder, or dissolvable tablet, all forms must be completely dissolved in at least one-half cup cold water or juice before drinking. Sip slowly over 5 to 10 minutes.

❑ *Extended-release tablets or capsules*: Although liquid supplements are safest, tablets and capsules are widely used to avoid the unpleasant taste of the liquids.[18] Rarely, but

often unpredictably, these tablets and capsules can cause stomach and intestinal ulcers, bleeding, blockage, and perforation when the potassium in the tablets and capsules does not dissolve and comes in contact with the lining of the digestive tract.[19] Abdominal pain, diarrhea, nausea, vomiting, and heartburn have also been reported.[20] Because the amount of time required for food to be digested and travel through the

Potassium Levels in Milliequivalents (mEq) of Selected Foods and Potassium Supplements		
Source	**Amount**	**mEq of Potassium**
peaches, dried, uncooked	1 cup	39
raisins, dried, uncooked	1 cup	31
dates, dried, cut	1 cup, pitted	29
apricots, dried, uncooked	17 large halves	25
figs, dried	7 medium	23
prune juice, canned	1 cup	15
watermelon	1 slice (1 1/2 inches)	15
banana	1 medium	14
beef round	4 ounces	14
cantaloupe	1/2 (5 inches in diameter)	13
orange juice, fresh	1 cup	13
turkey, roasted	3 1/2 ounces	13
Klotrix Tabs	1 tablet	10
Kaon Cl-10	1 tablet	10
Milk, whole, 3.5% fat	1 cup	9
Slow-K	1 tablet	8
Kaon-Cl	1 tablet	6.7

Foods High in Potassium		
All-bran cereals	Citrus fruits	Peas
Almonds	Coconut	Pork
Apricots (dried)	Crackers (rye)	Potatoes
Avocado	Dates and figs (dried)	Prunes (dried)
Bananas	Fish, fresh	Raisins
Beans	Ham	Shellfish
Beef	Lentils	Spinach
Broccoli	Liver, beef	Tomato juice
Brussels sprouts	Milk	Turkey
Cantaloupe	Molasses	Veal
Carrots (raw)	Peaches	Watermelon
Chicken	Peanut butter	Yams

digestive tract increases with age, older people are more likely to experience side effects with these tablets or capsules.[21,22] Increased transit time leaves more opportunity for an undissolved or partially dissolved tablet or capsule to damage mucous lining.

❑ *Enteric-coated tablets*: Avoid these. "Enteric-coated" tablets are not reliably absorbed and have frequently been blamed for intestinal ulceration.[23]

The last method for increasing potassium levels is with a class of drugs called potassium-sparing diuretics. Examples of these drugs are spironolactone (Aldactone), triamterene (Dyrenium), and amiloride (Midamor). Potassium-sparing diuretics are also found in combination products such as Moduretic and Aldactazide. **These should not be used for older adults**. These drugs can cause potentially fatal side effects such as kidney failure and the retention of too much potassium which causes irregular heartbeats and heart rhythm. Studies have shown that the potassium supplements discussed above are equally effective and less dangerous than potassium-sparing diuretics, if nondietary potassium replacement is required.

If you are taking a potassium-sparing diuretic, you should never also use a potassium supplement or salt-substitute containing potassium.[24] You should also not use an ACE inhibitor such as captopril (see p. 88) with potassium supplements because of the risk of high levels of potassium.[25] Too-high levels of potassium, a potentially fatal condition that may not produce warning symptoms, may develop rapidly.

Beta-blockers

Use

Beta-blockers are a class of drugs that are used to treat high blood pressure. Acebutolol, atenolol, labetalol, metoprolol, nadolol, pindolol, propranolol, and timolol are discussed in this book. A beta-blocker is often used as the drug of first choice for treating hypertension (high blood pressure) in young and middle-aged adults. A beta-blocker, however, is less effective in older adults. Therefore, hydrochlorothiazide (see p. 117), a diuretic (water pill), should be the drug of choice for treating hypertension in people 60 years old or older. If this drug is not sufficient to lower blood pressure, then a beta-blocker can be prescribed in addition to hydrochlorothiazide. (See p. 62 for a discussion of treatment strategies to lower blood pressure.) Some of the beta-blockers are also used to treat chest pain (angina), heart attacks, irregular heart rhythms, glaucoma, and migraine headaches.

Beta-blockers should not be taken if you have asthma, emphysema, chronic bronchitis, bronchospasm, allergies, congestive heart disease, or heart block. A baseline electrocardiogram (EKG) should be taken before a beta-blocker is first prescribed to be sure that you do not have heart block. Do not smoke while taking a beta-blocker (you shouldn't be smoking anyway!!). If you smoke, you might as well stop taking the beta-blocker because it just doesn't work satisfactorily. Not only will smoking aggravate some of the respiratory side effects, but it greatly reduces the level of drug in your body.

Beta-blockers may come as tablets or capsules in two forms. If you take the extended-release tablet or capsule, you should swallow them whole. Do not crush, break, or chew them before swallowing. If you do not take the extended-release form, the tablets may be crushed or the capsules opened and mixed with a teaspoon of applesauce or jelly to make them easier to swallow. It is important to schedule appointments regularly with your doctor so that he or she can check your progress and adjust your dosage. Make sure that you have enough medicine with you to last through weekends, holidays, or vacations. You may want to carry an extra prescription with you in case of emergency. **Do not stop taking this medicine without checking with your doctor.** Sudden withdrawal may cause a heart attack, chest pain (angina), or a rapid increase in your heart rate. If you are to reduce the amount of medicine you are taking, then your doctor should give you a schedule to help you gradually reduce the dosage.

Adverse Effects

Below are some general categories of adverse effects and a discussion of which beta-blockers are most or least likely to produce these effects. If you are having any of these adverse effects, ask your doctor about changing your prescription.

Effects On the Brain

Each of the beta-blockers has been reported to cause mental changes such as depression, nightmares, hallucinations, and insomnia in some people. These occur most frequently with people taking metoprolol, pindolol, or propranolol. Propranolol should be avoided by people who are depressed or have a past history of depression. Atenolol and nadolol may cause fewer of these reactions.

Breathing Difficulties

If you are experiencing breathing difficulty, call your doctor immediately. Beta-blockers can cause spasm in the air passages of the lungs (bronchospasm) and bring on asthmatic wheezing. Therefore, beta-blockers should not be used if you have asthma, bronchospasm, chronic bronchitis, or emphysema. Atenolol and metoprolol are less likely to cause difficulty with breathing, but they are not always completely free of respiratory side effects.

Low Blood Sugar

Beta-blockers may mask signs of low blood sugar (such as blood pressure changes, increased heart rate). Diabetics on beta-blockers must learn to recognize sweating as a sign of low blood sugar. For these reasons, beta-blockers are not often used in diabetics. If you are diabetic and must take a beta-blocker, atenolol may be the best choice, since it does not delay recovery of normal blood glucose levels.

Liver Function Impairment

Atenolol and nadolol are the best choices because their primary method of elimination from the body does not involve the liver. In older adults, the liver does not work as well in breaking down drugs and other compounds so that they can be eliminated safely from the body.

Kidney Function Impairment

Metoprolol, timolol, propranolol, and labetalol are the best choices because their primary method of elimination from the body does not depend on the kidneys.

Raynaud's Syndrome or Problems with Blood Supply to the Extremities (Hands and Feet)

In addition to its beta-blocking properties, labetalol also dilates blood vessels and increases blood supply to the extremities. Raynaud's syndrome is the only reason to prefer labetalol over the other beta-blockers.[26]

Dizziness, Lightheadedness, Low Blood Pressure

Labetalol causes these side effects most often. The high incidence of side effects makes labetalol a beta-blocker drug of second choice in uncomplicated high blood pressure.

Cholesterol-lowering Drugs

For People 70 or Older

It is clear that the relationship between moderately elevated cholesterol levels and increased risk of heart disease is not as clear as people get older. As geriatrician doctors Fran Kaiser and John Morely have recently written,

"Given the uncertainty of the effects of cholesterol manipulation in older individuals, what should be the approach of the prudent geriatrician to hypercholesterolemia [elevated blood cholesterol levels]? In persons over 70 years of age, life-long dietary habits are often difficult to change and overzealous dietary manipulation may lead to failure to eat and subsequent malnutrition. Thus in this group minor dietary manipulations such as the addition of some oatmeal [or other sources of oat bran or soluble fiber] and beans and modest increases in the amount of fish eaten, may represent a rational approach. Recommending a modest increase in exercise would also seem appropriate. Beyond this, it would seem best to remember that the geriatrician's dictum is to use no drug for which there is not a clear indication."[27]

The use of cholesterol-lowering drugs in people 70 or older should be limited to patients with very high cholesterol levels (greater than 300 milligrams) and those who manifest cardiovascular disease (previous history of heart attack or angina).[28]

Older Adults Younger than 70

Since no cholesterol-lowering drug has been shown to lower overall mortality — although cardiac deaths are lower, other deaths are higher — even in those who are under 70, drugs should not be the first choice for lowering cholesterol unless the levels are extremely high or other circumstances as discussed above exist.

To lower cholesterol the first, safer, and less costly measure is to eat a low-fat diet, using mostly polyunsaturated fats (such as canola, corn, safflower, and sunflower oils) or monounsaturated fats (such as olive oil). A change from animal to vegetable proteins often corrects high cholesterol. However, it is inadvisable to go on a very low-fat diet. The main focus on cholesterol-lowering diets has been on saturated fat and cholesterol content, not soluble fiber. (When added to the diet, psyllium or oat bran is a safe, effective way of lowering cholesterol.) Exercise is also recommended. Conditions that aggravate high cholesterol, such as dependence on alcohol or tobacco, diabetes, high blood pressure, low magnesium or potassium, and thyroid disease, should be corrected before adding a cholesterol-reducing drug. If cholesterol remains high despite diet, add 10 grams of psyllium a day (see p. 356). Numerous studies have shown that psyllium, for example five grams twice a day, can significantly lower total cholesterol and LDL cholesterol.[29] Psyllium, a naturally occurring vegetable fiber, is clearly safer than any of the cholesterol-lowering drugs.

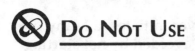 **DO NOT USE**

Alternative treatment: See Hydrochlorothiazide, p. 117.

Spironolactone and Hydrochlorothiazide (combined)
ALDACTAZIDE (Searle)

Family: Diuretics
Antihypertensives
(See High Blood Pressure, p. 62)

This product, a combination of spironolactone (see p. 72) and hydrochlorothiazide (see p. 117), is used to treat high blood pressure (hypertension). **Older adults should not use drugs that contain a fixed combination of spironolactone and hydrochlorothiazide.**

Spironolactone can cause severe side effects. It is especially dangerous for people with kidney disease.[30,31] It can cause kidney failure, retention of too much potassium,[32,33,34,35] muscular paralysis,[36] and mental confusion[37] in older adults. These are serious side effects that may be fatal. Spironolactone has also been found to cause leukemia and liver, thyroid, testicular, and breast cancer in rats.[38]

In addition to spironolactone's dangers, there are good reasons not to use any fixed-combination drug for high blood pressure. First, a single drug is often enough to control high blood pressure. If a combination drug like this one is controlling your high blood pressure, it is quite possible that one drug alone would do the same job. There is no reason to put yourself at extra risk by taking extra drugs you do not need.

If you have high blood pressure, the best way to reduce or eliminate your need for medication is through diet, weight loss, exercise, and less salt and alcohol. In mild hypertension, nutrition and hygenic measures can control high blood pressure. If these measures do not lower your blood pressure enough and you need medication, **hydrochlorothiazide, a water pill (see thiazide diuretics, p. 117), is the drug of**
choice for mild hypertension in people over 60 years old, starting with a low dose of 12.5 milligrams. It also costs less.

There is now good evidence that another benefit of thiazide diuretics such as hydrochlorothiazide is that they significantly decrease the rate of bone mineral loss in both men and women because they reduce the amount of calcium lost in the urine. An increasing number of researchers think that this will also decrease the number of fractures. [39]

Hydrochlorothiazide (a water pill) is one of the ingredients in this combination (see thiazide diuretics, p. 117). Spironolactone can cause severe side effects, as described above. If hydrochlorothiazide alone would control your blood pressure, there is no reason to take the extra risk of taking spironolactone as well.

If your high blood pressure is more severe and hydrochlorothiazide alone does not control it, there are still better drug treatments than this combination product. The best treatment in this case is a combination of hydrochlorothiazide and a second type of drug called a beta-blocker, such as propranolol (see p. 124). If you can't take a drug in the beta-blocker family, another drug called a calcium channel blocker may be used instead. In either case, your doctor would prescribe the hydrochlorothiazide and the second drug separately, with the dose of each drug adjusted to meet your needs, rather than using a product that combines the drugs in advance in a fixed combination.

If you are taking this fixed-combination drug, ask your doctor about changing your prescription.

Whatever drugs you take for high blood

pressure, once your blood pressure has been normal for a year or more, a cautious decrease in dose and renewed attention to non-drug treatment may be worth trying, according to *The Medical Letter*.[40]

"Treatment of hypertension is part of preventive medicine and like all preventive strategies, its progress should be regularly reviewed by whoever initiates it. Many problems could be avoided by not starting antihypertensive treatment until after prolonged observation. . . . Patients should no longer be told that treatment is necessarily for life: the possibility of reducing or stopping treatment should be mentioned at the outset."[41]

LIMITED USE

Spironolactone
ALDACTONE (Searle)

Generic: available

Family: Diuretics
Antihypertensives
(See High Blood Pressure, p. 62)

Spironolactone (speer on oh *lak* tone) is a water pill (diuretic) that removes less of the mineral potassium from your body than other types of diuretics do. Doctors sometimes prescribe it for high blood pressure, instead of another diuretic, in the hope that it will prevent a potassium imbalance, but there is no guarantee that this will work.

Spironolactone is a dangerous drug with many adverse effects, and it is especially dangerous for people with kidney disease.[42,43] **It can cause kidney failure, retention of too much potassium in your body,[44,45,46,47] muscle paralysis,[48] and mental confusion[49,50,51] in older adults.** These are serious side effects that may be fatal. Spironolactone has also been found to cause leukemia as well as liver, thyroid, testicular, and breast cancer in rats.[52]

Because of its dangers, spironolactone is not the best drug for treating high blood pressure or water retention. Older adults should not use spironolactone just for its ability to keep potassium in the body. If you need extra potassium, you can adjust your diet or take potassium supplements. Both methods are equally effective (see p. 66)[53] and are safer than using spironolactone. The only reason for an older adult to use this drug is to control a rare condition in which the body releases too much aldosterone (a hormone that regulates potassium and sodium levels).

If you have high blood pressure, the best way to reduce or eliminate your need for medication is through diet, weight loss, exercise, and less salt and alcohol. In mild hypertension, nutrition and hygenic measures can control high blood pressure. If these measures do not lower your blood pressure enough and you need medication, **hydrochlorothiazide, a water pill (see thiazide diuretics, p. 117), is the drug of choice for mild hypertension in people over 60 years old, starting with a low dose of 12.5 milligrams.** It also costs less.

There is now good evidence that another benefit of thiazide diuretics such as hydrochlorothiazide is that they significantly decrease the rate of bone mineral loss in both men and women because they reduce the amount of calcium lost in the urine. An increasing number of researchers think that this will also decrease the number of fractures. [54]

Whatever drugs you take for high blood

pressure, once your blood pressure has been normal for a year or more, a cautious decrease in dose and renewed attention to non-drug treatment may be worth trying, according to *The Medical Letter*.[55]

"Treatment of hypertension is part of preventive medicine and like all preventive strategies, its progress should be regularly reviewed by whoever initiates it. Many problems could be avoided by not starting antihypertensive treatment until after prolonged observation. . . . Patients should no longer be told that treatment is necessarily for life: the possibility of reducing or stopping treatment should be mentioned at the outset."[56]

Before You Use This Drug

Tell your doctor if you have or have had
- ❑ allergies to drugs
- ❑ diabetes
- ❑ kidney or liver disease
- ❑ heart disease
- ❑ breast enlargement

Tell your doctor about any other drugs you take, including aspirin, herbs, vitamins, and other non-prescription products.

When You Use This Drug

- ◆ Do not use potassium supplements, salt substitutes (potassium chloride), low-salt milk, or potassium-rich foods.

Heat Stress Alert

This drug can affect your body's ability to adjust to heat, putting you at risk of "heat stress." If you live alone, ask a friend to check on you several times during the day. Early signs of heat stress are dizziness, lightheadedness, faintness, and slightly high temperature. Call your doctor if you have any of these signs

Drink more fluids (water, fruit and vegetable juices) than usual even if you're not thirsty, unless your doctor has told you otherwise. Do not drink alcohol.

- ◆ If you plan to have any surgery, including dental, tell your doctor that you take this drug.
- ◆ **Do not take any other drugs without first talking to your doctor — especially nonprescription drugs for appetite control, asthma, colds, coughs, hay fever, or sinus problems.**

How To Use This Drug

- ◆ Take with food or milk to avoid stomach irritation.

Interactions With Other Drugs

The following drugs are listed in *Evaluations of Drug Interactions*, 1991 as causing "highly clinically significant" or "clinically significant" interactions when used together with this drug. There may be other drugs, especially those in the families of drugs listed below, that also will react with this drug to cause severe adverse effects. Make sure to ask your doctor for a complete listing of them and let her or him know if you are taking any of these interacting drugs:

digoxin; guanethidine; ISMELIN; K-LOR; K-LYTE TABLETS; KAOCHLOR; KAON-CL; KATO; KAY CIEL; KLOTRIX; LANOXIN; MICRO-K; potassium chloride; SLOW-K.

Adverse Effects

Call your doctor immediately:
- ❑ **signs of potassium imbalance:** confusion; anxiety; irregular heartbeat; numbness or tingling in hands, feet, lips; difficulty breathing; unusual tiredness or weakness; heavy legs
- ❑ sore throat and fever
- ❑ skin rash
- ❑ postmenopausal bleeding
- ❑ breast enlargement or tenderness

Call your doctor if these symptoms continue:
- ❑ drowsiness
- ❑ diarrhea, stomach cramps
- ❑ inability to get or keep an erection
- ❑ unusual sweating

- ❏ voice deepening in women
- ❏ dry mouth, increased thirst
- ❏ nausea, vomiting
- ❏ mental confusion
- ❏ stumbling, clumsiness

Periodic Tests
Ask your doctor which of these tests should

be done periodically while you are taking this drug:
- ❏ blood pressure
- ❏ complete blood counts
- ❏ kidney function tests
- ❏ blood levels of potassium and sodium (weekly when first starting to use the drug)

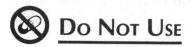 **Do Not Use**

Alternative treatment: See Hydrochlorothiazide, p. 117.

Methyldopa
ALDOMET (Merck)

Family: Antihypertensives
(See High Blood Pressure, p. 62)

Methyldopa (meth ill *doe* pa) **is an outdated medicine for treating high blood pressure (hypertension) in older adults.** It can cause severe depression and is particularly dangerous for anyone with a history of depression. It can also cause other severe side effects, including drug-induced parkinsonism (see p. 9), decreased mental sharpness, and "autoimmune effects" such as the destruction of blood cells and liver disease (hepatitis).

Many newer drugs are available that do not have methyldopa's severe side effects (see p. 62).

If you have high blood pressure, the best way to reduce or eliminate your need for medication is through diet, weight loss, exercise, and less salt and alcohol. In mild hypertension nutrition and hygenic measures can control high blood pressure. If these measures do not lower your blood pressure enough and you need medication, **hydrochlorothiazide, a water pill (see thiazide diuretics, p. 117), is the drug of choice for mild hypertension in people over 60 years old, starting with a low dose of 12.5 milligrams.** It also costs less.

There is now good evidence that another benefit of thiazide diuretics such as hydro-

chlorothiazide is that they significantly decrease the rate of bone mineral loss in both men and women because they reduce the amount of calcium lost in the urine. An increasing number of researchers think that this will also decrease the number of fractures. [57]

If this drug does not lower your blood pressure enough, your doctor can prescribe a second type of drug called a beta-blocker (see p. 68) to accompany the hydrochlorothiazide. If you cannot take a beta-blocker, a drug from another family (calcium channel blockers) can be used instead.

Whatever drugs you take for high blood pressure, once your blood pressure has been normal for a year or more, a cautious decrease in dose and renewed attention to non-drug treatment may be worth trying, according to *The Medical Letter*.[58]

"Treatment of hypertension is part of preventive medicine and like all preventive strategies, its progress should be regularly reviewed by whoever initiates it. Many problems could be avoided by not starting antihypertensive treatment until after prolonged observation. . . . Patients should no longer be told that treatment is necessarily for life: the possibility of reducing or stopping treatment should be mentioned at the outset."[59]

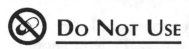 **DO NOT USE**

Alternative treatment: See Hydrochlorothiazide, p. 117.

Methyldopa and Hydrochlorothiazide (combined)
ALDORIL (Merck)

Family: Diuretics
Antihypertensives
(See High Blood Pressure, p. 62)

This product, a combination of methyldopa (see p. 74) and hydrochlorothiazide (see p. 117), is used to treat high blood pressure (hypertension). **Older adults should not use drugs that contain a fixed combination of methyldopa and hydrochlorothiazide.**

Methyldopa is an outdated drug for treating hypertension in older adults. Because of its serious side effects, including severe depression, we do not recommend that any older adult use methyldopa. It is particularly dangerous to anyone with a history of depression. In addition to depression, methyldopa can also cause autoimmune problems such as the destruction of blood cells and liver disease (hepatitis), drug-induced parkinsonism (see p. 9), and decreased mental sharpness.

In addition to methyldopa's dangers, there are good reasons not to use any fixed-combination drug for high blood pressure. First, a single drug is often enough to control high blood pressure. If a combination drug like this one is controlling your high blood pressure, it is quite possible that one drug alone would do the same job. There is no reason to put yourself at extra risk by taking extra drugs you do not need.

If you have high blood pressure, the best way to reduce or eliminate your need for medication is through diet, weight loss, exercise, and less salt and alcohol. In mild hypertension nutrition and hygenic measures can control high blood pressure. If these measures do not lower your blood pressure enough and you need medication, **hydrochlorothiazide, a water pill (see thiazide diuretics, p. 117) is the drug of choice for mild hypertension in people over 60 years old, starting with a low dose of 12.5 milligrams.** It also costs less.

There is now good evidence that another benefit of thiazide diuretics such as hydrochlorothiazide is that they significantly decrease the rate of bone mineral loss in both men and women because they reduce the amount of calcium lost in the urine. An increasing number of researchers think that this will also decrease the number of fractures. [60]

Hydrochlorothiazide, a water pill, is one of the ingredients in this combination (see thiazide diuretics, p.117). The other ingredient, methyldopa, can cause severe side effects, as described above. If hydrochlorothiazide alone would control your high blood pressure, there is no reason to take the extra risk of using methyldopa as well.

If your high blood pressure is more severe and hydrochlorothiazide alone does not control it, there are still better drug treatments than this combination product. The best treatment in this case is a combination of hydrochlorothiazide and a second type of drug called a beta-blocker, such as propranolol (see p. 124). If you can't take a drug in the beta-blocker family, another drug called a calcium channel blocker may be used instead. In either case, your doctor would prescribe the hydrochlorothiazide and the second drug separately, with the dose of each drug adjusted to meet your needs, rather than using a product that combines the drugs in advance in a fixed combination.

Whatever drugs you take for high blood pressure, once your blood pressure has been normal for a year or more, a cautious decrease in dose and renewed attention to non-drug treatment may be worth trying, according to *The Medical Letter*.[61]

"Treatment of hypertension is part of preventive medicine and like all preventive strategies, its progress should be regularly reviewed by whoever initiates it. Many problems could be avoided by not starting antihypertensive treatment until after prolonged observation. . . . Patients should no longer be told that treatment is necessarily for life: the possibility of reducing or stopping treatment should be mentioned at the outset."[62]

If you are taking this fixed-combination drug, ask your doctor about changing your prescription.

LIMITED USE

Hydralazine and Hydrochlorothiazide (combined)
APRESAZIDE (CIBA)
APRESOLINE-ESIDRIX (CIBA)

Generic: available

Family: Diuretics
Antihypertensives
(See High Blood Pressure, p. 62)

This product, a combination of hydralazine (see p. 78) and hydrochlorothiazide (see p. 117), is used to treat high blood pressure (hypertension). Drugs containing a fixed combination of hydralazine and hydrochlorothiazide offer limited benefit to older adults.

Hydralazine is not the first-choice drug for treating high blood pressure because of its side effects. People with heart failure should not take it.[63] Common side effects of this drug include rapid heartbeat and abnormally low blood pressure, which may cause lightheadedness, fainting, and falling.[64] Hydralazine may worsen chest pain (angina).[65]

In addition to hydralazine's dangers, there are good reasons not to use a fixed-combination drug for high blood pressure. First, a single drug is often enough to control high blood pressure. If a combination drug like this one is controlling your high blood pressure, it is quite possible that one drug alone would do the same job. There is no reason to put yourself at extra risk by taking extra drugs you do not need.

If you have high blood pressure, the best way to reduce or eliminate your need for medication is through diet, weight loss, exercise, and less salt and alcohol. In mild hypertension nutrition and hygenic measures can control high blood pressure. If these measures do not lower your blood pressure enough and you need medication, **hydrochlorothiazide, a water pill (see thiazide diuretics, p. 117), is the drug of choice for mild hypertension in people over 60 years old, starting with a low dose of 12.5 milligrams.** It also costs less.

There is now good evidence that another benefit of thiazide diuretics such as hydrochlorothiazide is that they significantly decrease the rate of bone mineral loss in both men and women because they reduce the amount of calcium lost in the urine. An increasing number of researchers think that this will also decrease the number of fractures. [66]

Hydrochlorothiazide is one of the ingredients in this combination (see thiazide diuretics, p. 117). Hydralazine can cause severe side effects, as described above. If hydrochlorothiazide alone would control your blood pressure, there is no reason to take the extra risk of taking the second drug as well.

If your high blood pressure is more severe and hydrochlorothiazide alone does not control it, the best treatment is a combination of hydrochlorothiazide and a second type of drug called a beta-blocker, such as propranolol (see p. 124). If you can't take a drug in the beta-blocker family, another drug called a calcium channel blocker may be used instead. In either case, your doctor would prescribe the hydrochlorothiazide and the second drug separately, with the dose of each drug adjusted to meet your needs, rather than using a product that combines the drugs in advance in a fixed combination.

If you are taking this fixed-combination drug, ask your doctor about changing your prescription.

Whatever drugs you take for high blood pressure, once your blood pressure has been normal for a year or more, a cautious decrease in dose and renewed attention to non-drug treatment may be worth trying, according to *The Medical Letter*.[67]

"Treatment of hypertension is part of preventive medicine and like all preventive strategies, its progress should be regularly reviewed by whoever initiates it. Many problems could be avoided by not starting anti-hypertensive treatment until after prolonged observation. . . . Patients should no longer be told that treatment is necessarily for life: the possibility of reducing or stopping treatment should be mentioned at the outset."[68]

This fixed-combination drug should not be the first drug used to treat your high blood pressure. You may not need more than one drug. If you do need two drugs, this product may not contain the dose of each drug that is right for you.

Your doctor has to regularly check your condition and reevaluate the effect of the drug(s) you take. This means adjusting doses and even changing drugs to ensure proper treatment. A fixed-combination drug may be the best drug for you, but it should be used only after you have tried each of its ingredients separately, in varying doses. If the doses that you need to control your high blood pressure match those in a fixed-combination product, use it. See Hydralazine, p. 78 and hydrochlorothiazide, p. 117, for more information on the use of these drugs and other drugs with which there is a potentially harmful interaction.

Heat Stress Alert
This drug can affect your body's ability to adjust to heat, putting you at risk of "heat stress." If you live alone, ask a friend to check on you several times during the day. Early signs of heat stress are dizziness, light-headedness, faintness, and slightly high temperature. Call your doctor if you have any of these signs.

Drink more fluids (water, fruit and vegetable juices) than usual even if you're not thirsty, unless your doctor has told you otherwise. Do not drink alcohol.

Hydralazine
APRESOLINE (CIBA)

Generic: available

Family: Antihypertensives
(See High Blood Pressure, p. 62)

Hydralazine (hye *dral* a zeen) is used to treat high blood pressure (hypertension), but it is not the first-choice drug for this purpose. People with coronary artery disease should not use hydralazine at all.[69]

If you have high blood pressure, the best way to reduce or eliminate your need for medication is through diet, weight loss, exercise, and less salt and alcohol. In mild hypertension, nutrition and hygenic measures can control high blood pressure. If these measures do not lower your blood pressure enough and you need medication, **hydrochlorothiazide, a water pill (see thiazide diuretics, p. 117), is the drug of choice for mild hypertension in people over 60 years old, starting with a low dose of 12.5 milligrams.** It also costs less.

There is now good evidence that another benefit of thiazide diuretics such as hydrochlorothiazide is that they significantly decrease the rate of bone mineral loss in both men and women because they reduce the amount of calcium lost in the urine. An increasing number of researchers think that this will also decrease the number of fractures. [70]

Whatever drugs you take for high blood pressure, once your blood pressure has been normal for a year or more, a cautious decrease in dose and renewed attention to non-drug treatment may be worth trying, according to *The Medical Letter*.[71]

"Treatment of hypertension is part of preventive medicine and like all preventive strategies, its progress should be regularly reviewed by whoever initiates it. Many problems could be avoided by not starting antihypertensive treatment until after prolonged observation. . . . .Patients should no longer be told that treatment is necessarily for life: the possibility of reducing or stopping treatment should be mentioned at the outset."[72]

A major problem with hydralazine is that after you take it for 4 to 24 months, you are likely to develop a "tolerance" for it.[73] This means that as time goes on, the same amount of the drug will have less and less effect. Because of this problem, your doctor should try other drugs — a combination of a water pill (diuretic) and a beta-blocker such as propranolol (see p. 124) — before prescribing hydralazine. Only if this combination fails to bring your blood pressure down enough (diastolic blood pressure below 100 millimeters of mercury) should your doctor consider hydralazine.[74]

Hydralazine commonly causes a rapid heartbeat and below normal blood pressure, which may lead to lightheadedness, fainting, and a risk of falling. It may also make chest pain (angina) worse.[75]

The starting dose of hydralazine should be between 10 and 12.5 milligrams (mg), four times a day. The total daily dose should not go over 150 to 200 milligrams.[76] **If you have impaired kidney function, you should be taking a smaller dose.**

Before You Use This Drug
Do not use if you have or have had
- ❏ aortic aneurysm
- ❏ disease of the arteries that nourish the heart
- ❏ disease of the blood vessels that nourish the brain
- ❏ rheumatic heart disease
- ❏ severe heart disease
- ❏ severe kidney disease

Tell your doctor if you have or have had
- ❏ allergies to drugs
- ❏ congestive heart failure
- ❏ kidney disease

Tell your doctor about any other drugs you take, including aspirin, herbs, vitamins, and other non-prescription products.

When You Use This Drug

◆ Until you know how you react to this drug, do not drive or perform other activities requiring alertness.

◆ **Do not stop taking this drug suddenly. Your doctor must give you a schedule to decrease your dose gradually.**

◆ You may feel dizzy when rising from a lying or sitting position. When getting out of bed, hang your legs over the side of the bed for a few minutes, then get up slowly. When getting up from a chair, get up slowly and stay beside the chair until you are sure that you are not dizzy. (See p. 14.)

◆ If you plan to have any surgery, including dental, tell your doctor that you take this drug.

◆ **Do not take other drugs without talking to your doctor first — especially non-prescription drugs for appetite control, asthma, colds, coughs, hay fever, or sinus problems.**

◆ You may need more vitamin B_6 (pyridoxine) than usual. Ask your doctor about getting more vitamin B_6 in your diet or about taking a supplement.

◆ Do not drink alcohol.

How To Use This Drug

◆ Take with food. Crush tablet and mix with food or drink, or swallow whole with water.

◆ Keep the liquid form in the refrigerator. Do not use it after 14 days or if its color changes. Replace it.

◆ If you miss a dose, take it as soon as you remember, but skip it if it is almost time for the next dose. **Do not take double doses.**

◆ Call your doctor if you miss two doses in a row.

Interactions With Other Drugs

Some other drugs that you may be taking (either over-the-counter or prescription drugs) can interact with this one, causing adverse effects. Find out from your doctor what these drugs are and let him or her know if you are taking any of them.

Adverse Effects

Call your doctor immediately:
❑ blisters on skin
❑ chest pain
❑ general discomfort or weakness
❑ joint pain
❑ numbness and tingling of hands and feet
❑ skin rash or itching
❑ sore throat and fever
❑ swelling of feet or lower legs
❑ swelling of lymph glands

Call your doctor if these symptoms continue:
❑ diarrhea or constipation
❑ loss of appetite
❑ nausea, vomiting
❑ rapid or irregular heartbeat
❑ shortness of breath on exertion
❑ dizziness, lightheadedness
❑ watering or irritated eyes
❑ headache
❑ stuffy nose (do not take any medication for this)

Periodic Tests

Ask your doctor which of these tests should be done done periodically while you are taking this drug:
❑ blood pressure
❑ antinuclear antibody titer
❑ complete blood counts
❑ direct Coombs' test
❑ lupus erythematosus (LE) cell preparation

Timolol
BLOCADREN (Merck)

Generic: available

Family: Beta-blockers (see p. 68)
Antihypertensives
(See High Blood Pressure, p. 62)

Timolol (*tim* oh lole) has two forms for different uses: tablets for the heart (Blocadren) and drops for the eyes (Timoptic). The tablet is used for high blood pressure (hypertension), chest pain (angina), and irregular heartbeats (arrhythmias), and to decrease the frequency of migraine headaches. **If you are over 60, you will generally need to take less than the usual adult dose of the tablet, especially if your liver function is impaired.** The eye drop is used for glaucoma.

Although this page discusses timolol primarily as a drug for heart and blood vessel disease, eye drop users may have some of the general side effects listed below, especially if the drops are used improperly. See p. 582 for instructions on using eye drugs properly.

For young adults with high blood pressure, doctors usually prescribe a drug in this family (a beta-blocker) before any other drug. But for blacks and older adults, these drugs are less effective as the sole treatment. For these groups of people, doctors usually prescribe another type of drug called a diuretic (water pill) to lower blood pressure, and add a beta-blocker, such as propranolol, as a second drug if the diuretic alone is not enough.

If you have high blood pressure, the best way to reduce or eliminate your need for medication is through diet, weight loss, exercise, and less salt and alcohol. In mild hypertension nutrition and hygenic measures can control high blood pressure. If these measures do not lower your blood pressure enough and you need medication,

hydrochlorothiazide, a water pill (see thiazide diuretics, p. 117), is the drug of choice for mild hypertension in people over 60 years old, starting with a low dose of 12.5 milligrams. It also costs less.

There is now good evidence that another benefit of thiazide diuretics such as hydrochlorothiazide is that they significantly decrease the rate of bone mineral loss in both men and women because they reduce the amount of calcium lost in the urine. An increasing number of researchers think that this will also decrease the number of fractures. [77]

Whatever drugs you take for high blood pressure, once your blood pressure has been normal for a year or more, a cautious decrease in dose and renewed attention to non-drug treatment may be worth trying, according to *The Medical Letter*.[78]

"Treatment of hypertension is part of preventive medicine and like all preventive strategies, its progress should be regularly reviewed by whoever initiates it. Many problems could be avoided by not starting antihypertensive treatment until after prolonged observation. . . . Patients should no longer be told that treatment is necessarily for life: the possibility of reducing or stopping treatment should be mentioned at the outset."[79]

All beta-blockers are similarly effective, although not necessarily interchangeable. Increased sensitivity to cold is one side effect. (See, glossary p. 689 for signs of hypothermia.) If you are bothered by side effects when taking timolol, talk to your doctor about switching to another beta-blocker, such as propranolol, which is available generically. The side effects of these drugs vary widely, and each individual responds differently to each one. See p. 68 for a discussion of alternatives to timolol.

Timolol has been shown to cause an

increased number of adrenal, lung, uterine, and breast cancers in rats.

Before You Use This Drug

Do not use if you have
- ❑ congestive heart failure
- ❑ asthma
- ❑ emphysema or chronic bronchitis

Tell your doctor if you have or have had
- ❑ allergies to drugs
- ❑ poor blood circulation
- ❑ diabetes
- ❑ difficulty breathing
- ❑ gout
- ❑ kidney, liver, lung, or pancreas disease
- ❑ lupus erythematosus
- ❑ mental depression
- ❑ alcohol dependence
- ❑ Raynaud's syndrome
- ❑ thyroid problems

Tell your doctor about any other drugs you take, including aspirin, herbs, vitamins, and other non-prescription products.

When You Use This Drug

- ◆ **Learn to take your pulse, and get immediate medical help if your pulse slows to 50 beats per minute or slower, even if you are feeling well. Some people have suffered from slowed heart rate and heart failure while taking timolol.**
- ◆ Until you know how you react to this drug, do not drive or perform other activities requiring alertness.
- ◆ Be careful not to overexert yourself, even though your chest pain may feel better.
- ◆ **Do not stop taking this drug suddenly. Your doctor must give you a schedule to decrease your dose gradually, to prevent chest pain and possible heart attack.**
- ◆ You may feel dizzy when rising from a lying or sitting position. When getting out of bed, hang your legs over the side of the bed for a few minutes, then get up slowly. When getting up from a chair, get up slowly and stay beside the chair until you are sure that you are not dizzy. (See p. 14.)
- ◆ **Caution diabetics:** see p. 516.

- ◆ If you plan to have any surgery, including dental, tell your doctor that you take this drug.
- ◆ **Do not take other drugs without talking to your doctor first — especially non-prescription drugs for appetite control, asthma, colds, coughs, hay fever, or sinus problems.**

Heat Stress Alert
This drug can affect your body's ability to adjust to heat, putting you at risk of "heat stress." If you live alone, ask a friend to check on you several times during the day. Early signs of heat stress are dizziness, light-headedness, faintness, and slightly high temperature. Call your doctor if you have any of these signs.

Drink more fluids (water, fruit and vegetable juices) than usual, even if you're not thirsty, unless your doctor has told you otherwise. Do not drink alcohol.

How To Use This Drug

- ◆ Crush tablets and mix with water, or swallow whole with water.
- ◆ If you miss a dose, take it as soon as you remember, unless it is less than 4 hours until your next scheduled dose. **Do not take double doses.**

Interactions With Other Drugs

The following drugs are listed in *Evaluations of Drug Interactions*, 1991 as causing "highly clinically significant" or "clinically significant" interactions when used together with this drug. There may be other drugs, especially those in the families of drugs listed below, that also will react with this drug to cause severe adverse effects. Make sure to ask your doctor for a complete listing of them and let her or him know if you are taking any of these interacting drugs:

ADRENALIN (also in bee sting kits); ALDOMET; amiodarone; CALAN; CATAPRES; chlorpromazine;

cimetidine; clonidine; cocaine;
CORDARONE; COUMADIN; epinephrine; ESKALITH; FLUOTHANE;
furosemide; halothane; INDERAL;
insulin; LASIX; levothyroxine;
lidocaine; lithium; methyldopa;
MINIPRESS; NEMBUTAL;
pentobarbital; prazosin; propranolol;
pseudoephedrine; RIFADIN; rifampin;
SUDAFED; SYNTHROID; TAGAMET;
THEO-DUR; theophylline;
THORACINE; thyroid; tobacco;
TUBARINE; tubocurarine; verapamil;
warfarin; XYLOCAINE.

Adverse Effects
Call your doctor immediately:
- ❏ headache
- ❏ anxiety, nervousness
- ❏ itching skin
- ❏ nausea, vomiting, diarrhea
- ❏ unusual tiredness or weakness
- ❏ disturbed sleep, nightmares
- ❏ decreased sexual ability
- ❏ numbness or tingling of limbs

Call your doctor if these symptoms continue:
- ❏ difficulty breathing
- ❏ chest pain
- ❏ hallucinations
- ❏ cold hands or feet
- ❏ mental depression
- ❏ skin rash
- ❏ swelling of ankles, feet, or legs
- ❏ slow pulse

More side effects information appears on p. 68.

Periodic Tests
Ask your doctor which of these tests should be done periodically while you are taking this drug:
- ❏ complete blood counts
- ❏ blood pressure and pulse rate
- ❏ heart function tests, such as electrocardiogram (EKG)
- ❏ kidney function tests
- ❏ liver function tests
- ❏ blood glucose levels
- ❏ eye pressure exams

LIMITED USE

Bumetanide
BUMEX (Roche)

Generic: not available

Family: Diuretics
Antihypertensives
(See High Blood Pressure, p. 62)

Bumetanide (byoo *met* a nide) is a very strong "water pill" (loop diuretic) with many side effects. It is used to treat fluid retention and high blood pressure. If you are over 60, you should use bumetanide only for reducing fluid retention, and then only if you have decreased kidney function[80] and have already tried a milder drug

such as hydrochlorothiazide (see p. 117) or the more proven and less expensive furosemide (see p. 136) without success.[81] People over 60 years old who have normal kidney function should rarely, if ever, use bumetanide.[82]

If you have high blood pressure, the best way to reduce or eliminate your need for medication is through diet, weight loss, exercise, and less salt and alcohol. In mild hypertension, nutrition and hygenic measures can control high blood pressure. If these measures do not lower your blood pressure enough and you need medication,

hydrochlorothiazide, a water pill (see thiazide diuretics, p. 117), is the drug of choice for mild hypertension in people over 60 years old, starting with a low dose of 12.5 milligrams. It also costs less.

There is now good evidence that another benefit of thiazide diuretics such as hydrochlorothiazide is that they significantly decrease the rate of bone mineral loss in both men and women because they reduce the amount of calcium lost in the urine. An increasing number of researchers think that this will also decrease the number of fractures. [83]

If hydrochlorothiazide alone does not work, your doctor should add a second drug such as a beta-blocker, propranolol for example, (see p. 124) rather than switching you to a strong diuretic like bumetanide.[84]

Older adults are more likely than others to develop blood clots, shock,[85] dizziness, confusion, and insomnia, and have an increased chance of falling, while taking bumetanide.[86]

Whatever drugs you take for high blood pressure, once your blood pressure has been normal for a year or more, a cautious decrease in dose and renewed attention to non-drug treatment may be worth trying, according to *The Medical Letter.*[87]

"Treatment of hypertension is part of preventive medicine and like all preventive strategies, its progress should be regularly reviewed by whoever initiates it. Many problems could be avoided by not starting antihypertensive treatment until after prolonged observation. . . . Patients should no longer be told that treatment is necessarily for life: the possibility of reducing or stopping treatment should be mentioned at the outset."[88]

Before You Use This Drug
Do not use if you have or have had
❑ a sensitivity to sulfa drugs (sulfonamides) or yellow dye #5
Tell your doctor if you have or have had
❑ allergies to drugs
❑ diabetes

❑ kidney, liver, or pancreas disease
❑ gout
❑ hearing loss
❑ lupus erythematosus
❑ salt- or sugar-restricted diet
Tell your doctor about any other drugs you take, including aspirin, herbs, vitamins, and other non-prescription products.

When You Use This Drug
◆ **Check with your doctor to make certain your fluid intake is adequate and appropriate. Because bumetanide is a very strong water pill, you are in danger of becoming dehydrated.**
◆ You may feel dizzy when rising from a lying or sitting position. When getting up from bed, hang your legs over the side of the bed for a few minutes, then get up slowly. When getting up from a chair, stay beside the chair until you are sure that you are not dizzy. (See p. 14.)
◆ **Bumetanide will cause your body to lose potassium, an important mineral.** See p. 66 for information on how to make sure you get enough potassium.
◆ Bumetanide can cause a loss of hearing, which is usually temporary but may be permanent. The risk of hearing loss is greater if you are also using amphotericin B or an antibiotic from the aminoglycoside family (see p. 594 for two examples).
◆ If you plan to have any surgery, includ-

Heat Stress Alert
This drug can affect your body's ability to adjust to heat, putting you at risk of "heat stress." If you live alone, ask a friend to check on you several times during the day. Early signs of heat stress are dizziness, lightheadedness, faintness, and slightly high temperature. Call your doctor if you have any of these signs.

Drink more fluids (water, fruit and vegetable juices) than usual even if you're not thirsty, unless your doctor has told you otherwise. Do not drink alcohol.

ing dental, tell your doctor that you take this drug.

◆ **Do not take other drugs without first talking to your doctor — especially nonprescription drugs for appetite control, asthma, colds, coughs, hay fever, or sinus problems.**

How To Use This Drug

◆ Take with food or milk to avoid stomach irritation. Tablet may be crushed and mixed with food or drink.

◆ If you are taking bumetanide more than once a day, try to take the last dose before 6 p.m. This will help you avoid interrupting your sleep to go to the bathroom.

◆ If you miss a dose, take it as soon as you remember, but skip it if it is almost time for the next dose. **Do not take double doses.**

Interactions With Other Drugs

The following drugs are listed in *Evaluations of Drug Interactions*, 1991 as causing "highly clinically significant" or "clinically significant" interactions when used together with this drug. There may be other drugs, especially those in the families of drugs listed below, that also will react with this drug to cause severe adverse effects. Make sure to ask your doctor for a complete listing of them and let her or him know if you are taking any of these interacting drugs:

CAPOTEN; captopril; cephalexin; charcoal; chlorpropamide; cholestyramine; cisplastin; DIABINESE; digoxin; ESKALITH; INDERAL; KEFLEX; LANOXIN; lithium; PLATINOL; propranolol; QUESTRAN; THEO-DUR; theophylline.

Adverse Effects

Call your doctor immediately:
❏ dry mouth, increased thirst
❏ irregular heartbeat
❏ mood or mental changes
❏ muscle cramps, pain
❏ nausea, vomiting
❏ unusual tiredness or weakness
❏ weak pulse
❏ skin rash
❏ chest pain
❏ nipple tenderness

Call your doctor if these symptoms continue:
❏ dizziness, lightheadedness
❏ diarrhea
❏ loss of appetite, upset stomach
❏ headache
❏ blurred vision
❏ premature ejaculation or difficulty with erection

Periodic Tests

Ask your doctor which of these tests should be done periodically while you are taking this drug:
❏ blood pressure
❏ complete blood counts
❏ blood levels of sodium, potassium, chloride, calcium, sugar, and uric acid
❏ liver function tests
❏ kidney function tests

Verapamil
CALAN, CALAN SR (sustained-release) (Searle)
ISOPTIN (Knoll)
VERELAN (Lederle)

Generic: available

Family: Calcium Channel Blockers
(See High Blood Pressure p. 62)

Verapamil (ver *ap* a mill) belongs to a family of drugs called calcium channel blockers. They are used primarily to treat chest pain (angina) and coronary artery disease, and also to lower blood pressure (hypertension) and improve irregular heartbeats (arrhythmias). Calcium channel blockers control, but do not cure high blood pressure. These drugs may improve capacity for exercise and delay the need for heart surgery.

Each calcium channel blocker differs in the likelihood of harmful side effects. Verapamil, more than other calcium channel blockers, commonly causes constipation. It is more apt to slow heart rate, depress heart contraction, and slow conduction than other calcium channel blockers, but is less likely to cause dizziness, flushing, headache, and swelling of legs and feet.[89]

Compared to other calcium channel blockers, certain individuals are more apt to get congestive heart failure from it.[90] Elderly people may be more sensitive to harmful effects. A dose of 40 milligrams of verapamil three times a day is recommended when older people, those with liver disease, or certain heart conditions start to take it. **People with decreased kidney function should avoid the long-acting forms of verapamil[91] and may require a low dose.** It is sometimes taken with other heart medications.

If you have high blood pressure, the best way to reduce or eliminate your need for medication is through diet, weight loss, exercise, and less salt and alcohol. In mild hypertension, nutrition and hygenic measures can control high blood pressure. If these measures do not lower your blood pressure enough and you need medication, **hydrochlorothiazide, a water pill (see thiazide diuretics, p. 117), is the drug of choice for mild hypertension in people over 60 years old, starting with a low dose of 12.5 milligrams.** It also costs less.

There is now good evidence that another benefit of thiazide diuretics such as hydrochlorothiazide is that they significantly decrease the rate of bone mineral loss in both men and women because they reduce the amount of calcium lost in the urine. An increasing number of researchers think that this will also decrease the number of fractures.[92]

Whatever drugs you take for high blood pressure, once your blood pressure has been normal for a year or more, a cautious decrease in dose and renewed attention to non-drug treatment may be worth trying, according to *The Medical Letter*.[93]

"Treatment of hypertension is part of preventive medicine and like all preventive strategies, its progress should be regularly reviewed by whoever initiates it. Many problems could be avoided by not starting antihypertensive treatment until after prolonged observation. . . . Patients should no longer be told that treatment is necessarily for life: the possibility of reducing or stopping treatment should be mentioned at the outset."[94]

Before You Use This Drug

In certain conditions use of verapamil is not only risky, but it is also less apt to work well.[95]

Do not use if you have or have had
- severe hypotension
- cardiogenic shock
- heart attack
- heartbeats which are too slow (bradycardia)
- heart block without a pacemaker
- heartbeats that are too rapid in association with Wolff-Parkinson-White syndrome
- heart failure[96]
- sick sinus syndrome

Tell your doctor if you have or have had
- allergies to drugs
- aortic stenosis
- diabetes[97]
- heart, kidney or liver problems
- low blood pressure
- muscular dystrophy
- myasthenia gravis[98]

Tell your doctor about any other drugs you take, including aspirin, herbs, vitamins, and other non-prescription products.

If you now take a beta-blocker, your doctor may gradually take you off of it before starting a calcium channel blocker.[99]

When You Use This Drug

◆ **Learn to take your pulse, and get immediate help if your pulse slows to 50 beats per minute or slower, even if you are feeling well.**

◆ Until you know how you react to this drug, do not drive or perform other activities requiring alertness.

◆ Follow a diet recommended by your doctor.

◆ Have your doctor suggest exercises which avoid overexertion.

◆ **Do not stop taking calcium channel blockers suddenly. Contact your doctor for a schedule to decrease your drug gradually.**

◆ You may feel dizzy when rising from a lying or sitting position. If you are lying down, hang your legs over the side of the bed for a few minutes, then get up slowly. When getting up from a chair, stay by the chair until you are sure that you are not dizzy. (See p. 14.)

◆ If you plan to have any surgery, including dental, tell your doctor that you take this drug.

◆ **Do not take other drugs without talking to your doctor first — especially drugs for asthma, colds, cough, diet, hay fever, or sinus problems.**

How To Use This Drug

◆ Swallow tablets whole or break in half. Do not break, chew, or crush the long-acting capsule or tablet forms.

◆ Take long-acting forms with food or milk.

◆ If you miss a dose, take it as soon as you remember, but skip it if it is almost time for the next dose. **Do not take double doses.**

◆ Do not store in the bathroom. Do not expose to heat, moisture or strong light.

◆ If you use a generic verapamil, request your pharmacist to dispense verapamil made by the same manufacturer each time.

Interactions With Other Drugs

The following drugs are listed in *Evaluations of Drug Interactions,* 1991 as causing "highly clinically significant" or "clinically significant" interactions when used together with this drug. There may be other drugs, especially those in the families of drugs listed below, that also will react with this drug to cause severe adverse effects. Make sure to ask your doctor for a complete listing of them and let her or him know if you are taking any of these interacting drugs:

alcohol; CALCIFEROL; calcium gluconate; carbamazepine; cimetidine; cyclosporine; DANTRIUM; dantrolene; digoxin; DILANTIN; ELIXOPHYLLIN; ergocalciferol; ESKALITH; INDERAL; LANOXIN; lithium; LITHOBID; NORCURON; phenytoin; propranolol; QUINAGLUTE; QUINIDEX; quinidine; RIFADIN; rifampin; RIMACTANE; SANDIMMUNE; TAGAMET; TEGRETOL; THEO-DUR; theophyllines; vecuronium.

Additionally, the *United States Pharmacopeia Drug Information*, 1992 lists these drugs as having interactions of major significance:

beta-blockers, optic; BETAGAN; BETOPTIC; disopyramide (If you stop taking verapamil wait at least 24 hours before starting disopyramide. If you are already on disopyramide, it should be stopped and you should wait 2 days before starting verapamil); NORPACE; timolol; TIMOPTIC.

If you stop taking verapamil, doses of interacting drugs may need to be adjusted.

Adverse Effects

Call your doctor immediately:
- breathing difficulties
- chest pain
- convulsions, jerking movements of limbs
- dizziness
- fever
- severe headache
- heartbeat changes
- low blood pressure
- skin rash
- swelling of legs or feet

Call your doctor if these symptoms continue:
- abdominal pain
- vivid or disturbing dreams
- dry mouth
- fatigue
- enlarged, bleeding, or tender gums[100]
- heartburn
- impotence
- muscle pain or tenderness
- nausea
- frequent urination
- blurred vision

Periodic Tests

Ask your doctor which of these tests should be done periodically while you are taking this drug:
- blood pressure
- electrocardiogram (EKG)
- kidney function tests
- liver functions tests
- pulse

LIMITED USE

Captopril
CAPOTEN (Squibb)
Lisinopril
PRINIVIL (Merck)
ZESTRIL (Stuart)
Enalapril
VASOTEC (Merck)

Generic: not available

Family: Antihypertensives
(See High Blood Pressure Drugs,
p. 62)

Captopril (*kap* toe pril), lisinopril (liss *sin* o prill) and enalapril (n *al* ap rill), belong to a group of drugs for high blood pressure called ACE inhibitors.

ACE inhibitors are effective drugs for the treatment of high blood pressure (hypertension) and congestive heart failure in older adults. **They can cause dangerous side effects such as bone marrow depression and kidney disease and, therefore, should be taken in lower doses by the elderly. This may amount to less than one-third the doses used in the past.**

You are more likely to suffer harmful effects from ACE inhibitors if you have decreased kidney function, especially if you are *dehydrated*. Since older adults generally have some decrease in kidney function, these drugs may be especially dangerous for them. For this reason, they should not be the first choice for patients with kidney disease. In addition, patients taking a diuretic (water pill) should be watched carefully or, at their physician's discretion, be taken off that medication when an ACE inhibitor is started. Patients using potassium-sparing drugs (see below) should not use ACE inhibitors.

At times when using ACE inhibitors, the blood pressure goes too low, especially with the first dose. Older people are more likely to be sensitive to low blood pressure. A rare but potentially life-threatening reaction is angioedema, a sudden swelling of the face, lips, and particularly the tongue, which may last three days.[101,102] While this reaction usually occurs with the first dose, it can occur years later. Once angioedema occurs, all ACE inhibitors should be stopped.[103] **In general, if you are over 60, you should be taking less than the usual adult dose.** Since enalapril stays in the body longer than captopril, its adverse effects may last longer.

If you have high blood pressure, the best way to reduce or eliminate your need for medication is through diet, weight loss, exercise, and less salt and alcohol. In mild hypertension nutrition and hygenic measures can control high blood pressure. If these measures do not lower your blood pressure enough and you need medication, **hydrochlorothiazide, a water pill (see thiazide diuretics, p. 117), is the drug of choice for mild hypertension in people over 60 years old, starting with a low dose of 12.5 milligrams.** It also costs less.

There is now good evidence that another benefit of thiazide diuretics such as hydrochlorothiazide is that they significantly decrease the rate of bone mineral loss in both men and women because they reduce the amount of calcium lost in the urine.

An increasing number of researchers think that this will also decrease the number of fractures. [104]

Whatever drugs you take for high blood pressure, once your blood pressure has been normal for a year or more, a cautious decrease in dose and renewed attention to non-drug treatment may be worth trying, according to *The Medical Letter*.[105]

"Treatment of hypertension is part of preventive medicine and like all preventive strategies, its progress should be regularly reviewed by whoever initiates it. Many problems could be avoided by not starting anti-hypertensive treatment until after prolonged observation. . . . .Patients should no longer be told that treatment is necessarily for life: the possibility of reducing or stopping treatment should be mentioned at the outset."[106]

Before You Use This Drug

Do not use if you have or have had
❑ angioedema[107,108]
❑ severe kidney disease
❑ or are taking a potassium-sparing drug such as spironolactone (Aldactone), triamterene (Dyrenium — a Do Not Use drug — or Dyazide/Maxzide

Tell your doctor if you have or have had
❑ allergies to drugs
❑ an autoimmune disease such as lupus or scleroderma
❑ renal artery stenosis or generalized arteriosclerosis[109]
❑ asthma or other lung problems
❑ bone marrow depression
❑ cerebrovascular accident
❑ diabetes
❑ salt-restricted diet
❑ heart problems
❑ high potassium levels
❑ kidney or liver problems

Tell your doctor about any other drugs you take, including aspirin, herbs, vitamins, and other non-prescription products.

When You Use This Drug

◆ If you take a diuretic, your doctor may taper you off of it, or lower your dose, a few days prior to starting one of these drugs. Take the first dose of enalapril under medical supervision. For hypertension, treatment supervision should last at least 2 hours and then an additional hour after your blood pressure has stabilized. Usually, this will be at a doctor's office. Have a companion stay with you until at least 6 hours has elapsed from your first dose.

◆ When taken for congestive heart failure, supervison should continue at least 6 hours. Many doctors prefer to start this drug in a hospital.[110] You should be watched closely for two weeks.

◆ Close supervision should also take place whenever your dose of either enalapril or diuretic is changed.

◆ You may feel dizzy when rising from a lying or sitting position. If you are lying down, hang your legs over the side of the bed for a few minutes, then get up slowly. When getting up from a chair, stay by the chair until you are sure that you are not dizzy. (See p. 14.)

◆ Drink plenty of fluids to avoid dehydration, especially when exercising, during spells of hot weather, or if you have nausea, vomiting or diarrhea. Call your doctor if it continues or becomes severe.

◆ **Do not take other drugs without talking to your doctor first — especially non-prescription drugs for appetite control, asthma, colds, coughs, hay fever, or sinus problems.**

◆ Be careful not to overexert yourself, even though your chest pain may feel better. Talk to your doctor about a safe exercise program.

◆ Until you know how you react to these drugs, do not drive or perform other activities requiring alertness. Do not drive after taking the first dose, or any time your dose changes.

◆ Maintain some sodium (salt) in your diet, but avoid excess salt. Do not use low-salt milk, or salt substitutes containing potassium. Check with your doctor before going on any kind of diet.[111] Avoid alcohol.

◆ Take your blood pressure periodically. Having your blood pressure checked away from the doctor's office is good practice. If possible have your own automatic blood pressure measuring device but be sure to have both your blood pressure and the device checked by your doctor.

◆ If you plan to have any surgery, including dental, tell your doctor that you take one of these drugs.

◆ **Do not stop taking this drug suddenly. Your doctor must give you a schedule to lower your dose gradually.**

Heat Stress Alert

This drug can affect your body's ability to adjust to heat, putting you at risk of "heat stress." If you live alone, ask a friend to check on you several times during the day. Early signs of heat stress are dizziness, lightheadedness, faintness, and slightly high temperature. Call your doctor if you have any of these signs.

Drink more fluids (water, fruit and vegetable juices) than usual, even if you're not thirsty, unless your doctor has told you otherwise. Do not drink alcohol.

Cough Alert

A common adverse effect, after taking ACE inhibitors a few weeks, is a dry, hacking cough, especially in women. Check with your doctor about a 4-day withdrawal from your ACE inhibitor to determine if this is the cause of your cough. This trial withdrawal can prevent unnecessary and sometimes costly tests and treatments.

How To Use This Drug

◆ Swallow tablets whole or break in half as prescribed. Take on an empty stomach at least one hour before meals.

◆ Take at the same time each day with the last dose at bedtime to control blood pressure overnight and decrease daytime drowsiness.

◆ Continue to take, even if you feel well.

◆ If you miss a dose, take it as soon as you remember but skip it if it is almost time for the next dose. **Do not take double doses.**

◆ Store at room temperature with lid on tightly.

◆ Do not store in the bathroom. Do not expose to heat, moisture or strong light.

Interactions With Other Drugs

The following drugs are listed in *Evaluations of Drug Interactions*, 1991 as causing "highly clinically significant" or "clinically significant" interactions when used together with this drug. There may be other drugs, especially those in the families of drugs listed below, that also will react with this drug to cause severe adverse effects. Make sure to ask your doctor for a complete listing of them and let her or him know if you are taking any of these interacting drugs:

aspirin; BUFFERIN; chlorpromazine; digoxin; ECOTRIN; ESKALITH; furosemide; INDOCIN; indomethacin; LANOXIN; LASIX; lithium; LITHOBID; MEASURIN; THORAZINE.

Additionally, the *United States Pharmacopeia Drug Information*, 1992 lists these drugs as having interactions of major significance: alcohol; ALDACTONE; diuretics, potassium-sparing type; DYRENIUM; K-TAB; MICRO-K; MIDAMOR; potassium; SLOW-K.

Adverse Effects

Seek emergency help:
❏ difficulty breathing
❏ sudden swelling of eyes, face, lips, throat, tongue

Call your doctor immediately:
❏ chest pain or angina
❏ confusion
❏ dizziness, lightheadedness
❏ fainting
❏ fever or chills

❏ irregular heartbeat
❏ hoarseness
❏ joint pain
❏ legs feel heavy, or weak, walking is awkward
❏ nervousness
❏ numbness or tingling in hands, feet, lips
❏ skin rash
❏ difficulty swallowing
❏ swelling of hands, ankles, feet

Call your doctor if these symptoms continue:
❏ diarrhea
❏ cough or dry, tickling sensation in throat
❏ fatigue, unusual tiredness
❏ headache

❏ itching
❏ nausea, vomiting
❏ taste sense is altered or lost, loss of appetite
❏ urinary pain, or change in frequency or quantity of urine

Periodic Tests
Ask your doctor which of these tests should be done periodically while you are taking this drug:
❏ blood pressure
❏ kidney function
❏ urinary protein
❏ white blood cell count

LIMITED USE

Captopril and Hydrochlorothiazide (combined)
CAPOZIDE (Squibb)
Lisinopril and Hydrochlorothiazide (combined)
PRINZIDE (Merck)
ZESTORETIC (Stuart)
Enalapril and Hydrochlorothiazide (combined)
VASERETIC (Merk, Sharp & Dohme)

Generic: not available

Family: Diuretics
Antihypertensives (See High Blood Pressure, p. 62) (See ACE inhibitors, p. 88)

ACE inhibitors are effective drugs for the treatment of high blood pressure (hypertension) and congestive heart failure in older adults. **They can cause dangerous side effects such as bone marrow depression and kidney disease and, therefore, should be taken in lower doses by the elderly. This may amount to less than one-third the doses used in the past.**

You are more likely to suffer harmful effects from ACE inhibitors if you have decreased kidney function, especially if you are *dehydrated*. Since older adults generally have some decrease in kidney function, these drugs may be especially dangerous for them. For this reason, they should not be the first choice for patients with kidney disease. In addition, patients taking a diuretic (water pill) should be watched carefully or, at their physician's discretion, be taken off that medication, when an ACE inhibitor is started. Patients using potassium-sparing drugs (see below) should not use ACE inhibitors.

These products, a combination of either

25 or 50 milligrams of captopril (see p. 88) with either 15 or 25 milligrams of hydrochlorothiazide (see p. 117), 20 milligrams of lisinopril (see p. 88) with either 12.5 or 25 milligrams of hydrochlorothiazide, or 10 milligrams of enalapril (see p. 88) with 25 milligrams of hydrochlorothiazide are used to treat high blood pressure (hypertension). Older adults should never use drugs that contain a fixed combination of one of these drugs and hydrochlorothiazide as a first choice. Captopril can cause kidney failure, bone marrow depression, and like all ACE inhibitors, can cause cough in 5 to 20% of users.[112]

There are good reasons not to use any fixed-combination drug for high blood pressure. First, a single drug is often enough to control high blood pressure. If a combination drug like this one is controlling your high blood pressure, it is quite possible that one drug alone would do the same job. There is no reason to put youself at extra risk by taking extra drugs you do not need.

If you have high blood pressure, the best way to reduce or eliminate your need for medication is through diet, weight loss, exercise, and less salt and alcohol. In mild hypertension nutrition and hygenic measures can control high blood pressure. If these measures do not lower your blood pressure enough and you need medication, **hydrochlorothiazide, a water pill (see thiazide diuretics, p. 117), is the drug of choice for mild hypertension in people over 60 years old, starting with a low dose of 12.5 milligrams.** It also costs less.

There is now good evidence that another benefit of thiazide diuretics such as hydrochlorothiazide is that they significantly decrease the rate of bone mineral loss in both men and women because they reduce the amount of calcium lost in the urine. An increasing number of researchers think that this will also decrease the number of fractures. [113]

If your high blood pressure is more severe and hydrochlorothiazide alone does not control it, the choice of a beta-blocker, (see p. 68), a calcium channel blocker (see p. 85), or an ACE inhibitor (see p. 88) depends on your condition. Whichever drug suits you, your doctor would prescribe the hydrochlorothiazide and the second drug separately with the dose of each drug adjusted to meet your needs, rather than using a product that combines the drugs in advance in this fixed combination. If you are taking both drugs, compare the total price of each drug separately. The separate drugs may prove less expensive than this combination product. The separate drugs are more flexible should your dose of either drug need to be changed. Whatever drugs you take for high blood pressure, once your blood pressure has been normal for a year or more, a cautious decrease in dose and

---

Warning

A fixed-combination drug should not be the first drug used to treat your high blood pressure. You may not need more than one drug. If you do need two drugs, this product may not contain the dose of each drug that is right for you. Your doctor has to regularly check your condition and reevaluate the effect of the drug(s) you take. This means adjusting doses and even changing drugs to ensure proper treatment. This fixed-combination drug may be the best drug for you, but it should be used only after you have tried each of its ingredients separately, in varying doses. If the doses that you need to control your high blood pressure match those in this fixed-combination product, use it if the combination drug is more convenient. See captopril, lisinopril, and enalapril (p. 88) and hydrochlorothiazide (p. 117) for more information about this drug and other drugs with which there is a potentially harmful interaction.

renewed attention to non-drug treatment may be worth trying, according to *The Medical Letter*.[114]

"Treatment of hypertension is part of preventive medicine and like all preventive strategies, its progress should be regularly reviewed by whoever initiates it. Many problems could be avoided by not starting antihypertensive treatment until after prolonged observation. . . . .Patients should no longer be told that treatment is necessarily for life: the possibility of reducing or stopping treatment should be mentioned at the outset."[115]

Heat Stress Alert

This drug can affect your body's ability to adjust to heat, putting you at risk of "heat stress." If you live alone, ask a friend to check on you several times during the day. Early signs of heat stress are dizziness, lightheadedness, faintness, and slightly high temperature. Call your doctor if you have any of these signs.

Drink more fluids (water, fruit and vegetable juices) than usual, even if you're not thirsty, unless your doctor has told you otherwise. Do not drink alcohol.

Cough Alert

A common adverse effect, after taking ACE inhibitors for a few weeks, is a dry, hacking cough, especially in women. Check with your doctor about a 4-day withdrawal from your ACE inhibitor to determine if this is the cause of your cough. This trial withdrawal can prevent unnecessary and sometimes costly tests and treatments.

LIMITED USE

Diltiazem
CARDIZEM (Marion Merrell Dow)
DILACOR (extended-release) (Rhone-Poulenc Rorer)

Generic: not available

Family: Calcium Channel Blockers (See High Blood Pressure, p. 62)

Diltiazem (dill *tie* a zem) belongs to a family of drugs called calcium channel blockers. They are used primarily to treat chest pain (angina) and coronary artery disease, and also to lower high blood pressure (hypertension) and improve irregular heartbeats (arrhythmias). Calcium channel blockers control, but do not cure high blood pressure. These drugs may improve capacity for exercise and delay the need for heart surgery.

Each calcium channel blocker differs in the likelihood of harmful side effects. Compared to other calcium channel blockers, diltiazem is midway in side effects. It is less likely than verapamil to cause constipation. Diltiazem is less likely than the nifedipine group of channel blockers to cause severe headaches, rapid heartbeat, and swelling of the legs and feet.[116]

If you have high blood pressure, the best way to reduce or eliminate your need for medication is through diet, weight loss, exercise, and less salt and alcohol. In mild hypertension nutrition and hygenic measures can control high blood pressure. If these measures do not lower your blood pressure enough and you need medication, hydrochlorothiazide, a water pill (see thiazide diuretics, p. 117), is the drug of choice for mild hypertension in people over 60 years old, starting with a low dose of 12.5 milligrams. It also costs less.

There is now good evidence that another benefit of thiazide diuretics such as hydrochlorothiazide is that they significantly decrease the rate of bone mineral loss in both men and women because they reduce the amount of calcium lost in the urine. An increasing number of researchers think that this will also decrease the number of fractures. [117]

Whatever drugs you take for high blood pressure, once your blood pressure has been normal for a year or more, a cautious decrease in dose and renewed attention to non-drug treatment may be worth trying, according to *The Medical Letter*.[118]

"Treatment of hypertension is part of preventive medicine and like all preventive strategies, its progress should be regularly reviewed by whoever initiates it. Many problems could be avoided by not starting antihypertensive treatment until after prolonged observation. . . . Patients should no longer be told that treatment is necessarily for life: the possibility of reducing or stopping treatment should be mentioned at the outset."[119]

Before You Use This Drug

Do not take if you have or have had
- ❑ aortic stenosis
- ❑ severe hypotension
- ❑ heart block without a pacemaker
- ❑ extremely low heart rate
- ❑ myocardial infarction (acute) and pulmonary congestion
- ❑ sick sinus syndrome

Tell your doctor if you have or have had
- ❑ allergies to drugs
- ❑ heart, kidney or liver problems
- ❑ low blood pressure
- ❑ lung condition or breathing problems

Tell your doctor about any other drugs you take, including aspirin, herbs, vitamins, and other non-prescription products.

When You Use This Drug
- ◆ Learn to take your pulse, and get immediate help if your pulse slows to 50 beats per minute or slower, even if you are feeling well.
- ◆ Until you know how you react to this drug, do not drive or perform other activities requiring alertness.
- ◆ Follow a diet recommended by your doctor.
- ◆ Have your doctor suggest exercises which avoid overexertion.
- ◆ **Do not stop taking calcium channel blockers suddenly. Contact your doctor for a schedule to decrease your drug gradually.**
- ◆ You may feel dizzy when rising from a lying or sitting position. If you are lying down, hang your legs over the side of the bed for a few minutes, then get up slowly. When getting up from a chair, stay by the chair until you are sure that you are not dizzy. (See p. 14.)
- ◆ If you plan to have any surgery, including dental, tell your doctor that you take this drug.
- ◆ Do not take other drugs without talking to your doctor first — especially drugs for asthma, colds, cough, diet, hay fever, or sinus problems.

How To Use This Drug
- ◆ Swallow capsule or tablet whole or break in half. Do not break, chew or crush the long-acting forms of the drug.
- ◆ Take on an empty stomach, at least 1 hour before or 2 hours after meals.
- ◆ If you miss a dose, take it as soon as you remember, but skip it if it is almost time for the next dose. **Do not take double doses.**
- ◆ Store this drug at room temperature with the lid on snuggly. Do not expose to light.

Interactions With Other Drugs

The following drugs are listed in *Evaluations of Drug Interactions*, 1991 as causing "highly clinically significant" or "clinically significant" interactions when used together with this drug. There may be other drugs, especially those in the families of drugs listed below, that also will react with this drug to cause severe adverse effects. Make sure to ask your doctor for a complete listing of them and let her or him know if you are taking any of these interacting drugs:

amiodarone; CALCIFEROL; calciums; carbamazepine; CORDARONE; cyclosporine; DANTRIUM; dantrolene; digoxin; DILANTIN; disopyramide; ELIXOPHYLLIN; ergocalciferol; ESKALITH; INDERAL; LANOXIN; lithium; LITHOBID; NORCURON; NORPACE; phenytoin; propranolol; QUINAGLUTE; QUINIDEX; quinidine; RIFADIN; rifampin; SANDIMMUNE; TEGRETOL; THEO-DUR; theophylline; vecuronium.

Additionally, the *United States Pharmacopeia Drug Information*, 1992 lists these drugs as causing interactions of major significance:

beta-blockers, optic; BETAGAN, TIMOPTIC.

Adverse Effects
Call your doctor immediately:
❑ difficulty breathing

❑ chest pain
❑ confusion, sleep disorder
❑ fainting
❑ severe headache
❑ irregular or pounding heartbeat
❑ slow pulse
❑ skin rash

Call your doctor if these symptoms continue:
❑ constipation, diarrhea
❑ dizziness, lightheadedness
❑ nausea, vomiting
❑ nervousness or mood changes
❑ swelling of ankles, feet, or legs
❑ thirst
❑ undesired weight change
❑ unusual tiredness or weakness

Periodic Tests
Ask your doctor which of these tests should be done periodically while you are taking this drug:
❑ blood pressure
❑ heart function tests, such as electrocardiogram (EKG)
❑ kidney function tests
❑ liver function tests
❑ pulse

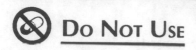 **DO NOT USE**

Alternative treatment: See Hydrochlorothiazide, p. 117.

Clonidine
CATAPRES (Boehringer Ingelheim)

Family: Antihypertensives
(See High Blood Pressure, p. 62)

Clonidine (*kloe* ni deen) is used to treat high blood pressure (hypertension). **It has severe side effects and should not be used.**

The main problem with clonidine is that missing only one or two doses of the drug can have serious effects, including sweating, tremor, flushing, and severe high blood pressure. Clonidine can also cause severe depression and is particularly dangerous for anyone with a history of depression. Nearly one-fourth of the people who use the patch form have a skin reaction.

If you have high blood pressure, the best way to reduce or eliminate your need for medication is through diet, weight loss, exercise, and less salt and alcohol. In mild hypertension nutrition and hygenic measures can control high blood pressure. If these measures do not lower your blood pressure enough and you need medication, **hydrochlorothiazide, a water pill (see thiazide diuretics, p. 117), is the drug of choice for mild hypertension in people over 60 years old, starting with a low dose of 12.5 milligrams.** It also costs less.

There is now good evidence that another benefit of thiazide diuretics such as hydrochlorothiazide is that they significantly decrease the rate of bone mineral loss in both men and women because they reduce the amount of calcium lost in the urine. An increasing number of researchers think that this will also decrease the number of fractures. [120]

If this does not lower your blood pressure enough, your doctor can prescribe a second type of drug called a beta-blocker, such as propranolol (see p. 124), to accompany the hydrochlorothiazide. If you cannot take a beta-blocker, a drug from another family (calcium channel blockers) can be used instead.

Whatever drugs you take for high blood pressure, once your blood pressure has been normal for a year or more, a cautious decrease in dose and renewed attention to non-drug treatment may be worth trying, according to *The Medical Letter*.[121]

"Treatment of hypertension is part of preventive medicine and like all preventive strategies, its progress should be regularly reviewed by whoever initiates it. Many problems could be avoided by not starting antihypertensive treatment until after prolonged observation. . . . Patients should no longer be told that treatment is necessarily for life: the possibility of reducing or stopping treatment should be mentioned at the outset."[122]

Do not suddenly stop using this drug. Ask your doctor for a schedule that lowers your dose gradually over at least 10 days, and more slowly if you begin to have withdrawal symptoms. Another drug for high blood pressure should be started at the same time.

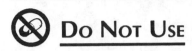 **DO NOT USE**

Papaverine
CERESPAN (USV) PAVABID (Marion)

Family: Vasodilators
(Blood Vessel Dilators)

Doctors prescribe papaverine (pa *pav* er een) to improve the blood circulation of people with certain types of blood vessel disease, in the hope that this will relieve pain that is caused by circulation problems (leg pain, for example) and improve mental functioning (by increasing blood flow to the brain). However, there is no evidence that papaverine prevents or relieves any disease of blood vessels to the brain, nor has it been shown to improve the mental or physical state of older or senile adults.[123] In fact, although this drug has been available for use and evaluation for many years, **it has not been proven effective for treating any condition.**[124,125] The American Medical Association's guide to drug therapy does not even suggest a dose for papaverine because "the role of this agent in the treatment of peripheral vascular disease [disease of the blood vessels in the arms or legs] has not been established."[126]

In addition to being ineffective, papaverine has serious dangers. There is strong evidence that it can cause liver damage; in one study, one out of five people taking the drug developed liver damage.[127] **We recommend that you do not use papaverine because it can cause harmful side effects and has not been proven to have any benefit.**

> Studies have failed to show that this drug is effective.

LIMITED USE

Cholestyramine
CHOLYBAR (Parke-Davis)
QUESTRAN, QUESTRAN LIGHT (Bristol)

Generic: not available

Family: Cholesterol-lowering Drugs (see p. 70)

Cholestyramine (coal es *tire* am ene) is used primarily to lower cholesterol, specifically low density lipoprotein (LDL). It works by binding bile acid in the intestines and therefore increasing the breakdown of cholesterol in the body. In middle-aged people it is clear that lowering cholesterol lessens the risk of coronary artery disease, but no cholesterol-lowering drug has been shown to lower overall death rates in this age group. In older adults the extent to which higher cholesterol levels contribute to heart disease and should be treated with drugs is much less clear. Cholestyramine helps control high cholesterol, but does not cure the condition. Besides removing cholesterol, cholestyramine may remove needed nutrients and medicines from your body, and actually increase triglycerides.[128] People over age 60 and those who take high doses are more likely to experience harmful effects from cholestyramine.[129]

The use of cholesterol-lowering drugs in people 70 or older should be limited to patients with very high cholesterol levels (greater than 300 milligrams) and those who manifest cardiovascular disease (previous history of heart attack or angina).[130]

For people under 70, if your cholesterol levels are high, the first, less costly measure is to eat a low-fat diet, using mostly polyunsaturated fats (such as canola, corn, safflower, and sunflower oils), or mono-unsaturated fats (such as olive oil). A change from animal to vegetable proteins often corrects high cholesterol. However, it is inadvisable to go on a very low-fat diet. The main focus on cholesterol-lowering diets has been on saturated fat and cholesterol content, not soluble fiber content. (When added to the diet, psyllium or oat bran is a safe, effective way of lowering cholesterol.) Exercise is also recommended. Conditions that aggravate high cholesterol, such as dependence on alcohol or tobacco, diabetes, high blood pressure, low magnesium or potassium and thyroid disease should be corrected before adding a cholesterol-reducing drug. If cholesterol remains high despite diet, add 10 grams of psyllium a day (see p. 356).

Before You Use This Drug
Do not use if you have or have had
❑ complete biliary obstruction
Tell your doctor if you have or have had
❑ allergies to drugs
❑ bleeding disorders
❑ chronic constipation
❑ diabetes
❑ gallbladder problems
❑ heart disease
❑ hemorrhoids
❑ kidney or liver problems
❑ osteoporosis
❑ phenylketonuria (PKU)
❑ thyroid disorder
❑ ulcers
Tell your doctor about any other drugs you take, including aspirin, herbs, vitamins, and other non-prescription products.

When taking cholestyramine it is important that your doctor knows all the drugs you take.

When You Use This Drug

◆ Tell any other doctor, dentist, nurse practitioner, or surgeon you see that you take cholestyramine.

◆ Tell your doctor whenever you start any new medication.

◆ If you take other medications, check with your doctor before you stop taking cholestyramine.

◆ Continue to follow a low-fat diet.

◆ Avoid constipation. Increase your fiber with more bran, fluids, fruits, or psyllium.[131] If constipation persists try a stool softener.

How To Use This Drug

◆ Take cholestyramine within half an hour of meals,[132] preferably before meals.[133]

❑ *If you take the bar form of cholestyramine*, chew thoroughly before swallowing. Drink plenty of fluids.

❑ *If you take the powder form of cholestyramine*, measure the dose unless you use premeasured packets. Color of the powder varies from batch to batch. Never swallow the dry form, but mix the powder in 2 or more ounces of water, milk, apple or orange juice. Stir vigorously, then shake. However, the mixture will not dissolve. To further improve flavor try stirring in a heavy fruit juice or pulpy fruits (applesauce, fruit cocktail, crushed pineapple), thin soups, or with milk in cold or hot cereal.[134] Chilling the mixture may aid the flavor. If you use a carbonated beverage stir slowly to reduce foaming.[135] Avoid taking with highly acidic drinks, such as Kool-Aid.[136] Swallow immediately. Do not hold or swish the mixture in your mouth.[137] To be sure all the medication is taken, rinse the container thoroughly and drink the remaining contents.[138]

❑ If you take any other medications, separate the times as far apart from cholestyramine as possible, but at least 1 hour before you take the cholestyramine, or 4 to 8 hours after you take the cholestyramine.

❑ If you miss a dose, take as soon as you remember but skip it if it is almost time for the next dose. **Do not take double doses**.

❑ Store at room temperature. Close lid of bulk powder tightly.

Interactions With Other Drugs

The following drugs are listed in *Evaluations of Drug Interactions*, 1991 as causing "highly clinically significant" or "clinically significant" interactions when used together with this drug. There may be other drugs, especially those in the families of drugs listed below, that also will react with this drug to cause severe adverse effects. Make sure to ask your doctor for a complete listing of them and let her or him know if you are taking any of these interacting drugs:

COUMADIN; CRYSTODIGIN; digitoxin; glipizide; GLUCOTROL; SYNTHROID; thyroid; thyroxine; warfarin.

Additionally, the *United States Pharmacopeia Drug Information*, 1992 lists these drugs as having interactions of major significance:

ACHROMYCIN; AZOLID; BUTAZOLIDIN; chlorothiazide; DIURIL; HYDRODIURIL; INDERAL; penicillin; PENTIDS; phenylbutazone; propranolol; tetracycline; VANCOCIN; vancomycin.

If you stop taking cholestyramine, your doctor will again review doses of your other drugs. Serious harm may occur if you stop taking cholestyramine while taking other medicines.

Adverse Effects

Call your doctor immediately:

❑ unusual bleeding or bruising

❑ black, tarry stools

❑ constipation

❑ inability to see as well at night

❑ severe stomach pain

❑ sudden weight loss

Call your doctor if these symptoms continue:

❑ belching or hiccups

- ❑ bloating
- ❑ diarrhea
- ❑ dizziness
- ❑ headache
- ❑ heartburn, indigestion, stomach pain
- ❑ irritation of skin, tongue, or anal area
- ❑ nausea or vomiting

Periodic Testing

Ask your doctor which of these tests should be done periodically while you are taking this drug:

- ❑ blood calcium, cholesterol, and triglyceride levels
- ❑ prothrombin time

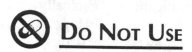 **DO NOT USE**

Alternative treatment: See Hydrochlorothiazide, p. 117.

Clonidine and Chlorthalidone (combined)
COMBIPRES (Boehringer Ingelheim)

Family: Diuretics
Antihypertensives
(See High Blood Pressure, p. 62)

This product, a combination of clonidine (see p. 96) and chlorthalidone (see p. 121), is used to treat high blood pressure. **Older adults should not use drugs containing a fixed combination of clonidine and chlorthalidone.**

Clonidine can cause severe depression, and can also cause a dangerous reaction if you miss only one or two doses (see box below). We do not recommend that any older adult use clonidine, and it is particularly dangerous for anyone with a history of depression.

Chlorthalidone puts the older adult user at such a high risk of side effects that the World Health Organization has said it should not be used by people over 60.

In addition to the risks of clonidine and chlorthalidone, there are good reasons not to use a fixed-combination drug for high blood pressure. First, a single drug is often enough to control high blood pressure. If a combination drug like this one is controlling your high blood pressure, it is quite possible that one drug alone would do the same job. There is no reason to put yourself at extra risk by taking extra drugs you do not need.

If you have high blood pressure, the best way to reduce or eliminate your need for medication is through diet, weight loss, exercise, and less salt and alcohol. In mild hypertension nutrition and hygenic measures can control high blood pressure. If these measures do not lower your blood pressure enough and you need medication, **hydrochlorothiazide, a water pill (see thiazide diuretics, p. 117), is the drug of choice for mild hypertension in people over 60 years old, starting with a low dose of 12.5 milligrams.** It also costs less.

There is now good evidence that another benefit of thiazide diuretics such as hydrochlorothiazide is that they significantly decrease the rate of bone mineral loss in both men and women because they reduce the amount of calcium lost in the urine. An increasing number of researchers think that this will also decrease the number of fractures. [139]

If your high blood pressure is more severe and hydrochlorothiazide alone does not control it, the best treatment is a combination of hydrochlorothiazide and a second type of drug called a beta-blocker, such as propranolol (see p. 124). If you can't take a drug in the beta-blocker family, another drug called a calcium channel blocker may be used instead. In either case, your doctor would prescribe the hydrochlorothiazide and the second drug separately, with the dose of each drug adjusted to meet your needs, rather than using a product that combines the drugs in advance in a fixed combination.

If you are taking this fixed-combination drug, ask your doctor about changing your prescription.

Whatever drugs you take for high blood pressure, once your blood pressure has been normal for a year or more, a cautious decrease in dose and renewed attention to non-drug treatment may be worth trying, according to *The Medical Letter*.[140]

"Treatment of hypertension is part of preventive medicine and like all preventive strategies, its progress should be regularly reviewed by whoever initiates it. Many problems could be avoided by not starting antihypertensive treatment until after prolonged observation. . . . Patients should no longer be told that treatment is necessarily for life: the possibility of reducing or stopping treatment should be mentioned at the outset."[141]

Do not stop using this drug suddenly. Sudden withdrawal from clonidine can cause sweating, tremors, flushing, and even severe high blood pressure. This dangerous reaction may occur after missing only one or two doses. Ask your doctor for a schedule that reduces your dose of clonidine gradually over at least 10 days, and more slowly if symptoms occur. At the same time as you are reducing your dose of clonidine, your doctor should start you on another drug for high blood pressure.

Nadolol
CORGARD (Squibb)

Generic: not available

Family: Beta-blockers (see p. 68)
Antihypertensives
(See High Blood Pressure, p. 62)

Nadolol (*nay* doe lole) is used to treat high blood pressure (hypertension), chest pain (angina), and irregular heartbeats (arrhythmias) and to decrease the frequency of migraine headaches. **If you are over 60, you will generally need to take less than the usual adult dose, especially if your kidney function is impaired.**

For young adults with high blood pressure, doctors usually prescribe a drug in this family (a beta-blocker) before any other drug. But for blacks and older adults, these drugs are less effective as the sole treatment. For these groups of people, doctors usually prescribe another type of drug called a diuretic (water pill) to lower blood pressure, and add a beta-blocker as a second drug if the diuretic alone is not enough.

If you have high blood pressure, the best way to reduce or eliminate your need for medication is through diet, weight loss, exercise, and less salt and alcohol. In mild hypertension nutrition and hygenic measures can control high blood pressure. If these measures do not lower your blood pressure enough and you need medication, **hydrochlorothiazide, a water pill (see thiazide diuretics, p. 117), is the drug of choice for mild hypertension in people**

over 60 years old, starting with a low dose of 12.5 milligrams. It also costs less.

There is now good evidence that another benefit of thiazide diuretics such as hydrochlorothiazide is that they significantly decrease the rate of bone mineral loss in both men and women because they reduce the amount of calcium lost in the urine. An increasing number of researchers think that this will also decrease the number of fractures. [142]

All beta-blockers are similarly effective, although not necessarily interchangeable. Increased sensitivity to cold is one side effect. (See, glossary p. 689 for signs of hypothermia.) If you are bothered by side effects when taking nadolol, talk to your doctor about switching to another beta-blocker, such as propranolol, which is available generically. The side effects of these drugs vary widely, and each individual responds differently to each one. See p. 68 for a discussion of alternatives to nadolol.

Whatever drugs you take for high blood pressure, once your blood pressure has been normal for a year or more, a cautious decrease in dose and renewed attention to non-drug treatment may be worth trying, according to *The Medical Letter*.[143]

"Treatment of hypertension is part of preventive medicine and like all preventive strategies, its progress should be regularly reviewed by whoever initiates it. Many problems could be avoided by not starting antihypertensive treatment until after prolonged observation. . . . Patients should no longer be told that treatment is necessarily for life: the possibility of reducing or stopping treatment should be mentioned at the outset."[144]

Before You Use This Drug
Do not use if you have
❑ congestive heart failure
❑ asthma
❑ emphysema or chronic bronchitis
Tell your doctor if you have or have had
❑ allergies to drugs
❑ gout
❑ alcohol dependence
❑ difficulty breathing
❑ kidney, liver, lung, or pancreas disease
❑ mental depression
❑ lupus erythematosus
❑ diabetes
❑ Raynaud's syndrome
❑ poor blood circulation
❑ thyroid problems
Tell your doctor about any other drugs you take, including aspirin, herbs, vitamins, and other non-prescription products.

When You Use This drug
◆ **Learn to take your pulse, and get immediate medical help if your pulse slows to 50 beats per minute or slower, even if you are feeling well. Some people have suffered from slowed heart rate and heart failure while taking nadolol.**
◆ Until you know how you react to this drug, do not drive or perform other activities requiring alertness.
◆ Be careful not to overexert yourself, even though your chest pain may feel better.
◆ **Do not stop taking this drug suddenly. Your doctor must give you a schedule to decrease your dose gradually, to prevent chest pain and possible heart attack.**
◆ You may feel dizzy when rising from a lying or sitting position. When getting out of bed, hang your legs over the side of the bed for a few minutes, then get up slowly. When getting up from a chair, get up slowly and stay beside the chair until you are sure that you are not dizzy. (See p. 14.)
◆ **Caution diabetics: see p. 516.**
◆ If you plan to have any surgery, including dental, tell your doctor that you take this drug.
◆ **Do not take other drugs without talking to your doctor first — especially non-prescription drugs for appetite control, asthma, colds, coughs, hay fever, or sinus problems.**

How To Use This Drug

◆ Crush tablets and mix with water, or swallow whole with water.
◆ If you miss a dose, take it as soon as you remember, but skip it if it is less than 8 hours before your next scheduled dose. **Do not take double doses.**

Interactions With Other Drugs

The following drugs are listed in *Evaluations of Drug Interactions*, 1991 as causing "highly clinically significant" or "clinically significant" interactions when used together with this drug. There may be other drugs, especially those in the families of drugs listed below, that also will react with this drug to cause severe adverse effects. Make sure to ask your doctor for a complete listing of them and let her or him know if you are taking any of these interacting drugs:

ALDOMET; amiodarone; ADRENALIN (also found in bee sting kits); CALAN; CATAPRES; chlorpromazine; cimetidine; clonidine; cocaine; CORDARONE; COUMADIN; epinephrine; ESKALITH; FLUOTHANE; halothane; INDOCIN; indomethacin; insulin; lidocaine; lithium; methyldopa; MINIPRESS; prazosin; TAGAMET; THORAZINE; TUBARINE; tubocurarine; verapamil; warfarin; XYLOCAINE.

Adverse Effects

Call your doctor immediately:
❏ difficulty breathing
❏ cold hands or feet
❏ mental depression
❏ skin rash
❏ swelling of ankles, feet, or legs
❏ slow pulse

Call your doctor if these symptoms continue:
❏ headache
❏ constipation or diarrhea
❏ nausea, vomiting
❏ unusual tiredness or weakness
❏ disturbed sleep, nightmares
❏ decreased sexual ability
❏ dry or sore eyes
❏ itching skin
❏ numbness or tingling of limbs

More side effects information appears on p. 68.

Periodic Tests

Ask your doctor which of these tests should be done periodically while you are taking this drug:
❏ complete blood counts
❏ blood pressure and pulse rate
❏ heart function tests, such as electrocardiogram (EKG)
❏ kidney function tests
❏ liver function tests
❏ blood glucose levels

Warfarin
COUMADIN (Du Pont)

Generic: available

Family: Anticoagulants

Warfarin (*war* far in) reduces the blood's ability to clot (coagulate) and prevents blood clots from forming in the arteries and veins. It is prescribed for people with a history of abnormal blood clots or who are at high risk of having abnormal clots. **If you are over 60, you should generally be taking less than the usual adult dose,** to lower the risk of heavy bleeding (hemorrhage). Once you have taken warfarin for three months, your need to remain on it should be reviewed.

If you do not take this drug properly, it can cause severe side effects (see Adverse Effects). **You must take warfarin exactly on schedule.** While taking warfarin, **you should visit your doctor regularly to monitor your progress with blood tests and to ensure that you are taking the most effective dose of the drug.**

Warfarin can interact with nearly all drugs. Its anti-clotting action is very difficult to control when other drugs are added or subtracted, or when another drug's dose is changed. Another medication may either increase or decrease warfarin's action. **While taking warfarin, do not take any other drugs, including non-prescription drugs** (such as aspirin, cold remedies, antacids, laxatives), **or change the dose of any drug that you currently take, without consulting your doctor first.**

Before You Use This Drug
Do not use if you have or have had
❑ recent surgery
❑ aneurysm or dissecting aorta
❑ blood disorders
❑ active bleeding
❑ severe, uncontrolled high blood pressure

Tell your doctor if you have or have had
❑ allergies to drugs
❑ heart problems including atrial fibrillation, myocardial infarction, or stroke
❑ thromboembolism
❑ severe allergies
❑ ulcers
❑ kidney or liver disease
❑ polyarthritis
❑ recent radiation therapy
❑ vitamin C or K deficiency
❑ alcohol dependence
❑ severe inflammation of blood vessels
❑ subacute bacterial endocarditis (infection of the heart)
❑ diabetes
❑ recent injury
Tell your doctor about any other drugs you take, including aspirin, herbs, vitamins, and other non-prescription products.

When You Use This Drug
◆ Wear a medical identification bracelet or carry a card stating that you take warfarin.
◆ Be very careful doing activities that may cause cuts or bleeding, such as shaving or cooking.
◆ Do not drink alcohol.
◆ Eat a normal, balanced diet. **Do not change your diet or take nutritional supplements or vitamins without first checking with your doctor.**
◆ If you plan to have any surgery, including dental, tell your doctor that you take this drug.
◆ **Do not take any other drugs, including non-prescription products (aspirin, cold remedies, antacids, laxatives), or change the dose of drugs you are taking, without consulting your doctor.**
◆ **Be sure to schedule regular doctor visits for blood tests.**

How To Use This Drug

◆ If you miss a dose, take it as soon as you remember, but skip it if you don't remember until the next day. **Do not take double doses.** Keep a record of missed doses and give the list to your doctor at each visit.

Interactions With Other Drugs

The following drugs are listed in *Evaluations of Drug Interactions*, 1991 as causing "highly clinically significant" or "clinically significant" interactions when used together with this drug. There may be other drugs, especially those in the families of drugs listed below, that also will react with this drug to cause severe adverse effects. Make sure to ask your doctor for a complete listing of them and let her or him know if you are taking any of these interacting drugs:

amiodarone; ANDROID; ANTABUSE; ANTURANE; AQUAMEPHYTON; aspirin; ATROMID-S; azathioprine; GENUINE BAYER ASPIRIN; BUTAZOLIDIN; cefamandole; chloral hydrate; cholestyramine; cimetidine; CLINORIL; clofibrate; CORDARONE; cyclosporine; DARVON; DARVON-N; disulfiram; DORIDEN; DURAQUIN; EES; E-MYCIN; EASPRIN; ECOTRIN; EMPIRIN; ERYTHROCIN; erythromycin; ESTRATEST H.S.; ethacrynic acid; ethchlorvynol; FLAGYL; flu shot; FULVICIN; glucagon; glutethimide; GRIFULVIN; GRISACTIN; GRIS-PEG; griseofulvin; ibuprofen; IFEX; ifosfamide; ILOSONE; IMURAN; INDERAL; INDOCIN; indomethacin; influenza virus vaccine; ketoconazole; KONAKION; lovastatin; LUMINAL; LYSODREN; MANDOL; METANDREN; methyltestosterone; metronidazole; MEVACOR; miconazole; mitotanc; MONISTAT DERM; MONISTAT 7; moricizine; MOTRIN; nafcillin; nalidixic acid; NIZORAL; NOCTEC; NOLVADEX; ORETON METHYL; PBR/12; phenobarbital; phenylbutazone; phytonadione; PLACIDYL; PREMARIN WITH METHYLTESTOSTERONE; propoxyphene; propranolol; QUESTRAN; QUINAGLUTE DURATABS; quinidine; RIFADIN; rifampin; RIMACTANE; SANDIMMUNE; SEPTRA; SOLFOTON; sulfamethoxazole; sulfinpyrazone; sulindac; TAGAMET; tamoxifen; TESTRED; thyroid; trimethoprim/sulfamethoxazole; UNIPEN; VINLON; vitamin E.

Adverse Effects

Call your doctor immediately:
❏ **if you experience signs of overdose or bleeding**: bleeding gums when brushing teeth; nosebleeds; unexplained bruising; heavy bleeding from cuts or wounds; abdominal pain or swelling; sudden lightheadedness; weakness; loss of consciousness; backaches; bloody or tarry stools; coughing up blood; vomiting blood or material that looks like coffee grounds
❏ abnormal bleeding
❏ bloody or cloudy urine
❏ difficult or painful urination or sudden decrease in amount of urine
❏ swelling of ankles, feet, or legs
❏ unusual weight gain
❏ blue/purple color of toes
❏ chills, fever, sore throat, or unusual tiredness
❏ dark urine, yellow eyes
❏ diarrhea, nausea, or vomiting
❏ skin rash, hives, or itching
❏ sores or white spots in mouth or throat
Call your doctor if these symptoms continue:
❏ bloated stomach or gas
❏ blurred vision
❏ unusual hair loss
❏ loss of appetite

Periodic Tests
Ask your doctor which of these tests should be done periodically while you are taking this drug:
❏ prothrombin time (measure of how long it takes your blood to clot): daily for the first week on warfarin, weekly for the next 3 months, and monthly thereafter
❏ complete blood counts
❏ stool tests for possible blood loss
❏ urine tests for possible blood loss

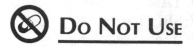 **DO NOT USE**

Alternative treatment: Mild exercise, no smoking, extreme cleanliness of legs and feet.

Cyclandelate
CYCLOSPASMOL (Wyeth)

Family: Vasodilators
(Blood Vessel Dilators)

Doctors prescribe cyclandelate (sye *klan* de late) to improve the blood circulation of people with certain types of blood vessel disease, in the hope that this will relieve pain that is caused by circulation problems (leg pain, for example) and improve mental functioning (by increasing blood flow to the brain). However, **there is no evidence that cyclandelate prevents or relieves any disease of blood vessels to the brain, nor has it been shown to improve the mental or physical state of older or senile adults.**[145] In fact, although this drug has been available for use and evaluation for many years, **it has not been proven effective for treating any condition.**[146] The American Medical Association's guide to drug therapy does not even suggest a dose for cyclandelate because "the role of this agent in the treatment of peripheral vascular disease [disease of the blood vessels in the arms or legs] has not been established."[147]

Cyclandelate's side effects include headache, nausea, chills, flushing, tingling and burning sensation of the skin, heart flutter, and stomach and intestinal problems. **We recommend that you do not use cyclandelate because it can cause harmful side effects and it has not been proven to have any benefit.**

The National Academy of Sciences has found that cyclandelate and a related drug called isoxsuprine lack evidence of effectiveness. The Food and Drug Administration has found that another drug in this family, nylidrin (Arlidin), also lacks evidence of effectiveness.

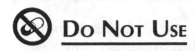 **DO NOT USE**

Alternative treatment: See Hydrochlorothiazide, p. 117.

Reserpine and Chlorothiazide (combined)
DIUPRES (Merck Sharp & Dohme)
CHLOROSERPINE (Schein)

Family: Diuretics
Antihypertensives
(See High Blood Pressure, p. 62)

This product, a combination of reserpine (see p. 165) and chlorothiazide (see p. 117), is used to treat high blood pressure (hypertension). **Older adults should not use drugs that contain a fixed combination of reserpine and chlorothiazide.**

Reserpine causes severe side effects that may occur during treatment and even months after you stop taking it. It has caused severe depression, in some cases leading to suicide. We do not recommend that any older adult use reserpine, and it is particularly dangerous for anyone who has had a depressive illness. It also decreases mental sharpness in older adults.

In addition to the risks of reserpine, there are good reasons not to use any fixed-combination drug for high blood pressure. First, a single drug is often enough to control high blood pressure. If a combination drug like this one is controlling your high blood pressure, it is quite possible that one drug alone would do the same job. There is no reason to put yourself at extra risk by taking extra drugs you do not need.

If you have high blood pressure, the best way to reduce or eliminate your need for medication is through diet, weight loss, exercise, and less salt and alcohol. In mild hypertension nutrition and hygenic measures can control high blood pressure. If these measures do not lower your blood pressure enough and you need medication, **hydrochlorothiazide, a water pill (see thiazide diuretics, p. 117), is the drug of** choice for mild hypertension in people over 60 years old, starting with a low dose of 12.5 milligrams. It also costs less.

There is now good evidence that another benefit of thiazide diuretics such as hydrochlorothiazide is that they significantly decrease the rate of bone mineral loss in both men and women because they reduce the amount of calcium lost in the urine. An increasing number of researchers think that this will also decrease the number of fractures. [148]

If your high blood pressure is more severe and hydrochlorothiazide alone does not control it, there are still better drug treatments than this combination product. The best treatment in this case is a combination of hydrochlorothiazide and a second type of drug called a beta-blocker such as propranolol (see p. 124). If you can't take a drug in the beta-blocker family, another drug called a calcium channel blocker may be used instead. In either case, your doctor would prescribe the hydrochlorothiazide and the second drug separately, with the dose of each drug adjusted to meet your needs, rather than using a product that combines the drugs in advance in a fixed combination.

If you are taking this fixed-combination drug, ask your doctor about changing your prescription.

Whatever drugs you take for high blood pressure, once your blood pressure has been normal for a year or more, a cautious decrease in dose and renewed attention to non-drug treatment may be worth trying, according to *The Medical Letter*. [149]

"Treatment of hypertension is part of

preventive medicine and like all preventive strategies, its progress should be regularly reviewed by whoever initiates it. Many problems could be avoided by not starting antihypertensive treatment until after prolonged observation. . . . Patients should no longer be told that treatment is necessarily for life: the possibility of reducing or stopping treatment should be mentioned at the outset."[150]

LIMITED USE

Quinidine
DURAQUIN (Parke-Davis)
QUINAGLUTE DURA-TABS (Berlex)

Generic: available

Family: Antiarrhythmics

Quinidine (*kwin* i deen) slows the heart rate and decreases irregular heartbeats (arrhythmias). It is often the first drug used to treat an irregular heartbeat. **If your kidney function is impaired, you will need to take less than the usual dose.**

Many people who are taking quinidine or another drug in its family have relatively mild disturbances in their heart rhythm and no symptoms of underlying heart disease. The vast majority of these people do not need these drugs, and there is no evidence that using them improves health. In fact, most of the drugs in this family have severe side effects that are sometimes worse and even more life-threatening than the irregular heartbeats they treat. All of these drugs can also cause new irregularities in your heartbeat.

If you have an irregular heartbeat without any symptoms of underlying heart disease, you should not be exposed to the dangers of a drug that has no health benefit for your condition.[151] If you are taking quinidine or another drug in its family for an irregular heartbeat (arrhythmia), talk to your doctor and find out whether you also have symptoms of underlying heart disease. If not, discuss the possibility of stopping the drug.

Some people are very sensitive to quinidine and may have breathing difficulty, changes in vision, dizziness, fever, headache, ringing in ears, or skin rash when taking this drug. Since there is a narrow range between a helpful and a harmful amount of this drug, call your doctor immediately if you experience these side effects (as well as any of those listed under Adverse Effects).

Before You Use This Drug
Do not use if you have or have had
❑ complete heart block
❑ digitalis toxicity with heart block
Tell your doctor if you have or have had
❑ allergies to drugs
❑ asthma or emphysema
❑ incomplete heart block
❑ digitalis toxicity
❑ liver function impairment
❑ kidney disease
❑ increased secretion of thyroid hormones
❑ low blood potassium
❑ myasthenia gravis
❑ psoriasis
❑ difficulty stopping bleeding
Tell your doctor about any other drugs you take, including aspirin, herbs, vitamins, and other non-prescription products.

When You Use This Drug

- ◆ **Do not stop taking this drug suddenly. Your doctor must give you a schedule to lower your dose gradually, to prevent serious changes in heart function.**
- ◆ Wear a medical identification bracelet or carry a card stating that you take quinidine.
- ◆ If you plan to have any surgery, including dental, tell your doctor that you take this drug.

How To Use This Drug

- ◆ Swallow extended-release tablets whole. Do not crush or break them. Take with **a full glass (8 ounces) of water.** Take your last dose of the day **with a full glass of water** at least an hour before bedtime. If your stomach gets irritated when you take this drug, you can take it with food or milk to help prevent that.
- ◆ If you miss a dose, take it as soon as you remember, but skip it if it is within 2 hours of your next scheduled dose. **Do not take double doses.**

Interactions With Other Drugs

The following drugs are listed in *Evaluations of Drug Interactions*, 1991 as causing "highly clinically significant" or "clinically significant" interactions when used together with this drug. There may be other drugs, especially those in the families of drugs listed below, that also will react with this drug to cause severe adverse effects. Make sure to ask your doctor for a complete listing of them and let her or him know if you are taking any of these interacting drugs:

CALAN; cimetidine; COUMADIN; cyclosporine; digoxin; DILANTIN; ISOPTIN; ketoconazole; LANOXICAPS; LANOXIN; LUMINAL; NIZORAL; PBR/12; phenobarbital; phenytoin; propafenone; RIFADIN; rifampin; RIMACTANE; RYTHMOL; SANDIMMUNE; SOLFOTON; TAGAMET; tubocurarine; verapamil; warfarin.

Adverse Effects

Call your doctor immediately:
- ❑ blurred vision
- ❑ dizziness or fainting
- ❑ fever
- ❑ severe headache
- ❑ ringing in ears or loss of hearing
- ❑ skin rash, hives, or itching
- ❑ painful joints
- ❑ wheezing, shortness of breath
- ❑ unusual bleeding or bruising
- ❑ unusually fast heartbeat
- ❑ unusual tiredness or weakness
- ❑ confusion

Call your doctor if these symptoms continue:
- ❑ bitter taste in mouth
- ❑ diarrhea
- ❑ flushing of skin or itching
- ❑ loss of appetite
- ❑ nausea, vomiting, stomach pain

Periodic Tests

Ask your doctor which of these tests should be done periodically while you are taking this drug:
- ❑ complete blood counts
- ❑ heart function tests, such as electrocardiogram (EKG)
- ❑ kidney function tests
- ❑ liver function tests
- ❑ blood levels of potassium and quinidine

LIMITED USE

Isradipine
DYNACIRC (Sandoz)
Nicardipine
CARDENE (Syntex)
Nifedipine
ADALAT (Miles) PROCARDIA (Pfizer)

Generic: in some strengths of nifedipine only

Family: Calcium Channel Blockers, (see High Blood Pressure, p. 62)

Isradipine (is *rad* ip ene), nicardipine (nick *card* ip ene), and nifedipine (nye *fed* i peen), belong to a family of drugs called calcium channel blockers. They are used primarily to treat chest pain (angina) and coronary artery disease and also to lower blood pressure (hypertension). Calcium channel blockers control, but do not cure high blood pressure. These drugs may improve capacity for exercise and delay the need for heart surgery.

Each calcium channel blocker differs in the likelihood of harmful side effects. Although this group of calcium channel blockers is less likely than verapamil to cause constipation it is more apt to cause dizziness, flushing, headaches, rapid heartbeat, and swelling of legs and feet compared to other calcium channel blockers.[152] These adverse effects can seriously limit use.

Elderly people are more apt to have decreased kidney function, and may require a low dose of calcium channel blockers. Sometimes calcium channel blockers are used with a water pill or beta-blocker (see p. 68) .

For angina, improvement can occur with exercise training.[153] The American Medical Association reports nifedipine and nicardipine are more effective for angina than verapamil and diltiazem.[154]

If you have high blood pressure, the best way to reduce or eliminate your need for medication is through diet, weight loss, exercise, and less salt and alcohol. In mild hypertension nutrition and hygenic measures can control high blood pressure. If these measures do not lower your blood pressure enough and you need medication, **hydrochlorothiazide, a water pill (see thiazide diuretics, p. 117), is the drug of choice for mild hypertension in people over 60 years old, starting with a low dose of 12.5 milligrams.** It also costs less.

There is now good evidence that another benefit of thiazide diuretics such as hydrochlorothiazide is that they significantly decrease the rate of bone mineral loss in both men and women because they reduce the amount of calcium lost in the urine. An increasing number of researchers think that this will also decrease the number of fractures. [155]

Whatever drugs you take for high blood pressure, once your blood pressure has been normal for a year or more, a cautious decrease in dose and renewed attention to non-drug treatment may be worth trying, according to *The Medical Letter*.[156]

"Treatment of hypertension is part of preventive medicine and like all preventive strategies, its progress should be regularly reviewed by whoever initiates it. Many problems could be avoided by not starting antihypertensive treatment until after

prolonged observation. . . . Patients should no longer be told that treatment is necessarily for life: the possibility of reducing or stopping treatment should be mentioned at the outset."[157]

Before You Use This Drug
Do not use if you have or have had
❑ severe hypotension
Tell your doctor if you have or have had
❑ allergies to drugs
❑ aortic stenosis
❑ diabetes
❑ heart, kidney or liver problems
❑ low blood pressure
Tell your doctor about any other drugs you take, including aspirin, herbs, vitamins, and other non-prescription products. Be sure to include the name of any eyedrops which you use.

If you now take a beta-blocker, your doctor may gradually take you off of it before starting a calcium channel blocker.[158]

When You Use This Drug
◆ **Learn to take your pulse, and get immediate help if your pulse slows to 50 beats per minute or slower, even if you are feeling well.**
◆ Periodically check your blood pressure one or two hours after you take a dose, and again eight hours after your last dose.
◆ Until you know how you react to this drug, do not drive or perform other activities requiring alertness.
◆ Follow a diet recommended by your doctor.
◆ Have your doctor suggest exercises which avoid overexertion.
◆ **Do not stop taking calcium channel blockers suddenly. Contact your doctor for a schedule to decrease your drug gradually.**
◆ You may feel dizzy when rising from a lying or sitting position. If you are lying down, hang your legs over the side of the bed for a few minutes, then get up

slowly. When getting up from a chair, stay by the chair until you are sure that you are not dizzy. (See p. 14.)
◆ If you plan to have any surgery, including dental, tell your doctor that you take this drug.
◆ **Do not take other drugs without talking to your doctor first — especially drugs for asthma, colds, cough, diet, hay fever, or sinus problems.**

How To Use This Drug
◆ Swallow capsule or tablet whole. Do not break, chew or crush long-acting forms of this drug.
◆ Be aware that the shell, empty of the drug, of some forms will pass in your stool.
◆ If you miss a dose, take it as soon as you remember, but skip it if it is almost time for the next dose. **Do not take double doses.**
◆ Do not store in the bathroom. Do not expose to heat, moisture or strong light.

Interactions With Other Drugs
The following drugs are listed in *Evaluations of Drug Interactions*, 1991 as causing "highly clinically significant" or "clinically significant" interactions when used together with this drug. There may be other drugs, especially those in the families of drugs listed below, that also will react with this drug to cause severe adverse effects. Make sure to ask your doctor for a complete listing of them and let her or him know if you are taking any of these interacting drugs:

amiodarone; CALCIFEROL; calcium; carbamazepine; CORDARONE; cyclosporine; DANTRIUM; dantrolene; digoxin; DILANTIN; ELIXOPHYLLIN; ergocalciferol; ESKALITH; INDERAL; LANOXIN; lithium; LITHIONATE; LITHOBID; NORCURON; phenytoin; propranolol; QUINAGLUTE; QUINIDEX; quinidine; RIFADIN; rifampin; SANDIMMUNE; TEGRETOL; THEO-DUR; theophylline; vecuronium.

Additionally, the *United States Pharmacopeia Drug Information*, 1992 lists these drugs as causing interactions of major significance: beta-blockers, optic; BETAGAN; disopyramide; NORPACE; timolol; TIMOPTIC.

Adverse Effects

Call your doctor immediately:
- chest pain
- dizziness
- irregular heartbeat
- pounding headache[159]
- fiery red discoloration of knees or ankles[160]
- swelling of legs and feet
- yellowing of skin or eyes
- problems urinating[161]

Call your doctor if these symptoms continue:
- coughing, wheezing
- drowsiness
- dry mouth
- flushed face
- headache
- indigestion
- muscle cramps
- nausea
- numbness
- redness, heat, or pain in the fingers (This is more apt to happen during warm weather or while in bed at night.[162] If this occurs, dip your hands in cold water.)
- skin rash
- feeling of weakness

Periodic Tests

Ask your doctor which of these tests should be done periodically while you are taking this drug:
- blood pressure
- heart function tests, such as electrocardiogram (EKG)
- kidney function tests
- liver function tests

LIMITED USE

Triamterene and Hydrochlorothiazide (combined)
DYAZIDE (Smith Kline & French)
MAXZIDE (Lederle)

Generic: available

Family: Diuretics
Antihypertensives
(See High Blood Pressure, p. 62)

This product, a combination of triamterene (see p. 115) and hydrochlorothiazide (see p. 117), is used to treat high blood pressure (hypertension). **Older adults should never use drugs that contain a fixed combination of triamterene and hydrochlorothiazide as a first choice drug.** Triamterene can cause kidney stones, kidney failure, and retention of too much potassium (especially if potassium supplements are also given), side effects which may be fatal.[163,164] Because of these effects, we do not recommend that any older adult use triamterene, alone.

In addition to triamterene's dangers, there are good reasons not to use any fixed-combination drug for high blood pressure. First, a single drug is often enough to control high blood pressure. If a combination drug like this one is controlling your high blood pressure, it is quite possible that one drug alone would do the same job. There is no reason to put yourself at extra risk by taking extra drugs you do not need.

If you have high blood pressure, the best way to reduce or eliminate your need for medication is through diet, weight loss, exercise, and less salt and alcohol. In mild hypertension nutrition and hygenic measures can control high blood pressure. If these measures do not lower your blood pressure enough and you need medication, **hydrochlorothiazide, a water pill (see thiazide diuretics, p. 117) is the drug of choice for mild hypertension in people** over 60 years old, starting with a low dose of 12.5 milligrams. It also costs less.

There is now good evidence that another benefit of thiazide diuretics such as hydrochlorothiazide is that they significantly decrease the rate of bone mineral loss in both men and women because they reduce the amount of calcium lost in the urine. An increasing number of researchers think that this will also decrease the number of fractures. [165]

Since Dyazide and Maxzide contain 25 milligrams and 50 milligrams of hydrochlorothiazide respectively, it is therefore not possible for older adults to start with a lower starting dose of 12.5

This fixed-combination drug should not be the first drug used to treat your high blood pressure. You may not need more than one drug. If you do need two drugs, this product may not contain the dose of each drug that is right for you.

Your doctor has to regularly check your condition and reevaluate the effect of the drug(s) you take. This means adjusting doses and even changing drugs to ensure proper treatment. A fixed-combination drug may be the best drug for you, but it should be used only after you have tried each of its ingredients separately, in varying doses. If the doses that you need to control your high blood pressure match those in a fixed-combination product, use it. See hydrochlorothiazide, p. 117, for more information about this drug and other drugs with which there is a potentially harmful interaction.

milligrams if either of these products are used. People responding to 12.5 milligrams of hydrochlorothiazide alone will have a lower risk of adverse effects and less need to use potassium supplements or a potassium-saving drug such as triamterene.

If hydrochlorothiazide alone would control your high blood pressure, there is no reason to take the extra risk of using triamterene as well.

If your high blood pressure is more severe and hydrochlorothiazide alone does not control it, there are still better drug treatments than this combination product. The best treatment in this case is a combination of hydrochlorothiazide and a second type of drug called a beta-blocker such as propranolol (see p. 124). If you can't take a drug in the beta-blocker family, another drug called a calcium channel blocker may be used instead. In either case, your doctor would prescribe the hydrochlorothiazide and the second drug separately, with the dose of each drug adjusted to meet your needs, rather than using a product that combines the drugs in advance in a fixed combination.

If you are taking this fixed-combination drug, ask your doctor about changing your prescription.

Whatever drugs you take for high blood pressure, once your blood pressure has been normal for a year or more, a cautious decrease in dose and renewed attention to non-drug treatment may be worth trying, according to *The Medical Letter*.[166]

"Treatment of hypertension is part of preventive medicine and like all preventive strategies, its progress should be regularly reviewed by whoever initiates it. Many problems could be avoided by not starting antihypertensive treatment until after prolonged observation. . . . Patients should no longer be told that treatment is necessarily for life: the possibility of reducing or stopping treatment should be mentioned at the outset."[167]

Heat Stress Alert

This drug can affect your body's ability to adjust to heat, putting you at risk of "heat stress." If you live alone, ask a friend to check on you several times during the day. Early signs of heat stress are dizziness, lightheadedness, faintness, and slightly high temperature. Call your doctor if you have any of these signs.

Drink more fluids (water, fruit and vegetable juices) than usual, even if you're not thirsty, unless your doctor has told you otherwise. Do not drink alcohol.

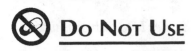 **DO NOT USE**

Alternative treatment: See Hydrochlorothiazide, p. 117.

Triamterene
DYRENIUM (Smith Kline & French)

Family: Diuretics
Antihypertensives
(See High Blood Pressure, p. 62)

Triamterene (trye *am* ter een) is a water pill (diuretic) that removes less of the mineral potassium from your body than other types of diuretics do. Doctors sometimes prescribe it for high blood pressure, instead of another diuretic, in the hope that it will prevent a potassium imbalance. **It should not be used by older adults.** It can cause serious and sometimes fatal side effects such as kidney stones, kidney failure, retention of too much potassium in your body, and a drop in your body's production of blood cells (bone marrow depression).[168,169]

If you have high blood pressure, the best way to reduce or eliminate your need for medication is through diet, weight loss, exercise, and less salt and alcohol. In mild hypertension nutrition and hygenic measures can control high blood pressure. If these measures do not lower your blood pressure enough and you need medication, **hydrochlorothiazide, a water pill (see thiazide diuretics, p. 117), is the drug of choice for mild hypertension in people over 60 years old, starting with a low dose of 12.5 milligrams.** It also costs less.

There is now good evidence that another benefit of thiazide diuretics such as hydrochlorothiazide is that they significantly decrease the rate of bone mineral loss in both men and women because they reduce the amount of calcium lost in the urine. An increasing number of researchers think that this will also decrease the number of fractures. [170]

If you are taking triamterene, ask your doctor about switching to hydrochlorothiazide (see p. 117). If you need to replace potassium in your body because of potassium losses from other drugs, certain potassium supplements are less dangerous than a drug such as triamterene and are equally effective[171] (see p. 66).

Whatever drugs you take for high blood pressure, once your blood pressure has been normal for a year or more, a cautious decrease in dose and renewed attention to non-drug treatment may be worth trying, according to *The Medical Letter*.[172]

"Treatment of hypertension is part of preventive medicine and like all preventive strategies, its progress should be regularly reviewed by whoever initiates it. Many problems could be avoided by not starting antihypertensive treatment until after prolonged observation. . . . Patients should no longer be told that treatment is necessarily for life: the possibility of reducing or stopping treatment should be mentioned at the outset."[173]

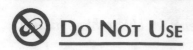 **DO NOT USE**

Alternative treatment: See Hydrochlorothiazide, p. 117.

Deserpidine and Methyclothiazide (combined)
ENDURONYL (Abbott)

Family: Diuretics
Antihypertensives
(See High Blood Pressure, p. 62)

This product, a combination of deserpidine (de *ser* pi deen) and methyclothiazide (see p. 117), is used to treat high blood pressure. **Older adults should not use drugs containing a fixed combination of deserpidine and methyclothiazide.**

Deserpidine is in the same family of drugs as reserpine (see p. 165) and should not be used by older adults. Drugs in this family cause severe side effects during treatment and sometimes months after treatment has ended. Some people taking these drugs have suffered severe depression, in some cases leading to suicide. Deserpidine is particularly dangerous for anyone with a history of depression.[174] This drug can also cause decreased mental sharpness in older adults.

In addition to the risks of deserpidine, there are good reasons not to use any fixed-combination drug for high blood pressure. First, a single drug is often enough to control high blood pressure. If a combination drug like this one is controlling your high blood pressure, it is quite possible that one drug alone would do the same job. There is no reason to put yourself at extra risk by taking extra drugs you do not need.

If you have high blood pressure, the best way to reduce or eliminate your need for medication is through diet, weight loss, exercise, and less salt and alcohol. In mild hypertension nutrition and hygenic measures can control high blood pressure. If these measures do not lower your blood pressure enough and you need medication, **hydrochlorothiazide, a water pill (see thiazide diuretics, p. 117), is the drug of choice for mild hypertension in people over 60 years old, starting with a low dose of 12.5 milligrams.** It also costs less.

There is now good evidence that another benefit of thiazide diuretics such as hydrochlorothiazide is that they significantly decrease the rate of bone mineral loss in both men and women because they reduce the amount of calcium lost in the urine. An increasing number of researchers think that this will also decrease the number of fractures. [175]

If your high blood pressure is more severe and hydrochlorothiazide alone does not control it, there are still better drug treatments than this combination product. The best treatment in this case is a combination of hydrochlorothiazide and a second type of drug called a beta-blocker such as propranolol (see p. 124). If you can't take a drug in the beta-blocker family, another drug called a calcium channel blocker may be used instead. In either case, your doctor would prescribe the hydrochlorothiazide and the second drug separately, with the dose of each drug adjusted to meet your needs, rather than using a product that combines the drugs in advance in a fixed combination.

If you are taking this fixed-combination drug, ask your doctor about changing your prescription.

Whatever drugs you take for high blood pressure, once your blood pressure has been normal for a year or more, a cautious decrease in dose and renewed attention to non-drug treatment may be worth trying, according to *The Medical Letter.*[176]

"Treatment of hypertension is part of preventive medicine and like all preventive strategies, its progress should be regularly reviewed by whoever initiates it. Many problems could be avoided by not starting antihypertensive treatment until after prolonged observation. . . . Patients should

no longer be told that treatment is necessarily for life: the possibility of reducing or stopping treatment should be mentioned at the outset."[177]

THIAZIDE DIURETICS
Hydrochlorothiazide (hye droe klor oh *thye* a zide)
ESIDRIX (CIBA) HYDRODIURIL (Merck)

LIMITED USE

Chlorothiazide (klor oh *thye* a zide)
DIURIL (Merck)
Trichlormethiazide (trye klor meth *eye* a zide)
METAHYDRIN (Merrell Dow)
NAQUA (Schering)
Methyclothiazide (meth ee kloe *thye* a zide)
ENDURON (Abbott)
Metolazone (me *tole* a zone)
DIULO (Searle) ZAROXOLYN (Pennwalt)
Indapamide (in *dap* a mide)
LOZOL (USV)

Generic: available

Family: Diuretics
Antihypertensives
(See High Blood Pressure, p. 62)

Diuretics, commonly called "water pills," are used to treat high blood pressure (hypertension), congestive heart failure, and other conditions in which the body holds too much fluid.[178] All diuretics have potential side effects, commonly including loss of potassium and sodium from the body, harmful interactions with other drugs, and allergic reactions. Older adults also may

suffer blood clots and shock, but this is rare.[179] Diuretics in this family (thiazide diuretics) are mild, which reduces the risk of dizziness, falling, and other side effects that you may suffer if your body loses too much fluid. It has recently been stated by an expert on hypertension in older adults that "thiazide diuretics [as the ones discussed on this page] are almost certainly safer than any of the other drugs available to treat hypertension." [180]

If you have high blood pressure, the best way to reduce or eliminate your need for medication is through diet, weight loss, exercise, and less salt and alcohol. In mild hypertension nutrition and hygenic measures can control high blood pressure. If these measures do not lower your blood pressure enough and you need medication, **hydrochlorothiazide, a water pill, is the drug of choice for mild hypertension in people over 60 years old, starting with a low dose of 12.5 milligrams.** It also costs less.

There is now good evidence that another benefit of thiazide diuretics such as hydrochlorothiazide is that they significantly decrease the rate of bone mineral loss in both men and women because they reduce the amount of calcium lost in the urine. An increasing number of researchers think that this will also decrease the number of fractures. [181]

Hydrochlorothiazide has been studied more than the other diuretics in this family, is available in a generic form, usually costs less, and is just as effective as the other thiazide diuretics. If you are taking a thiazide diuretic other than hydrochlorothiazide, compare cost and then ask your doctor about switching.

If you are taking hydrochlorothiazide, you should in most cases not be taking more than 50 milligrams per day. Daily doses higher than 50 milligrams do not significantly improve blood pressure control and can make side effects worse.[182]

If your hypertension is severe rather than mild and has not responded to a drug in this family, you may need a stronger drug. See p. 62 for a discussion of the alternatives.

Whatever drugs you take for high blood pressure, once your blood pressure has been normal for a year or more, a cautious decrease in dose and renewed attention to non-drug treatment may be worth trying, according to *The Medical Letter.*[183]

"Treatment of hypertension is part of preventive medicine and like all preventive strategies, its progress should be regularly reviewed by whoever initiates it. Many problems could be avoided by not starting antihypertensive treatment until after prolonged observation. . . . Patients should no longer be told that treatment is necessarily for life: the possibility of reducing or stopping treatment should be mentioned at the outset."[184]

Before You Use This Drug
Do not use if you have or have had
❑ a sensitivity to sulfa drugs (sulfonamides) or thiazide drugs
Tell your doctor if you have or have had
❑ allergies to drugs
❑ diabetes
❑ gout
❑ kidney, liver, or pancreas disease
❑ lupus erythematosus
❑ salt- or sugar-restricted diet
Tell your doctor about any other drugs you take, including aspirin, herbs, vitamins, and other non-prescription products.

When You Use This Drug
◆ **Because these drugs help you lose water, you may become dehydrated. Check with your doctor to make certain your fluid intake is adequate and appropriate.**
◆ Stay out of the sun as much as possible, and call your doctor if you get a rash, hives, or skin reaction. These drugs can make you more sensitive to the sun.
◆ **These drugs may cause your body to lose potassium, an important mineral.** Potassium loss is worse when there is too much salt in your diet. See p. 66 for information on how to make sure you get enough potassium.
◆ You may feel dizzy when rising from a lying or sitting position. When getting out of bed, hang your legs over the side of the bed for a few minutes, then get up slowly. When getting up from a chair, stay beside the chair until you are sure that you are not dizzy. (See p. 14.)
◆ If you plan to have any surgery, including dental, tell your doctor that you take a thiazide diuretic.
◆ **Do not take any other drugs without first talking to your doctor — especially non-prescription drugs for appetite**

control, asthma, colds, coughs, hay fever, or sinus problems.

Heat Stress Alert

These drugs can affect your body's ability to adjust to heat, putting you at risk of "heat stress." If you live alone, ask a friend to check on you several times during the day. Early signs of heat stress are dizziness, lightheadedness, faintness, and slightly high temperature. Call your doctor if you have any of these signs.

Drink more fluids (water, fruit and vegetable juices) than usual, even if you're not thirsty, unless your doctor has told you otherwise. Do not drink alcohol.

How To Use This Drug

◆ Take with food or milk to avoid stomach irritation. Tablet may be crushed and mixed with food or drink.

◆ If you are taking a thiazide diuretic more than once a day, try to take the last dose before 6 p.m. This will help you avoid interrupting your sleep to go to the bathroom.

◆ If you miss a dose, take it as soon as you remember, but skip it if it is almost time for the next dose. **Do not take double doses.**

Interactions With Other Drugs

The following drugs are listed in *Evaluations of Drug Interactions*, 1991 as causing "highly clinically significant" or "clinically significant" interactions when used together with this drug. There may be other drugs, especially those in the families of drugs listed below, that also will react with this drug to cause severe adverse effects. Make sure to ask your doctor for a complete listing of them and let her or him

know if you are taking any of these interacting drugs:

calcium carbonate; CAPOTEN; captopril; chlorpropamide; DIABINESE; digoxin; ESKALITH; guanethidine; INDOCIN; indomethacin; ISMELIN; LANOXIN; lithium; TUMS.

These drugs are listed as interacting with hydrochlorothiazide only.

Adverse Effects

Call your doctor immediately:
❑ coughing, wheezing
❑ breathing difficulty
❑ dry mouth or increased thirst that does not go away quickly after you take a drink
❑ fever, chills
❑ irregular heartbeat, chest pain
❑ weak pulse
❑ mood or mental changes
❑ muscle cramps, pain
❑ nausea, vomiting
❑ unusual tiredness or weakness

Call your doctor if these symptoms continue:
❑ dizziness, lightheadedness
❑ diarrhea
❑ loss of appetite, upset stomach
❑ headache
❑ blurred vision or "halo" effect
❑ premature ejaculation or difficulty with erection

Periodic Tests

Ask your doctor which of these tests should be done periodically while you are taking this drug:
❑ blood pressure
❑ complete blood counts
❑ blood levels of sodium, potassium, chloride, calcium, sugar, and uric acid
❑ liver function tests
❑ kidney function tests

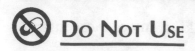 **DO NOT USE**

Alternative treatment: See Hydrochlorothiazide, p. 117.

Reserpine and Hydrochlorothiazide (combined)
HYDROPRES (Merck)
HYDROSERPINE (Schein)

Family: Diuretics
Antihypertensives
(See High Blood Pressure, p. 62)

This product, a combination of reserpine (see p. 165) and hydrochlorothiazide (see p. 117), is used to treat high blood pressure (hypertension). **Older adults should not use drugs that contain a fixed combination of reserpine and hydrochlorothiazide.**

Reserpine causes severe side effects that may occur during treatment and even months after you stop taking it. It has caused severe depression, in some cases leading to suicide. We do not recommend that any older adult use reserpine, and it is particularly dangerous for anyone who has had a depressive illness.[185] It also decreases mental sharpness in older adults.

In addition to the risks of reserpine, there are good reasons not to use any fixed-combination drug for high blood pressure. First, a single drug is often enough to control high blood pressure. If a combination drug like this one is controlling your high blood pressure, it is quite possible that one drug alone would do the same job. There is no reason to put yourself at extra risk by taking extra drugs you do not need.

If you have high blood pressure, the best way to reduce or eliminate your need for medication is through diet, weight loss, exercise, and less salt and alcohol. In mild hypertension nutrition and hygenic measures can control high blood pressure. If these measures do not lower your blood pressure enough and you need medication, **hydrochlorothiazide, a water pill (see thiazide diuretics, p. 117), is the drug of choice for mild hypertension in people over 60 years old, starting with a low** dose of 12.5 milligrams. It also costs less.

There is now good evidence that another benefit of thiazide diuretics such as hydrochlorothiazide is that they significantly decrease the rate of bone mineral loss in both men and women because they reduce the amount of calcium lost in the urine. An increasing number of researchers think that this will also decrease the number of fractures. [186]

Hydrochlorothiazide is one of the ingredients in this combination (see thiazide diuretics, p. 117). Reserpine can cause severe side effects, as described above. If hydrochlorothiazide alone would control your blood pressure, there is no reason to take the extra risk of taking the second drug as well.

If your high blood pressure is more severe and hydrochlorothiazide alone does not control it, there are still better drug treatments than this combination product. The best treatment in this case is a combination of hydrochlorothiazide and a second type of drug called a beta-blocker, such as propranolol (see p. 124). If you can't take a drug in the beta-blocker family, another drug called a calcium channel blocker may be used instead. In either case, your doctor would prescribe the hydrochlorothiazide and the second drug separately, with the dose of each drug adjusted to meet your needs, rather than using a product that combines the drugs in advance in a fixed combination.

If you are taking this fixed-combination drug, ask your doctor about changing your prescription.

Whatever drugs you take for high blood pressure, once your blood pressure has been normal for a year or more, a cautious decrease in dose and renewed attention to non-drug treatment may be worth trying, according to *The Medical Letter*.[187]

"Treatment of hypertension is part of preventive medicine and like all preventive strategies, its progress should be regularly reviewed by whoever initiates it. Many problems could be avoided by not starting antihypertensive treatment until after prolonged observation. . . . Patients should no longer be told that treatment is necessarily for life: the possibility of reducing or stopping treatment should be mentioned at the outset."[188]

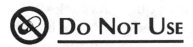 **Do Not Use**

Alternative treatment: See Hydrochlorothiazide, p. 117.

Chlorthalidone
HYGROTON (USV)

Family: Diuretics

Chlorthalidone (klor *thal* i doan) is used to remove water and salt from the body in order to lower blood pressure. **It should not be used by people over 60.** It can make you urinate more often, so that you may lose too much water, potassium, and magnesium which can be dangerous; it can also cause you to lose bladder control, which is both inconvenient and embarrassing. The risk of serious side effects is so high that the World Health Organization has said chlorthalidone should not be used by older adults.[189]

If you have high blood pressure, the best way to reduce or eliminate your need for medication is through diet, weight loss, exercise, and less salt and alcohol. In mild hypertension nutrition and hygenic measures can control high blood pressure. If these measures do not lower your blood pressure enough and you need medication, **hydrochlorothiazide, a water pill (see thiazide diuretics, p. 117), is the drug of choice for mild hypertension in people over 60 years old, starting with a low dose of 12.5 milligrams.** It also costs less.

There is now good evidence that another benefit of thiazide diuretics such as hydrochlorothiazide is that they significantly decrease the rate of bone mineral loss in both men and women because they reduce the amount of calcium lost in the urine. An increasing number of researchers think that this will also decrease the number of fractures.

If you use chlorthalidone, ask your doctor about changing your prescription to hydrochlorothiazide (see p. 117).

Whatever drugs you take for high blood pressure, once your blood pressure has been normal for a year or more, a cautious decrease in dose and renewed attention to non-drug treatment may be worth trying, according to *The Medical Letter*.[187]

"Treatment of hypertension is part of preventive medicine and like all preventive strategies, its progress should be regularly reviewed by whoever initiates it. Many problems could be avoided by not starting antihypertensive treatment until after prolonged observation. . . . Patients should no longer be told that treatment is necessarily for life: the possibility of reducing or stopping treatment should be mentioned at the outset."[188]

LIMITED USE

Terazosin
HYTRIN (Abbott/Burroughs Wellcome)

Generic: not available

Family: Antihypertensives
(See High Blood Pressure, p. 62)

Terazosin (tair *az* o sin) is used to control high blood pressure (hypertension) and is in a group of drugs called alpha adrenergic blocking agents. It does not cure hypertension.[190] According to *The Medical Letter*, this group of drugs is not a good first choice for hypertension.[191]

When taken for high blood pressure, terazosin is sometimes combined with a water pill (thiazide diuretic, see p. 117) or a drug called a beta-blocker (see p. 68). The water pill works with terazosin to lower your blood pressure and helps decrease your body's retention of salt and water, but it also increases your risk of becoming dizzy or lightheaded.

Occasionally, a person will collapse and lose consciousness for a few minutes up to an hour after taking his or her first dose. This is more likely to happen to older adults, but several measures decrease the risk of fainting.[192,193] Your doctor should prescribe a first dose of no more than one milligram. Before you take the first dose, remove any object that would be dangerous if you fell onto it. It is wise to have a companion stay with you for a couple of hours after taking the first dose. Do not drive or attempt any hazardous task for 24 hours after the first dose.

Eat some food. If your diet allows, include a moderate amount of salt. Do not stand for a prolonged time. It is best to take your dose at bedtime.[194] Repeat these precautions any time your dose is increased, or you restart the drug after an interruption in

therapy, or an additional blood pressure drug is prescribed for you. It may take 8 weeks to reach the desired control of blood pressure with terazosin. Some individuals develop palpitation and rapid heartbeat with this medication. Be sure to report this to your doctor if it occurs.

If you have high blood pressure, the best way to reduce or eliminate your need for medication is through diet, weight loss, exercise, and less salt and alcohol. In mild hypertension nutrition and hygenic measures can control high blood pressure. If these measures do not lower your blood pressure enough and you need medication, **hydrochlorothiazide, a water pill (see thiazide diuretics, p. 117), is the drug of choice for mild hypertension in people over 60 years old, starting with a low dose of 12.5 milligrams.** It also costs less.

There is now good evidence that another benefit of thiazide diuretics such as hydrochlorothiazide is that they significantly decrease the rate of bone mineral loss in both men and women because they reduce the amount of calcium lost in the urine. An increasing number of researchers think that this will also decrease the number of fractures. [195]

Whatever drugs you take for high blood pressure, once your blood pressure has been normal for a year or more, a cautious decrease in dose and renewed attention to non-drug treatment may be worth trying, according to *The Medical Letter*.[196]

"Treatment of hypertension is part of preventive medicine and like all preventive strategies, its progress should be regularly reviewed by whoever initiates it. Many problems could be avoided by not starting antihypertensive treatment until after

prolonged observation. . . . Patients should no longer be told that treatment is necessarily for life: the possibility of reducing or stopping treatment should be mentioned at the outset."[197]

Before You Use This Drug
Tell your doctor if you have or have had
❑ allergies to drugs
❑ angina (chest pain)
❑ heart disease
❑ kidney function impairment
❑ liver function impairment (dose should be decreased)
❑ a low-salt diet
Tell your doctor about any other drugs you take, including aspirin, herbs, vitamins, and other non-prescription products.

When You Use This Drug
◆ You may feel dizzy when rising from a lying or sitting position. If you are lying down, hang your legs over the side of the bed for a few minutes, then get up slowly. When getting up from a chair, stay by the chair until you are sure that that you are not dizzy. (See p. 14.)
◆ If you plan to have any surgery, including dental, tell your doctor that you take this drug.
◆ Do not take other drugs without talking to your doctor first — especially non-prescription drugs for appetite control,

---

Heat Stress Alert
This drug can affect your body's ability to adjust to heat, putting you at risk of "heat stress." If you live alone, ask a friend to check on you several times during the day. Early signs of heat stress are dizziness, lightheadedness, faintness, and slightly high temperature. Call your doctor if you have any of these signs.

Drink more fluids (water, fruit, and vegetable juices) than usual, even if you're not thirsty, unless your doctor has told you otherwise. Do not drink alcohol.

---

asthma, colds, coughs, hay fever, sinus problems, pain, or sleep.

How To Use This Drug
◆ Swallow tablets whole. Do not fast while taking this drug.
◆ Take at the same time every day, preferably at bedtime.
◆ Take even when you feel well.
◆ If your doctor directs taking terazosin twice a day, space your doses 10 to 12 hours apart.
◆ If you miss a dose, take it as soon as you remember, but skip it if it is almost time for the next dose. **Do not take double doses**.
◆ Store at room temperature with cap on snuggly. Do not store in the bathroom. Do not expose to heat.
◆ Monitor your blood pressure periodically, both standing and lying down.[198]

Interactions With Other Drugs
The following drugs are listed in *Evaluations of Drug Interactions*, 1991 as causing "highly clinically significant" or "clinically significant" interactions when used together with this drug. There may be other drugs, especially those in the families of drugs listed below, that also will react with this drug to cause severe adverse effects. Make sure to ask your doctor for a complete listing of them and let her or him know if you are taking any of these interacting drugs:
    digoxin; INDOCIN; indomethacin; LANOXIN.

Adverse Effects
Call your doctor immediately:
❑ dizziness, lightheadedness
❑ fainting
❑ chest pain (angina)
❑ irregular heartbeat
❑ shortness of breath
❑ swelling of feet and lower legs
❑ inability to control urination
❑ numbness and tingling of hands and feet
❑ skin rash

Call your doctor if these symptoms continue:
- ❑ drowsiness
- ❑ headache
- ❑ lack of energy
- ❑ nausea, vomiting
- ❑ decreased sexual ability
- ❑ diarrhea or constipation
- ❑ dry cough
- ❑ nasal congestion

- ❑ pain in arms, back, or legs
- ❑ unusual tiredness
- ❑ undesired weight gain
- ❑ blurred vision

Periodic Tests
Ask your doctor which of these tests should be done periodically while you are taking this drug:
- ❑ blood pressure

Propranolol
INDERAL (Ayerst)

Generic: available

Family: Beta-blockers (see p. 68)
Antihypertensives
(See High Blood Pressure, p. 62)

Propranolol (proe *pran* oh lole) is used to treat high blood pressure (hypertension), chest pain (angina), and irregular heartbeats (arrhythmias) and to decrease the frequency of migraine headaches. **If you are over 60, you will generally need less than the usual adult dose, especially if your liver function is impaired.**

For young adults with high blood pressure, doctors usually prescribe a drug in this family (a beta-blocker) before any other drug. But for blacks and older adults, these drugs are less effective as the sole treatment. For these groups of people, doctors usually prescribe another type of drug called a diuretic (water pill) to lower blood pressure, and add a beta-blocker as a second drug if the diuretic alone is not enough.

If you have high blood pressure, the best way to reduce or eliminate your need for medication is through diet, weight loss, exercise, and less salt and alcohol. In mild hypertension nutrition and hygenic measures can control high blood pressure. If these measures do not lower your blood pressure enough and you need medication, **hydrochlorothiazide, a water pill (see thiazide diuretics, p. 117), is the drug of choice for mild hypertension in people over 60 years old, starting with a low dose of 12.5 milligrams.** It also costs less.

There is now good evidence that another benefit of thiazide diuretics such as hydrochlorothiazide is that they significantly decrease the rate of bone mineral loss in both men and women because they reduce the amount of calcium lost in the urine. An increasing number of researchers think that this will also decrease the number of fractures. [199]

All beta-blockers are similarly effective, although not necessarily interchangeable. Increased sensitivity to cold is one side effect. (See, glossary p. 689 for signs of hypothermia.) If you are bothered by side effects when taking propranolol, talk to your doctor about switching to another beta-blocker. The side effects of these drugs vary widely, and each individual responds differently to each one. See p. 68 for a discussion of alternatives to propranol.

Whatever drugs you take for high blood pressure, once your blood pressure has been normal for a year or more, a cautious decrease in dose and renewed attention to non-drug treatment may be worth trying, according to *The Medical Letter*. [200]

"Treatment of hypertension is part of preventive medicine and like all preventive strategies, its progress should be regularly reviewed by whoever initiates it. Many problems could be avoided by not starting antihypertensive treatment until after prolonged observation. . . . Patients should no longer be told that treatment is necessarily for life: the possibility of reducing or stopping treatment should be mentioned at the outset."[201]

Before You Use This Drug

Do not use if you have or have had
❑ congestive heart failure
❑ asthma
❑ emphysema or chronic bronchitis
Tell your doctor if you have or have had
❑ allergies to drugs
❑ difficulty breathing
❑ gout
❑ kidney, liver, lung, or pancreas disease
❑ lupus erythematosus
❑ mental depression
❑ alcohol dependence
❑ poor blood circulation
❑ Raynaud's syndrome
❑ diabetes
❑ thyroid problems
Tell your doctor about any other drugs you take, including aspirin, herbs, vitamins, and other non-prescription products.

When You Use This Drug

◆ **Learn to take your pulse, and get immediate medical help if your pulse slows to 50 beats per minute or less, even if you are feeling well.** Some people have suffered slowed heart rate and heart failure while taking propranolol.
◆ Until you know how you react to this drug, do not drive or perform other activities requiring alertness.
◆ Be careful not to overexert yourself, even though your chest pain may feel better.
◆ **Do not stop taking this drug suddenly. Your doctor must give you a schedule to decrease your dose gradually, to prevent chest pain and possible heart attack.**

◆ You may feel dizzy when rising from a lying or sitting position. When getting out of bed, hang your legs over the side of the bed for a few minutes, then get up slowly. When getting up from a chair, stay beside the chair until you are sure that you are not dizzy. (See p. 14.)
◆ **Caution diabetics: see p. 516.**
◆ If you plan to have any surgery, including dental, tell your doctor that you take this drug.
◆ **Do not take other drugs without talking to your doctor first — especially non-prescription drugs for appetite control, asthma, colds, coughs, hay fever, or sinus problems.**

Heat Stress Alert

This drug can affect your body's ability to adjust to heat, putting you at risk of "heat stress." If you live alone, ask a friend to check on you several times during the day. Early signs of heat stress are dizziness, lightheadedness, faintness, and slightly high temperature. Call your doctor if you have any of these signs.

Drink more fluids (water, fruit and vegetable juices) than usual, even if you're not thirsty, unless your doctor has told you otherwise. Do not drink alcohol.

How To Use This Drug

◆ Take with food. Crush tablets and mix with food or drink, or swallow whole.
◆ Swallow extended-release capsules whole.
◆ If you miss a dose, take it as soon as you remember, unless it is less than 4 hours until your next scheduled dose. **Do not take double doses.**

Interactions With Other Drugs

The following drugs are listed in *Evaluations of Drug Interactions*, 1991 as causing "highly clinically significant" or "clinically significant" interactions when used to-

gether with this drug. There may be other drugs, especially those in the families of drugs listed below, that also will react with this drug to cause severe adverse effects. Make sure to ask your doctor for a complete listing of them and let her or him know if you are taking any of these interacting drugs:

ADRENALIN (also in bee sting kits); amiodarone; ALDOMET; BRONKODYL; CALAN; CATAPRES; chlorpromazine; cimetidine; clonidine; cocaine; CONSTANT-T; CORDARONE; COUMADIN; ELIXOPHYLLIN; epinephrine; ESKALITH; FLUOTHANE; furosemide; halothane; INDOCIN; indomethacin; insulin; LASIX; lidocaine; lithium; methyldopa; NEMBUTAL; pentobarbital; QUIBRON-T-SR; SLO-BID; SLO-PHYLLIN; SUSTAIRE; TAGAMET; THEO-24; THEOLAIR; theophylline; THORAZINE; thyroid; tobacco; tubocurarine; verapamil; warfarin; XYLOCAINE.

Adverse Effects
Call your doctor immediately:
❑ difficulty breathing
❑ cold hands or feet
❑ mental depression
❑ confusion, hallucinations
❑ skin rash
❑ swelling of ankles, feet, or legs
❑ slow pulse
Call your doctor if these symptoms continue:
❑ headache
❑ anxiety, nervousness
❑ constipation or diarrhea
❑ nausea, vomiting
❑ unusual tiredness or weakness
❑ disturbed sleep, nightmares
❑ dry or sore eyes or mouth
❑ numbness or tingling of limbs
❑ decreased sexual ability
More side effects information appears on p. 68.

Periodic Tests
Ask your doctor which of these tests should be done periodically while you are taking this drug:
❑ complete blood counts
❑ blood pressure and pulse rate
❑ heart function tests, such as electrocardiogram (EKG)
❑ kidney function tests
❑ liver function tests
❑ blood glucose levels

LIMITED USE

Propranolol and Hydrochlorothiazide (combined)
INDERIDE (Ayerst)

Generic: available

Family: Diuretics
Antihypertensives
(See High Blood Pressure, p. 62)

This product, a combination of propranolol (see p. 124) and hydrochlorothiazide (see p. 117), is used to treat high blood pressure (hypertension). Drugs containing a fixed combination of propranolol and hydrochlorothiazide offer limited benefit to older adults.

In general, there are good reasons not to use a fixed-combination drug for high blood pressure. First, a single drug is often enough to control high blood pressure. If a combination drug like this one is controlling your high blood pressure, it is quite possible that one drug alone would do the same job. There is no reason to put yourself at extra risk by taking extra drugs you do not need.

If you have high blood pressure, the best way to reduce or eliminate your need for medication is through diet, weight loss, exercise, and less salt and alcohol. In mild hypertension nutrition and hygenic measures can control high blood pressure. If these measures do not lower your blood pressure enough and you need medication, **hydrochlorothiazide, a water pill (see thiazide diuretics, p. 117), is the drug of choice for mild hypertension in people over 60 years old, starting with a low dose of 12.5 milligrams.** It also costs less.

There is now good evidence that another benefit of thiazide diuretics such as hydrochlorothiazide is that they significantly decrease the rate of bone mineral loss in both men and women because they reduce the amount of calcium lost in the urine. An increasing number of researchers think that this will also decrease the number of fractures. [202]

Hydrochlorothiazide, a water pill, is one of the ingredients in this combination (see thiazide diuretics, p. 117). If you can't take propranolol or any other drug in the beta-blocker family, another drug called a calcium channel blocker may be used instead. In either case, your doctor would prescribe the hydrochlorothiazide and the second drug separately, with the dose of each drug adjusted to meet your

---

This fixed-combination drug should not be the first drug used to treat your high blood pressure. You may not need more than one drug. If you do need two drugs, this product may not contain the dose of each drug that is right for you.

Your doctor has to regularly check your condition and reevaluate the effect of the drug(s) you take. This means adjusting doses and even changing drugs to ensure proper treatment. A fixed-combination drug may be the best drug for you, but it should be used only after you have tried each of its ingredients separately, in varying doses. If the doses that you need to control your high blood pressure match those in a fixed-combination product, use it. See propranolol, p. 124, and hydrochlorothiazide, p. 117, for further information on the use of these drugs and other drugs with which there is a potentially harmful interaction.

needs, rather than using a product that combines the drugs in advance in a fixed combination.

If you are taking this fixed-combination drug, ask your doctor about changing your prescription.

Whatever drugs you take for high blood pressure, once your blood pressure has been normal for a year or more, a cautious decrease in dose and renewed attention to non-drug treatment may be worth trying, according to *The Medical Letter*.[203]

"Treatment of hypertension is part of preventive medicine and like all preventive strategies, its progress should be regularly reviewed by whoever initiates it. Many problems could be avoided by not starting antihypertensive treatment until after prolonged observation. . . . Patients should no longer be told that treatment is necessarily for life: the possibility of reducing or stopping treatment should be mentioned at the outset."[204]

Heat Stress Alert

This drug can affect your body's ability to adjust to heat, putting you at risk of "heat stress." If you live alone, ask a friend to check on you several times during the day. Early signs of heat stress are dizziness, lightheadedness, faintness, and slightly high temperature. Call your doctor if you have any of these signs.

Drink more fluids (water, fruit, and vegetable juices) than usual, even if you're not thirsty, unless your doctor has told you otherwise. Do not drink alcohol.

Isosorbide Dinitrate
ISORDIL (Wyeth)
SORBITRATE (Stuart)
Nitroglycerin
DEPONIT (Schwarz Pharma K-U)
MINITRAN (3-M)
NITRO-BID (Marion)*
NITRODISC (Searle)*
NITRO-DUR (Key)
NITROSTAT (Parke-Davis)
TRANSDERM-NITRO (CIBA)
* (see box below)

Generic: available

Family: Nitrates

Isosorbide dinitrate (eye soe *sor* bide dye *nye* trate) and nitroglycerin (nye troe *gli* ser in) are used to treat sudden severe attacks of chest pain (acute angina). They come in several different forms: tablets that dissolve under the tongue (sublingual), chewable tablets, tablets and capsules to be swallowed, and ointments and patches to be applied to the skin. For treating sudden attacks of chest pain, only the sublingual tablets, and certain chewable tablets are effective. The other dosage forms are used on a regular basis to prevent angina attacks from occurring, although the high doses of oral tablets and capsules needed to be effective make them less useful.

Topical forms of nitroglycerin are conditionally approved by the Food and Drug Administration (FDA). Wearing nitroglycerin patches continuously can lead to tolerance to nitroglycerin, which can be prevented or slowed by wearing patches 10 to 12 hours, instead of continuously.

However, the nitrate-free interval may be associated with decreased tolerance to exercise, and the possibility of increased angina. A final evaluation of effectiveness of these products is underway by the FDA.

Before You Use This Drug
Tell your doctor if you have or have had
❑ allergies to any adhesives, drugs, or other materials
❑ glaucoma
❑ hemorrhage of a blood vessel supplying the head
❑ food absorption problem
❑ recent heart attack
❑ severe anemia
❑ trauma to the head
Tell your doctor about any other drugs you take, including aspirin, herbs, vitamins, and other non-prescription products.

When You Use This Drug
◆ You may feel dizzy for a time, or faint, after taking these drugs, especially if you are upright and standing still. If you feel dizzy, put your head between your knees, breathe deeply, and move your arms and legs.
◆ Be careful not to overexert yourself, even though your chest pain may feel better.
◆ Do not drink alcohol.
◆ **If you are taking this drug regularly, do not stop taking it suddenly.** Your doctor

must give you a schedule to lower your dose gradually, to prevent chest pain and possible heart attack.

◆ Until you know how you react to this drug, do not drive or perform other activities requiring alertness.

◆ *For patch*: Carry identification that you use nitroglycerin patches.

◆ If you seek emergency care, or have surgery, including dental, tell your doctor that you take nitroglycerin and the form you use.

Heat Stress Alert

This drug can affect your body's ability to adjust to heat, putting you at risk of "heat stress." If you live alone, ask a friend to check on you several times during the day. Early signs of heat stress are dizziness, lightheaded-ness, faintness, and slightly high tem-perature. Call your doctor if you have any of these signs.

Drink more fluids (water, fruit and vegetable juices) than usual even if you're not thirsty, unless your doctor has told you otherwise. Do not drink alcohol.

How To Use This Drug

For sublingual form:

◆ Place tablet under tongue and allow it to dissolve. Do not chew, crush, or swal-low. While tablet is dissolving, do not eat, drink, or smoke.

◆ Store tablets only in the original con-tainer with the lid on tightly. Nitroglyc-erin is very sensitive and can lose strength rapidly if not stored properly. Do not add any other drug, material, or object to the container that was not there originally. Protect from air, heat, mois-ture, and sunlight. This includes times you carry nitroglycerin with you, or otherwise store it away from home. Special stainless steel containers are available to wear for emergency supplies of nitroglycerin. Once any container of

nitroglycerin is opened, the supply should be replaced within six months.

◆ *For isosorbide dinitrate*: You should feel the drug's effect in 5 minutes. If the pain does not go away in 5 to 10 minutes, take a second tablet. If you still have chest pain after 3 tablets in 15 minutes, call your doctor or go to an emergency room immediately.

◆ *For nitroglycerin*: You should feel the drug's effect in 5 minutes. If the pain does not go away in 5 minutes, take a second tablet. If you still have chest pain after 3 tablets in 10 to 15 minutes, call your doctor or go to an emergency room immediately.

◆ **Do not take other drugs without talking to your doctor first — especially non-prescription drugs for appetite control, asthma, colds, coughs, hay fever, or sinus problems.**

For patch form:

◆ Open and prepare patch according to package instructions. Do not cut or trim the patch to adjust the dose.

◆ Select a site that is dry, on the chest, upper arm, or shoulders. Avoid areas that are broken, calloused, hairy, irri-tated, shaved, sites below the knee or elbow, or areas where movement or clothing is apt to dislodge the patch. The need to rotate sites has recently been questioned.

◆ Press adhesive side of patch to skin firmly.

◆ Replace patch if it loosens, or falls off.

◆ Leave on the amount of time specified by your doctor, then remove.

◆ Apply new patch at the same time each day.

◆ Discard used patch.

◆ Store unopened patches at room tem-perature. Do not expose to high tempera-tures or moisture. Do not store in a bathroom or refrigerator.

Interactions With Other Drugs

The following drugs are listed in *Evalua-tions of Drug Interactions*, 1991 as causing

"highly clinically significant" or "clinically significant" interactions when used together with this drug. There may be other drugs, especially those in the families of drugs listed below, that also will react with this drug to cause severe adverse effects. Make sure to ask your doctor for a complete listing of them and let her or him know if you are taking any of these interacting drugs:

DHE; dihydroergotamine (with nitroglycerin); disopyramide; heparin; imipramine; NORPACE; TOFRANIL.

Adverse Effects
Call your doctor immediately:
- ❑ **if you experience signs of overdose:** bluish lips, fingernails, or palms; dizziness or fainting; feeling of pressure in head; shortness of breath; unusual tiredness or weakness; weak and unusually fast heartbeat; fever; seizures
- ❑ blurred vision
- ❑ dry mouth
- ❑ skin rash

Call your doctor if these symptoms continue:
- ❑ severe or prolonged headache
- ❑ dizziness, lightheadedness
- ❑ nausea or vomiting
- ❑ flushed face and neck
- ❑ rapid pulse
- ❑ burning, itching, or reddened skin

Periodic Tests
Ask your doctor which of these tests should be done periodically while you are taking this drug:
- ❑ blood pressure and pulse
- ❑ heart function tests, such as electrocardiogram (EKG)

---

* Nitro-Bid and Nitrodisc topical dosage forms have been conditionally approved by the Food and Drug Administration (FDA) and may be marketed while further investigation continues. A final evaluation of their effectiveness will be announced by the FDA.

Potassium Supplements
(Nondietary)
Oral solution: KAY CIEL (Forest) KAOCHLOR, KAON-CL (Adria)
Powder for oral solution: K-LOR (Abbott) KATO (ICN) K-LYTE TABLETS (Mead Johnson)

Generic: available for oral solution

LIMITED USE

Extended-release capsules: MICRO-K (Robins)
Extended-release tablets: KLOTRIX (Mead Johnson) SLOW-K (CIBA)

Generic: available for extended-release capsules

If you need to get more of the mineral potassium (poe *tass* ee um), the safest and least expensive way is to eat more potassium-rich foods *daily* (see p. 66 for a discussion of dietary potassium). When researchers compared people eating a potassium-rich diet, people taking potassium supplements, and people taking drugs designed to keep potassium in the body, they found the following: (1) diet is the safest way to replace potassium and (2) potassium supplements and potassium-sparing drugs return potassium levels to normal in only half the people who use them.

Potassium supplements can cause stomach and intestinal ulcers, bleeding, blockage, and perforation. Because of these serious potential side effects, you should only take supplements if you have been eating plenty of potassium-rich foods yet still have a low level of potassium in your blood (less than 3.0 millimoles per liter of blood).[205] Also, you should only take potassium supplements if you have adequate kidney function. The safest form of potassium supplement is an oral solution (liquid) of potassium chloride, and you should only use other forms if you cannot tolerate the liquid. However, enteric-coated potassium products should never be taken.

Before You Use This Drug
Do not use if you have or have had
- ❑ Addison's disease
- ❑ diarrhea, prolonged and severe
- ❑ heart disease
- ❑ intestinal blockage
- ❑ kidney disease or decreased urine production
- ❑ stomach ulcer

Tell your doctor about any other drugs you take, including aspirin, herbs, vitamins, and other non-prescription products.

When You Use This Drug
- ◆ **If you have black, tarry stools or bloody vomit, call your doctor immediately.** These are signs of stomach or intestinal bleeding.
- ◆ Schedule regular appointments with your doctor to check your progress.

◆ Check with your doctor before using salt substitutes, low-salt milk, or other low-salt foods. Because these foods often contain potassium, your potassium supplement dose may have to be adjusted to avoid getting dangerously high levels of potassium in your blood.

◆ Ask your doctor whether you should supplement your diet with vitamin B_{12}. Your body may not be able to absorb this vitamin as well while you are taking potassium supplements.

How To Use This Drug

◆ Take with or immediately after meals. If you are taking extended-release tablets or capsules, swallow them whole, without chewing or crushing them. Take tablets with **a full glass (8 ounces) of water**. Take your last dose of the day with a full glass of water at least an hour before bedtime. If your stomach gets irritated when you take this drug, you can take it with food to help prevent that. If you are taking a solution, dissolvable tablet, or powder, dissolve it completely in at least 1/2 glass (4 ounces) of juice or cold water, then sip slowly over a 5 to 10 minute period. Do not use tomato juice, which has a high salt content.

◆ Do not store in the bathroom, and do not expose to heat, strong light, or moisture. Do not allow the liquid form to freeze.

◆ If you miss a dose, take it if you remember it within 2 hours of the time you were supposed to take it. Skip it if it is almost time for the next dose. **Do not take double doses.**

Interactions With Other Drugs

The following drugs are listed in *Evaluations of Drug Interactions*, 1991 as causing "highly clinically significant" or "clinically significant" interactions when used together with this drug. There may be other drugs, especially those in the families of drugs listed below, that also will react with this drug to cause severe adverse effects. Make sure to ask your doctor for a complete listing of them and let her or him know if you are taking this interacting drug:

ALDACTONE; spironolactone.

Adverse Effects

Call your doctor immediately:
❑ confusion
❑ irregular heartbeat
❑ numbness or tingling in hands, feet, or lips
❑ unusual tiredness or weakness
❑ weakness or heaviness of legs

Call your doctor if these symptoms continue:
❑ diarrhea*
❑ nausea or vomiting*
❑ stomach pain*

Periodic Tests

Ask your doctor which of these tests should be done periodically while you are taking this drug:
❑ heart function tests, such as electrocardiogram (EKG)
❑ kidney function tests
❑ blood potassium levels
❑ blood pH and bicarbonate levels

---

*These side effects can be reduced by taking potassium with food or by using more liquid (water or juice) to dilute it.

Digoxin
LANOXIN, LANOXICAPS (Burroughs Wellcome)

Generic: available

Family: Digitalis Glycosides
     Antiarrhythmics

Digoxin (di *jox* in) is usually used to treat heart failure, a condition in which the heart cannot pump enough blood through the body. The symptoms of heart failure are fatigue, difficulty breathing, swelling (especially in the legs and ankles), and rapid or "galloping" heartbeats. Digoxin is also used to slow certain kinds of abnormally fast heartbeats and to stabilize certain kinds of irregular heartbeats (arrhythmias).

Before prescribing digoxin for heart failure, your doctor should first try giving you another type of drug called a thiazide diuretic (water pill). You should only switch to digoxin if the diuretic does not control your symptoms well enough. **In general, if you are over 60, you should be taking a smaller daily dose than the usual 0.25 milligram,[206] especially if you have impaired kidney function.**

Anyone taking digoxin is at risk of toxic effects (digitalis toxicity). While you are taking digoxin, your doctor should regularly check the levels of the drug in your blood. You and your doctor should also watch for the subtle symptoms of toxicity: fatigue, loss of appetite, nausea and vomiting, problems with vision, bad dreams, nervousness, drowsiness, and hallucinations.[207] Other signs of toxicity are changes in heart rhythm, slow pulse, and lethargy. Since there is a narrow range between a helpful and a harmful amount of digoxin in your body, you should take the drug daily in the exact amount prescribed. If you get too much digoxin in your body, you may develop the effects listed above; if you get too little, you may develop symptoms of heart failure or a rapid heart rate.

Digoxin is often overprescribed for older adults.[208] One study of people using digoxin outside the hospital found that 4 out of 10 people were getting no benefit from the drug.[209] Because of digoxin's toxic effects, taking the drug when it has no benefit is not only wasteful but also dangerous. As many as 1 out of 5 digoxin users develops signs of toxic effects,[210] and much of this could be prevented if the people who did not need digoxin were taken off the drug. Evidence shows that **up to 8 out of 10 long-term digoxin users can stop using the drug successfully, under close supervision by a doctor, with no harmful results.**[211] This is partly due to digoxin being wrongly prescribed in the first place.

If you have used digoxin regularly for some time, ask your doctor if you might be able to try withdrawing from the drug. You are more likely to be able to stop taking digoxin if you meet the following conditions:
1. You have used digoxin for a long time without your initial symptoms of heart failure coming back.
2. You have a normal heart rhythm.
3. You are not using digoxin to control an irregular heart rhythm.

There is no good way of knowing in advance who can stop taking digoxin. People taking digoxin to correct an irregular heart rhythm should not attempt to stop taking the drug, but most other people will benefit from a trial of withdrawal under close supervision by a doctor.

Before You Use This Drug
Do not use if you have or have had
❑ toxic effects from other digitalis preparations
❑ ventricular fibrillation
Tell your doctor if you have or have had
❑ allergies to drugs

❏ high blood calcium level
❏ decreased thyroid hormones
❏ rheumatic fever
❏ heart block
❏ carotid sinus hypersensitivity
❏ high or low blood potassium level
❏ insufficient oxygen supply to the heart
❏ irregular or rapid heartbeat
❏ kidney disease
❏ low blood magnesium level
❏ heart attack
❏ severe lung disease
❏ heart disease in which enlargement of the heart muscle decreases the heart's ability to pump blood (IHSS)

Tell your doctor about any other drugs you take, including aspirin, herbs, vitamins, and other non-prescription products.

When You Use This Drug

◆ **Learn to take your pulse, and get immediate medical help if your pulse slows to 60 beats per minute or less. Some people have suffered a slow heart rate and heart failure while using digoxin.**

◆ **Do not stop taking this drug suddenly.** Your doctor must give you a schedule to lower your dose gradually, to prevent serious changes in your heart function.

◆ Wear a medical identification bracelet or carry a card saying that you take digoxin.

◆ Eat a diet that is rich in potassium, adequate in magnesium, and low in salt and dietary fiber (see p. 66).

◆ **Do not take other drugs without talking to your doctor first — especially non-prescription drugs for appetite control, asthma, colds, coughs, hay fever, or sinus problems.**

◆ If you plan to have any surgery, including dental, tell your doctor that you take this drug.

How To Use This Drug

◆ Crush tablets and mix with water, or swallow whole with water. Take on an empty stomach, at least 1 hour before or 2 hours after meals.

◆ Measure the liquid form only with the specially marked dropper.

◆ If you miss a dose, do not take it. Wait until your next scheduled dose. **Do not take double doses.** If you miss 2 or more doses in a row, call your doctor.

Interactions With Other Drugs

The following drugs are listed in *Evaluations of Drug Interactions* 1991, as causing "highly clinically significant" or "clinically significant" interactions when used together with this drug. There may be other drugs, especially those in the families of drugs listed below, that also will react with this drug to cause severe adverse effects. Make sure to ask your doctor for a complete listing of them and let her or him know if you are taking any of these interacting drugs:

ACROMYCIN; ALAGEL; ALDACTONE; ALTERNAGEL; aluminum hydroxide; amiodarone; AMPHOJEL; AZULFIDINE; CALAN; calcium chloride injection; capoten; CAPTOPRIL; cholestyramine; CORDARONE; CUPRIMINE; cyclophosphamide; cyclosporine; DELTASONE; DEPEN; diazepam; DILANTIN; DURAQUIN; E-MYCIN; ERYC; erythromycin base; furosemide; GAVISCON; hydroxychloroquine; ibuprofen; ISOPTIN; kaolin; KAOLIN-PECTIN; LASIX; M.O.M.; magnesium hydroxide; magnesium trisilicate; MATULANE; metoclopramide; MINIPRESS; MOTRIN; neomycin; ONCOVIN; PANMYCIN; PAREPECTOLIN; penicillamine; phenytoin; PHILLIPS MILK OF MAGNESIA; prazosin; prednisone; PRO-BANTHINE; procarbazine; propantheline; QUESTRAN; quinidine; QUINIGLUTE DURA-TABS; RYTHMOL; SANDIMMUNE; SK PROPANTHELINE BROMIDE; spironolactone; succinylcholine; sulfasalazine; tetracycline; thyroid; VALIUM; verapamil; vincristine.

Adverse Effects
Call your doctor immediately:
❑ **if you experience signs of overdose:** loss of appetite; nausea; vomiting; diarrhea; irregular heartbeats; slow pulse; unusual tiredness or weakness; blurred vision or colored "halos"; mental depression or confusion; drowsiness; headache; bad dreams; hallucinations; nervousness
❑ skin rash or hives

Periodic Tests
Ask your doctor which of these tests should be done periodically while you are taking this drug:
❑ blood pressure and pulse rate
❑ heart function tests, such as electrocardiogram (EKG)
❑ kidney function tests
❑ liver function tests
❑ blood levels of potassium, magnesium and calcium
❑ blood levels of digoxin

LIMITED USE

Furosemide
LASIX (Hoechst-Roussel)

Generic: available

Family: Diuretics
Antihypertensives
(See High Blood Pressure, p. 62)

Furosemide (fur *oh* se mide) is a very strong "water pill" (loop diuretic) with many side effects. It is used to treat fluid retention and high blood pressure. If you are over 60, you should be taking this drug only to reduce fluid retention, and then only if you have decreased kidney function and have tried milder drugs such as hydrochlorothiazide (see p.117) without success. People over 60 years old who have normal kidney function should not use furosemide for any reason.[212]

If you are taking furosemide to reduce fluid retention, the initial dose should be 20 milligrams daily, adjusted as needed.[213] Older adults are more likely than others to develop blood clots, shock,[214] dizziness, confusion, and insomnia, and to have an increased risk of falling, while taking furosemide.[215]

If you have high blood pressure, the best way to reduce or eliminate your need for medication is through diet, weight loss, exercise, and less salt and alcohol. In mild hypertension nutrition and hygenic measures can control high blood pressure. If these measures do not lower your blood pressure enough and you need medication, **hydrochlorothiazide, a water pill (see thiazide diuretics, p. 117), is the drug of choice for mild hypertension in people over 60 years old, starting with a low dose of 12.5 milligrams.** It also costs less.

There is now good evidence that another benefit of thiazide diuretics such as hydrochlorothiazide is that they significantly decrease the rate of bone mineral loss in both men and women because they reduce the amount of calcium lost in the urine. An increasing number of researchers think that this will also decrease the number of fractures. [216]

If hydrochlorothiazide alone does not work, your doctor should add a second drug such as a beta-blocker, for example propranolol (see p. 124) rather than switching you to a strong diuretic like furosemide.

Warning: Thiamine Deficiency With Furosemide

Recent studies have shown that significant amounts of thiamine (vitamin B_1) are lost in the urine of people using furosemide (Lasix) and that patients therefore become thiamine deficient. The researchers found that replenishing thiamine, by taking one 100 milligram pill of thiamine hydrochloride daily for 7 weeks, significantly improved heart function in patients who were using furosemide.[217,218] It is likely that after replacing the significant thiamine losses with these larger doses, the daily maintainance dose will be less. For now, however, **we recommend the use of 100 milligrams a day of thiamine hydrochloride for at least 7 weeks in people who have used furosemide chronically.**

In consultation with your physician, if there seems to be an improvement in your heart status, you should continue with a daily dose of about 50 milligrams of thiamine as long as you are taking furosemide.

Whatever drugs you take for high blood pressure, once your blood pressure has been normal for a year or more, a cautious decrease in dose and renewed attention to non-drug treatment may be worth trying, according to *The Medical Letter*.[219]

"Treatment of hypertension is part of preventive medicine and like all preventive strategies, its progress should be regularly reviewed by whoever initiates it. Many problems could be avoided by not starting antihypertensive treatment until after prolonged observation. . . . Patients should no longer be told that treatment is necessarily for life: the possibility of reducing or stopping treatment should be mentioned at the outset."[220]

Before You Use This Drug
Do not use if you have or have had
❑ a sensitivity to sulfa drugs (sulfonamides) or yellow dye #5
Tell your doctor if you have or have had
❑ allergies to drugs
❑ diabetes
❑ gout
❑ kidney, liver, or pancreas disease
❑ hearing loss
❑ lupus erythematosus
❑ salt- or sugar-restricted diet
Tell your doctor about any other drugs you take, including aspirin, herbs, vitamins, and other non-prescription products.

When You Use This Drug
◆ **Check with your doctor to make certain your fluid intake is adequate and appropriate. Because furosemide is a very strong water pill, you are in danger of becoming dehydrated.**
◆ Stay out of the sun as much as possible, and call your doctor if you get a rash, hives, or any other skin reaction. Furosemide makes you more sensitive to the sun.
◆ **Furosemide will cause your body to lose potassium, an important mineral.** See p. 66 for a discussion of how to make sure you get enough.
◆ You may feel dizzy when rising from a lying or sitting position. When getting up from bed, hang your legs over the side of the bed for a few minutes, then get up slowly. When getting up from a chair, stay beside the chair until you are sure that you are not dizzy. (See p. 14.)
◆ Furosemide can cause a loss of hearing, which is usually temporary but may be permanent. The risk of hearing loss is greater if you are also using amphotericin B or an antibiotic from the aminoglycoside family (see p. 594 for two examples).
◆ If you plan to have any surgery, including dental, tell your doctor that you take this drug.
◆ **Do not take other drugs without first talking to your doctor — especially**

non-prescription drugs for appetite control, asthma, colds, coughs, hay fever, or sinus problems.

Heat Stress Alert

This drug can affect your body's ability to adjust to heat, putting you at risk of "heat stress." If you live alone, ask a friend to check on you several times during the day. Early signs of heat stress are dizziness, lightheadedness, faintness, and slightly high temperature. Call your doctor if you have any of these signs.

Drink more fluids (water, fruit and vegetable juices) than usual, even if you're not thirsty, unless your doctor has told you otherwise. Do not drink alcohol.

How To Use This Drug

◆ Take with food or milk to avoid stomach irritation. Tablets may be crushed and mixed with food or drink.

◆ If you are taking furosemide more than once a day, try to take the last dose before 6 p.m. This will help you avoid interrupting your sleep to go to the bathroom.

◆ If you miss a dose, take it as soon as you remember, but skip it if it is almost time for the next dose. **Do not take double doses.**

Interactions With Other Drugs

The following drugs are listed in *Evaluations of Drug Interactions*, 1991 as causing "highly clinically significant" or "clinically significant" interactions when used together with this drug. There may be other drugs, especially those in the families of drugs listed below, that also will react with this drug to cause severe adverse effects. Make sure to ask your doctor for a complete listing of them and let her or him know if you are taking any of these interacting drugs:

CAPOTEN; captopril; cephalothin; charcoal; cholestyramine; cisplatin; digoxin; ELIXOPHYLLIN; ESKALITH; INDERAL; KEFLIN; LANOXICAPS; LANOXIN; lithium; PLATINOL; propranolol; QUESTRAN; THEO-DUR; theophylline.

Adverse Effects

Call your doctor immediately:
❑ dry mouth, increased thirst
❑ irregular heartbeat
❑ mood or mental changes
❑ muscle cramps, pain
❑ nausea, vomiting
❑ unusual tiredness or weakness
❑ weak pulse
❑ yellow vision

Call your doctor if these symptoms continue:
❑ dizziness, lightheadedness
❑ diarrhea
❑ loss of appetite, upset stomach
❑ headache
❑ blurred vision
❑ premature ejaculation or difficulty with erection

Periodic Tests

Ask your doctor which of these tests should be done periodically while you are taking this drug:
❑ blood pressure
❑ complete blood counts
❑ blood levels of sodium, potassium, chloride, calcium, sugar, and uric acid
❑ liver function tests
❑ kidney function tests

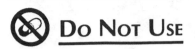 **DO NOT USE**

Alternative treatment: See Cholesterol-lowering Drugs, p. 70

Gemfibrozil
LOPID (Parke-Davis)

Family: Cholesterol-lowering Drugs
(See p. 70)
See psyllium, p. 356

Gemfibrozil (gem *fi* broe zil) is given to people who have high levels of cholesterol or fats in their blood, to lower those levels in the hope of preventing heart disease. Although gemfibrozil does lower the level of fats in your blood, it has little effect on cholesterol levels. More importantly, there is no evidence that it decreases your risk of sickness or death from heart disease. **In fact, there is no proof that gemfibrozil has any health benefit, such as lowering the chance of having a heart attack, for most people with high blood cholesterol or fat levels.**

A Food and Drug Administration physician recently summarized the results of human studies on gemfibrozil: referring to a study in which some patients who had had a previous heart attack were given gemfibrozil, and some were given a placebo, the study

"showed adverse trends with higher total mortality, higher coronary deaths and higher coronary heart disease events in the gemfibrozil (Lopid) group compared to the placebo group. . . . Studies have repeatedly shown increased gallbladder toxicity and statistically increased appendectomies with gemfibrozil. . . . We are concerned about the potential for human carcinogenesis induced by long-term treatment with fibrates [such as gemfibrozil] based on animal findings at doses equal to those used with humans."[221]

Other serious problems with this drug are seen if it is used in combination with lovastatin (Mevacor, see p. 144) or pravastatin (Pravachol, see p. 154). There are numerous reports of severe muscle damage sometimes accompanied by life-threatening destruction of muscle and subsequent kidney damage.[222] Therefore, gemfibrozil and lovastatin (or pravastatin) should never be used together.

The use of cholesterol-lowering drugs in people 70 or older should be limited to patients with very high cholesterol levels (greater than 300 milligrams) and those who manifest cardiovascular disease (previous history of heart attack or angina).[223]

For people under 70, to lower cholesterol the first, safer, and less costly measure is to eat a low-fat diet, using mostly polyunsaturated fats (such as canola, corn, safflower, and sunflower oils) or monounsaturated fats (such as olive oil). A change from animal to vegetable proteins often corrects high cholesterol. However, it is inadvisable to go on a very low-fat diet. The main focus on cholesterol-lowering diets has been on saturated fat and cholesterol content, not soluble fiber. (When added to the diet, psyllium or oat bran is a safe, effective way of lowering cholesterol.) Exercise is also recommended. Conditions that aggravate high cholesterol, such as dependence on alcohol, or tobacco, diabetes, high blood pressure, low magnesium or potassium, and thyroid disease, should be corrected before adding a cholesterol-reducing drug. If cholesterol remains high despite diet, add 10 grams of psyllium a day (see p. 356).

Metoprolol
LOPRESSOR (Geigy)

Generic: not available

Family: Beta-blockers (See p. 68)
Antihypertensives
(See High Blood Pressure, p. 62)

Metoprolol (me *toe* proe lole) is used to treat high blood pressure (hypertension), chest pain (angina), and irregular heartbeat (arrhythmias) and to decrease the frequency of migraine headaches.

For young adults with high blood pressure, doctors usually prescribe a drug in this family (a beta-blocker) before any other drug. But for blacks and older adults, these drugs are less effective as the sole treatment. For these groups of people, doctors usually prescribe another type of drug called a diuretic (water pill) to lower blood pressure, and add a beta-blocker as a second drug if the diuretic alone is not enough.

If you have high blood pressure, the best way to reduce or eliminate your need for medication is through diet, weight loss, exercise, and less salt and alcohol. In mild hypertension nutrition and hygenic measures can control high blood pressure. If these measures do not lower your blood pressure enough and you need medication, **hydrochlorothiazide, a water pill (see thiazide diuretics, p. 117), is the drug of choice for mild hypertension in people over 60 years old, starting with a low dose of 12.5 milligrams.** It also costs less.

There is now good evidence that another benefit of thiazide diuretics such as hydrochlorothiazide is that they significantly decrease the rate of bone mineral loss in both men and women because they reduce the amount of calcium lost in the urine. An increasing number of researchers think that this will also decrease the number of fractures. [224]

Metoprolol frequently causes sleep disturbances. If you are bothered by side effects when using this drug, talk with your doctor about switching to another drug in this family (beta-blockers). Increased sensitivity to cold is one side effect. (See, glossary p. 689 for signs of hypothermia.) The side effects of drugs in this family vary widely, and each individual responds differently to each one. See p. 68 for a discussion of alternatives to metoprolol.

A low dose of metoprolol (50 milligrams per day, for example) taken once a day may not keep your blood pressure down for a full 24 hours. If you are on a once-a-day schedule, your blood pressure should be checked almost 24 hours after you have taken a dose (just before you take the next dose), to make sure that the drug is working for the entire day. If it is not, you may need to take more than one dose a day.

Whatever drugs you take for high blood pressure, once your blood pressure has been normal for a year or more, a cautious decrease in dose and renewed attention to non-drug treatment may be worth trying, according to *The Medical Letter*. [225]

"Treatment of hypertension is part of preventive medicine and like all preventive strategies, its progress should be regularly reviewed by whoever initiates it. Many problems could be avoided by not starting antihypertensive treatment until after prolonged observation. . . . Patients should no longer be told that treatment is necessarily for life: the possibility of reducing or stopping treatment should be mentioned at the outset." [226]

Before You Use This Drug
Do not use if you have
❑ emphysema or chronic bronchitis
❑ congestive heart failure
❑ asthma
Tell your doctor if you have or have had
❑ allergies to drugs

❑ poor blood circulation
❑ thyroid problems
❑ gout
❑ kidney, liver, lung, or pancreas disease
❑ difficulty breathing
❑ lupus erythematosus
❑ mental depression
❑ alcohol dependence
❑ Raynaud's syndrome
❑ diabetes

Tell your doctor about any other drugs you take, including aspirin, herbs, vitamins, and other non-prescription products.

When You Use This Drug

◆ **Learn to take your pulse, and get immediate medical help if your pulse slows to 50 beats per minute or less, even if you are feeling well. Some people have suffered a slow heart rate and heart failure while taking metoprolol.**

◆ Until you know how you react to this drug, do not drive or perform other activities that require alertness.

◆ Be careful not to overexert yourself, even though your chest pain may feel better.

◆ **Do not stop taking this drug suddenly. Your doctor must give you a schedule to decrease your dose gradually, to prevent chest pain and possible heart attack.**

◆ You may feel dizzy when rising from a lying or sitting position. If you are lying down, hang your legs over the side of the bed for a few minutes, then get up slowly. When getting up from a chair, stay beside the chair until you are sure that you are not dizzy. (See p. 14.)

◆ **Caution diabetics: see p. 516.**

◆ If you plan to have any surgery, including dental, tell your doctor that you take this drug.

◆ **Do not take other drugs without talking to your doctor first — especially non-prescription drugs for appetite control, asthma, colds, coughs, hay fever, or sinus problems.**

How To Use This Drug

◆ Take with food. Crush tablet unless you are taking the extended-release tablet and mix with food or drink, or swallow whole with water.

◆ If you miss a dose, take it as soon as you remember, unless it is less than 4 hours until your next dose. **Do not take double doses.**

Interactions With Other Drugs

The following drugs are listed in *Evaluations of Drug Interactions,* 1991 as causing "highly clinically significant" or "clinically significant" interactions when used together with this drug. There may be other drugs, especially those in the families of drugs listed below, that also will react with this drug to cause severe adverse effects. Make sure to ask your doctor for a complete listing of them and let her or him know if you are taking any of these interacting drugs:

amiodarone; CALAN; CATAPRES; chlorpromazine; cimetidine; clonidine; cocaine; CORDARONE; ESKALITH; FLUOTHANE; halothane; INDOCIN; indomethacin; lidocaine; lithium carbonate; LITHOBID; LITHONATE; MINIPRESS; NEMBUTAL; pentobarbital; prazosin; SYNTHROID; TAGAMET; THORAZINE; thyroid; tubocurarine; verapamil; XYLOCAINE.

Heat Stress Alert

This drug can affect your body's ability to adjust to heat, putting you at risk of "heat stress." If you live alone, ask a friend to check on you several times during the day. Early signs of heat stress are dizziness, lightheadedness, faintness, and slightly high temperature. Call your doctor if you have any of these signs.

Drink more fluids (water, fruit and vegetable juices) than usual even if you're not thirsty, unless your doctor has told you otherwise. Do not drink alcohol.

Adverse Effects

Call your doctor immediately:
- ❑ difficulty breathing
- ❑ cold hands or feet
- ❑ mental depression
- ❑ hallucinations
- ❑ confusion, memory loss
- ❑ skin rash
- ❑ swelling of ankles, feet, or legs
- ❑ slow pulse

Call your doctor if these symptoms continue:
- ❑ headache
- ❑ constipation or diarrhea
- ❑ nausea, vomiting
- ❑ unusual tiredness or weakness
- ❑ disturbed sleep, nightmares

- ❑ itching skin
- ❑ decreased sexual ability

More side effects information appears on p. 68.

Periodic Tests

Ask your doctor which of these tests should be done periodically while you are taking this drug:
- ❑ complete blood counts
- ❑ blood pressure and pulse rate
- ❑ heart function tests, such as electrocardiogram (EKG)
- ❑ kidney function tests
- ❑ liver function tests
- ❑ blood glucose levels

LIMITED USE

Probucol
LORELCO (Marion Merrell-Dow)

Generic: not available

Family: Cholesterol-lowering Drugs
(See p. 70)
See psyllium, p. 356

Probucol (pro *biew* call) lowers cholesterol, especially low-density lipoprotein (LDL) cholesterol. It helps control high cholesterol, but does not cure any condition. In middle-aged people, it is clear that lowering cholesterol lessens the risk of coronary artery disease, but no cholesterol-lowering drug has been shown to lower overall death rates in this age group. In older adults the extent to which higher cholesterol levels contribute to heart disease and should be treated with drugs is much less clear.

Unfortunately, probucol also lowers desirable high density lipoprotein (HDL) cholesterol. While taking probucol, heart arrhythmias and prolonged QT interval can occur which may cause serious harm, and can even be fatal.

Probucol is not as effective at lowering LDL cholesterol as other drugs, such as niacin, cholestyramine, and lovastatin. It takes a few weeks to work.

The use of cholesterol-lowering drugs in people 70 or older should be limited to patients with very high cholesterol levels (greater than 300 milligrams) and those who manifest cardiovascular disease (previous history of heart attack or angina).[227]

For people under 70, to lower cholesterol the first, safer, and less costly measure is to eat a low-fat diet, using mostly polyunsaturated fats (such as canola, corn, safflower, and sunflower oils) or monounsaturated fats (such as olive oil). A change from animal to vegetable proteins often corrects high cholesterol.[228] However, it is inadvisable to go on a very low-fat diet.[229] The main focus on cholesterol-lowering diets has been on saturated fat and cholesterol content, not soluble fiber content. (When added to the diet, psyllium or oat bran is a safe, effective way of lowering cholesterol.) Exercise is also recommended. Conditions that aggravate high cholesterol, such as dependence on alcohol or tobacco, diabetes, high blood pressure, low magnesium or potassium, and thyroid disease, should be corrected before adding a cholesterol-reducing drug. If cholesterol remains high despite diet add 10 grams of psyllium a day (see p. 356). Probucol should be discontinued if there is no response after four months.

Before You Use This Drug

Do not use if you have or have had
- ❏ primary biliary cirrhosis
- ❏ unexplained fainting
- ❏ prolonged QT interval
- ❏ myocardial infarction
- ❏ pulse rate below 60

Tell your doctor if you have or have had
- ❏ allergies to other drugs
- ❏ congestive heart failure
- ❏ diabetes[230,231]
- ❏ gallstones
- ❏ goiter
- ❏ heart problems, including arrhythmias
- ❏ liver problems
- ❏ low magnesium or potassium
- ❏ thyroid problems

Tell your doctor about any other drugs you take, including aspirin, herbs, vitamins, and other non-prescription products.

When You Use This Drug
- ◆ Continue to follow a low-fat diet.
- ◆ Check with your doctor before deciding to stop taking probucol.

How To Use This Drug
- ◆ Swallow tablets whole. Take with meals.
- ◆ If you miss a dose, take it as soon as you remember but skip it if it is almost time for the next dose. **Do not take double doses.**
- ◆ Store tablets at room temperature with lid on firmly.

- ◆ Do not store in the bathroom. Do not expose to heat, moisture or strong light.

Interactions With Other Drugs
Some other drugs that you may be taking (either over-the-counter or prescription drugs) can interact with this one, causing adverse effects. Find out from your doctor what these drugs are and let him or her know if you are taking any of them.

Adverse Effects
Since probucol stays in the body six months or longer after stopping the drug, these adverse effects can happen even six months after stopping probucol.
Call your doctor immediately:
- ❏ unusual bleeding or bruising
- ❏ chest pain
- ❏ dizziness, fainting
- ❏ irregular heartbeat
- ❏ skin rash
- ❏ swelling of face, hands, feet, or mouth
- ❏ unusual tiredness or weakness

Call your doctor if these symptoms continue:
- ❏ diarrhea
- ❏ stomach pain or gas
- ❏ headache
- ❏ impotence
- ❏ insomnia
- ❏ nausea or vomiting
- ❏ numbness or tingling of face, fingers, or toes
- ❏ ringing in ears
- ❏ sense of taste becomes metallic
- ❏ sweat with foul odor
- ❏ urinary frequency at night
- ❏ blurred vision

Periodic Tests
Ask your doctor which of these tests should be done periodically while you are taking this drug:
- ❏ cholesterol tests
- ❏ electrocardiogram (EKG)
- ❏ triglyceride tests

LIMITED USE

Lovastatin
MEVACOR (Merck, Sharpe & Dohme)

Generic: not available

Family: Cholesterol-lowering Drugs (See p. 70)

Lovastatin (low vah *stat* in) lowers cholesterol by preventing the body from making as much cholesterol, specifically low-density lipoprotein (LDL) cholesterol. In middle-aged people it is clear that lowering cholesterol lessens the risk of coronary artery disease, but no cholesterol-lowering drug has been shown to lower overall death rates in this age group. In older adults, the extent to which higher cholesterol levels contribute to heart disease and should be treated with drugs is much less clear.

Lovastatin belongs to the same family of drugs as pravastatin. This family of drugs are generally better tolerated than other cholesterol-lowering drugs, according to *The Medical Letter.*[232] Still, these drugs commonly cause gastrointestinal problems. Of particular concern is the possibility of liver toxicity, including hepatitis. Therefore, liver function tests should be done every 6 weeks in patients on therapy. In animals these drugs have produced cancers. Severe inflammation and pain in the muscles can occur, especially when lovastatin is combined with gemfibrozil. In people simultaneously using gemfibrozil and lovastatin, there are also numerous reports of severe muscle damage sometimes accompanied by life-threatening destruction of muscle and subsequent kidney damage. Therefore, gemfibrozil and lovastatin should never be used together.[233]

Long-term effects of interfering with the body's making of cholesterol are not known.[234,235,236] This family of drugs is not effective for the homozygous familial type of high blood cholesterol.[237]

The use of cholesterol-lowering drugs in people 70 or older should be limited to patients with very high cholesterol levels (greater than 300 milligrams) and those who manifest cardiovascular disease (previous history of heart attack or angina).[238]

For people under 70, to lower cholesterol the first, safer, and less costly measure is to eat a low-fat diet, using mostly polyunsaturated fats (such as canola, corn, safflower, and sunflower oils) or monounsaturated fats (such as olive oil). A change from animal to vegetable proteins often corrects high cholesterol. However, it is inadvisable to go on a very low-fat diet. The main focus on cholesterol-lowering diets has been on saturated fat and cholesterol content, not soluble fiber. (When added to the diet, psyllium or oat bran is a safe, effective way of lowering cholesterol.) Exercise is also recommended. Conditions that aggravate high cholesterol, such as dependence on alcohol or tobacco, diabetes, high blood pressure, low magnesium or potassium, and thyroid disease, should be corrected before adding a cholesterol-reducing drug. If cholesterol remains high despite diet, add 10 grams of psyllium a day (see p. 356).

Lovastatin is usually reserved for people who do not respond to other drugs.[239] However, choice of a drug in the elderly must be individualized.[240]

Before You Use This Drug
Do not use this drug if you have
❑ liver disease, active
Tell your doctor if you have or have had
❑ allergies to drugs
❑ alcohol dependence
❑ cataracts
❑ low blood pressure

❑ metabolic, hormone or mineral imbalances
❑ severe infections
❑ severe injuries
❑ kidney problems
❑ prior liver problems such as hepatitis or jaundice
❑ organ transplant or other major surgery
❑ seizures

Tell your doctor about any other drugs you take, including aspirin, herbs, vitamins, and other non-prescription products.

When You Use This Drug
◆ Continue to eat a low-fat diet
◆ If you plan to have any surgery, including dental, tell your doctor that you take this drug.

How To Use This Drug
◆ Swallow the tablet whole. Take the first dose with an evening meal. If you take once daily, take it with the evening meal. If you take more than one dose a day take with meals or snacks.
◆ If you miss a dose, take it as soon as you remember but skip it it it is almost time for the next dose. **Do not take double doses.**
◆ Do not store in the bathroom. Do not expose to heat, moisture or strong light. Store at room temperature, with the lid on snuggly.
◆ Check with your doctor before you stop taking lovastatin.

Interactions With Other Drugs
The following drugs are listed in *Evaluations of Drug Interactions*, 1991 as causing "highly clinically significant" or "clinically significant" interactions when used together with this drug. There may be other drugs, especially those in the families of drugs listed below, that also will react with this drug to cause severe adverse effects.

Make sure to ask your doctor for a complete listing of them and let her or him know if you are taking any of these interacting drugs:
gemfibrozil; LOPID; niacin (vitamin B₃) (this only refers to very large doses of niacin used to lower cholesterol, not ordinary niacin in your diet).

Additionally, the *United States Pharmacopeia Drug Information*, 1992 lists this drug as having interactions of major significance:
cyclosporine; SANDIMMUNE.

Adverse Effects
Call your doctor immediately:
❑ breathing difficulty
❑ fever or chills
❑ muscle aches
❑ numbness
❑ skin rash or yellowing of skin or eyes
❑ swelling of face, lips, legs
❑ unusual tiredness
❑ blurred vision
Call your doctor if these symptoms continue:
❑ anxiety
❑ constipation
❑ diarrhea
❑ dizziness
❑ gas, heartburn, stomach pain
❑ headache
❑ impotence
❑ insomnia
❑ itching
❑ nausea

Periodic Tests
Ask your doctor which of these tests should be done periodically done while you are taking this drug:
❑ blood test for cholesterol and for creatine kinsase
❑ eye exam
❑ liver function tests

LIMITED USE

Mexiletine
MEXITIL (Boehringer Ingelheim)

Generic: not available

Family: Antiarrhythmics

Mexiletine (mex *ill* et een) slows rapid heartbeat and stabilizes irregular heartbeats (arrhythmias). Mexiletine prevents recurrence of ventricular arrhythmias, such as premature heartbeats. It can prevent sudden death. Mexiletine belongs to the same family of drugs as lidocaine (Xylocaine).

It is as effective as quinidine for some, but not all, arrthymias[241] and sometimes is used beneficially with quinidine.[242] Mexiletine has little risk of organ toxicity but has a high risk of noncardiac adverse effects.[243] However, these adverse effects often cause people to stop taking mexiletine.[244,245] Lower doses can reduce unwanted effects. People with decreased liver function should take a lower dose. At times mexiletine actually worsens some types of arrhythmias. It is not for use in minor arrhythmias. Use of mexiletine with procainamide (Pronestyl) is of little or no value.[246]

Before You Use This Drug
Do not use if you have or have had
❏ cardiogenic shock
❏ heart block of 2nd or 3rd degree without a pacemaker
Tell your doctor if you have or have had
❏ allergies to drugs
❏ angina
❏ congestive heart failure[247]
❏ heart block or other heart problems
❏ kidney[248] or liver problems
❏ low blood pressure
❏ myocardial infarction
❏ pacemaker
❏ seizures

Tell your doctor about any other drugs you take, including aspirin, herbs, vitamins, and other non-prescription products.

When You Use This Drug
◆ Until you know how you react to this drug, do not drive or perform other activities requiring alertness. This drug may cause blurred vision and drowsiness.
◆ You may feel dizzy when rising from a lying or sitting position. If you are lying down, hang your legs over the side of the bed for a few minutes, then get up slowly. When getting up from a chair, stay by the chair until you are sure that you are not dizzy. (See p. 14.)
◆ Ask your doctor to recommend exercises suitable to your condition.
◆ Quit smoking, or at least try to cut down on smoking.
◆ Carry identification stating that you take mexiletine
◆ If you plan to have any surgery, including dental, tell your doctor that you take this drug.

How To Use This Drug
◆ Swallow capsule whole. Take with food, milk, or antacids to lessen stomach upset. Space doses evenly apart. Antacids with calcium or magnesium may slow absorption of mexiletine. If you use these antacids, be consistent in usage, and avoid large doses.
◆ If you miss a dose, take it as soon as you remember but skip it if it is less than 4 hours until your next scheduled dose. **Do not take double doses.**
◆ Store at room temperature with lid on firmly. Do not expose to heat.

Interactions With Other Drugs

The following drugs are listed in *Evaluations of Drug Interactions*, 1991 as causing "highly clinically significant" or "clinically significant" interactions when used together with this drug. There may be other drugs, especially those in the families of drugs listed below, that also will react with this drug to cause severe adverse effects. Make sure to ask your doctor for a complete listing of them and let her or him know if you are taking any of these interacting drugs:

amiodarone; CORDARONE; cimetidine;[249] cyclosporine; SANDIMMUNE; SLOPHYLLIN; TAGAMET; THEO-DUR; theophyllines (all brands)[250,251,252]; UNIPHYL.

Mexiletine intensifies the effect of caffeine. Eliminate or reduce your intake of beverages containing caffeine.

Adverse Effects

Call your doctor immediately:
- unusual bleeding or bruising
- difficulty breathing
- chest pains
- fainting
- fever, chills
- unusually fast or slow heartbeat
- seizures
- sore throat

Call your doctor if these symptoms continue:
- abdominal pain
- confusion
- constipation, diarrhea
- depression
- dizziness, lightheadedness
- dry mouth
- headache
- heartburn
- impotence
- nausea, vomiting, loss of appetite
- nervousness
- numbness or tingling of fingers, toes
- pain in joints
- ringing in ears
- skin rash, yellowing of skin
- sleeping problems
- slurred speech
- swelling of hands or feet
- trembling of hands
- unsteadiness, trouble walking
- unusual tiredness or weakness
- urination decreases
- blurred vision

Periodic Tests

Ask your doctor which of these tests should be done periodically while you are taking this drug:
- blood aspartate aminotranferase (AST {SGOT}) tests
- blood mexiletine levels
- electrocardiogram (EKG)

LIMITED USE

Prazosin
MINIPRESS (Pfizer)

Generic: available

Family: Antihypertensives
(See High Blood Pressure, p. 62)

Prazosin (*pra* zoe sin) is used to treat sudden congestive heart failure and to reduce high blood pressure (hypertension). It is effective for sudden congestive heart failure but is not the best drug for high blood pressure.[253] After a few days of taking prazosin, you are likely to develop a "tolerance" for it, which means that the same dose has less and less effect.[254] This problem limits prazosin's usefulness for long-term therapy. Some long-term studies have found that prazosin is no more effective than a sugar pill (placebo).[255]

When taken for high blood pressure, prazosin is most effective when combined with a water pill (thiazide diuretic, see p. 117) or a drug called a beta-blocker (see p. 68). The water pill or beta-blocker works with the prazosin to lower your blood pressure and helps to decrease your body's retention of salt and water, but it also increases your risk of becoming dizzy or lightheaded.[256]

Occasionally, a person will collapse and lose consciousness for a few minutes to an hour after taking his or her first dose of prazosin.[257] This is more likely to happen to older adults, people on a low-salt diet, and people who are taking other high blood pressure drugs.[258] To decrease your risk of fainting, your doctor should prescribe a first dose of no more than one milligram, and you should take that dose at bedtime.[259,260] After taking the first dose, wait at least 4 hours before driving or doing anything else that requires alertness.

In general, your daily dose of prazosin should be no more than 6 to 10 milligrams.

Some doctors prescribe daily doses as high as 20 to 40 milligrams, but doses higher than 6 to 10 milligrams increase the risk of harmful side effects without increasing the drug's benefit.[261]

If you have high blood pressure, the best way to reduce or eliminate your need for medication is through diet, weight loss, exercise, and less salt and alcohol. In mild hypertension nutrition and hygenic measures can control high blood pressure. If these measures do not lower your blood pressure enough and you need medication, **hydrochlorothiazide, a water pill (see thiazide diuretics, p. 117), is the drug of choice for mild hypertension in people over 60 years old, starting with a low dose of 12.5 milligrams.** It also costs less.

There is now good evidence that another benefit of thiazide diuretics such as hydrochlorothiazide is that they significantly decrease the rate of bone mineral loss in both men and women because they reduce the amount of calcium lost in the urine. An increasing number of researchers think that this will also decrease the number of fractures. [262]

Whatever drugs you take for high blood pressure, once your blood pressure has been normal for a year or more, a cautious decrease in dose and renewed attention to non-drug treatment may be worth trying, according to *The Medical Letter*.[263]

"Treatment of hypertension is part of preventive medicine and like all preventive strategies, its progress should be regularly reviewed by whoever initiates it. Many problems could be avoided by not starting antihypertensive treatment until after prolonged observation. . . . Patients should no longer be told that treatment is necessarily for life: the possibility of reducing or stopping treatment should be mentioned at the outset."[264]

Before You Use This Drug
Tell your doctor if you have or have had
- allergies to drugs
- angina (chest pain)
- heart disease
- kidney function impairment
- liver function impairment (dose should be decreased)
- a low-salt diet

Tell your doctor about any other drugs you take, including aspirin, herbs, vitamins, and other non-prescription products.

When You Use This Drug
- You may feel dizzy when rising from a lying or sitting position. When getting out of bed, hang your legs over the side of the bed for a few minutes, then get up slowly. When getting up from a chair, get up slowly and stay beside the chair until you are sure that you are not dizzy. (See p. 14.)
- If you plan to have any surgery, including dental, tell your doctor that you take this drug.
- **Do not take other drugs without talking to your doctor first — especially non-prescription drugs for appetite control, asthma, colds, coughs, hay fever, or sinus problems.**

Heat Stress Alert
This drug can affect your body's ability to adjust to heat, putting you at risk of "heat stress." If you live alone, ask a friend to check on you several times during the day. Early signs of heat stress are dizziness, lightheadedness, faintness, and slightly high temperature. Call your doctor if you have any of these signs.

Drink more fluids (water, fruit and vegetable juices) than usual, even if you're not thirsty, unless your doctor has told you otherwise. Do not drink alcohol.

How To Use This Drug
- Crush tablet and mix with water, or swallow whole with water.
- If you miss a dose, take it as soon as you remember, but skip it if it is almost time for the next dose. **Do not take double doses.**

Interactions With Other Drugs
The following drugs are listed in *Evaluations of Drug Interactions*, 1991 as causing "highly clinically significant" or "clinically significant" interactions when used together with this drug. There may be other drugs, especially those in the families of drugs listed below, that also will react with this drug to cause severe adverse effects. Make sure to ask your doctor for a complete listing of them and let her or him know if you are taking any of these interacting drugs:

digoxin; INDERAL; INDOCIN; indomethacin; LANOXIN; propranolol.

Adverse Effects
Call your doctor immediately:
- dizziness, lightheadedness
- fainting
- chest pain (angina)
- irregular heartbeat
- shortness of breath
- swelling of feet and lower legs
- weight gain from salt and water retention
- inability to control urination
- numbness and tingling of hands and feet
- skin rash

Call your doctor if these symptoms continue:
- drowsiness
- headache
- lack of energy
- nausea, vomiting
- decreased sexual ability
- diarrhea or constipation

Periodic Tests
Ask your doctor which of these tests should be done periodically while you are taking this drug:
- blood pressure

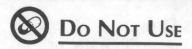 **DO NOT USE**

Alternative treatment: See Hydrochlorothiazide, p. 117.

Amiloride and Hydrochlorothiazide (combined)
MODURETIC (Merck)

Family: Diuretics
Antihypertensives
(See High Blood Pressure, p. 62)

This product, a combination of amiloride (a *mill* oh ride) and hydrochlorothiazide (see p. 117), is used to treat high blood pressure (hypertension). **Older adults should not use drugs that contain a fixed combination of amiloride and hydrochlorothiazide.**

Thiazides with amiloride may produce high potassium in the blood and substantial sodium depletion.[265]

There are good reasons not to use any fixed-combination drug for high blood pressure. First, a single drug is often enough to control high blood pressure. If a combination drug like this one is controlling your high blood pressure, it is quite possible that one drug alone would do the same job. There is no reason to put yourself at extra risk by taking extra drugs you do not need.

If you have high blood pressure, the best way to reduce or eliminate your need for medication is through diet, weight loss, exercise, and less salt and alcohol. In mild hypertension nutrition and hygenic measures can control high blood pressure. If these measures do not lower your blood pressure enough and you need medication, **hydrochlorothiazide, a water pill (see thiazide diuretics, p. 117), is the drug of choice for mild hypertension in people over 60 years old, starting with a low dose of 12.5 milligrams.** It also costs less.

There is now good evidence that another benefit of thiazide diuretics such as hydrochlorothiazide is that they significantly decrease the rate of bone mineral loss in both men and women because they reduce the amount of calcium lost in the urine. An increasing number of researchers think that this will also decrease the number of fractures. [266]

Hydrochlorothiazide, a water pill, is one of the ingredients in this combination (see thiazide diuretics, p. 117). If your high blood pressure is more severe and hydrochlorothiazide alone does not control it, there are still better drug treatments than this combination product. The best treatment in this case is a combination of hydrochlorothiazide and a second type of drug called a beta-blocker like propranolol (see p. 124). If you can't take a drug in the beta-blocker family, another drug called a calcium channel blocker may be used instead. In either case, your doctor would prescribe the hydrochlorothiazide and the second drug separately, with the dose of each drug adjusted to meet your needs, rather than using a product that combines the drugs in advance in a fixed combination.

If you are taking this fixed-combination drug, ask your doctor about changing your prescription.

Whatever drugs you take for high blood pressure, once your blood pressure has been normal for a year or more, a cautious decrease in dose and renewed attention to non-drug treatment may be worth trying, according to *The Medical Letter*.[267]

"Treatment of hypertension is part of preventive medicine and like all preventive strategies, its progress should be regularly reviewed by whoever initiates it. Many problems could be avoided by not starting antihypertensive treatment until after

prolonged observation. . . . Patients should no longer be told that treatment is necessarily for life: the possibility of reducing or stopping treatment should be mentioned at the outset."[268]

Disopyramide
NORPACE (Searle)

Generic: available

Family: Antiarrhythmics

Disopyramide (dye soe *peer* a mide) slows the heart rate and stabilizes irregular heartbeats (arrhythmias). Because it has serious side effects, your doctor should not prescribe disopyramide unless you have already tried safer antiarrhythmic drugs such as quinidine (see p. 108) without success.

Disopyramide is linked to a high incidence of congestive heart failure and problems with urination, so people with these medical problems should not use the drug.[269] Since there is a narrow range between a helpful and a harmful amount of this drug in your body, call your doctor immediately if you experience these side effects or any of those listed under Adverse Effects. **If you have decreased kidney function, you should be taking less than the usual dose of disopyramide.**[270]

Many people who are taking disopyramide or another drug in its family have relatively mild disturbances in their heart rhythm and no symptoms of underlying heart disease. The vast majority of these people do not need these drugs, and there is no evidence that using them improves health. In fact, most of the drugs in this family have severe side effects that are sometimes worse and even more life-threatening than the irregular heartbeats they treat. All of these drugs can also cause new irregularities in your heartbeat.

If you have an irregular heartbeat without any symptoms of underlying heart disease, you should not be exposed to the dangers of a drug that has no health benefit for your condition.[271] If you are taking disopyramide or another drug in its family for an irregular heartbeat (arrhythmia), talk to your doctor and find out whether you also have symptoms of underlying heart disease. If not, discuss the possibility of stopping the drug.

Warning: Special Mental and Physical Adverse Effects

Older adults are especially sensitive to the harmful anticholinergic effects of disopyramide. Drugs in this family should not be used unless absolutely necessary.

Mental Effects: confusion, delirium, short-term memory problems, disorientation, and impaired attention.

Physical Effects: dry mouth, constipation, difficulty urinating (especially for a man with an enlarged prostate), blurred vision, decreased sweating with increased body temperature, sexual dysfunction, and worsening of glaucoma.

Before You Use This Drug
Do not use if you have or have had
❑ complete heart block
❑ shock due to heart failure
Tell your doctor if you have or have had
❑ allergies to drugs

❑ diabetes
❑ any heart problems
❑ enlarged prostate gland
❑ glaucoma
❑ kidney function impairment
❑ liver function impairment
❑ too much or too little blood potassium
❑ myasthenia gravis
❑ urinary obstruction

Tell your doctor about any other drugs you take, including aspirin, herbs, vitamins, and other non-prescription products.

When You Use This Drug

Until you know how you react to this drug, do not drive or perform other activities requiring alertness. Disopyramide may cause dizziness.

◆ You may feel dizzy when rising from a lying or sitting position. When getting out of bed, hang your legs over the side of the bed for a few minutes, then get up slowly. When getting up from a chair, get up slowly and stay beside the chair until you are sure that you are not dizzy. (See p. 14.)

Do not stop taking this drug suddenly. Your doctor must give you a schedule to lower your dose gradually, to prevent serious changes in heart function.

Wear a medical identification bracelet or carry a card stating that you take disopyramide.

If you plan to have any surgery, including dental, tell your doctor that you take this drug.

How To Use This Drug

Swallow extended-release tablets whole. Do not crush or break.

Take with food or milk to decrease stomach upset.

If you miss a dose, take it as soon as you remember, but skip it if it is less than 4 hours (8 hours if you are taking extended-release capsules) until your next scheduled dose. **Do not take double doses.**

Interactions With Other Drugs

The following drugs are listed in *Evaluations of Drug Interactions*, 1991 as causing "highly clinically significant" or "clinically significant" interactions when used together with this drug. There may be other drugs, especially those in the families of drugs listed below, that also will react with this drug to cause severe adverse effects. Make sure to ask your doctor for a complete listing of them and let her or him know if you are taking any of these interacting drugs:

charcoal; DILANTIN; E-MYCIN; erythromycin; ISORDIL; isosorbide (sublingual); phenytoin; SORBITRATE.

Adverse Effects

Call your doctor immediately:
❑ difficulty urinating
❑ chest pains
❑ confusion
❑ dizziness or fainting
❑ muscle weakness
❑ shortness of breath
❑ swelling of feet or lower legs
❑ unusually fast or slow heartbeat
❑ rapid weight gain
❑ eye pain
❑ mental depression
❑ sore throat and fever
❑ yellow eyes and skin
❑ **signs of low blood sugar:** anxious feeling; chills; cold sweats; confusion; cool pale skin; drowsiness; headache; hunger; nausea; nervousness; rapid heartbeat; shakiness; unsteady walk; unusual tiredness or weakness

Call your doctor if these symptoms continue:
❑ dry mouth, throat, eyes, or nose (relieve by sucking ice or chewing sugarless gum)
❑ bloating or stomach pain
❑ blurred vision
❑ decreased sexual ability
❑ loss of appetite
❑ frequent urge to urinate
❑ constipation

Periodic Tests
Ask your doctor which of these tests should be done periodically while you are taking this drug:
- ❏ heart function tests, such as electrocardiogram (EKG)
- ❏ kidney function tests
- ❏ liver function tests
- ❏ blood levels of glucose and potassium
- ❏ eye pressure exams

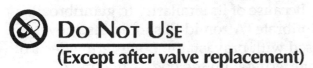 **DO NOT USE**
(Except after valve replacement)

Alternative treatment for angina: See Propranolol, p. 124.

Dipyridamole
PERSANTINE (Boehringer Ingelheim)

Family: Blood-clotting Inhibitor

Dipyridamole (dye peer *id* a mole) is used to reduce blood-clot formation and for other heart and blood conditions. **This drug has not been proven to have any health benefit** except in one study involving a certain type of heart surgery, heart valve replacement. It is also sometimes given in combination with aspirin to prevent a stroke, but there is no proof that this combination works any better than aspirin alone.

There is no convincing evidence that dipyridamole will prevent or relieve any disease of the blood vessels supplying the brain, decrease the severity or frequency of chest pain (angina), or improve the mental or physical state of older or senile people.

> The National Academy of Sciences has determined that this drug lacks evidence of effectiveness.

LIMITED USE

Pravastatin
PRAVACHOL (Bristol-Myers)

Generic: not available

Family: Cholesterol-lowering Drugs
(See p. 70)

Pravastatin (prav ah *stat* in) lowers cholesterol by preventing the body from making as much cholesterol, specifically low-density lipoprotein (LDL) cholesterol. In middle-aged people it is clear that lowering cholesterol lessens the risk of coronary artery disease, but no cholesterol-lowering drug has been shown to lower overall death rates in this age group. In older adults, the extent to which higher cholesterol levels contribute to heart disease and should be treated with drugs is much less clear. Pravastatin controls high cholesterol, but does not cure any condition. It may prevent atherosclerosis.[272]

Pravastatin belongs to the same family of drugs as lovastatin. although unlike lovastatin, pravastatin does not cross into your brain. This family of drugs is generally better tolerated than other cholesterol-lowering drugs, according to *The Medical Letter*.[273] Still, these drugs commonly cause gastrointestinal problems. Of particular concern is the possibility of liver toxicity, including hepatitis. Therefore, liver function tests should be done every 6 weeks in patients on therapy. In animals these drugs have produced cancers. Severe inflammation and pain in the muscles can occur, especially when combined with gemfibrozil. In people simultaneously using gemfibrozil and lovastatin, there are numerous reports of severe muscle damage sometimes accompanied by life-threatening destruction of muscle and subsequent kidney damage.[274] Similar problems have occurred with the combination of pravastatin and gemfibrozil. Therefore, gemfibrozil and pravastatin should never be used together.

Because of its similarity to gemfibrozil, clofibrate (Atromid-S) should also never be used with pravastatin. Long-term effects of interfering with the body's making of cholesterol are not known.[275,276,277] This family of drugs is not effective for the homozygous familial type of high blood cholesterol.[278]

The use of cholesterol-lowering drugs in people 70 or older should be limited to patients with very high cholesterol levels (greater than 300 milligrams) and those who manifest cardiovascular disease (previous history of heart attack or angina).[279]

For people under 70, to lower cholesterol the first, safer, and less costly measure is to eat a low-fat diet, using mostly polyunsaturated fats (such as canola, corn, safflower, and sunflower oils) or monounsaturated fats (such as olive oil). A change from animal to vegetable proteins often corrects high cholesterol. However, it is inadvisable to go on a very low-fat diet. The main focus on cholesterol-lowering diets has been on saturated fat and cholesterol content, not soluble fiber. (When added to the diet, psyllium or oat bran is a safe, effective way of lowering cholesterol.) Exercise is also recommended. Conditions that aggravate high cholesterol, such as dependence on alcohol or tobacco, diabetes, high blood pressure, low magnesium or potassium, and thyroid disease, should be corrected before adding a cholesterol-reducing drug. If cholesterol remains high despite diet, add 10 grams of psyllium a day (see p. 356). Pravastatin is usually reserved for people who do not respond to other drugs. However, choice of a drug in the elderly must be individualized.

Before You Use This Drug

Do not use if you have
❑ liver disease, active
Tell your doctor if you have or have had
❑ allergies to drugs
❑ alcohol dependence
❑ cataracts
❑ low blood pressure
❑ metabolic, hormone or mineral imbalance
❑ severe infections
❑ serious injuries
❑ kidney problems
❑ liver problems such as hepatitis or jaundice
❑ organ transplant or other major surgery
❑ seizures
Tell your doctor about any other drugs you take, including aspirin, herbs, vitamins, and other non-prescription products.

When You Use This Drug

◆ Continue to eat a low-fat diet.
◆ If you plan to have any surgery, including dental, tell your doctor that you take this drug.

How To Use This Drug

◆ Swallow tablet whole.
◆ If you take pravastatin once daily, take it with the evening meal. If you are taking more than one dose a day take it with meals or snacks.
◆ If you miss a dose, take it as soon as you remember but skip it if it is almost time for the next dose. **Do not take double doses.**
◆ Do not store in the bathroom. Do not expose to heat, moisture or strong light. Store tablets at room temperature.
◆ If you also take cholestyramine (Questran, Cholybar) or colestipol (Colestid), take the pravastatin at least 1 hour before, or 4 hours after taking the other drugs.[280]

Interactions With Other Drugs

The following drugs are listed in *Evaluations of Drug Interactions*, 1991 as causing "highly clinically significant" or "clinically significant" interactions when used together with this drug. There may be other drugs, especially those in the families of drugs listed below, that also will react with this drug to cause severe adverse effects. Make sure to ask your doctor for a complete listing of them and let her or him know if you are taking any of these interacting drugs:

gemfibrozil; LOPID; niacin (vitamin B$_3$) (this only refers to very large doses of niacin used to lower cholesterol, not usual dietary amounts of niacin).

Additionally, the *United States Pharmacopeia Drug Information*, 1992 lists this drug as having interactions of major significance:

cyclosporine; SANDIMMUNE.

Adverse Effects

Call your doctor immediately:
❑ fever
❑ muscle aches, cramps
❑ unusual tiredness or weakness
❑ blurred vision
Call your doctor if these symptoms continue:
❑ constipation or diarrhea
❑ dizziness
❑ gas, heartburn
❑ headache
❑ nausea
❑ skin rash

Periodic Tests

Ask your doctor which of these tests should be done periodically while you are taking this drug:
❑ blood cholesterol and creatine kinase tests
❑ eye exam
❑ liver function tests

Procainamide
PRONESTYL (Squibb)
PROCAN SR (Parke-Davis)

Generic: available

Family: Antiarrhythmics

Procainamide (proe *kane* a mide) slows the heart rate and stabilizes irregular heartbeats (arrhythmias). Since this drug frequently causes a disease called lupus erythematosus, as well as other side effects, it is not the best choice for long-term treatment of irregular heartbeats.[281] For long-term use, your doctor should first try quinidine, a safer drug in this family (see p. 108). **If your kidney or liver function is impaired, you should be taking less than the usual dose.**[282]

Many people who are taking procainamide or another drug in its family have relatively mild disturbances in their heart rhythm and no symptoms of underlying heart disease. The vast majority of these people do not need these drugs, and there is no evidence that using them improves health. In fact, most of the drugs in this family have severe side effects that are sometimes worse and even more life-threatening than the irregular heartbeats they treat. All of these drugs can also cause new irregularities in your heartbeat.

If you have an irregular heartbeat without any symptoms of underlying heart disease, you should not be exposed to the dangers of a drug that has no health benefit for your condition.[283] If you are taking procainamide or another drug in its family for an irregular heartbeat (arrhythmia), talk to your doctor and find out whether you also have symptoms of underlying heart disease. If not, discuss the possibility of stopping the drug.

Since there is a narrow range between a helpful and a harmful amount of this drug in your body, call your doctor immediately if you experience side effects (see Adverse Effects).

Before You Use This Drug
Do not use if you have or have had
❑ complete heart block
❑ digitalis toxicity with heart block
Tell your doctor if you have or have had
❑ allergies to drugs
❑ asthma or emphysema
❑ digitalis toxicity
❑ incomplete heart block
❑ kidney disease
❑ liver function impairment
❑ lupus erythematosus
❑ myasthenia gravis
Tell your doctor about any other drugs you take, including aspirin, herbs, vitamins, and other non-prescription products.

When You Use This Drug
◆ Until you know how you react to this drug, do not drive or perform other activities requiring alertness. Procainamide may cause dizziness.
◆ **Do not stop taking this drug suddenly. Your doctor must give you a schedule to lower your dose gradually, to prevent serious changes in heart function.**
◆ Wear a medical identification bracelet or carry a card stating that you take procainamide.
◆ If you plan to have any surgery, including dental, tell your doctor that you take this drug.

How To Use This Drug
◆ Swallow extended-release tablets whole. Do not crush or break them.
◆ Take with food or milk to decrease stomach upset.

◆ Store procainamide in a dry place. Do not store in the bathroom or refrigerator.

◆ If you miss a dose, take it as soon as you remember, but skip it if it is less than 2 hours until your next scheduled dose. **Do not take double doses.**

Interactions With Other Drugs

The following drugs are listed in *Evaluations of Drug Interactions*, 1991 as causing "highly clinically significant" or "clinically significant" interactions when used together with this drug. There may be other drugs, especially those in the families of drugs listed below, that also will react with this drug to cause severe adverse effects. Make sure to ask your doctor for a complete listing of them and let her or him know if you are taking any of these interacting drugs:

amiodarone; cimetidine; CORDARONE; cyclosporine; SANDIMMUNE; TAGAMET.

Adverse Effects

Call your doctor immediately:

❑ **if you experience signs of overdose:** confusion; dizziness; fainting; drowsiness; nausea and vomiting; unusual

decrease in urination; unusually fast or irregular heartbeat

❑ **signs of lupus-like syndrome:** fever; chills; joint pain or swelling; pain with breathing; skin rash or itching

❑ confusion, hallucinations, or mental depression

❑ sore mouth, gums, or throat

❑ unusual bleeding or bruising

❑ unusual tiredness or weakness

Call your doctor if these symptoms continue:

❑ diarrhea

❑ loss of appetite

Periodic Tests

Ask your doctor which of these tests should be done periodically while you are taking this drug:

❑ complete blood counts

❑ heart function tests, such as electrocardiogram (EKG)

❑ blood pressure

❑ liver function tests

❑ blood levels of procainamide and NAPA (a metabolite of procainamide)

❑ antinuclear antibody test (if this is positive ask your doctor about changing your drug, since a positive value is often linked with a lupus-like syndrome)

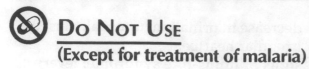

Do Not Use
(Except for treatment of malaria)

Alternative treatment: Exercise and painkillers.

Quinine
QUINAMM (Merrell Dow)
QUINITE (Reid Rowell)
STREMA (Foy)

Family: Leg Cramp Treatment

Quinine (*kwye* nine) **is used to treat night-time leg cramps, but there is no convincing evidence that it is safe and effective for this purpose.**[284] Repeated use of quinine can cause a group of side effects (cinchonism) including ringing in the ears, headache, nausea, and abnormal vision. It can also affect the gastrointestinal tract, the nervous system, the cardiovascular system, and the skin. It can cause fatal bleeding disorders due to low levels of blood platelets. Because of its risks and its lack of proven effectiveness, quinine should not be used to treat leg cramps.

Quinine is useful for malaria, but it is not often prescribed in the United States for this purpose.

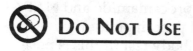

Do Not Use

Alternative treatment: See Hydrochlorothiazide, p. 117.

Reserpine and Chlorthalidone (combined)
REGROTON (USV)
DEMI-REGROTON (USV)

Family: Diuretics
Antihypertensives
(See High Blood Pressure, p. 62)

This product, a combination of reserpine (see p. 165) and chlorthalidone (see p. 121), is used to treat high blood pressure (hypertension). **Older adults should not use drugs that contain a fixed combination of reserpine and chlorthalidone.**

Reserpine causes severe side effects that may occur during treatment and even months after you stop taking it. It has caused severe depression, in some cases leading to suicide. We do not recommend that any older adult use reserpine, and it is particularly dangerous for anyone who has had a depressive illness.[285] It also decreases mental sharpness in older adults.

Chlorthalidone puts the older adult user at such a high risk of side effects that the World Health Organization has said it should not be used by people over 60.[286] We do not recommend that any older adult use chlorthalidone.

In addition to the risks of reserpine and chlorthalidone, there are good reasons not to use any fixed-combination drug for high blood pressure. First, a single drug is often enough to control high blood pressure. If a combination drug like this one is controlling your high blood pressure, it is quite possible that one drug alone would do the same job. There is no reason to put yourself at extra risk by taking extra drugs you do not need.

If you have high blood pressure, the best way to reduce or eliminate your need for medication is through diet, weight loss, exercise, and less salt and alcohol. In mild hypertension nutrition and hygenic measures can control high blood pressure. If these measures do not lower your blood pressure enough and you need medication, **hydrochlorothiazide, a water pill (see thiazide diuretics, p. 117), is the drug of choice for mild hypertension in people over 60 years old, starting with a low dose of 12.5 milligrams.** It also costs less.

There is now good evidence that another benefit of thiazide diuretics such as hydrochlorothiazide is that they significantly decrease the rate of bone mineral loss in both men and women because they reduce the amount of calcium lost in the urine. An increasing number of researchers think that this will also decrease the number of fractures. [287]

If your high blood pressure is more severe and hydrochlorothiazide alone does not control it, there are still safer drug treatments than this combination product. The best treatment in this case is a combination of hydrochlorothiazide and a second type of drug called a beta-blocker, such as propranolol (see p. 124). If you can't take a drug in the beta-blocker family, another drug called a calcium channel blocker may be used instead. In either case, your doctor would prescribe the hydrochlorothiazide and the second drug separately, with the dose of each drug adjusted to meet your needs, rather than using a product that combines the drugs in advance in a fixed combination.

If you are taking this fixed-combination drug, ask your doctor about changing your prescription.

Whatever drugs you take for high blood pressure, once your blood pressure has been normal for a year or more, a cautious decrease in dose and renewed attention to non-drug treatment may be worth trying, according to *The Medical Letter*.[288]

"Treatment of hypertension is part of preventive medicine and like all preventive strategies, its progress should be regularly reviewed by whoever initiates it. Many problems could be avoided by not starting antihypertensive treatment until after prolonged observation. . . . Patients should no longer be told that treatment is necessarily for life: the possibility of reducing or stopping treatment should be mentioned at the outset."[289]

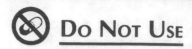 **Do Not Use**

Alternative treatment: See Hydrochlorothiazide, p. 117.

Reserpine and Hydroflumethiazide (combined)
SALUTENSIN (Bristol)

Family: Diuretics
Antihypertensives
(See High Blood Pressure, p. 62)

This product, a combination of reserpine (see p. 165) and hydroflumethiazide (hye droe floo meth *eye* a zide), is used to treat high blood pressure. **Older adults should not use drugs containing a fixed combination of reserpine and hydroflumethiazide.**

Reserpine causes severe side effects that may occur during treatment and even months after you stop taking it. It has caused severe depression, in some cases leading to suicide. We do not recommend that any older adult use reserpine, and it is particularly dangerous for anyone who has had a depressive illness.[290] It also decreases mental sharpness in older adults.

In addition to the risks of reserpine, there are good reasons not to use any fixed-combination drug for high blood pressure. First, a single drug is often enough to control high blood pressure. If a combination drug like this one is controlling your high blood pressure, it is quite possible that one drug alone would do the same job. There is no reason to put yourself at extra risk by taking extra drugs you do not need.

If you have high blood pressure, the best way to reduce or eliminate your need for medication is through diet, weight loss, exercise, and less salt and alcohol. In mild hypertension nutrition and hygenic measures can control high blood pressure. If these measures do not lower your blood pressure enough and you need medication, **hydrochlorothiazide, a water pill (see thiazide diuretics, p. 117), is the drug of choice for mild hypertension in people over 60 years old, starting with a low dose**

of 12.5 milligrams. It also costs less.

There is now good evidence that another benefit of thiazide diuretics such as hydrochlorothiazide is that they significantly decrease the rate of bone mineral loss in both men and women because they reduce the amount of calcium lost in the urine. An increasing number of researchers think that this will also decrease the number of fractures. [291]

Hydrochlorothiazide is a better choice than hydroflumethiazide because it is equally effective, less expensive, and milder. If your high blood pressure is more severe and hydrochlorothiazide alone does not control it, there are still better drug treatments than this combination product. The best treatment in this case is a combination of hydrochlorothiazide and a second type of drug called a beta-blocker, such as propranolol (see p. 124). If you can't take a drug in the beta-blocker family, another drug called a calcium channel blocker may be used instead. In either case, your doctor would prescribe the hydrochlorothiazide and the second drug separately, with the dose of each drug adjusted to meet your needs, rather than using a product that combines the drugs in advance in a fixed combination.

If you are taking this fixed-combination drug, ask your doctor about changing your prescription.

Whatever drugs you take for high blood pressure, once your blood pressure has been normal for a year or more, a cautious decrease in dose and renewed attention to non-drug treatment may be worth trying, according to *The Medical Letter*.[292]

"Treatment of hypertension is part of preventive medicine and like all preventive strategies, its progress should be regularly reviewed by whoever initiates it. Many problems could be avoided by not starting antihypertensive treatment until after prolonged observation. . . . Patients should

no longer be told that treatment is necessarily for life: the possibility of reducing or stopping treatment should be mentioned at the outset."[293]

Acebutolol
SECTRAL (Wyeth-Ayerst)

Generic: not available

Family: Beta-blockers (see p. 68)
Antihypertensives (See High Blood Pressure, p. 62)

Acebutolol (ace ah *butte* o lall) is used to treat high blood pressure and heart arrhythmias. It lowers blood pressure, reduces the number of premature ventricular heartbeats, and decreases the frequency of angina attacks. Acebutolol controls, but does not cure, these conditions. **If you are over age 60, you will generally need less than the usual adult dose, especially if your kidney or liver function is impaired.**

For young adults with high blood pressure, doctors usually prescribe a drug in this family (a beta-blocker) before any other drug. But for blacks and older adults, these drugs are less effective as the sole treatment. For these groups of people, doctors usually prescribe another type of drug called a diuretic (water pill) to lower blood pressure, and add a beta-blocker as a second drug if the diuretic alone is not enough. Increased sensitivity to cold is one side effect. (See glossary p. 689 for signs of hypothermia.)

If you have high blood pressure, the best way to reduce or eliminate your need for medication is through diet, weight loss, exercise, and less salt and alcohol. In mild hypertension nutrition and hygenic measures can control high blood pressure. If these measures do not lower your blood pressure enough and you need medication,

hydrochlorothiazide, a water pill (see thiazide diuretics, p. 117), is the drug of choice for mild hypertension in people over 60 years old, starting with a low dose of 12.5 milligrams. It also costs less.

There is now good evidence that another benefit of thiazide diuretics such as hydrochlorothiazide is that they significantly decrease the rate of bone mineral loss in both men and women because they reduce the amount of calcium lost in the urine. An increasing number of researchers think that this will also decrease the number of fractures.[294]

Whatever drugs you take for high blood pressure, once your blood pressure has been normal for a year or more, a cautious decrease in dose and renewed attention to non-drug treatment may be worth trying, according to *The Medical Letter*.[295]

"Treatment of hypertension is part of preventive medicine and like all preventive strategies, its progress should be regularly reviewed by whoever initiates it. Many problems could be avoided by not starting antihypertensive treatment until after prolonged observation. . . . Patients should no longer be told that treatment is necessarily for life: the possibility of reducing or stopping treatment should be mentioned at the outset."[296]

Before You Use This Drug
Do not take if you have or have had
❏ allergies to beta-blockers or dyes
❏ cardiogenic shock
❏ congestive heart failure, uncontrolled
❏ heart block

If other treatments have not worked, and you have the following conditions, acebutolol may be tried with great caution in low doses.

❑ allergies to drugs or a history of allergies
❑ asthma
❑ autoimmune disease[297]
❑ bronchitis, chronic
❑ congestive heart failure controlled by digitalis and a diuretic
❑ coronary heart disease
❑ diabetes prone to low blood sugar
❑ emphysema
❑ liver problems
❑ myasthenia gravis[298]
❑ peripheral vascular disease

Tell your doctor if you have or have had
❑ angina
❑ bronchitis
❑ depression
❑ diabetes
❑ kidney problems
❑ low blood pressure
❑ lupus
❑ adrenal gland tumor
❑ psoriasis
❑ smoked
❑ thyroid problems

Tell your doctor about any other drugs you take, including aspirin, herbs, vitamins, and other non-prescription products.

When You Use This Drug

◆ **Learn to take your pulse, and get immediate medical help if your pulse slows to 50 beats per minute or slower, even if you are feeling well. Some people have suffered from slowed heart rate and heart failure while taking acebutolol.**

◆ Until you know how you react to this drug, do not drive or perform other activities requiring mental alertness.

◆ You may feel dizzy when rising from a lying or sitting position. If you are lying down, hang your legs over the side of the bed for a few minutes, then get up slowly. When getting up from a chair, stay by the chair until you are sure that you are not dizzy. (See p. 14.)

◆ Be careful not to overexert yourself, even though your chest pain may feel better.

◆ **Do not suddenly stop taking acebutolol. Abruptly stopping could be fatal. Check with your doctor for a schedule to taper you off the acebutolol. This is especially important if you have angina or coronary artery disease, or also take clonidine or guanabenz. Limit physical activity during the tapering period.**

◆ If you have emergency treatment or plan to have any surgery, including dental, tell your doctor that you take this drug. Some surgeons prefer to taper you off beta-blockers, both oral and eye forms, before surgery.

◆ Carry medical identification stating your condition and that you take acebutolol.

Heat Stress Alert
This drug can affect your body's ability to adjust to heat, putting you at risk of "heat stress." If you live alone, ask a friend to check on you several times during the day. Early signs of heat stress are dizziness, lightheadedness, faintness, and slightly high temperature. Call your doctor if you have any of these signs.

Drink more fluids (water, fruit, and vegetable juices) than usual, even if you're not thirsty, unless your doctor has told you otherwise. Do not drink alcohol.

How To Use This Drug

◆ Swallow capsule whole.

◆ Try not to miss doses. Take at the same time each day. Keep enough medication on hand to last through weekends, holidays, vacations, and storms. Carry a supply of acebutolol with you at all times. **Do not take double doses**.

◆ If you do miss a dose take it as soon as you remember unless it is less than 4 hours until your next scheduled dose.

◆ Store at room temperature with lid on firmly. Do not expose to heat.

Interactions With Other Drugs

The following drugs are listed in *Evaluations of Drug Interactions*, 1991 as causing "highly clinically significant" or "clinically significant" interactions when used together with this drug. There may be other drugs, especially those in the families of drugs listed below, that also will react with this drug to cause severe adverse effects. Make sure to ask your doctor for a complete listing of them and let her or him know if you are taking any of these interacting drugs:

ADRENALIN (also in bee sting kits); amiodarone; CALAN; chlorpromazine; cimetidine; cocaine; CORDARONE; COUMADIN; DIABETA; ELIXOPHYLLIN; epinephrine; furosemide; glyburide; ILETIN; INDOCIN; indomethacin; insulin; ISOPTIN; LASIX; lidocaine; MINIPRESS; NICODERM; nicotine; NOVOLIN; prazosin; SLOPHYLLIN; SYNTHROID; TAGAMET; THEO-DUR; theophylline; THORAZINE; thyroid; thyroxine; tobacco; TUBARINE; tubocurarine; verapamil; warfarin; XYLOCAINE.

Additionally, the *United States Pharmacopeia Drug Information*, 1992 lists these drugs as having interactions of major significance:

CATAPRES; clonidine; guanabenz; sympathomimetic drugs (often an ingredient in over-the-counter drugs such as nasal decongestants); WYTENSIN.

Monoamine oxidase (MAO) inhibitors should not be taken at the same time, or for 14 days after you stop taking any beta-blocker. These include:

deprenyl; ELDEPRYL; EUTONYL; furazolidone; FUROXONE; isocarboxazid; MARPLAN; MATULANE; NARDIL; pargyline; PARNATE; phenelzine; procarbazine; selegiline; trancylpromine.

Adverse Effects

Call your doctor immediately:

- ❑ unusual bleeding or bruising
- ❑ difficulty breathing especially on exertion or lying down
- ❑ confusion
- ❑ dizziness, lightheadedness
- ❑ fever
- ❑ hallucinations
- ❑ irregular heartbeat
- ❑ muscle weakness
- ❑ pain in abdomen, back, joints, or feet
- ❑ slow pulse
- ❑ skin rash
- ❑ sore throat
- ❑ swelling of legs, ankles, or feet
- ❑ thoughts of suicide
- ❑ vision change

Call your doctor if these symptoms continue:

- ❑ anxiety
- ❑ cold hands or feet
- ❑ constipation or diarrhea
- ❑ cough at night
- ❑ depression
- ❑ dry or sore eyes
- ❑ forgetfulness
- ❑ gas
- ❑ headache
- ❑ disturbed sleep or nightmares
- ❑ itching
- ❑ nasal congestion
- ❑ nausea or vomiting
- ❑ psoriasis
- ❑ sensitivity to touch increases or decreases
- ❑ decreased sexual ability
- ❑ unusual tiredness
- ❑ painful, dark or frequent urination

Periodic Tests

Ask your doctor which of these tests should be done periodically while you are taking this drug:

- ❑ blood cell counts
- ❑ blood pressure
- ❑ blood glucose
- ❑ heart function monitoring, such as electrocardiogram (EKG)
- ❑ kidney function tests
- ❑ liver function tests
- ❑ pulse

⊘ **DO NOT USE**

Alternative treatment: See Hydrochlorothiazide, p. 117.

Reserpine, Hydralazine, and Hydrochlorothiazide (combined)
SER-AP-ES (CIBA)

Family: Diuretics
Antihypertensives
(See High Blood Pressure, p. 62)

This product, a combination of reserpine (see p. 165), hydralazine (see p. 78), and hydrochlorothiazide (see p. 117), is used to treat high blood pressure (hypertension). **Older adults should not use drugs that contain a fixed combination of reserpine, hydralazine, and hydrochlorothiazide.**

Reserpine causes severe side effects that may occur during treatment and even months after you stop taking it. It has caused severe depression, in some cases leading to suicide. We do not recommend that any older adult use reserpine, and it is particularly dangerous for anyone who has had a depressive illness.[299] It also decreases mental sharpness in older adults.

Hydralazine is not the first-choice drug for treating hypertension because of its side effects. Common ones are rapid heartbeat and below normal blood pressure, which may cause lightheadedness, fainting, and falls. Hydralazine may worsen chest pain (angina).[300]

In addition to the risks of reserpine and hydralazine, there are good reasons not to use any fixed-combination drug for high blood pressure. First, a single drug is often enough to control high blood pressure. If a combination drug like this one is controlling your high blood pressure, it is quite possible that one drug alone would do the same job. There is no reason to put yourself at extra risk by taking extra drugs you do not need.

If you have high blood pressure, the best way to reduce or eliminate your need for medication is through diet, weight loss, exercise, and less salt and alcohol. In mild hypertension nutrition and hygenic measures can control high blood pressure. If these measures do not lower your blood pressure enough and you need medication, **hydrochlorothiazide, a water pill (see thiazide diuretics, p. 117) is the drug of choice for mild hypertension in people over 60 years old, starting with a low dose of 12.5 milligrams.** It also costs less.

There is now good evidence that another benefit of thiazide diuretics such as hydrochlorothiazide is that they significantly decrease the rate of bone mineral loss in both men and women because they reduce the amount of calcium lost in the urine. An increasing number of researchers think that this will also decrease the number of fractures. [301]

Hydrochlorothiazide, a water pill, is one of the ingredients in this combination (see thiazide diuretics, p. 117). Reserpine and hydralazine can cause severe side effects, as described above. If hydrochlorothiazide alone would control your blood pressure, there is no reason to take the extra risk of taking the other two drugs as well.

If your high blood pressure is more severe and hydrochlorothiazide alone does not control it, there are still better drug treatments than this combination product. The best treatment in this case is a combination of hydrochlorothiazide and a second type of drug called a beta-blocker such as propranolol (see p. 124). If you can't take a drug in the beta-blocker family, another drug called a calcium channel blocker may be used instead. In either case, your doctor would prescribe the hydrochlorothiazide and the second drug separately, with the dose of each drug adjusted to meet your needs, rather than using a product that combines the drugs in advance in a fixed combination.

If you are taking this fixed-combination drug, ask your doctor about changing your prescription.

Whatever drugs you take for high blood pressure, once your blood pressure has been normal for a year or more, a cautious decrease in dose and renewed attention to non-drug treatment may be worth trying, according to *The Medical Letter.*[302]

"Treatment of hypertension is part of preventive medicine and like all preventive strategies, its progress should be regularly reviewed by whoever initiates it. Many problems could be avoided by not starting antihypertensive treatment until after prolonged observation. . . . Patients should no longer be told that treatment is necessarily for life: the possibility of reducing or stopping treatment should be mentioned at the outset."[303]

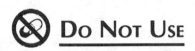 **DO NOT USE**

Alternative treatment: See Hydrochlorothiazide, p. 117.

Reserpine
SERPASIL (CIBA) SANDRIL (Lilly)

Family: Antihypertensives
(See High Blood Pressure, p. 62)

Reserpine (re *ser* peen) is sometimes used to treat severe high blood pressure (hypertension) in older adults. **It should not be used because it has severe side effects, including depression, dizziness, drowsiness, flushed skin, and slow pulse. These may occur while taking reserpine and can last or even begin many months after treatment has ended.** Some people taking reserpine have become so severely depressed that they have committed suicide. People who have suffered from any depressive illness should never take reserpine.[304] The drug can also cause decreased mental sharpness in older adults.

Mental depression caused by reserpine can be difficult to recognize because it occurs very gradually. Symptoms of depression include feelings of hopelessness, helplessness, and rejection; lack of self-worth; inability to sleep in the morning; vivid dreams; nightmares; and loss of appetite.

Stop taking reserpine and contact your doctor immediately if you have any of these symptoms.

If you have high blood pressure, the best way to reduce or eliminate your need for medication is through diet, weight loss, exercise, and less salt and alcohol. In mild hypertension nutrition and hygenic measures can control high blood pressure. If these measures do not lower your blood pressure enough and you need medication, **hydrochlorothiazide, a water pill (see thiazide diuretics, p. 117), is the drug of choice for mild hypertension in people over 60 years old, starting with a low dose of 12.5 milligrams.** It also costs less.

There is now good evidence that another benefit of thiazide diuretics such as hydrochlorothiazide is that they significantly decrease the rate of bone mineral loss in both men and women because they reduce the amount of calcium lost in the urine. An increasing number of researchers think that this will also decrease the number of fractures. [305]

Whatever drugs you take for high blood

pressure, once your blood pressure has been normal for a year or more, a cautious decrease in dose and renewed attention to non-drug treatment may be worth trying, according to *The Medical Letter*.[306]

"Treatment of hypertension is part of preventive medicine and like all preventive strategies, its progress should be regularly reviewed by whoever initiates it. Many problems could be avoided by not starting antihypertensive treatment until after prolonged observation. . . . Patients should no longer be told that treatment is necessarily for life: the possibility of reducing or stopping treatment should be mentioned at the outset."[307]

LIMITED USE

Guanfacine
TENEX (Robins)

Generic: not available

Family: Antihypertensives
(See High Blood Pressure, p. 62.)

Guanfacine (gwawn *fas* seen) helps lower high blood pressure. It is not the first or second choice, but is reserved for use when other high blood pressure drugs do not work. In most studies with guanfacine, it is used along with diuretics (water pills), and no studies have yet established the appropriate dose of guanfacine when used alone.[308] Guanfacine controls, but does not cure high blood pressure. Nor does guanfacine improve your memory.[309,310]

A report in the *The American Journal of Medical Sciences* states that adrenergic blockers, such as guanfacine, should be used sparingly.[311] The same article finds any value of guanfacine over clonidine (a Do Not Use drug, see p. 96) to be marginal, and the cost of guanfacine compared to generic clonidine to be considerably higher. Tolerance to guanfacine can develop within a year, requiring an increased dose (and expense) for the same effect. Tolerance slows somewhat after the second year. Unfortunately, adverse effects increase with an increased dose. Guanfacine is not the drug of choice for people with congestive heart failure.[312]

In older people guanfacine tends to stay in the body longer. Elderly people also may be more sensitive to drowsiness and a low blood pressure when taking guanfacine.

If you have high blood pressure, the best way to reduce or eliminate your need for medication is through diet, weight loss, exercise, and less salt and alcohol. In mild hypertension nutrition and hygenic measures can control high blood pressure. If these measures do not lower your blood pressure enough and you need medication, **hydrochlorothiazide, a water pill (see thiazide diuretics, p. 117), is the drug of choice for mild hypertension in people over 60 years old, starting with a low dose of 12.5 milligrams.** It also costs less.

There is now good evidence that another benefit of thiazide diuretics such as hydrochlorothiazide is that they significantly decrease the rate of bone mineral loss in both men and women because they reduce the amount of calcium lost in the urine. An increasing number of researchers think that this will also decrease the number of fractures.[313]

If a diuretic does not lower your blood pressure enough, your doctor can prescribe a beta-blocker, such as propranolol (see p. 124) to accompany the hydrochlorothiazide. If you cannot take a beta-blocker, a calcium channel blocker or other alternative can be used instead.

Whatever drugs you take for high blood pressure, once your blood pressure has been normal for a year or more, a cautious decrease in dose and renewed attention to non-drug treatment may be worth trying, according to *The Medical Letter*.[314]

"Treatment of hypertension is part of preventive medicine and like all preventive strategies, its progress should be regularly reviewed by whoever initiates it. Many problems could be avoided by not starting antihypertensive treatment until after prolonged observation. . . . Patients should no longer be told that treatment is necessarily for life: the possibility of reducing or stopping treatment should be mentioned at the outset."[315]

Before You Use This Drug
Do not use if you have or have had
❑ sick sinus node syndrome[316]
Tell your doctor if you have or have had
❑ allergies to drugs
❑ cerebrovascular disease
❑ depression
❑ diabetes[317,318]
❑ heart, liver or kidney problems
❑ myocardial infarction
Tell your doctor about any other drugs you take, including aspirin, herbs, vitamins, and other non-prescription products.

When You Use This Drug
◆ You may feel dizzy when rising from a lying or sitting position. If you are lying down, hang your legs over the side of the bed for a few minutes, then get up slowly. When getting up from a chair, stay by the chair until you are sure that you are not dizzy. (See p. 14.)
◆ Until you know how you react to this drug, do not drive or perform other tasks requiring mental alertness. Drowsiness is especially common when first starting guanfacine.
◆ Have your blood pressure taken periodically, including just before your daily dose.

◆ Eat a diet low in salt. Restrict calories if overweight.
◆ Check with your doctor before using non-prescription drugs to assure that the ingredients do not interact with guanfacine.
◆ If you have emergency medical care, or plan to have any surgery, including dental, tell your doctor that you take this drug.

How To Use This Drug
◆ Swallow tablet whole. Take at bedtime since it may cause drowsiness.
◆ Continue to take guanfacine, even if you feel well.
◆ If you miss a dose, take it as soon as you remember, but skip it if it is almost time for the next dose. **Do not take double doses.**
◆ **Do not suddenly stop taking this drug. Ask your doctor for a schedule to lower your dose gradually.**
◆ Store at room temperature with the lid on tightly. Do not expose to heat and light.

Interactions With Other Drugs
Some other drugs that you may be taking (either over-the-counter or prescription drugs) can interact with this one, causing adverse effects. Find out from your doctor what these drugs are and let him or her know if you are taking any of them.

Adverse Effects
Get emergency help if you have signs of overdose:
❑ breathing difficulty
❑ extreme dizziness, faintness
❑ slow heartbeat
❑ unusually severe tiredness, weakness
Call your doctor immediately:
❑ confusion
❑ depression
❑ numbness
❑ skin rash
Call your doctor if these symptoms continue:
❑ constipation, diarrhea

❑ dizziness
❑ drowsiness
❑ dry mouth
❑ burning, dry, or itching eyes
❑ headache
❑ leg cramps
❑ itching
❑ nausea, vomiting
❑ ringing in ears
❑ sexual problems, impotence
❑ insomnia
❑ sweating
❑ swelling of legs or eyes[319]
❑ thirst[320]
❑ unusual tiredness, weakness
❑ urinary incontinence
❑ vision changes
❑ weight change[321,322]

Also call your doctor if signs of withdrawal occur. This usually happens 2 to 7 days after more than one dose is missed, or guanfacine is suddenly stopped. Withdrawal may be aggravated if your dose was large, or you also took a beta-blocker along with guanfacine.[323] Withdrawal symptoms include:

❑ anxiety, nervousness, restlessness, tenseness
❑ blood pressure rises
❑ chest pain
❑ irregular heartbeat
❑ nausea, vomiting
❑ saliva increases
❑ shaking or trembling of fingers and hands
❑ sleep disturbed
❑ stomach cramps
❑ sweating

Periodic Tests

Ask your doctor which tests should be done periodically while you are taking this drug:
❑ blood pressure

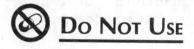 **Do Not Use**

Alternative treatment: See Hydrochlorothiazide, p. 117.

Atenolol and Chlorthalidone (combined)
TENORETIC (Stuart)

Family: Diuretics
Antihypertensives
(See High Blood Pressure, p. 62)

This product, a combination of atenolol (see p. 169) and chlorthalidone (see p. 121), is used to treat high blood pressure. **Older adults should not use drugs containing a fixed combination of atenolol and chlorthalidone.**

Chlorthalidone puts the older adult user at such a high risk of side effects that the World Health Organization has said it should not be used by people over 60.[324]

In addition to the risks of chlorthalidone, there are good reasons not to use a fixed-combination drug for high blood pressure. First, a single drug is often enough to control high blood pressure. If a combination drug like this one is controlling your high blood pressure, it is quite possible that one drug alone would do the same job. There is no reason to put yourself at extra risk by taking extra drugs you do not need.

If you have high blood pressure, the best way to reduce or eliminate your need for medication is through diet, weight loss, exercise, and less salt and alcohol. In mild hypertension nutrition and hygenic measures can control high blood pressure. If these measures do not lower your blood pressure enough and you need medication, **hydrochlorothiazide, a water pill (see thiazide diuretics, p. 117), is the drug of choice for mild hypertension in people**

over 60 years old, starting with a low dose of 12.5 milligrams. It also costs less.

There is now good evidence that another benefit of thiazide diuretics such as hydrochlorothiazide is that they significantly decrease the rate of bone mineral loss in both men and women because they reduce the amount of calcium lost in the urine. An increasing number of researchers think that this will also decrease the number of fractures. [325]

If your high blood pressure is more severe and hydrochlorothiazide alone does not control it, the best treatment is a combination of hydrochlorothiazide and a second type of drug called a beta-blocker, such as propranolol (see p. 124). If you can't take a drug in the beta-blocker family, another drug called a calcium channel blocker may be used instead. In either case, your doctor would prescribe the hydrochlorothiazide and the second drug separately, with the dose of each drug adjusted to meet your needs, rather than using a product that combines the drugs in advance in a fixed combination. Increased sensitivity to cold is one side effect. (See glossary p. 689 for signs of hypothermia.)

If you are taking this fixed-combination drug, ask your doctor about changing your prescription.

Whatever drugs you take for high blood pressure, once your blood pressure has been normal for a year or more, a cautious decrease in dose and renewed attention to non-drug treatment may be worth trying, according to *The Medical Letter*.[326]

"Treatment of hypertension is part of preventive medicine and like all preventive strategies, its progress should be regularly reviewed by whoever initiates it. Many problems could be avoided by not starting antihypertensive treatment until after prolonged observation. . . . Patients should no longer be told that treatment is necessarily for life: the possibility of reducing or stopping treatment should be mentioned at the outset."[327]

Atenolol
TENORMIN (Stuart)

Generic: available

Family: Beta-blockers (see p. 68)
Antihypertensives
(See High Blood Pressure, p. 62)

Atenolol (a *ten* oh lole) is used to treat high blood pressure (hypertension), chest pain (angina), and irregular heartbeats (arrythmias) and to decrease the frequency of migraine headaches. **If you are over 60, you will generally need to take less than the usual adult dose, especially if your kidney function is impaired.**

For young adults with high blood pressure, doctors usually prescribe a drug in this family (a beta-blocker) before any other drug. But for blacks and older adults, these drugs are less effective as the sole treatment. For these groups of people, doctors usually prescribe another type of drug called a diuretic (water pill) to lower blood pressure, and add a beta-blocker as a second drug if the diuretic alone is not enough.

If you have high blood pressure, the best way to reduce or eliminate your need for medication is through diet, weight loss, exercise, and less salt and alcohol. In mild hypertension nutrition and hygenic measures can control high blood pressure. If these measures do not lower your blood pressure enough and you need medication, **hydrochlorothiazide, a water pill (see** thiazide diuretics, p. 117), is the drug of choice for mild hypertension in people over 60 years old, starting with a low dose of 12.5 milligrams. It also costs less.

There is now good evidence that another benefit of thiazide diuretics such as hydrochlorothiazide is that they significantly decrease the rate of bone mineral loss in both men and women because they reduce the amount of calcium lost in the urine. An increasing number of researchers think that this will also decrease the number of fractures. [328]

All beta-blockers are similarly effective, although not necessarily interchangeable. If you are bothered by side effects when taking atenolol, talk to your doctor about switching to another beta-blocker, such as propranolol, which is available generically. The side effects of these drugs vary widely, and each individual responds differently to each one. See p. 68 for a discussion of alternatives to atenolol.

Whatever drugs you take for high blood pressure, once your blood pressure has been normal for a year or more, a cautious decrease in dose and renewed attention to non-drug treatment may be worth trying, according to *The Medical Letter*.[329]

"Treatment of hypertension is part of preventive medicine and like all preventive strategies, its progress should be regularly reviewed by whoever initiates it. Many problems could be avoided by not starting antihypertensive treatment until after prolonged observation. . . . Patients should no longer be told that treatment is necessarily for life: the possibility of reducing or stopping treatment should be mentioned at the outset."[330]

Before You Use This Drug

Do not use if you have
❏ congestive heart failure
❏ asthma
❏ emphysema or chronic bronchitis
Tell your doctor if you have or have had
❏ allergies to drugs
❏ gout

❏ alcohol dependence
❏ mental depression
❏ kidney, liver, lung, or pancreas disease
❏ diabetes
❏ lupus erythematosus
❏ difficulty breathing
❏ poor blood circulation
❏ Raynaud's syndrome
❏ thyroid problems
Tell your doctor about any other drugs you take, including aspirin, herbs, vitamins, and other non-prescription products.

When You Use This Drug

◆ **Learn to take your pulse, and get immediate medical help if your pulse slows to 50 beats per minute or slower, even if you are feeling well. Some people have suffered from slowed heart rate and heart failure while taking atenolol.**
◆ Until you know how you react to this drug, do not drive or perform other activities requiring alertness.
◆ Be careful not to overexert yourself, even though your chest pain may feel better.
◆ **Do not stop taking this drug suddenly. Your doctor must give you a schedule to decrease your dose gradually, to prevent chest pain and possible heart attack.**
◆ You may feel dizzy when rising from a

Heat Stress Alert

This drug can affect your body's ability to adjust to heat, putting you at risk of "heat stress." If you live alone, ask a friend to check on you several times during the day. Early signs of heat stress are dizziness, lightheadedness, faintness, and slightly high temperature. Call your doctor if you have any of these signs.

Drink more fluids (water, fruit and vegetable juices) than usual, even if you're not thirsty, unless your doctor has told you otherwise. Do not drink alcohol.

lying or sitting position. When getting out of bed, hang your legs over the side of the bed for a few minutes, then get up slowly. When getting up from a chair, get up slowly and stay beside the chair until you are sure that you are not dizzy. (See p. 14.)

◆ **Caution diabetics:** see p. 516.
◆ If you plan to have any surgery, including dental, tell your doctor that you take this drug.
◆ **Do not take other drugs without talking to your doctor first — especially non-prescription drugs for appetite control, asthma, colds, coughs, hay fever, or sinus problems.**

How To Use This Drug
◆ Crush tablets and mix with water, or swallow whole with water.
◆ If you miss a dose, take it as soon as you remember, but skip it if it is less than 8 hours until your next scheduled dose. **Do not take double doses.**

Interactions With Other Drugs
The following drugs are listed in *Evaluations of Drug Interactions*, 1991 as causing "highly clinically significant" or "clinically significant" interactions when used together with this drug. There may be other drugs, especially those in the families of drugs listed below, that also will react with this drug to cause severe adverse effects. Make sure to ask your doctor for a complete listing of them and let her or him know if you are taking any of these interacting drugs:

amiodarone; CATAPRES; chlorpromazine; clonidine; cocaine; CORDARONE; ESKALITH; FLUOTHANE; halothane; INDOCIN; indomethacin; lithium; MINIPRESS; prazosin; THORAZINE; tubocurarine.

Adverse Effects
Call your doctor immediately:
❑ difficulty breathing
❑ cold hands or feet
❑ mental depression
❑ skin rash
❑ swelling of ankles, feet, or legs
❑ slow pulse
Call your doctor if these symptoms continue:
❑ headache
❑ dizziness, lightheadedness
❑ nausea, vomiting, diarrhea
❑ unusual tiredness or weakness
❑ disturbed sleep, nightmares
❑ decreased sexual ability
More side effects information appears on p. 68.

Periodic Tests
Ask your doctor which of these tests should be done periodically while you are taking this drug:
❑ complete blood counts
❑ blood pressure and pulse rate
❑ heart function tests, such as electrocardiogram (EKG)
❑ kidney function tests
❑ liver function tests
❑ blood glucose levels

Tocainide
TONOCARD (Merck Sharp & Dohme)

Generic: not available

Family: Antiarrhythmics

Tocainide (toe *kay* nide) slows the heart rate and stabilizes irregular heartbeats (arrhythmias). Because it has severe side effects, your doctor should not prescribe tocainide unless you have already tried safer drugs in its family, such as quinidine (see p. 108), without success. **If you have impaired liver or kidney function, you should be taking less than the usual dose.**

Tocainide most commonly causes harmful effects in the digestive tract and central nervous system. These effects include nausea, vomiting, dizziness, tremor, confusion, and a "pins-and-needles" sensation on the skin.[331] Three of the most serious possible side effects are bone marrow depression, hepatitis (liver disease), and inflammation of the lungs.[332]

Many people who are taking tocainide or another drug in its family have relatively mild disturbances in their heart rhythm and no symptoms of underlying heart disease. The vast majority of these people *do not need these drugs*, and there is no evidence that using them improves health. In fact, most of the drugs in this family have severe side effects that are sometimes worse and even more life-threatening than the irregular heartbeats they treat. All of these drugs can also cause *new* irregularities in your heartbeat.

If you have an irregular heartbeat without any symptoms of underlying heart disease, you should not be exposed to the dangers of a drug that has no health benefit for your condition.[333] If you are taking tocainide or another drug in its family for an irregular heartbeat (arrhythmia), talk to your doctor and find out whether you also have symptoms of underlying heart dis-

ease. If not, discuss the possibility of stopping the drug.

Before You Use This Drug
Do not use if you have or have had
❑ allergic reaction to lidocaine (see p. 323)
❑ complete heart block
Tell your doctor if you have or have had
❑ allergies to drugs
❑ congestive heart failure
❑ kidney or liver disease
Tell your doctor about any other drugs you take, including aspirin, herbs, vitamins, and other non-prescription products.

When You Use This Drug
◆ Until you know how you react to this drug, do not drive or perform other activities requiring alertness. Tocainide may cause dizziness.
◆ You may feel dizzy when rising from a lying or sitting position. When getting out of bed, hang your legs over the side of the bed for a few minutes, then get up slowly. When getting up from a chair, get up slowly and stay beside the chair until you are sure that you are not dizzy. (See p. 14.)
◆ **Do not stop taking this drug suddenly. Your doctor must give you a schedule to lower your dose gradually, to prevent serious changes in heart function.**
◆ Wear a medical identification bracelet or carry a card stating that you take tocainide.
◆ If you plan to have any surgery, including dental, tell your doctor that you take this drug.

How To Use This Drug
◆ Take with food or milk to reduce stomach upset.
◆ If you miss a dose, take it as soon as you remember, but skip it if it is less

than 4 hours until your next scheduled dose. **Do not take double doses.**

◆ Store away from heat and light.

Interactions With Other Drugs

The following drugs are listed in *Evaluations of Drug Interactions*, 1991 as causing "highly clinically significant" or "clinically significant" interactions when used together with this drug. There may be other drugs, especially those in the families of drugs listed below, that also will react with this drug to cause severe adverse effects. Make sure to ask your doctor for a complete listing of them and let her or him know if you are taking any of these interacting drugs:

amiodarone; cimetidine; CORDARONE; cyclosporine; ELIXOPHYLLIN; INDERAL; propranolol; SANDIMMUNE; TAGAMET; theophylline.

Adverse Effects

Call your doctor immediately:
❏ trembling or shaking
❏ cough or shortness of breath
❏ fever, chills, or sore throat
❏ unusual bleeding or bruising
❏ irregular heartbeats

Call your doctor if these symptoms continue:
❏ dizziness or lightheadedness
❏ loss of appetite
❏ nausea or vomiting
❏ blurred vision
❏ confusion
❏ headache
❏ nervousness
❏ numbness or tingling of fingers or toes
❏ skin rash
❏ sweating

Periodic Tests

Ask your doctor which of these tests should be done periodically while you are taking this drug:
❏ complete blood counts
❏ heart function tests, such as electrocardiogram (EKG)
❏ chest X-ray

LIMITED USE

Labetalol
TRANDATE (Glaxo)

Generic: not available

Family: Beta-blockers (see p. 68)
Antihypertensives
(See High Blood Pressure, p. 62)

Labetalol (la *bet* a lole) is used to lower high blood pressure (hypertension). It is no better than generic propranolol, which is also less expensive[334] (see p. 124). In addition, it has a high incidence of side effects, so it is not the best drug in its family (beta-blockers) for treating uncomplicated high

blood pressure. Increased sensitivity to cold is one side effect. (See glossary p. 689 for signs of hypothermia.) However, because people react differently to different drugs in this family, labetalol may be the best drug for some individuals who have tried other drugs without success. See p. 68 for a discussion of alternatives to labetalol.

If you are over 60, you will generally need to take less than the usual adult dose, especially if your liver function is impaired.

If you have high blood pressure, the best way to reduce or eliminate your need for medication is through diet, weight loss, exercise, and less salt and alcohol. In mild hypertension nutrition and hygenic measures can control high blood pressure. If these measures do not lower your blood pressure enough and you need medication, **hydrochlorothiazide, a water pill (see thiazide diuretics, p. 117) is the drug of choice for mild hypertension in people over 60 years old, starting with a low dose**

Warning

A recent study found 11 cases, including three deaths, of liver damage induced by labetalol.[335] According to one of the authors of the study, Dr. Hyman Zimmerman, a world-renowned authority on drug-induced liver damage, the evidence for serious, sometimes fatal liver damage from labetalol is stronger than for any other drug in the beta-blocker family. The authors recommended that "Because of the seriousness of the present cases of labetalol-induced hepatocellular necrosis [death of liver cells], we believe that physicians should adopt a preventive approach. . . . This approach involves several steps: administering baseline liver function tests at least once before starting therapy; periodically retesting liver function beginning at one month and changing to an alternative agent if abnormalities are found; informing patients of the signs and symptoms of liver involvement and that they must seek further medical evaluation should these signs or symptoms occur [symptoms of labetalol-induced liver damage seen in the study included jaundice [yellowish skin or eyeballs], dark urine, nausea, vomiting, loss of appetite, rash, and itching]; and avoiding further exposure of persons with liver abnormalities to labetalol. If laboratory evidence of liver injury or jaundice is noted labetalol therapy should be stopped and never restarted."

---

of 12.5 milligrams. It also costs less.

There is now good evidence that another benefit of thiazide diuretics such as hydrochlorothiazide is that they significantly decrease the rate of bone mineral loss in both men and women because they reduce the amount of calcium lost in the urine. An increasing number of researchers think that this will also decrease the number of fractures. [336]

Whatever drugs you take for high blood pressure, once your blood pressure has been normal for a year or more, a cautious decrease in dose and renewed attention to non-drug treatment may be worth trying, according to *The Medical Letter*.[337]

"Treatment of hypertension is part of preventive medicine and like all preventive strategies, its progress should be regularly reviewed by whoever initiates it. Many problems could be avoided by not starting anti-hypertensive treatment until after prolonged observation. . . . Patients should no longer be told that treatment is necessarily for life: the possibility of reducing or stopping treatment should be mentioned at the outset."[338]

Before You Use This Drug
Do not use if you have
❑ congestive heart failure
❑ asthma
❑ emphysema or chronic bronchitis
Tell your doctor if you have or have had
❑ allergies to drugs
❑ gout
❑ thyroid problems
❑ kidney, liver, lung, or pancreas disease
❑ alcohol dependence
❑ lupus erythematosus
❑ mental depression
❑ diabetes
❑ difficulty breathing
Tell your doctor about any other drugs you take, including aspirin, herbs, vitamins, and other non-prescription products.

When You Use This Drug
◆ Learn to take your pulse, and get immediate medical help if your pulse slows

to 50 beats per minute or slower, even if you are feeling well. Some people have suffered from slowed heart rate and heart failure while taking labetalol.

◆ Until you know how you react to this drug, do not drive or perform other activities requiring alertness.

◆ Be careful not to overexert yourself, even though your chest pain may feel better.

◆ **Do not stop taking this drug suddenly. Your doctor must give you a schedule to decrease your dose gradually, to prevent chest pain and possible heart attack.**

◆ You may feel dizzy when rising from a lying or sitting position. When getting out of bed, hang your legs over the side of the bed for a few minutes, then get up slowly. When getting up from a chair, get up slowly and stay beside the chair until you are sure that you are not dizzy. (See p. 14.)

◆ **Caution diabetics:** see p. 516.

◆ If you plan to have any surgery, including dental, tell your doctor that you take this drug.

◆ **Do not take other drugs without talking to your doctor first — especially non-prescription drugs for appetite control, asthma, colds, coughs, hay fever, or sinus problems.**

Heat Stress Alert

This drug can affect your body's ability to adjust to heat, putting you at risk of "heat stress." If you live alone, ask a friend to check on you several times during the day. Early signs of heat stress are dizziness, lightheadedness, faintness, and slightly high temperature. Call your doctor if you have any of these signs.

Drink more fluids (water, fruit and vegetable juices) than usual, even if you're not thirsty, unless your doctor has told you otherwise. Do not drink alcohol.

How To Use This Drug

◆ Crush tablet and mix with food or drink, or swallow whole with water.

◆ If you miss a dose, take it as soon as you remember, but skip it if it is less than 8 hours until your next scheduled dose. **Do not take double doses.**

Interactions With Other Drugs

The following drugs are listed in *Evaluations of Drug Interactions*, 1991 as causing "highly clinically significant" or "clinically significant" interactions when used together with this drug. There may be other drugs, especially those in the families of drugs listed below, that also will react with this drug to cause severe adverse effects. Make sure to ask your doctor for a complete listing of them and let her or him know if you are taking any of these interacting drugs:

ADRENALIN (also in bee sting kits); amiodarone; CALAN; chlorpromazine; cimetidine; cocaine; CORDARONE; COUMADIN; epinephrine; FLUOTHANE; furosemide; halothane; INDOCIN; indomethacin; insulin; LASIX; lidocaine; MINIPRESS; NEMBUTAL; pentobarbital; prazosin; SYNTHROID; TAGAMET; THEO-DUR; theophylline; THORAZINE; thyroid; tobacco; tubocurarine; verapamil; warfarin; XYLOCAINE.

Adverse Effects
Call your doctor immediately:
❑ difficulty breathing
❑ cold hands or feet
❑ mental depression
❑ skin rash
❑ swelling of ankles, feet, or legs
❑ slow pulse
Call your doctor if these symptoms continue:
❑ headache
❑ dizziness, lightheadedness
❑ nausea, vomiting, diarrhea
❑ unusual tiredness or weakness
❑ disturbed sleep, nightmares

❑ decreased sexual ability
More side effects information appears on p. 68.

Periodic Tests
Ask your doctor which of these tests should be done periodically while you are taking this drug:
❑ complete blood counts

❑ blood pressure and pulse rate
❑ heart function tests, such as electrocardiogram (EKG)
❑ kidney function tests
❑ liver function tests
❑ blood glucose levels
❑ eye exams to check for drug accumulation (in the choroid)

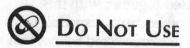 **DO NOT USE**

Alternative treatment: Mild exercise, no smoking, extreme cleanliness of legs and feet.

Pentoxifylline
TRENTAL (Hoechst-Roussel)

Family: Blood Flow Improvers

Pentoxifylline (pen tox *if* i lin) is advertised as a drug to relieve leg cramps caused by poor blood circulation (intermittent claudication). The manufacturer claims that the drug improves the flow of blood through the blood vessels by making red blood cells more flexible. Studies have shown, however, that exercise is more effective than pentoxifylline in reducing these cramps.[339] There is no convincing evidence that pentoxifylline is very effec-

tive in improving blood circulation.

Pentoxifylline may also have serious dangers. **One medical center recently reported two cases in which pentoxifylline caused fatal damage to patients' bone marrow.**[340] Animal studies have shown that rats develop benign breast tumors when taking this drug.

According to the Hospital Pharmacy Therapeutics Committee at the University of California, San Francisco Medical Center, studies are inconclusive as to the benefit of this drug.[341]

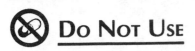 **DO NOT USE**

Alternative treatment: Mild exercise, no smoking, extreme cleanliness of legs and feet.

Isoxsuprine
VASODILAN (Mead Johnson)

Family: Vasodilators
(Blood Vessel Dilators)

Doctors prescribe isoxsuprine (eye *sox* syoo preen) to improve the blood circulation of people with certain types of blood vessel disease, in the hope that this will relieve pain that is caused by circulation problems (leg pain, for example) and improve mental functioning (by increasing blood flow to the brain). However, **isoxsuprine has not been proven effective for these problems**. It does not improve the flow of blood to calf muscles in people with diseased blood vessels, nor does it help leg cramps caused by poor blood circulation (intermittent claudication).[342] In fact, although this drug has been available for use and evaluation for many years, **it has not been proven effective for treating any condition**.[343] The American Medical Association's guide to drug therapy does not even suggest a dose for isoxsuprine because "the role of this agent in the treatment of peripheral vascular disease [disease of the blood vessels in the arms or legs] has not been established."[344]

Isoxsuprine's side effects include headache, nausea, chills, flushing, tingling and burning sensation of the skin, heart flutter, and stomach and intestinal problems. **We recommend that you do not use isoxsuprine because it can cause harmful side effects and has not been proven to have any benefit.**

The National Academy of Sciences has found that isoxsuprine and a related drug called cyclandelate lack evidence of effectiveness. The Food and Drug Administration has found that another drug in this family, nylidrin (Arlidin), also lacks evidence of effectiveness.

Warning
Isoxsuprine can cause or worsen high blood pressure. It is especially dangerous for people who have high blood pressure, heart disease, diabetes, or thyroid disease. People over 60 are more likely than younger people to experience effects on the heart and blood pressure, restlessness, nervousness, and confusion.

Pindolol
VISKEN (Sandoz)

Generic: not available

Family: Beta-blockers (see p. 68)
Antihypertensives
(See High Blood Pressure, p. 62)

Pindolol (*pin* doe lole) is used to treat high blood pressure (hypertension), chest pain (angina), and irregular heartbeats (arrhythmias) and to decrease the frequency of migraine headaches. **In general, people over 60 require less than the usual adult dose, especially if kidney or liver function is impaired.**

If you have high blood pressure, the best way to reduce or eliminate your need for medication is through diet, weight loss, exercise, and less salt and alcohol. In mild hypertension nutrition and hygenic measures can control high blood pressure. If these measures do not lower your blood pressure enough and you need medication, **hydrochlorothiazide, a water pill (see thiazide diuretics, p. 117) is the drug of choice for mild hypertension in people over 60 years old, starting with a low dose of 12.5 milligrams.** It also costs less.

There is now good evidence that another benefit of thiazide diuretics such as hydrochlorothiazide is that they significantly decrease the rate of bone mineral loss in both men and women because they reduce the amount of calcium lost in the urine. An increasing number of researchers think that this will also decrease the number of fractures. [345]

For young adults with high blood pressure, doctors usually prescribe a drug in this family (a beta-blocker) before any other drug. But for blacks and older adults, these drugs are less effective as the sole treatment. For these groups of people, doctors usually prescribe another type of drug called a diuretic (water pill) to lower blood pressure, and add a beta-blocker as a second drug if the diuretic alone is not enough.

If you are bothered by side effects when using pindolol, talk with your doctor about switching to another drug in this family (beta-blocker). The side effects of these drugs vary widely, and each individual responds differently to each one. Increased sensitivity to cold is one side effect. (See glossary p. 689 for signs of hypothermia.) See p. 68 for a discussion of alternatives to pindolol.

Whatever drugs you take for high blood pressure, once your blood pressure has been normal for a year or more, a cautious decrease in dose and renewed attention to non-drug treatment may be worth trying, according to *The Medical Letter*.[346]

"Treatment of hypertension is part of preventive medicine and like all preventive strategies, its progress should be regularly reviewed by whoever initiates it. Many problems could be avoided by not starting antihypertensive treatment until after prolonged observation. . . . Patients should no longer be told that treatment is necessarily for life: the possibility of reducing or stopping treatment should be mentioned at the outset."[347]

Before You Use This Drug
Do not use if you have
❑ congestive heart failure
❑ asthma
❑ emphysema or chronic bronchitis
Tell your doctor if you have or have had
❑ allergies to drugs
❑ gout
❑ mental depression
❑ difficulty breathing
❑ kidney, liver, lung, or pancreas disease
❑ alcohol dependence
❑ lupus erythematosus

❑ diabetes
❑ poor blood circulation
❑ Raynaud's syndrome
❑ thyroid problems
Tell your doctor about any other drugs you take, including aspirin, herbs, vitamins, and other non-prescription products.

When You Use This Drug

Heat Stress Alert

This drug can affect your body's ability to adjust to heat, putting you at risk of "heat stress." If you live alone, ask a friend to check on you several times during the day. Early signs of heat stress are dizziness, lightheadedness, faintness, and slightly high temperature. Call your doctor if you have any of these signs.

Drink more fluids (water, fruit and vegetable juices) than usual, even if you're not thirsty, unless your doctor has told you otherwise. Do not drink alcohol.

◆ **Learn to take your pulse, and get immediate medical help if your pulse slows to 50 beats per minute or slower, even if you are feeling well. Some people have suffered from slowed heart rate and heart failure while taking pindolol.**
◆ Until you know how you react to this drug, do not drive or perform other activities requiring alertness.
◆ Be careful not to overexert yourself, even though your chest pain may feel better.
◆ **Do not stop taking this drug suddenly. Your doctor must give you a schedule to decrease your dose gradually, to prevent chest pain and possible heart attack.**
◆ You may feel dizzy when rising from a lying or sitting position. When getting out of bed, hang your legs over the side of the bed for a few minutes, then get up slowly. When getting up from a chair, get up slowly and stay beside the chair until you are sure that you are not dizzy. (See p. 14.)
◆ **Caution diabetics:** see p. 516.
◆ If you plan to have any surgery, including dental, tell your doctor that you take this drug.
◆ **Do not take other drugs without talking to your doctor first — especially non-prescription drugs for appetite control, asthma, colds, coughs, hay fever, or sinus problems.**

How To Use This Drug
◆ Mix crushed tablets or swallow whole with water.
◆ If you miss a dose, take it as soon as you remember, but skip it if it is less than 4 hours until your next scheduled dose. **Do not take double doses.**

Interactions With Other Drugs
The following drugs are listed in *Evaluations of Drug Interactions,* 1991 as causing "highly clinically significant" or "clinically significant" interactions when used together with this drug. There may be other drugs, especially those in the families of drugs listed below, that also will react with this drug to cause severe adverse effects. Make sure to ask your doctor for a complete listing of them and let her or him know if you are taking any of these interacting drugs:

ALDOMET; CATAPRES; clonidine; cocaine; COUMADIN; ESKALITH; FLUOTHANE; halothane; INDOCIN; indomethacin; insulin; lithium; methyldopa; MINIPRESS; prazosin; THEO-DUR; theophylline; warfarin.

Adverse Effects
Call your doctor immediately:
❑ difficulty breathing
❑ back or joint pain
❑ chest pain
❑ cold hands or feet
❑ mental depression, hallucinations
❑ skin rash
❑ swelling of ankles, feet, or legs

❑ slow pulse, irregular heartbeat
Call your doctor if these symptoms continue:
❑ nausea, vomiting, diarrhea
❑ unusual tiredness or weakness
❑ disturbed sleep
❑ anxiety, nervousness
❑ decreased sexual ability
❑ itching skin
❑ dry or sore eyes
More side effects information appears on p. 68.

Periodic Tests
Ask your doctor which of these tests should be done periodically while you are taking this drug:
❑ complete blood counts
❑ blood pressure and pulse rate
❑ heart function tests, such as electrocardiogram (EKG)
❑ kidney function tests
❑ liver function tests
❑ blood glucose levels

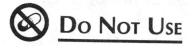 **DO NOT USE**

Alternative treatment: See Hydrochlorothiazide, p. 117.

Guanabenz
WYTENSIN (Wyeth)

Family: Antihypertensives
  (See High Blood Pressure, p. 62)

Guanabenz (*gwahn* a benz) is used to treat high blood pressure (hypertension).
It has severe side effects and should not be used.

The main problem with guanabenz is that missing only *one* or *two* doses of the drug can have serious effects, including sweating, tremor, flushing, and severe high blood pressure. Guanabenz can also cause severe depression and is particularly dangerous for anyone with a history of depression.

If you have high blood pressure, the best way to reduce or eliminate your need for medication is through diet, weight loss, exercise, and less salt and alcohol. In mild hypertension nutrition and hygenic measures can control high blood pressure. If these measures do not lower your blood pressure enough and you need medication, **hydrochlorothiazide, a water pill (see thiazide diuretics, p. 117), is the drug of choice for mild hypertension in people over 60 years old, starting with a low dose**

of 12.5 milligrams. It also costs less.

There is now good evidence that another benefit of thiazide diuretics such as hydrochlorothiazide is that they significantly decrease the rate of bone mineral loss in both men and women because they reduce the amount of calcium lost in the urine. An increasing number of researchers think that this will also decrease the number of fractures. [348]

If this does not lower your blood pressure enough, your doctor can prescribe a second type of drug called a beta-blocker (see p. 68) to accompany the hydrochlorothiazide. If you cannot take a beta-blocker, a drug from another family (calcium channel blockers) can be used instead.

Whatever drugs you take for high blood pressure, once your blood pressure has been normal for a year or more, a cautious decrease in dose and renewed attention to non-drug treatment may be worth trying, according to *The Medical Letter*. [349]

"Treatment of hypertension is part of preventive medicine and like all preventive strategies, its progress should be regularly reviewed by whoever initiates it. Many problems could be avoided by not starting antihypertensive treatment until after prolonged observation. . . . Patients should no longer be told that treatment is necessarily for life: the possibility of reducing or stopping treatment should be mentioned at the outset."[350]

Do not suddenly stop using this drug. Ask your doctor for a schedule that lowers your dose gradually over at least 10 days, and more slowly if you begin to have withdrawal symptoms. Another drug for high blood pressure should be started at the same time.[345]

Notes for Heart, Blood Pressure, and Blood Vessel Drugs

1. Squires S. Medical pressure cooker: doctors debate what to do about hypertension, *Washington Post* Health Section, February 10, 1987.

2. Hansen AG, Jensen H, Langesen LP, Peterson A. Withdrawal of antihypertensive drugs in the elderly. *Acta Medica Scandivica* 1982; 676:178-85.

3. Cohobanian A. Antihypertensive therapy in evolution. *New England Journal of Medicine* 1986; 314:1701-2.

4. Rowe J. Systolic hypertension in the elderly. *New England Journal of Medicine* 1983; 309:1246-7.

5. Stamler R. et al. Nutritional therapy for high blood pressure. *Journal of the American Medical Association* 1987; 257:1484-91.

6. 1984 Joint National Committee on Detection, Evaluation, and Treatment of High Blood Pressure. Nonpharmacological approaches to the control of high blood pressure: final report of the Subcommittee on Nonpharmacological Therapy. *Hypertension* 1986; 8:454-5.

7. Schlamowitz P, et al. Treatment of mild to moderate hypertension with dietary fibre. *The Lancet* 1987; 8559:622-3.

8. Eichner E. Nonpharmacological therapy of hypertension. *Internal Medicine* 1987; 8:155-61.

9. Vestal RE, ed. *Drug Treatment in the Elderly*. Sydney, Australia: ADIS Health Science Press, 1984:77-88.

10. Burton R. Withdrawing antihypertensive treatment: hypertension may settle with time. *British Medical Journal* 1991; 303:324-5.

11. Ibid.

12. *The Medical Letter on Drugs and Therapeutics*. New York: The Medical Letter Inc., 1991; 33:33-8.

13. *The Medical Letter on Drugs and Therapeutics*. New York: The Medical Letter Inc., 1981; 23:3.

14. *The Medical Letter on Drugs and Therapeutics*. New York: The Medical Letter Inc., 1978; 20:30.

15. Ibid.

16. Harrington JT, Isner JM, Kassirer JP. Our national obsession with potassium. *American Journal of Medicine* 1982; 73:155-9.

17. *The Medical Letter on Drugs and Therapeutics*, 1981, op. cit., p. 71.

18. *The Medical Letter on Drugs and Therapeutics*, 1981, op. cit., p. 3.

19. *The Medical Letter on Drugs and Therapeutics*, 1981, op. cit., p. 71.

20. *The Medical Letter on Drugs and Therapeutics*, 1981, op. cit., p. 3.

21. Ibid.

22. Kastrup EK, ed. *Facts and Comparisons*. St. Louis: J.B. Lippincott Co., July 1987:15a.

23. AMA Department of Drugs. *AMA Drug Evaluations*. 5th ed. Chicago: American Medical Association, 1983:1111.

24. *The Medical Letter on Drugs and Therapeutics*, 1981, op. cit., p. 3.

25. *Drug and Therapeutics Bulletin*, 1992; 29:87-91.

26. Conversation with Dr. Andrew Herxheimer, Charing Cross Hospital, Editor, *Drug and Therapeutics Bulletin*, October 21, 1986.

27. Kaiser FE, Morley JE. Cholesterol can be lowered in older persons: should we care? *Journal of the American Geriatric Society* 1990; 38:84-5.

28. American College of Physicians. Geriatrics: nutritional issues. Medical Knowledge Self-Assessment Program IX, 1991.

29. Levin WEG, Miller VT, Muesing RA, Stoy DB, Balm TK, LaRosa JC. Comparison of psyllium hydrophilic mucilloid and cellulose as adjuncts to a prudent diet in the treatment of mild to moderate hypercholesterolemia. *Archives of Internal Medicine* 1990; 150:1822-7.

30. Greenblatt DJ, Koch-Weser J. Adverse reactions to spironolactone. *Journal of the American Medical Association* 1973; 225:40-3.

31. Neal TJ, Lynn KL, Bailey RR. Spironolactone-associated aggravation of renal function impairment. *New Zealand Medical Journal* 1976. 83:147-9.

32. Greenblatt, op. cit.

33. Pongpaew C, Songkhla RN, Kozam RL. Hyperkalemic cardiac arrythmia secondary to spironolactone. *Chest* June 1973; 63:1023-5.

34. Yap V, Patel A, Thomsen J. Hyperkalemia with cardiac arrythmia: induction by salt substitutes, spironolactone and azotemia. *Journal of the American Medical Association* 1976; 236:2775-6.

35. Davies DM, ed. *Textbook of Adverse Drug Reactions*. Oxford: Oxford University Press, 1977:237.

36. Udezue EO, Harrold BP. Hyperkalaemic paralysis due to spironolactone. *Postgraduate Medical Journal* 1980; 56:254-5.

37. *Physicians' Desk Reference*. 41st ed. Oradell, N.J.: Medical Economics Company, 1987:1540-1.

38. *Physicians' Desk Reference*. 40th ed. Oradell, N.J.: Medical Economics Company, 1986:1675.

39. Wasnich R, Davis J, Ross P, Vogel J. Effect of thiazide on rates of bone mineral loss: a longitudinal study. *British Medical Journal* 1991; 301:1303-5.

40. *The Medical Letter on Drugs and Therapeutics*, 1991, op. cit., p. 33-8.

41. Burton, op. cit.

42. Greenblatt, op. cit.

43. Neal, op. cit.

44. Greenblatt, op. cit.

45. Pongpaew, op. cit.

46 Yap, op. cit.

47. Davies, op. cit.

48. Udezue, op. cit.

49. Greenblatt, op. cit.

50. *Physicians' Desk Reference*, 1987, op. cit., p. 1540-1.

51. *Physicians' Desk Reference*, 1986, op. cit., p. 1677.

52. *Physicians' Desk Reference*, 1986, op. cit., p. 1675.

53. Papademetriou V, Burris J, Kukich S, Freis ED. Effectiveness of potassium chloride or triamterene in thiazide hypokalemia. *Archives of Internal Medicine*, 1985; 145:1986-90.

54. Wasnich, op. cit.

55. *The Medical Letter on Drugs and Therapeutics*, 1991, op. cit., p. 33-8.

56. Burton, op. cit.

57. Wasnich, op. cit.

58. *The Medical Letter on Drugs and Therapeutics*, 1991, op. cit., p. 33-8.

59. Burton, op. cit.

60. Wasnich, op. cit.

61. *The Medical Letter on Drugs and Therapeutics*, 1991, op. cit., p. 33-8.

62. Burton, op. cit.

63. Orland MJ, Saltman RJ eds. *Manual of Medical Therapeutics*. 25th ed. Boston: Little Brown and Company, 1986:57-69.

64. Orland, op. cit., p. 89-104.

65. Ibid.

66. Wasnich, op. cit.

67. *The Medical Letter on Drugs and Therapeutics*, 1991, op. cit., p. 33-8.

68. Burton, op. cit.

69. Orland, op. cit., p. 57-69.

70. Wasnich, op. cit.

71. *The Medical Letter on Drugs and Therapeutics*, 1991, op. cit., p. 33-8.

72. Burton, op. cit.

73. *The Medical Letter on Drugs and Therapeutics*. New York: The Medical Letter Inc., 1984; 26:116.

74. Vestal, op. cit., p. 77-88.

75. Orland, op. cit., p. 89-104.

76. Vestal, op. cit., p. 77-88.

77. Wasnich, op. cit.

78. *The Medical Letter on Drugs and Therapeutics*, 1991, op. cit., p. 33-8.

79. Burton, op. cit.

80. Lynn KL, Bailey RR, Swainson CP, Sainsbury R, Low WI. Renal failure with potassium-sparing diuretics. *New Zealand Medical Journal* 1985; 98:629-33.

81. *The Medical Letter on Drugs and Therapeutics*. New York: The Medical Letter, Inc., 1983; 25:62.

82. Vestal, op. cit., p. 77-88.

83. Wasnich, op. cit.

84. Conversation with Dr. Andrew Herxheimer, op. cit.

85. *USP DI, Drug Information for the Health Care Provider.* 6th ed. Rockville MD: The United States Pharmacopeial Convention, Inc., 1986:704.

86. *Drug Intelligence and Clinical Pharmacy* July/August 1983; 17:539.

87. *The Medical Letter on Drugs and Therapeutics*, 1991, op. cit., p. 33-8.

88. Burton, op. cit.

89. Laverenne J. Effets indesirables des inhibiteurs calciques. *Therapie* 1989; 44:197.

90. AMA Department of Drugs. *AMA Drug Evaluations Annual* 1992. Chicago: American Medical Association, 1992:541.

91. Pritza DR, Bierman MH, Hammeke MD. Acute toxic effects of sustained-release verapamil in chronic renal failure. *Archives of Internal Medicine* 1991; 151:2081-4.

92. Wasnich, op. cit.

93. *The Medical Letter on Drugs and Therapeutics*, 1991, op. cit., p. 33-8.

94. Burton, op. cit.

95. Kuhn M, Schriger DL. Verapamil administration to patients with contraindications: is it associated with adverse outcomes? *Annals of Emergency Medicine* 1991; 20:1094-9.

96. Gheorghiade M. Calcium channel blockers in the management of myocardial infarction patients. *Henry Ford Hospital Medical Journal* 1991; 39:210-6.

97. Ferrier C, Ferrari P, Weidmann P, Keller U, Beretta-Piccoli C, Riesen WF. Antihypertensive therapy with Ca2+. *Diabetes Care* 1991; 14:911-4.

98. Swash M, Ingram DA. Adverse effect of verapamil in myasthenia gravis. *Muscle & Nerve* 1992; 15:396-8.

99. *USP DI, Drug Information for the Health Care Professional.* 12th ed. Rockville MD: The United States Pharmacopeial Convention, Inc., 1992:779-90.

100. Tam IM, Wandres DL. Calcium-channel blockers and gingival hyperplasia. *The Annals of Pharmacotherapy* 1992; 26:213-4.

101. Gannon TH, Eby TL. Angioedema from angiotensin converting enzyme inhibitors: a cause of upper airway obstruction. *Laryngoscope* 1990; 100:1156-60.

102. Roberts JR, Wuerz RC. Clinical characteristics of angiotensin-converting enzyme inhibitor-induced angioedema (abstract). *Annals of Emergency Medicine* 1991; 20:555-8.

103. Ibid.

104. Wasnich, op. cit.

105. *The Medical Letter on Drugs and Therapeutics*, 1991, op. cit., p. 33-8.

106. Burton, op. cit.

107. American Society of Hospital Pharmacists. *American Hospital Formulary Service Drug Information*, Bethesda, MD, 1992:866-74.

108. Roberts, op. cit.

109. Sterner G. Renal artery stenosis and ACE inhibitor (letter). *Journal of Internal Medicine* 1990; 228:541.

110. American Society of Hospital Pharmacists, op. cit., p. 866-74.

111. Stoltz ML, Andrews CE. Severe hyperkalemia during very low-calorie diets and angiotensin converting enzyme use (letter). *Journal of the American Medical Association* 1990; 264:2737-8.

112. *The Medical Letter on Drugs and Therapeutics*, 1991, op. cit., p. 33-8.

113. Wasnich, op. cit.

114. *The Medical Letter on Drugs and Therapeutics*, 1991, op. cit., p. 33-8.

115. Burton, op. cit.

116. Laverenne, op. cit.

117. Wasnich, op. cit.

118. *The Medical Letter on Drugs and Therapeutics*, 1991, op. cit., p. 33-8.

119. Burton, op. cit.

120. Wasnich, op. cit.

121. *The Medical Letter on Drugs and Therapeutics*, 1991, op. cit., p. 33-8.

122. Burton, op. cit.

123. *The Medical Letter on Drugs and Therapeutics*. New York: The Medical Letter, Inc., 1976, 18:38-9.

124. AMA, 1983, op. cit., p. 678-9.

125. Gilman AG, Goodman LS, Rall TW, Murad F, eds. *The Pharmacological Basis of Therapeutics*. 7th ed. New York: Macmillan, 1985: 823.

126. AMA, 1983, op. cit., p. 678-9.

127. *New England Journal of Medicine* 1969; 281:1333-5 and 1364-5.

128. Jay RH, Rampling MW, Betteridge DJ. Abnormalities of blood rheology in familial hypercholesterolaemia: effects of treatment. *Atherosclerosis* 1990; 85:249-56.

129. *USP DI*, 1992, op. cit., p. 921-3.

130. American College of Physicians, op. cit.

131. *The Medical Letter on Drugs and Therapeutics*, 1991, op. cit., p. 1-4.

132. Orland MJ, Saltmar RF, eds. *Manual of Medical Therapeutics*, 26th Edition, Washington University, St. Louis, MO, 1989:421.

133. *The Medical Letter on Drugs and Therapeutics*, 1991, op. cit., p. 1-4.

134. *USP DI*, 1992, op. cit., p. 921-3.

135. American Society of Hospital Pharmacists, op. cit., p. 939-42.

136. Curtis DM, Driscoll DJ, Goldman DH, Weidman WH. Loss of dental enamel in a patient taking cholestyramine. *Mayo Clinic Proceedings* 1991; 66:1131.

137. Ibid.

138. *USP DI*, 1992, op. cit., p. 921-3.

139. Wasnich, op. cit.

140. *The Medical Letter on Drugs and Therapeutics*, 1991, op. cit., p. 33-8.

141. Burton, op. cit.

142. Wasnich, op. cit.

143. *The Medical Letter on Drugs and Therapeutics*, 1991, op. cit., p. 33-8.

144. Burton, op. cit.

145. *The Medical Letter on Drugs and Therapeutics*, 1976, op. cit.

146. Gilman, 1985, op. cit., p. 823.

147. AMA, 1983, op. cit., p. 678-9.

148. Wasnich, op. cit.

149. *The Medical Letter on Drugs and Therapeutics*, 1991, op. cit., p. 33-8.

150. Burton, op. cit.

151. Nygaard TW, Sellers TD, Cook TS, Marco JP. Adverse reactions to antiarrythmic drugs during therapy for ventricular arrythmias. *Journal of the American Medical Association* 1986; 256:57.

152. Laverenne, op. cit.

153. Thomas MG, Sander GE, Given MB, Quiroz AC, Roffidal LE, Giles TD. Efficacy of nicardipine in angina pectoris. *Journal of Clinical Pharmacology* 1990; 30:24-8.

154. AMA, 1992, op. cit., p. 511.

155. Wasnich, op. cit.

156. *The Medical Letter on Drugs and Therapeutics*, 1991, op. cit., p. 33-8.

157. Burton, op. cit.

158. *USP DI*, 1992, op. cit., p. 779-90.

159. Webster J, Petrie JC, Jeffers TA, Roy-Chaudhury P, Crichton W, Witte K, Jamieson M, MacDonald FC, Beard M, Dow RJ, Murray GR. Nicardipine sustained release in hypertension. *British Journal of Clinical Pharmacology* 1991; 32:433-9.

160. Ibid.

161. Dukes MNG, Beeley L. *Side Effects of Drugs Annual* 13, Amsterdam: Elsevier, 1989:158.

162. Dukes MNG, Beeley L. *Side Effects of Drugs Annual* 14, Amsterdam: Elsevier, 1990:165.

163. Lynn, op. cit.

164. Davies, op. cit.

165. Wasnich, op. cit.

166. *The Medical Letter on Drugs and Therapeutics*, 1991, op. cit., p. 33-8.

167. Burton, op. cit.

168. Davies, op. cit.

169. Lynn, op. cit.

170. Wasnich, op. cit.

171. Papademetriou, op. cit.

172. *The Medical Letter on Drugs and Therapeutics*, 1991, op. cit., p. 33-8.

173. Burton, op. cit.

174. *Physicians' Desk Reference*, 1987, op. cit., p. 516.

175. Wasnich, op. cit.

176. *The Medical Letter on Drugs and Therapeutics*, 1991, op. cit., p. 33-8.

177. Burton, op. cit.

178. *Physicians' Desk Reference*, 1986, op. cit., p. 1353.

179. *USP DI*, 1986, op. cit.

180. Morgan T, Adam W, Hodgson M. Adverse reactions to long-term diuretic therapy for hypertension. *Journal of Cardiovascular Pharmacology* 1984; 6:S269.

181. Wasnich, op. cit.

182. *The Medical Letter on Drugs and Therapeutics*, 1984, op. cit., p. 107.

183. *The Medical Letter on Drugs and Therapeutics*, 1991, op. cit., p. 33-8.

184. Burton, op. cit.

185. Gilman, 1985, op. cit., p. 209.

186. Wasnich, op. cit.

187. *The Medical Letter on Drugs and Therapeutics*, 1991, op. cit., p. 33-8.

188. Burton, op. cit.

189. Vestal, op. cit., p. 40

190. Cohen JD. Long-term efficacy and safety of terazosin alone and in combination with other antihypertensive agents. *American Heart Journal* 1991; 122:919-25.

191. *The Medical Letter on Drugs and Therapeutics*, 1991, op. cit., p. 15-6.

192. Gilman, AG, Rall TW, Nies AS, Taylor, P, eds. *The Pharmacological Basis of Therapuetics.* 8th ed. New York: Pergamon Press 1990: 226-7.

193. *USP DI*, 1992, op. cit., p. 2591-3.

194. Titmarsh S, Monk JP. Terazosin: a review of its pharmacodynamic and pharmacokinetic properties, and therapeutic efficacy in essential hypertension. *Drugs* 1987; 33:461-77.

195. Wasnich, op. cit.

196. *The Medical Letter on Drugs and Therapeutics*, 1991, op. cit., p. 33-8.

197. Burton, op. cit.

198. Gilman, 1990, op. cit.

199. Wasnich, op. cit.

200. *The Medical Letter on Drugs and Therapeutics*, 1991, op. cit., p. 33-8.

201. Burton, op. cit.

202. Wasnich, op. cit.

203. *The Medical Letter on Drugs and Therapeutics*, 1991, op. cit., p. 33-8.

204. Burton, op. cit.

205. Harrington, op. cit.

206. Vestal, op. cit., p. 66.

207. *The Medical Letter on Drugs and Therapeutics*. New York: The Medical Letter Inc., 1979, 21:44.

208. Carlson KJ. An analysis of physicians' reasons for prescribing long-term digitalis therapy in outpatients. *Journal of Chronic Diseases* 1985; 389: 733-9.

209. Lee DC. Heart failure in outpatients: A randomized trial of digoxin versus placebo. *New England Journal of Medicine* 1982; 306:699-705.

210. AMA, 1983, op. cit., p. 606.

211. Fleg J, Lakatta E. How useful is digitalis in patients with congestive heart failure and sinus rhythm? *International Journal of Cardiology* 1984; 6:295-305.

212. Vestal, op. cit., p. 77-8.

213. *Drugs for the Elderly*. Denmark: World Health Organization, 1985.

214. *USP DI*, 1986, op. cit.

215. *Drug Intelligence and Clinical Pharmacy*, op. cit.

216. Wasnich, op. cit.

217. Seligmann H, Halkin H, Rauchfleisch S, Kaufmann N, Motro M, Vered Z, David E. Thiamine deficiency in patients with congestive heart failure receiving long-term furosemide therapy: a pilot study. *American Journal of Medicine* 1991; 91:151-5.

218. Shimon I, Seligmann H, Vered Z, Steinmetz A, Almog S, Halkin H, Ezra D. Thiamine supplements improve left ventricular function in patients with chronic heart failure. *Journal of the American College of Cardiology* 1993; 21:366A.

219. *The Medical Letter on Drugs and Therapeutics*, 1991, op. cit., p. 33-8.

220. Burton, op. cit.

221. Statement by Ross Pierce, M.D., FDA Supervisory Medical Officer to NIH Consensus Development Conference Panel on Triglycerides, High Density Lipoprotein and Coronary Heart Disease, February, 25, 1992.

222. Pierce LR, Wysowski DK, Gross TP. Myopathy and rhabdomyolysis associated with lovastatin-gemfibrozil combination therapy. *Journal of the American Medical Association* 1990; 264:71-5.

223. American College of Physicians, op. cit.

224. Wasnich, op. cit.

225. *The Medical Letter on Drugs and Therapeutics*, 1991, op. cit., p. 33-8.

226. Burton, op. cit.

227. American College of Physicians, op. cit.

228. Sirtori CR, Manzoni C, Lovati MR. Mechanisms of lipid-lowering agents. *Cardiology* 1991; 78:226-35.

229. D'Amico G, Gentile MG. Pharmacological and dietary treatment of lipid abnormalities in nephrotic patients. *Kidney International* 1991; 39 (Suppl. 31):S-65-9.

230. Babiy AV, Gebicki JM, Sullivan DR, Willey K. Increased oxidizability of plasma lipoproteins in diabetic patients can be decreased by probucol therapy and is not due to glycation. *Biochemical Pharmacology* 1992; 43:995-1000.

231. Lane JT, Subbaiah PV, Otto ME, Bagdade JD. Lipoprotein composition and HDL particle size distribution in women with non-insulin-dependent diabetes mellitus and the effects of probucol treatment. *Journal of Laboratory and Clinical Medicine* 1991; 118:120-8.

232. *The Medical Letter on Drugs and Therapeutics*, 1991, op. cit., p. 1-4.

233. Pierce, op. cit.

234. Illingworth DR. Clinical implications of new drugs for lowering plasma cholesterol concentrations. *Drugs* 1991; 41:151-60.

235. McTavish D, Sorkin EM. Pravastatin: a review of its pharmacological properties and therapeutic potential in hypercholesterolaemia. *Drugs* 1991; 42:65-89.

236. *The Medical Letter on Drugs and Therapeutics*, 1991, op. cit., p. 18-20.

237. McTavish, op. cit.

238. American College of Physicians, op. cit.

239. *Manual of Medical Therapeutics*, op. cit., p. 422.

240. American Society of Hospital Pharmacists, op. cit., p. 955-61.

241. Frank MJ, Watkins LO, Prisant LM, Smith MS, Russell SL, Abdulla AM, Manwaring RL. Mexiletine versus quinidine as first-line antiarrhythmia therapy: results from consecutive trials. *Journal of Clinical Pharmacology* 1991; 31:222-8.

242. Dukes MNG, Beeley L. *Side Effects of Drugs Annual 15*, Amsterdam: Elsevier, 1991:178-80.

243. Podrid PJ, Kowey PR, Frishman WH, Arnold RJG, Kaniecki DJ, Beck JR, Beshansky JR. Comparative cost-effectiveness analysis of quinidine, procainamide and mexiletine. *The American Journal of Cardiology* 1991; 68:1662-7.

244. Frank, op. cit.

245. Dukes, 1991, op. cit.

246. Widerhorn J, Sager PT, Rahimtoola SH, Bhandari AK. The role of combination therapy with mexiletine and procainamide in patients with inducible sustained ventricular tachycardia refractory to intravenous procainamide (abstract). *PACE* 1991; 14:420.

247. Gottlieb SS, Weinberg M. Comparative hemodynamic effects of mexiletine and quinidine in patients with severe left ventricular dysfunction (abstract). *American Heart Journal* 1991; 122:1368.

248. Dukes, 1991, op. cit.

249. Olin BR, ed. *Facts and Comparisons*. St. Louis: J.B. Lippincott Co., September 1992: 610-3.

250. Hurwitz A, Vacek JL, Botteron GW, Sztern MI, Hughes EM, Jayaraj A. Mexiletine effects on theophylline disposition. *Clinical Pharmacology and Therapeutics* 1991; 50:299-307.

251. Stoysich AM, Mohiuddin SM, Destache CJ, Nipper HC, Hilleman DE. Influence of mexiletine on the pharmacokinetics of theophylline in healthy volunteers. *Journal of Clinical Pharmacology* 1991; 31:354-7.

252. Ueno K, Miyai K, Kato M, Kawaguchi Y, Suzuki T. Mechanism of interaction between theophylline and mexiletine. *DICP, The Annals of Pharmacotherapy* 1991; 25:727-30.

253. *The Medical Letter on Drugs and Therapeutics*, 1984, op. cit., p. 116.

254. Orland, op. cit., p. 89-104.

255. *The Medical Letter on Drugs and Therapeutics*, 1984, op. cit., p. 116.

256. Kastrup, op. cit., p.160-70.

257. *The Medical Letter on Drugs and Therapeutics*. New York: The Medical Letter, Inc., 1977; 19:1.

258. Gilman, 1985, op. cit., p. 793.

259. Orland, op. cit., p. 57-69.

260. Kastrup, op. cit., p. 160-170.

261. *Drugs for the Elderly*, op. cit.

262. Wasnich, op. cit.

263. *The Medical Letter on Drugs and Therapeutics*, 1991, op. cit., p. 33-8.

264. Burton, op. cit.

265. *Drugs for the Elderly*, op. cit.

266. Wasnich, op. cit.

267. *The Medical Letter on Drugs and Therapeutics*, 1991, op. cit., p. 33-8.

268. Burton, op. cit.

269. Vestal, op. cit., p. 77-88.

270. Ibid.

271. Nygaard, op. cit.

272. Illingworth, op. cit.

273. *The Medical Letter on Drugs and Therapeutics.* New York, The Medical Letter, Inc. 1992; 34:57-8.

274. Pierce, op. cit.

275. Illingworth, op. cit.

276. McTavish, op. cit.

277. *The Medical Letter on Drugs and Therapeutics*, 1991, op. cit., p. 18-20.

278. McTavish, op. cit.

279. American College of Physicians, op. cit.

280. *The Medical Letter on Drugs and Therapeutics*, 1991, op. cit., p. 18-20.

281. AMA, 1983, op. cit., p. 637.

282. Vestal, op. cit., p. 66.

283. Nygaard, op. cit.

284. AMA, 1983, op. cit., p. 638.

285. Gilman, 1985, op. cit., p. 209.

286. Vestal, op. cit., p. 40.

287. Wasnich, op. cit.

288. *The Medical Letter on Drugs and Therapeutics*, 1991, op. cit., p. 33-8.

289. Burton, op. cit.

290. Gilman, 1985, op. cit., p. 209.

291. Wasnich, op. cit.

292. *The Medical Letter on Drugs and Therapeutics*, 1991, op. cit., p. 33-8.

293. Burton, op. cit.

294. Wasnich, op. cit.

295. *The Medical Letter on Drugs and Therapeutics*, 1991, op. cit., p. 33-8.

296. Burton, op. cit.

297. Confavreux C, Charles N, Aimard G. Fulminant myasthenia gravis soon after initiation of acebutolol therapy. *Europeon Neuorology* 1990; 30:279-81.

298. Ibid.

299. Gilman, 1985, op. cit., p. 209.

300. Orland, op. cit., p. 89-104.

301. Wasnich, op. cit.

302. *The Medical Letter on Drugs and Therapeutics*, 1991, op. cit., p. 33-8.

303. Burton, op. cit.

304. Gilman, 1985, op. cit., p. 209.

305. Wasnich, op. cit.

306. *The Medical Letter on Drugs and Therapeutics*, 1991, op. cit., p. 33-8.

307. Burton, op. cit.

308. Olin, op. cit., p. 738.

309. McEntee WJ, Crook T, Jenkyn LR, Petrie W, Larrabee GJ, Coffey DJ. Treatment of age-associated memory impairment with guanfacine. *Psychopharmacology Bulletin* 1991; 27:41-6.

310. Wilson MF, Blackshear J, Parsons OA, Lovallo WR, Mathur P. Antihypertensive efficacy of guanfacine and methyldopa in patients with mild to moderate essential hypertension. *Journal of Clinical Pharmacology* 1991; 31:318-26.

311. Mosqueda-Garcia R. Guanfacine: a second generation alpha 2-adrenergic blocker. *The American Journal of the Medical Sciences* 1990; 299:73-6.

312. Oster JR, Epstein M. Use of centrally acting sympatholytic agents in the management of hypertension. *Archives of Internal Medicine* 1991; 151:1638-44.

313. Wasnich, op. cit.

314. *The Medical Letter on Drugs and Therapeutics*, 1991, op. cit., p. 33-8.

315. Burton, op. cit.

316. Oster, op. cit.

317. O'Byrne S, Feely J. Effects of drugs on glucose tolerance in non-insulin-dependent diabetics (part I). *Drugs* 1990; 40:6-18.

318. Oster, op. cit.

319. Ibid.

320. San L, Cami J, Peri JM, Mata R, Porta M. Efficacy of clonidine, guanfacine and methadone in the rapid detoxification of heroin addicts: a controlled clinical trial. *British Journal of Addiction* 1990; 85:141-7.

321. Levin, op. cit.

322. Mosqueda-Garcia, op. cit.

323. Oster, op. cit.

324. Vestal, op. cit., p. 40.

325. Wasnich, op. cit.

326. *The Medical Letter on Drugs and Therapeutics*, 1991, op. cit., p. 33-8.

327. Burton, op. cit.

328. Wasnich, op. cit.

329. *The Medical Letter on Drugs and Therapeutics*, 1991, op. cit., p. 33-8.

330. Burton, op. cit.

331. Roden DM, Woosley RL. Drug therapy tocainide. *New England Journal of Medicine* 1986; 315:41.

332. *The Medical Letter on Drugs and Therapeutics*. New York: The Medical Letter Inc., 1985; 27:10.

333. Nygaard, op. cit.

334. *The Medical Letter on Drugs and Therapeutics*. New York: The Medical Letter Inc., 1984; 26:85.

335. Clark JA, Zimmerman HJ, Tanner LA. Labetalol hepatotoxicity. *Annals of Internal Medicine* 1990; 113:210-13.

336. Wasnich, op. cit.

337. *The Medical Letter on Drugs and Therapeutics*, 1991, op. cit., p. 33-8.

338. Burton, op. cit.

339. *The Medical Letter on Drugs and Therapeutics,* 1984, op. cit., p. 103.

340. Mass RD, Venook AP, Linker CA. Pentoxiphylline and aplastic anemia. *Annals of Internal Medicine* 1987; 107:428.

341. *Pharmacy and Therapeutics Forum* 1987:4.

342. AMA, 1983, op. cit., p. 678-9.

343. Gilman, 1985, op. cit., p. 823.

344. AMA, 1983, op. cit., p. 678-9.

345. Wasnich, op. cit.

346. *The Medical Letter on Drugs and Therapeutics,* 1991, op. cit., p. 33-8.

347. Burton, op. cit.

348. Wasnich, op. cit.

349. *The Medical Letter on Drugs and Therapeutics,* 1991, op. cit., p. 33-8.

350 Burton, op. cit.

351. Gilman, 1985, op. cit., p. 792.

Mind Drugs:
Tranquilizers and Sleeping Pills, Antipsychotics and Antidepressants

Tranquilizers and Sleeping Pills

Tranquilizers and Sleeping Pills: Two Other Groups of Dangerously Overprescribed Drugs for Older Adults

Tranquilizers (minor tranquilizers or antianxiety pills) and sleeping pills are discussed together because the most commonly used drugs in both classes belong to the same family of chemicals, called *benzodiazepines*.

In 1986, more than 86% of prescriptions filled in retail drugstores for minor tranquilizers or antianxiety pills, were for *benzodiazepines* such as Valium (diazepam), Librium (chlordiazepoxide), Xanax (alprazolam), and Tranxene (clorazepate). Similarly, about 75% of prescriptions for sleeping pills were for *benzodiazepines* such as Dalmane (flurazepam), Restoril (temazepam), or Halcion (triazolam).[1] In addition, many of the tranquilizers, such as Valium, are used as sleeping pills.

Because older adults have a much more difficult time clearing benzodiazepines and similar drugs from their bodies and are more sensitive to the effects of many of these drugs than are younger adults, there are significantly increased risks of serious adverse drug effects. These include: unsteady gait; dizziness; falling, causing an increased risk of hip fractures; increased risk of an injurious auto accident; drug-induced or drug-worsened impairment of thinking; memory loss; and addiction.

Despite these significantly increased risks to older adults, sleeping pills and minor tranquilizers are prescribed much more often than they are for younger adults, for much longer periods of time, and usually not at the reduced dose that could decrease the risks.

Other commonly used sleeping pills or tranquilizers include the following:
❑ Buspirone (*BuSpar*)
❑ Barbiturates: According to the World Health Organization, these drugs should never be used by older adults.[2] (The exception is phenobarbital for the treatment of convulsions or seizures.)
❑ Meprobamate (*Miltown, Equanil*)
❑ Hydroxyzine (*Atarax, Vistaril*) as a sleeping pill or tranquilizer
❑ Glutethimide (*Doriden*)
❑ Chloral hydrate
❑ Methyprylon (*Noludar*)
❑ Diphenhydramine (*Benadryl*)

How Often Are These Drugs Prescribed For Older Adults?

Minor Tranquilizers

Three surveys have determined what percentage of noninstitutionalized older adults use minor tranquilizers. Although one is regional (the west coast of Florida), one is statewide (Tennessee), and one is national, they came up with remarkably similar findings on overall minor tranquilizer use:

❑ In Florida, 15.6% of people 65 and older had used minor tranquilizers during the year the study was done. Of these, 39% had used them daily and 78% had used the pills for more than a year.[3]
❑ In Tennessee, 21% of Medicaid patients 65 and older living in the community had used minor tranquilizers during the year of the study.[4]
❑ A national study found that 16.9% of people 65 and older had used a minor tranquilizer during the previous year, and that 5.2% of all people 65 and older had used minor tranquilizers daily for at least a year.[5]

If we apply the national figure of 16.9% users (which falls between the other two) to the entire U.S. population 65 and over (28.53 million people in 1985),[6] there are 4.82 million people 65 and older using minor tranquilizers. **One and a half million people are using these drugs every day for at least a year.**

One of the most striking findings of the

national study was that a much larger proportion of older tranquilizer-users (30%) were using the drugs on a long-term (longer than one year) daily basis than were users in the younger age groups (14% of people age 35-49 using tranquilizers used them daily for one year or more). The authors of the study attribute this finding to more physical health problems in older people. They said, however, that this does not "necessarily justify the long-term duration of use."[7]

This seriously understates a major public health problem: *Even though 1.5 million older adults (65 and older) use minor tranquilizers daily for at least one year continuously, there is no evidence that any of these drugs are effective for more than four months.* **Furthermore, most, if not all, people using these drugs for more than several months become addicted. Therefore, drug-induced falls, impairment of memory and thinking, and other adverse effects, especially in older adults, also occur with these drugs that have no proven long-term benefits.** (See later sections for more information on benefits and risks.)

In 1985, for example, patients 60 and older filled approximately 21.3 million prescriptions for benzodiazepine minor tranquilizers (Valium, Librium, Tranxene, Serax, Centrax, Paxipam, Ativan, and Xanax) in retail pharmacies. Since the number of people 60 and over using benzodiazepine minor tranquilizers is approximately 5.8 million (39.53 million people 60 and over, 16.9% using minor tranquilizers of which 86% are benzodiazepines, assuming that the rate of use in people 60 to 64 is the same as in the 65 and older group), this means that **the average person 60 and older who used benzodiazepine tranquilizers filled more than three prescriptions a year.** This totals approximately 160 pills a year, enough for one month's to five months' use.[8]

Older people are clearly being "tranquilized" far more frequently than younger adults. Whereas people 60 and older make up 16.5% of the U.S. population, 35.7% of the prescriptions for minor tranquilizers are for people in this age group.[9]

Sleeping Pills

Two of the studies mentioned above reported on prescription sleeping pill use among the elderly and again came to the same conclusions about the extraordinary rate of use.

In Florida, 6.3% of people 65 years or older used sleeping pills during the year of the study. Of these users, 32% took them daily, almost 90% of these daily users had been using the drugs for a year or longer. Thus, 1.77% of all people 65 or older had been taking sleeping pills daily for at least a year.[10]

The study in Tennessee found that 5% of noninstitutionalized people 65 to 84 years of age had used a sleeping pill in the past year, agreeing closely with the 6.3% rate of use in Florida.[11]

Again applying these findings on a national basis, if 6.3% of all those 65 or older are using sleeping pills, this amounts to 1.76 million prescription sleeping-pill users, including 496,000 who have been using these pills daily for at least a year. An even larger number has been using sleeping pills daily for at least one month, based on the Florida findings. **Thus, it is estimated that more than half a million people 65 or older are using prescription sleeping pills for one month or longer, although there is no evidence that these drugs are effective for more than two to four weeks at the longest.**[12,13]

The use of these medications in institutions is even higher: 16% of patients 65 to 84 years old in Tennessee nursing homes received sleeping pills.[14] In another nursing home study,[15] 25.2% received them, and the percentage of older adults on sleeping pills in the hospital is even higher.

A study in the prestigious New York Hospital, of Cornell Medical School, found that 46% of patients on the medical wards had prescriptions written specifically for sleep, and that 31% actually were given a dose at least once during their hospitalization. On the surgical service an even larger percentage, 96% of patients, not varying according to age, had prescriptions written, and 88% actually were given the drugs.[16]

In short, although people 60 and older make up one-sixth (16.6%) of the population, they are prescribed more than one-half (51%) of the sleeping medications. Most of these (75%) are the benzodiazepine sleeping pills such as Dalmane, Halcion, and Restoril.[17]

How Much Use Is Justified in View of the Significant Risks?

Minor Tranquilizers

Although minor tranquilizers are prescribed more often and for longer periods of time for older adults than for younger adults, studies have shown that, if anything, older adults have lower levels of "psychic distress" or serious "life crisis" than younger adults. Worse yet, since older adults usually take more prescription drugs for the direct treatment of physical diseases, the prescribing of tranquilizers is all the more dangerous because of possibly dangerous interactions.

In 1979, Roche, maker of Valium, Librium, and Dalmane, sent doctors brochures encouraging the use of Valium for older adults as "an important component of treatment programs for the relief of excessive geriatric anxiety and psychic tension."[18]

Faced with falling sales of Valium, the early 1980s saw Roche (and other drug makers, in order to widen their market shares) escalate the war on older adults. A series of handsomely illustrated brochures entitled "Roche Seminars on Aging," was mailed to doctors in 1982. Roche recommended Valium as appropriate for the elderly with "limited" coping skills, facing "not only the constraints brought about by their own reduced capabilities, but also those imposed by the social structure and environment."

The campaign worked because the rate of use of minor tranquilizers in people 60 and over increased significantly between 1980 and 1985, especially in older women.[19]

The fact that 1.5 million people 65 and older use minor tranquilizers daily for at least a year is the best evidence that they are being overprescribed.[20] Given that there is no evidence that any of these drugs are effective for more than four months, the number of older adults whose use of these drugs exceeds four months is even greater. As mentioned above, **the average number of pills, 160, that each of the 10 million minor tranquilizer users 60 and over gets per year, is enough for one to five months of use.**

In a discussion about the use of tranquilizers and sleeping pills by older adults, World Health Organization (WHO) experts said the following:

"Anxiety is a normal response to stress and only when it is severe and disabling should it lead to drug treatment. Long-term treatment . . . is rarely effective and should be avoided . . . . Short-term use (less than two weeks) will minimize the risk of dependence."

They concluded by saying that *"discussion of the problems of sleeplessness and anxiety and the drawbacks of drug therapy will often help the patient to come to terms with his or her problem without the need to resort to drugs."*[21]

Two studies on alternatives to the use of minor tranquilizers, applying the WHO ideas further, highlight how much of the present use is unnecessary. Ninety patients, mainly suffering from anxiety, were randomly divided into two groups when they went to see their family doctors. The first group was given the usual dose of one of the benzodiazepine tranquilizers. The other group was given a small dose of a much safer treatment consisting solely of "listening, explanation, advice, and reassurance." The two treatments were equally effective in relieving the anxiety, but those receiving the informal counselling were more satisfied with their treatment than those given minor tranquilizers.[22]

In a second study, patients with anxiety were either given one of three different tranquilizers or a placebo (sugar pill). At the end of a month, with weekly evaluations of their anxiety levels being made by the patients themselves and by professional evaluators, the results showed "all four treatments to be efficacious in their therapeutic effects on relieving anxiety."[23] That is, placebos worked as well as tranquilizers.

Sleeping Pills

As seen with minor tranquilizers, the clearest evidence that there is dangerous overprescribing and misprescribing of sleeping medications to older adults comes from the estimated one-half million people who have been taking these drugs daily for at least a month. Since there is no evidence of effectiveness for longer than this period of time, all of these people are getting the full risks of these drugs without the benefits.

In addition, as discussed above, the average number of benzodiazepine sleeping pills obtained per user is enough for five months, five to ten times longer than the drugs have been shown to be effective. Conservatively then, 80 to 90% of the use of these pills is a dangerous waste.

The increases in the use of these drugs by older adults, noted above, flies strongly in the face of the conclusions and recommendations of an exhaustive study by the National Academy of Sciences' Institute of Medicine in 1979.[24]

Speaking generally about the use of these drugs, the study concluded that:

"hypnotics (sleeping medications) should have only a limited place in contemporary medical practice: it is difficult to justify much of the current prescribing of sleeping medication. As a standard of prudent ambulatory medical care, the committee favors the prescription of only very limited numbers of sleeping pills for use for a few

nights at a time. . . . Hypnotic drugs should be selected carefully and prescribed cautiously, if at all, for patients . . . who are old."

Commenting specifically on sleeping pill use by older adults, the authors said:

"Of particular concern is the regular and prolonged use by this group of sleep-inducing medications that are of dubious value, and that add new hazards to their already complicated drug intake regimens."

Although older people tend to complain more than younger people about sleeping problems, the study found that the time it takes to fall asleep does not increase with age, and that the **total sleep time decreases very little, if at all. Older people who go to bed early and take cat naps during the daytime often do have sleeping problems. But, the study concluded, "it is this pattern of daytime sleep that must be changed instead of treating the night time insomnia that results from it."**

According to Dr. Marshall Folstein, a Johns Hopkins psychiatrist and expert in Alzheimer's disease, *"it is extraordinarily rare to find an older person who actually requires them [sleeping pills]."*[25]

A further threat is posed by high doses. A recent study of sleeping pill dose and age found that a majority (almost 80%) of people 65 and over were using the "overdose" amount of 30 milligrams a night of Dalmane even though 15 milligrams is recommended for older adults. (In this book we list Dalmane as a "Do Not Use" drug.) In view of the limited use of these drugs recommended by the National Academy of Sciences, the current and increasing prescribing of sleeping medications for older adults — especially the extensive prolonged-use patterns discussed above — poses a serious threat to their health.

What Are the Main Risks of Sleeping Pills and Tranquilizers?

Addiction, daytime sedation, confusion, memory loss, increased risk of an injurious auto accident, poor coordination causing falls and hip fractures, impaired learning ability, slurred speech, and even death are adverse effects of these drugs. They are more likely to occur when these drugs are taken in combination with alcohol or other depressant drugs. They can happen to anyone at any age.

Older adults, however, cannot clear many of these drugs from their systems as rapidly as younger people can. They are also more sensitive to the drugs' adverse effects. Despite this evidence, older adults (1) are more likely to be given a prescription for tranquilizers or sleeping pills, (2) are not usually given the reduced dose that would at least diminish the odds of serious adverse effects, and (3) are prescribed these drugs for longer periods of time than are younger people. Therefore, it is not surprising that older adults are at much greater risk of suffering from adverse effects, and, when they occur, they are much more serious.

One of the biggest impediments to discovering and eliminating these drug-induced problems is their frequent attribution to the aging process instead of to the drugs. The onset of impaired intelligence with memory loss, confusion, or impaired learning, or the onset of loss of coordination in a younger person will more likely prompt an inquiry leading to the drug as culprit. But the same symptoms in an older person, especially if they develop more slowly, are often dismissed with a familiar remark, "Well, he (or she) is just growing old, what do you expect?" This lack of suspicion allows the drug to keep doing damage because the doctor keeps up the prescription.

Hip Fractures

A study of 1,021 older adults with hip fractures found that 14% of these life-threatening injuries are attributable to the use of mind-affecting drugs, including sleeping pills and minor tranquilizers, antipsychotics, and antidepressants.[26]

There are approximately 227,000 hip fractures each year in the United States, virtually all in older adults.[27] Since the above study found that 14% of hip fractures are drug-induced, this means that if the results of the study are projected nationally, approximately **32,000 hip fractures a year in older adults are caused by the use of mind-affecting drugs.** Of these, about 30%, or almost 10,000 hip fractures a year, are caused by sleeping pills and minor tranquilizers, particularly the long-acting drugs such as Valium, Librium, and Dalmane.

Another study on fractures in older adults found that the increased occurrence of falls resulting in such fractures could often be reduced by removing the offending drug.[28]

Injurious Automobile Crashes

A recent study involving 495 automobile crashes in older drivers in which an injury occurred found that a significant number of such crashes in older adults aged 65-84 were attributable to the use of benzodiazepine tranquilizers and cyclic antidepressants. The study was particularly impressive because its findings were strengthened by observing that the rate of injurious crashes increased in the same group of people when they were using these drugs as opposed to when they were not using the drugs. The majority of the excess number of injurious auto crashes were attributable to the benzodiazepines. The authors, stating that the study findings may be generalizable to the population at large, found that if the association is causal, **at least 16,000 injurious auto crashes each year in older drivers are attributable to psychoactive drug use (specifically benzodiazepines and tricyclic antidepressants)** out of the 217,000 injurious crashes that occur each year among elderly drivers.[29]

Drug-induced or Drug-worsened Senility (Decreased Mental Functioning)

Drug-induced impairment of thinking is one of the most reversible, or treatable, forms of dementia. It is a by-product of the increased use of drugs during the past few decades. Among the 28.5 million people 65 and over in the United States,[30] approximately five out of every hundred have dementia, with an estimated one of these five due to "reversible" conditions such as treatable diseases (thyroid disease, for example) or adverse effects of drugs.[31]

A study of 308 older adults with significant intellectual impairment found that in 11.4% of these people the problem was caused or worsened by a drug.[32] This study, the first to ever systematically analyze this problem, revealed that after stopping the use of the dementia-causing drugs, all persons had long-term improvement of their mental function. The most common class of drugs to cause the impairment of mental function was the sleeping pill/tranquilizer group. It accounted for 46% of the drug-induced or drug-worsened dementia.

The University of Washington researchers who did the study had two further observations:

1. *"Most patients had used these drugs for years, and the side effect of cognitive (mental) impairment developed insidiously as a 'late' complication of a drug begun at an earlier age.*
2. *The improvement experienced by patients in this study was usually surprising to family and caregivers. The patients noted an improved sense of wellbeing and were better able to care for themselves."*

If these important findings are applied to all of the estimated 1.43 million Americans 65 and over who have dementia, there are 163,000 people whose mental impairment has either been entirely caused by or worsened by drugs. **For approximately 75,000 older adults, their worsened mental functioning is caused by sleeping pills or minor tranquilizers.**

Addiction

By addiction we mean the regular use of a substance for a long enough period of time so that, upon stopping the use, especially stopping suddenly, the person develops physical signs and symptoms of withdrawal. These physical problems include sweating, nervousness or, when more severe, hallucinations or seizures which are often accompanied by psychological addiction.

The myth used to be that only people who were prone to addiction, as judged by a prior history of alcoholism or other drug problems, would possibly become addicted to benzodiazepine tranquilizers or sleeping pills. What is more, said the drugmakers to the doctors, even then you had to use very large doses of these drugs for a long period of time before addiction could occur.

This attitude, intended to cover up a major national problem, was "pushed" by the president of Hoffman-La Roche, the world's biggest benzodiazepine-maker (Valium, Librium, and Dalmane). Testifying in 1979 before U.S. Senate hearings on the abuse of these drugs, President Robert Clark said that "true addiction is probably exceedingly unusual and, when it occurs, is probably confined to those individuals with abuse-prone personalities who ingest very large amounts."[33]

It was then quite clear and is now even clearer that a large fraction, probably the overwhelming majority, of people who use any of the benzodiazepines at the recommended dose for more than one or two months will become addicted.

Another study showed that a large proportion of people became addicted to these drugs and experienced an unpleasant withdrawal syndrome when they suddenly stopped taking the drug (as opposed to gradually tapering the dose to reduce, if not eliminate, the withdrawal symptoms). The only difference between addiction to the longer-acting drugs such as Valium and Dalmane, and the shorter-acting drugs such as Ativan and Serax was the time, after the drug was suddenly stopped, that it took before withdrawal symptoms occurred. With the longer-acting drugs the day of worst symptoms was the tenth; for the shorter-acting drugs it was the first. Withdrawal symptoms included anxiety, headache, insomnia, tension, sweating, difficulty concentrating, tremor, fear, and fatigue.

The authors concluded that "when withdrawal was abrupt, symptoms were more frequent and more severe than when a gradual tapering technique was used. . . . there is little justification for abrupt withdrawal."[34]

Using the estimates cited earlier in this chapter concerning long-term use, **the majority of the 2 million older adults in this country who regularly use these pills have become addicted to benzodiazepine tranquilizers and sleeping pills,** thanks to their doctors and the drug industry.

Serious Breathing Problems

Another serious adverse effect of the benzodiazepines is their effect on respiration, which occurs in two different ways. The first has to do with *sleep apnea*, a common condition in older adults in which, for varying periods of time while asleep, breathing stops. Dr. William Dement, an expert in sleep research, has found that older people with sleep apnea who use sleeping medications can stop breathing for much longer — dangerously longer — periods of time as a result of the respiration-suppressing effects of the drugs. He told a government task force on sleeping problems that people over 65 should not use Dalmane because of the risk of worsening sleep apnea.[35]

A second problem in this category is in people with *severe lung disease*. Anyone with severe lung disease should not use benzodiazepines because they decrease the urge to breathe, which can be life-threatening.[36] **Asthmatics should also avoid benzodiazepine sleeping pills and tranquilizers.**

Other Adverse Effects[37]

Frequent: drowsiness and lack of coordination that can affect walking or driving a car.

Occasional: confusion, forgetfulness, excitement instead of sedation, rebound insomnia (more difficulty sleeping) when the drug wears off), or, especially with Halcion (triazolam), excitement instead of sedation.

Rare: low blood pressure, bone marrow toxicity, liver disease, allergies and rage reactions.

Reducing the Risks from Sleeping Pills and Tranquilizers

The best way to reduce the risks of these powerful drugs is not to use them for most of the conditions for which they are now being used, especially in older adults.

Alternatives for Anxiety

According to noted British psychiatrist, Dr. Malcolm Lader:

"Until recently most anxious patients in the United Kingdom were treated with tranquillizers, usually a benzodiazepine. However, recognition that these drugs can cause dependence even at normal therapeutic dosages has led to a re-evaluation of drug therapy, and the value of non-pharmacologic treatments is increasingly being recognized."[38]

Two British doctors use a nondrug alternative for the treatment of mild to moderate anxiety (and similar problems). They say that *"the best treatment is likely to be brief counselling provided by the general practitioner or by another professional working in the practice. Such counselling need not be intensive or specially skilled. It should always include careful assessment of the causes of the patient's distress. Once these have been identified, anxiety may often be reduced to tolerable levels by means of explanation, exploration of feelings, reassurance, and encouragement."*[39]

What else can be done? Talking to nonmedical people — a friend, a spouse, a relative, a member of the clergy, may help to identify causes of anxiety and potential solutions, as well as allow for sharing of feelings and reassurance. Gathering the courage to talk about difficult concerns will generally be a better solution than taking pills. Getting regular exercise can also help relieve anxiety.

In addition, the use of foods, beverages, and over-the-counter (nonprescription) or prescription drugs that have significant stimulant effects can also cause a chemically-induced anxiety that can be remedied. (See the list of such substances below, under alternatives for sleeping problems.)

Alternatives for Sleeping Problems

Experts in sleep and aging have recently stated that:

- ❑ *Many old people have exaggerated expectations of what sleep should be like and they "spend too much time in bed chasing sleep";*
- ❑ *Many older people use sleep as an escape from boredom;*
- ❑ *"It's extraordinarily rare to find an old person who actually requires [sleeping pills]."* [40]

If the cause of the sleeping problem is depression (see p. 215 for other problems that go along with depression), the depression should be addressed instead of using sleeping medication to treat its symptoms. If the cause is a medical condition with pain as one of the components, the pain has to be treated rather than using a sleeping pill to induce sleep despite the pain. In the case of senile brain disease, such as Alzheimer's, the sleep disturbance will probably not respond to sleeping medications.[41]

Other causes of sleeping problems that can also be "treated" without using drugs include the following:

- ❑ Daytime napping or going to bed too early.
- ❑ Inaccurate idea of how much sleep you require each night. If you do not feel tired during the day, you had enough sleep the night before.
- ❑ Environmental factors such as light and noise. A quieter, darker room may promote a more restful sleep.

- ❑ Drinking stimulants — coffee, tea, or cola beverages — or eating chocolate within 8 hours of when you want to sleep.
- ❑ Lack of a nighttime routine. A warm bath, a pleasant book, a light but bland snack, no working just before going to bed or while in bed are ways to encourage sleep.

Drugs can produce stimulating effects and a chemically-induced anxiety:

- ❑ *Over-the-counter (nonprescription) drugs:* sleeplessness can be caused by caffeine, found in Anacin and other drugs; PPA (phenylpropanolamine), the stimulants found in Actifed, Contac, Sudafed and other decongestant products; and the ingredients in many asthma drugs.
- ❑ *Prescription drugs* — asthma drugs containing theophylline or aminophylline such as Amoline and Bronkodyl; amphetamines such as Benzidrine and diet pills; steroids such as cortisone and prednisone; thyroid drugs; and the withdrawal from the use of sleeping pills, tranquilizers, and antidepressants. (See p. 29 in Chapter 2 for a list of drugs that can cause insomnia.)

If you have a sleeping problem and use one of these drugs, or if the problem began when you started using another drug, talk to your doctor. Tell him or her all the drugs (over-the-counter and prescription) you are taking. It might be possible to change the drug or lower the dosage to help you sleep. Returning to sleeping pills to get past withdrawal effects will only place you in a vicious cycle.

Which Tranquilizers or Sleeping Pills Should You Use, If Any?

Although we strongly discourage the use of these drugs in most situations, especially for older adults, there are some perfectly competent physicians who, in very well-defined circumstances and for very short periods of time, will prescribe them. **But even the labeling approved by the Food and Drug Administration for all of the** tranquilizers has to state, "Anxiety or tension associated with the stress of everyday life usually does not require treatment with an anxiolytic [tranquilizer]."[42] (See the seven rules for safer use, below.)

As mentioned at the beginning of this chapter, **older adults should never use barbiturates as sleeping pills or tranquilizers.** Other drugs such as meprobamate (Miltown, Equanil), hydroxyzine (Vistaril, Atarax) for sleep, glutethimide (Doriden), chloral hydrate and methyprylon (Noludar) should also not be used.[43]

This leaves buspirone (BuSpar, see p. 224) and the benzodiazepines, with the possibly bewildering list of eight benzodiazepine drugs marketed primarily as tranquilizers and five as sleeping pills. All of these drugs are equally effective in tranquilizing or promoting sleep. "Calling some anti-anxiety drugs and others hypnotics (sleeping pills) has more to do with marketing than with pharmacology."[44]

These 13 benzodiazepine drugs are different from each other, and the difference has to do with the different ways in

which they are dangerous for older adults. WHO specifically recommends that older adults should not use the most widely prescribed sleeping pill, Dalmane (flurazepam), "owing to a high incidence of adverse effects."[45]

Seven other benzodiazepines are also more slowly cleared out of the body, especially in older adults, and can therefore accumulate, leading to increased risks. These drugs, which also should be avoided by older adults, include Valium (diazepam), Librium (chlordiazepoxide), Tranxene (chlorazepate), Centrax (prazepam), Paxipam (halazepam), Doral (quazepam) and Prosom (estazolam).

Another widely used sleeping pill, Halcion (triazolam), should also be avoided by older adults because it is so short-acting that it can cause rebound insomnia (increased sleeping problems when the drug effect has worn off), anxiety, serious amnesia (forgetfulness or memory loss) and violent, aggressive behavior. In 1992, Public Citizen's Health Research Group petitioned the Food and Drug Administration to ban Halcion. The new sleeping pill Prosom (estazolam) is in the same class as Halcion and, according to *The Medical Letter*, there is no reason to use it.[46] It also has the disadvantage of slow clearance from the body.

In a discussion of which of these drugs are best for older adults, it was stated that Serax (oxazepam) and Restoril (temazepam) were the drugs of choice.[47] But it has also been stated that **"oxazepam (Serax) may be the safest benzodiazepine for the older patient"** because **"oxazepam may offer the advantages of a short half-life and the absence of active metabolites"** (that is, chemicals the body converts the drug into which can also have adverse effects).[48] In addition, studies have shown that oxazepam has much less of a "street" drug abuse potential than, for example, diazepam (Valium).[49,50]

In a recent article on how 11 of these benzodiazepines compare with one another as far as memory loss, a serious problem especially in

---

We do not recommend the use of any benzodiazepines other than Oxazepam. Here is how the large proportion of older adults who are using these drugs to their physical and mental detriment can stop using them, more safely.

If you have been taking any of these drugs for longer than several weeks continuously, there is a good chance that you have become addicted. Stopping the drugs suddenly (going "cold turkey") is a bad idea. With the help of your doctor, work out a schedule for slowly tapering down the amount of tranquilizer or sleeping pill by an average of 5 to 10% each day. Keep a written record of the dosage reduction schedule with you. This will greatly reduce the difficulty of stopping the use of these drugs.

older adults, geriatric drug expert Dr. Peter Lamy stated that oxazepam had less memory impairment than all other benzodiazepines except chlorazepate,[51] a long-acting tranquilizer which should not be used by older adults for reasons mentioned above.

In summary, the only prescription tranquilizers or sleeping pills that we advise for use, albeit limited use, in the older adult are buspirone (BuSpar) and oxazepam, available generically, and under the brand name of Serax.

Rules for Safer Use of Oxazepam
(This is the only benzodiazepine we believe older adults should be prescribed.)

1. The dose should be one-third to one-half the dose for younger people.[52] This means that the highest starting dose for older adults should be 7.5 milligrams, 1 to 3 times a day, if used as a tranquilizer, or 7.5 milligrams at bedtime, if used as a sleeping pill. (This is 1/2 of a 15 milligram tablet, generically available.

2. Ask your doctor to limit the size of the prescription to seven days' worth of pills.

3. Ask your doctor to write *NO REFILL* on the prescription so that you will not be inclined (because of the "good chemical feelings" these pills may provide) to refill the prescription 5 times without seeing the doctor again. This dangerously lax refill policy is perfectly legal because oxazepam and other similar drugs are not very carefully controlled by the government. By urging your doctor to write *NO REFILL* you are making sure that he or she will reevaluate your condition after you use oxazepam for a short time. You want to discuss how you are doing with your anxiety or sleeping problem, rather than continuing to take the drug without a reevaluation. Continuing to take oxazepam without talking to your doctor could be the first step to addiction or other drug-induced problems.

4. At the end of the first day, and every day you use oxazepam, evaluate what you have done, on your own or by talking to others, to find out what is making you anxious. This includes evaluation of what you have done to alter the internal or external circumstances causing your anxiety. Keep a record of these evaluations. As soon as possible, try reducing the dose, in consultation with your doctor. Since you only have enough medication for one week, it is unlikely that you will have become addicted this quickly.

5. Do not drive a car or operate dangerous machinery while using oxazepam.

6. Do not drink alcohol. The combination of this drug with alcohol dangerously increases the effects of both. An overdose of oxazepam in combination with alcohol can be fatal.

7. Before using oxazepam, make sure that your doctor knows if you are taking other drugs with a sedative or "downer" effect, such as antidepressants, antipsychotics, antihistamines, narcotic painkillers, epilepsy medications, barbiturates, or other sleeping medications. Oxazepam taken with other drugs with sedative effects dangerously increases the risks of both.

Antipsychotic Drugs:
Another Group of Dangerously Overused Drugs for Older People

Antipsychotic drugs, also called neuroleptic drugs or major tranquilizers, are properly and successfully used to treat serious psychotic mental disorders, the most common of which is schizophrenia. Schizophrenia is a disease in which people have lost touch with reality, often see or hear things which are not there (hallucinations), believe things which are not true (delusions), often have severe problems with their mood such as being depressed, lose their expressiveness of feeling ("flat affect"), and in general, have disorders of thinking. Psychoses include other mental disorders which involve abnormal perceptions of reality such as hallucinations and delusions. Schizophrenia and the other psychoses are much less common in older adults than in younger adults, according to studies done by the National Institute of Mental Health.

Whereas about 1.12% of people aged 18 to 44 have been found to have active schizophrenia (symptoms in last six months) and 0.6% of 45- to 64-year-olds have this diagnosis, only 0.1% of people 65 and older are diagnosed as having active schizophrenia.[53] In other words, active schizophrenia is only one-fifth to one-tenth as common in older adults as in younger adults.

In younger adults, an alarming number of those with schizophrenia who could and often have previously benefited from antipsychotic drugs are not receiving them. They are seen, among other places, on the streets and in homeless shelters. In older adults, the problem is gross overuse by people who are not psychotic, not underuse.

Drugs That Can Cause Psychoses (Hallucinations) or Delirium

For anyone of any age who has recently become psychotic (has hallucinations, for example) or developed delirium, there should be careful questioning to see if this serious mental problem might have been drug-induced before the person is started on antipsychotic drugs. **In someone who is 60 years old or older, there is a strong likelihood that the recent onset of hallucinations, delirium, or other behavior which is like schizophrenia is due either to the effects of the drugs listed below or withdrawal from addiction to alcohol, barbiturates, or other sleeping pills or tranquilizers.** Commonly used drugs which cause psychotic symptoms such as hallucinations include the following:[54]

❑ Analgesics/Narcotics such as indomethacin (Indocin), ketamine (Ketalar), morphine (Roxanol), pentazocine (Talwin), propoxyphene (Darvon), and salicylates (aspirin)

❑ Antibiotics and other anti-infective agents such as acyclovir (Zovirax), amantadine (Symmetrel), amphotericin B (Fungizone), chloroquine (Aralen), cycloserine (Seromycin), dapsone, ethionamide (Trecator-SC), isoniazid (INH), nalidixic acid (NegGram), niridazole (Ambilhar), penicillin G, procaine, podophyllum, quinacrine (Atabrine), and thiabendazole (Mintezol)

❑ Anticonvulsants such as ethosuximide (Zarontin), phenytoin (Dilantin), and primidone (Mysoline)

❑ Allergy drugs such as antihistamines (Chlor-Trimetron, Dimetane, etc.)

❑ Antiparkinsonians such as carbidopa-levodopa (Sinemet), bromocriptine (Parlodel), and levodopa (Dopar)

❑ Asthma drugs such as albuterol (Proventil, Ventolin)

❑ Drugs for depression such as trazodone (Desyrel) and tricyclic antidepressants such as amitriptyline (Elavil) and doxepin (Adapin, Sinequan)

❏ Heart drugs such as digitalis preparations (Lanoxin, etc.), lidocaine (Xylocaine), procainamide (Pronestyl), and tocainide (Tonocard)

❏ High blood pressure drugs such as clonidine (Catapres), methyldopa (Aldomet), prazosin (Minipress), and propranolol (Inderal)

❏ Nasal decongestants such as ephedrine, oxymetazoline (Afrin and others), phenylephrine (Neo-Synephrine), and pseudoephedrine (Sudafed)

❏ Drugs such as amphetamines, PCP, barbiturates, cocaine, and crack

❏ Sedatives/Tranquilizers such as alprazolam (Xanax), diazepam (Valium), ethchlorvynol (Placidyl), and triazolam (Halcion)

❏ Other drugs such as atropine, aminocaproic acid (Amicar), baclofen (Lioresal), cimetidine (Tagamet), ranitidine (Zantac), corticosteroids, disulfiram (Antabuse), methylphenidate (Ritalin), methysergide (Sansert), metrizamide (Amipaque), phenelzine (Nardil), thyroid hormones, and vincristine (Oncovin)

How Often Are Antipsychotic Drugs Used in Older Adults?

Although schizophrenia, the most common justifiable use for antipsychotic drugs, is much less common in older adults than younger adults, in the community and especially in nursing homes, older adults are prescribed a dangerously excessive amount of these powerful drugs. This has resulted in hundreds of thousands of cases of severe, disabling, and often irreversible adverse reactions which should never have occurred. People under 60 get about four prescriptions a year per hundred people of the antipsychotic drugs. But people over 60, with much less schizophrenia and other psychoses, get more than 10 prescriptions per 100 people a year.[55]

A study of older adults (ages 65 to 84) on Medicaid found that about 5% of those in the community and 39% of those in nursing homes had received a prescription for antipsychotic drugs during the previous year.[56] An earlier study by the same researchers [57] found that 30.1% of Medicaid nursing home patients had received at least three months' worth of antipsychotic drugs during the year of the study.

Even if a more recent and lower estimate of the percentage of nursing home residents who are chronically prescribed antipsychotic drugs is used — 22.9% — this means that approximately 300,000 of the 1.3 million U.S. nursing home residents 65 and over (*Health: United States 1987*) take these drugs for at least three or four months continuously.[58] In addition, one-third of noninstitutionalized people getting these drugs are estimated to be using them for at least three or four months continuously,[59] adding another 450,000 older adults to the number of potential victims.[60] **Thus, an estimated 750,000 people 65 or older,** *not even including those older people in mental hospitals,* **are regularly using antipsychotic drugs, even though the total number of people 65 and over with schizophrenia (not in mental hospitals) is only approximately 92,000.**[61] **Thus, 92,000 of the 750,000 older adults regularly using antipsychotic drugs — less than one-eighth (12.3%) — actually have schizophrenia.** Put another way, over 80% of the use of antipsychotic drugs in older adults is unnecessary.

In addition to these 750,000 people over 65 chronically using antipsychotic drugs (although fewer than 100,000 are schizophrenic), there are more than one million additional people 65 and over in nursing homes and in the community getting prescriptions for antipsychotic drugs for less than three or four months continuously.[62] **Thus, a total of approximately 1.7 million people 65 and over get a prescription for an antipsychotic drug each year,** according to these estimates.

What Are These Antipsychotic Drugs Being Prescribed For, If Not for Schizophrenia and Other Psychoses?

A group of physicians and other health professionals who specialize in geriatric pharmacology have recently stated that:

"The usefulness of antipsychotic medications in nonpsychotic, elderly patients has been questioned. . . . The high frequency of toxic reactions to these drugs is well documented, with many older patients who take them experiencing orthostatic hypotension [low blood pressure on sitting or standing], Parkinson's syndrome, tardive dyskinesia (see p. 211), akathisia (see p. 212), worsened confusion, dry mouth, constipation, oversedation, and urinary incontinence." [63]

One of the more common purposes for which antipsychotic drugs are blatantly misused is as a sedative in nursing home patients.[64] Other unjustifiable uses include controlling the overall level of disturbance in older demented (nonpsychotic) patients,[65] and for treating chronic anxiety.[66] Two different studies concluded that often the most mentally alert and least physically disabled people are given these drugs.[67,68] This is consistent with the charge that these drugs are being used more for the convenience of the nursing home staff or other caretaker than for the needs of the patients.

Another study found that *"80% of elderly demented persons are receiving tranquilizers (antipsychotic drugs) unnecessarily."*[69] Other researchers concluded that antipsychotics are "frequently prescribed inappropriately as sedatives to elderly patients" and that "using these drugs incorrectly or for unnecessarily prolonged periods enhances the probability of developing this virtually untreatable, disfiguring syndrome" (referring to tardive dyskinesia).[70]

After finding that overall there were no significant benefits for antipsychotic drugs in elderly demented patients, one group of researchers concluded that "because of the apparently limited therapeutic efficacy of antipsychotic medication, it is especially important to search for possible social and environmental solutions for behavioural disturbances in this population."[71]

In other words, find out what it is in the environment that may be causing or contributing to the problems older people are having and change it, if possible, rather than endanger their health with these powerful drugs. A perfect example is the use of antipsychotic drugs at the end of the day to treat the so-called sundowner syndrome. As the end of the day approaches, some patients become agitated, restless, confused, and may wander about. A careful study of the characteristics of people with this problem found that they were much more likely than those without sundowner syndrome to have been in their present room for less than one month, to have come to the nursing home more recently, and to be awakened much more on the evening shift. The implication was that changes in the management of these patients by nurses and other staff could reduce the problem without resorting to the use of antipsychotic drugs.[72]

A recent review of the use of antipsychotic drugs in older adults confirmed that their most common use was to control agitation, wandering, belligerence, and sleeplessness. But this "disturbed" behavior is sometimes an appropriate response to changes in the environment or physical changes in the older adult. Treating the physical problem or changing the environment may lessen the need to resort to the antipsychotic drugs.[73]

A recent study of older adults found that in those for whom antipsychotic drugs were prescribed as treatment for depression there was an alarmingly high incidence of tardive dyskinesia (see p. 211) and the authors recommended that doctors "should be cautious in prescribing neuroleptic [antipsychotic] drugs for these patients." Thus, another important category of misprescribing of antipsychotic drugs in older adults — especially worrisome because of the high risk of serious adverse effects in this age group — is for depression, instead of, or in addition to antidepressants.[74]

Two other drugs — prochlorperazine (Compazine) and promethazine (Phenergan), which are from the same family as the antipsychotics (phenothiazines) — are mainly used for treating nonpsychotic (especially gastrointestinal) disorders and both are significantly overused. Discussions of their use appear on p. 343 and 361.

Benefits and Risks of Antipsychotic Drugs

For the small fraction of older adults taking antipsychotic drugs appropriately, that is for the treatment of psychotic illnesses such as schizophrenia, the significant risks are more than balanced out by the proven benefits for those people who respond. But at least 80% of the use of these drugs in older adults is inappropriate. Either the drugs are ineffective, as in the treatment of senile dementia, or unnecessary, as in their frequent uses to sedate or control nonpsychotic behavior that is often responsive to nondrug approaches.

Thus, well over 1 million older adults are being prescribed antipsychotic drugs, often for months or years continuously, for unjustified purposes, and they are suffering the consequences of risks without benefits.

What Are the Main Adverse Effects of Antipsychotic Drugs?
Falls and hip fractures

16,000 older adults a year suffer from drug-induced hip fractures, attributable to the use of antipsychotic drugs. In one study, the main category of drugs responsible for falls leading to hip fractures was antipsychotic drugs.[75] Fifty-two percent of those hip fractures attributable to the use of mind-affecting drugs were due to antipsychotic drug use. (Also, see chapter on minor tranquilizers and sleeping pills, p. 198.)

Nerve problems
Tardive dyskinesia

This is the most common, serious, and often irreversible adverse effect of antipsychotic drugs. It is characterized by involuntary movements of the lips, tongue, and sometimes the fingers, toes, and trunk.[76] Older adults are at increased risk for this adverse effect, and it may occur in as many as 40% of people over the age of 60 taking antipsychotic drugs.[77]

Tardive dyskinesia is more common and more severe in older adults. The majority of cases are irreversible and often result in immobility, difficulty chewing and swallowing, and eventually weight loss and dehydration. None of the antipsychotic drugs has a lower chance of causing this problem than others.[78]

In most studies of elderly patients, the incidence of tardive dyskinesia in people taking antipsychotic medications is between 30 and 35%. However, a recent study found that in those elderly patients who had never before been given an antipsychotic drug, the incidence of tardive dyskinesia was 60% in those patients given the drugs for depression, significantly higher than in older adults getting these drugs for other purposes.[79]

Another study estimated that there were 192,718 people in the United States who had developed tardive dyskinesia attributable to antipsychotic drugs.[80] Of these, 54,284 cases occurred in nursing homes. If 80% of these exposures to antipsychotic drugs were unnecessary, more than 43,000 people in nursing homes developed tardive dyskinesia unnecessarily because they should not have been given these drugs. An additional 112,854 people not in an institution also suffered from tardive dyskinesia induced by antipsychotic drugs. According to national drug prescribing data, approximately 33% of the prescriptions for the drugs were in people over the age of 60.[81] Thus, an additional 37,000 noninstitutionalized older adults appear to have developed tardive dyskinesia from these drugs. If the prescriptions for 80% of these people are unnecessary, another 30,000 cases of tardive dyskinesia which should have been avoided, have occurred. **Thus, there are approximately 73,000 cases of tardive dyskinesia, in older adults which are the result of poor prescribing practices by physicians.**

To date, no drug has been found to be effective in treating tardive dyskinesia, thus making its prevention extremely important.

Drug-induced parkinsonism

Drug-induced parkinsonism involves the following symptoms: difficulty speaking or swallowing; loss of balance; mask-like face; muscle spasms; stiffness of arms or legs; trembling and shaking; unusual twisting movements of body.

Although many people believe that parkinsonism is one of the inevitable consequences of growing old, a large proportion of the cases seen in older adults are caused by drugs. A study found that 51% of 93 patients referred for evaluation of newly developed parkinsonism had drug-induced diseases.[82] One-fourth of patients with drug-induced parkinsonism could not walk when first seen by their doctors, and 45% required hospital admission. The parkinsonism cleared in 66% of the patients, but 11% continued to have the disease a year after the drug was stopped. An additional 25% who had cleared initially went on to develop classic Parkinson's disease, leading the authors to speculate that, for this latter 25%, these drugs were "unmasking" a disease which might have showed up later.

Even more disturbing is the finding in another study in which **36% of patients with drug-induced parkinsonism had been started on antiparkinson drugs to treat the disease! Because the doctors had not considered the possibility that a drug was responsible for the disease, they assumed that the patients had classic Parkinson's disease and treated the parkinsonism with another drug instead** of stopping the one responsible for the disease in the first place.[83]

Another way of looking at this serious problem is to ask what proportion of patients who take antipsychotic drugs or other drugs which can also cause these problems (Phenergan, Compazine, and Reglan) get drug-induced parkinsonism. In various groups of patients in whom this has been studied, the range is from 15 to 52%.[84] In a recent study, 26% of older adults (60 and over) taking haloperidol (Haldol) developed drug-induced parkinsonism.[85] Other studies have shown an overall incidence of 15.4% but, among patients over 60, the incidence was approximately 40%.[86] In the same study, 90% of the cases of drug-induced parkinsonism began within 72 days after starting the drug.

Restless leg (akathisia)

Another very common adverse effect of these drugs is the restless leg syndrome, in which the person restlessly paces around and describes having the "jitters." When seated, the patient often taps his or her feet. Not infrequently, this might be interpreted as needing *more* antipsychotic medicine. Instead of reducing the dose of the drug or stopping it entirely, more of the drug causing the problem may be used.

Weakness and muscular fatigue (akinesia)

The most common of this group of drug-induced nerve problems (extrapyramidal reactions) is when the patient appears listless, disinterested, and depressed. This drug-induced problem is often misdiagnosed as primary depression, and the patient is put on antidepressant drugs. Giving these drugs along with the antipsychotic drugs even further increases the risk of serious adverse effects. Once again, instead of recognizing a drug-induced problem and either stopping or lowering the dose of the drug, another drug is added making things even worse.

Although seen as a component of parkinsonism, akinesia can also occur on its own. Additional problems can include infrequent blinking, slower swallowing of saliva with subsequent drooling, and a lack of facial expression.

As a general rule, if any elderly person on psychoactive medication — sleeping pills, antianxiety tranquilizers, antidepressants, or antipsychotic drugs appears to be doing poorly, first think about reducing the dose or stopping the drug rather than adding another drug.

Anticholinergic adverse effects

The two types of anticholinergic effects are those affecting the brain, such as confusion, delirium, short-term memory problems, disorientation, and impaired attention and those affecting the rest of the body. The latter type includes dry mouth, constipation, retention of urine (especially in men with an enlarged prostate), blurred vision, decreased sweating with increased body temperature, sexual dysfunction, and worsening of glaucoma. These adverse effects are much more common in the so-called high-dose antipsychotic drugs (see chart below).

Sedation

Sedation is one of the most common adverse effects of the antipsychotic drugs, especially with the high-dose drugs. Since these drugs are often improperly prescribed as sleeping pills, older adults will often have a decreased level of functioning during the day. In nonpsychotic older adults, the largest group being given these drugs, the quality of sleep is extremely unpleasant. The frightening aspects of this drug-induced disturbed sleep can last up to 24 hours after a single dose.

Generic /Brand Name	Sedative	Anticholinergic (dry mouth, urine retention, confusion)	Extrapyramidal (parkinsonism)	Hypotensive
chlorpromazine/ Thorazine	strong	strong	moderate	strong
thioridazine/ Mellaril	strong	strong	mild	moderate
trifluoperazine/ Stelazine	mild	mild	strong	moderate
fluphenazine/ Prolixin	mild	mild	strong	mild
haloperidol/ Haldol	mild	mild	strong	mild
loxapine/ Loxitane	mild	mild	strong	mild
thiothixene/ Navane	mild	mild	strong	moderate

Adverse Effects of Antipsychotic Drugs Commonly Used For Older Adults

mild = mild adverse effects
moderate = moderate adverse effects
strong = strong adverse effects[87]

Hypotension: lowering of blood pressure to levels that are too low

Orthostatic (postural) hypotension, or the fall in blood pressure which occurs when someone stands up suddenly, is a common side effect of antipsychotic drugs, especially in older adults. It can be even more troublesome if the person is already at increased risk for this problem because he or she is taking other drugs to treat high blood pressure. As a result of such a drug-induced drop in blood pressure, falls which result in injury, heart attacks, and strokes can occur. For this reason, before starting one of these drugs, the person's blood pressure should be taken both in the lying position and after standing for two minutes. This should be repeated after the person has used the drug for several weeks. People taking these drugs should rise slowly from a lying position and wear supportive stockings to help prevent hypotension. This adverse effect is also seen more often with the use of the higher dose drugs, such as chlorpromazine (Thorazine), but occurs with all of the antipsychotic drugs.

Other adverse effects

Other adverse effects include weight gain, poor ability to withstand high or low temperatures (because these drugs affect the body's temperature regulation center), increased sensitivity to sunlight and other skin problems, bone marrow toxicity, and abnormal heart rhythms.

How To Reduce The Risks of These Antipsychotic Drugs

❑ **Give antipsychotic drugs only to people who need them.** The majority, at least 80%, of older adults being prescribed these drugs should not be getting them, and the serious adverse effects are just as harmful in them as in the small fraction of people for whom the drugs are appropriate (people with schizophrenia). Thus, the most effective way of reducing the risk of these drugs for most older adults is to stop using them. Unless the patient

has schizophrenia or another psychotic condition, beginning to use them or continuing to use them provides significant risks without compensating benefits. These drugs are also not effective for psychoses seen with senile dementia.[88] As discussed on p. 211, the use of these powerful drugs for older people who have depression is fraught with a high incidence — 60% — of tardive dyskinesia.

Antipsychotic drugs should never be used as sleeping pills or to treat anxiety.

❑ **Start with the lowest possible dose: usually one-tenth to two-fifths the dose for younger adults. Use the drug for as short a period of time as possible.**[89] If, however, the use of antipsychotic drugs is indicated, the first thing to realize is that as is the case for many drugs for older adults, the starting dose and, very likely, the eventually used dose should be lower than the dose for younger adults. These are three of the reasons why this is so for the antipsychotic drugs:

First, kidney function in older adults decreases, which means that the drugs last longer in the body. To put it another way, you get more "mileage" out of a given dose. Second, because of a decrease in an important brain chemical, dopamine, as people age, there is an increased risk in older adults of the adverse effects, such as drug-induced parkinsonism or akinesia. Third, because of another change in brain metabolism with aging, there is an increased sensitivity to the anticholinergic effects of these drugs, such as confusion, delirium, dry mouth, difficulty urinating, constipation and worsening of glaucoma.[90]

❑ **Pay attention to the adverse effect profile of the drugs (see comparison chart on p. 213).** As mentioned previously, the antipsychotic drugs are all quite similar in their effectiveness for treating psychoses, but differ mainly in the spectrum of their adverse effects. The chart shows a great difference in the severity of the adverse reactions, depending on whether the drug is a less potent or more potent one.

At the top of the list is the less potent, higher dose chlorpromazine (Thorazine). It causes more sedative, anticholinergic, and hypotensive effects, but has a relatively lower risk of the extrapyramidal effects, such as restless leg and drug-induced parkinsonism. At the bottom of the list are more potent, lower dose drugs, such as haloperidol (Haldol) and thiothixene (Navane). They cause fewer sedative, anticholinergic, and hypotensive adverse effects, but have a higher risk of the extrapyramidal side effects, such as drug-induced parkinsonism.

Since all of these drugs are equally effective, the choice depends on which adverse effects would likely be or are most intolerable. For a person with a tendency to become faint or dizzy upon standing (orthostatic, postural hypotension), the addition of Thorazine with its high risk of lowering blood pressure would not be a good idea. Instead, if drug treatment is really necessary, one of the more potent drugs with fewer hypotensive and sedative effects might be a better choice. Similarly, people who already have trouble walking or who have trouble with their posture would be at much greater risk if they developed one of the extrapyramidal adverse effects of Haldol, Navane, or the other more potent antipsychotic drugs. Therefore, these people would probably do better on one of the less potent drugs with fewer extrapyramidal side effects. The most important consideration is to adjust the dose or change or discontinue drugs when and if adverse effects occur. **This is especially true when the side effects are as bad or worse than the original reason for starting the drug.**

Depression: When Are Drugs Called For and Which Ones Should You Use?

Should Everyone Who Is Sad or Depressed Take Antidepressants?

Although depression is the most common mental illness in older adults, everyone who is sad or depressed is not a candidate for these powerful drugs.

Kinds of Depression
Drug-induced depression

Ironically, one of the kinds of depression that should not be treated with drugs is depression *caused* by other kinds of drugs. If someone is depressed and the depression started after beginning a new drug, it may well be drug-caused. Commonly used drugs known to cause depression include the following:

❑ Barbiturates such as phenobarbital
❑ Tranquilizers such as diazepam (Valium) and triazolam (Halcion)
❑ Heart drugs containing reserpine (Serpasil and others)
❑ Beta-blockers such as propranolol (Inderal)
❑ High blood pressure drugs such as clonidine (Catapres), methyldopa (Aldomet), and prazosin (Minipress)
❑ Drugs for treating abnormal heart rhythms such as disopyramide (Norpace)
❑ Ulcer drugs such as cimetidine (Tagamet) and ranitidine (Zantac)
❑ Antiparkinsonians such as levodopa (Dopar) and bromocriptine (Parlodel)
❑ Corticosteroids such as cortisone and prednisone

❑ Anticonvulsants such as phenytoin (Dilantin), ethosuximide (Zarontin), and primidone (Mysoline)

❑ Antibiotics such as cycloserine (Seromycin), isoniazid (INH), ethionamide (Trecator-SC), and metronidazole (Flagyl)

❑ Diet drugs such as amphetamines (during withdrawal from the drug)

❑ Painkillers or arthritis drugs such as pentazocine (Talwin), indomethacin (Indocin), and ibuprofen (Motrin, Rufen, Advil, Nuprin)

❑ Other drugs including metrizamide (Ampaque), a drug used for diagnosing slipped discs, and disulfiram (Antabuse), the alcoholism treatment drug.[91]

The remedy for this kind of depression is to reduce the dose of the drug or stop it altogether if possible. If necessary, switch to another drug that does not cause depression.

Another major cause of drug-induced depression is alcoholism, the treatment of which is difficult.

Situational or reactive depression

Other causes of depression which should not be treated with antidepressant drugs are the "normal" reactions to life problems, such as the loss of a spouse, friend, relative, or job, or other situations that normally make almost anyone sad. If the depression is clearly a response to overwhelming life crises, antidepressants have little value. Other options such as support from family and friends, psychotherapy, or a change in your environment, are worth exploring.[92] Doing something nice for yourself, talking with a friend, and exercising every day can help you get through these difficult situations.

Medical conditions that can cause depression

Older adults (or anyone) who appear depressed may have a thyroid disorder; a type of cancer, such as pancreatic, bowel, brain, or lymph node (lymphoma); viral pneumonia; or hepatitis.[93,94] In addition, there is evidence that people who have had a stroke or who have Parkinson's disease or Alzheimer's disease may become depressed and, in some cases, may respond to antidepressant drugs.[95]

Endogenous depression: the kind that will usually respond to drugs

If a depressed mood accompanied by several of the following problems has been present for at least several weeks, and a careful history, physical exam, and lab tests have ruled out specific causes of depression, true primary depression is probably the diagnosis. The problems are sadness that impairs normal functioning, difficulty concentrating, low self-esteem, guilt, suicidal thoughts, extreme fatigue, low energy level or agitation, sleep disturbances (increased or decreased), or appetite disturbance (increased or decreased) with associated weight change.[96] Since suicidal thoughts and attempts often characterize depression, the possibility of suicide using antidepressant drugs has to be kept in mind and only a small number of pills (see p. 220) prescribed at one time. Another way of describing the pervasive nature of this kind of severe depression is that the person displays — and relates if asked — a sense of "helplessness, hopelessness, worthlessness and uselessness . . . as well as intense feelings of guilt over real or imagined shortcomings or indiscretions."[97]

Although depression in older adults is usually unipolar (depression alone), occasionally there is a bipolar pattern with alternation of depression and mania. The latter shows up as an elated mood, rapid flow of ideas, and increased "energy." The patient, often seeming hyperactive during this manic phase, can be intrusive, have an infectious sense of humor, and may show poor judgment in business or personal affairs, not infrequently going on spending sprees.[98] Lithium is often used successfully to treat people with bipolar disease (see p. 229).

Serious depressive illness is far less frequent in the elderly. According to data from the National Institute of Mental

Health, while nearly 4% of people age 25 to 44 have had a major depression recently, fewer than 1% of people 65 and over have had this misfortune. In spite of this, about one-third of antidepressants are prescribed for people 60 and over even though they make up just one-sixth of the population.

Some of this apparent "overtreatment" may be due to failing to diagnose drug-induced depression and, instead, the use of a second drug to treat the depression caused by the first.

Other Uses — Usually Inappropriate — for Antidepressants

In addition to drug-induced depression, medical conditions which can cause depression and situational or reactive depression — none of which merit treatment with antidepressants — there are other circumstances in which antidepressants are inappropriately dished out. In one community-based study, more than 50% of older people who had been taking antidepressants for a year or more had been started without a clear history of depression. Of these, one-half (or one out four of all people using antidepressants) were using antidepressants as a sleeping pill and others were given the drugs as alternatives to tranquilizers.[99] In view of the significant adverse effects of these drugs, their use for such purposes will cause risks which will outweigh the benefits.

What Is the Best and Worst Treatment for Severe Depression?

Everyone with the kind of severe depression described above should be evaluated by a mental health professional to determine what kind of psychotherapy would be best to supplement the antidepressant drugs that are going to be used.

The decision as to which drug is best will depend largely on choosing one with the fewest adverse effects, since all of the so-called tricyclic antidepressants are equally effective.[100] If depression has occurred previously and responded to one of the

drugs without too many adverse effects, that would be the best one to try first. Otherwise, the table below compares the eight tricyclic antidepressants that are listed in this book and fluoxetine (Prozac) and bupropion (Wellbutrin).

The Main Risks of Antidepressant Drugs

The four most common groups of adverse effects are anticholinergic, sedative, hypotensive (blood-pressure-lowering), and those effects on heart rate or rhythm. Two serious risks arising from the adverse effects are hip fractures and injurious automobile crashes.

Hip fractures

A study of 1,021 older adults with hip fractures found that 14% of these life-threatening injuries are attributable to the use of mind-affecting drugs, including sleeping pills and minor tranquilizers, antipsychotics, and antidepressants.[101]

There are approximately 227,000 hip fractures each year in the United States, virtually all in older adults.[102] Since the above study found that 14% of hip fractures are drug-induced, this means that if the results of the study are projected nationally, approximately **32,000 hip fractures a year in older adults are caused by the use of mind-affecting drugs.** Approximately 60% of these hip fractures are caused by antidepressant drugs.

Injurious automobile crashes

A recent study involving 495 automobile crashes in older drivers in which an injury occurred found that a significant number of such crashes in older adults aged 65-84 were attributable to the use of benzodiazepine tranquilizers and tricyclic antidepressants. The study was particularly impressive because its findings were strengthened by observing that the rate of injurious crashes increased in the same group of people when they were using these drugs as opposed to when they were not using the drugs. The majority of the excess number of injurious auto crashes were attributable to the benzodiazepines. The authors, stating that the study findings may be generalizable to the population at large, found that if the association is causal, **at least 16,000 injurious auto crashes each year in older drivers are attributable to psychoactive drug use (specifically benzodiazepines and tricyclic antidepressants)** out of the 217,000 injurious crashes that occur each year among elderly drivers.[103]

Anticholinergic effects

> *Warning: Special Mental and Physical Adverse Effects*
> Older adults are especially sensitive to the harmful anticholinergic effects of tricyclic antidepressants. Drugs in this family should not be used unless absolutely necessary.
> *Mental Effects:* confusion, delirium, short-term memory problems, disorientation, and impaired attention.
> *Physical Effects:* dry mouth, constipation, difficulty urinating (especially for a man with an enlarged prostate), blurred vision, decreased sweating with increased body temperature, sexual dysfunction, and worsening of glaucoma.

Sedative effects

Most older adults who think they have a sleeping problem do not have the kind of severe depression that justifies the use of these drugs. (See p. 205 for a discussion of nondrug treatments for sleeplessness.) Nevertheless, if the sleep disorder is a consequence of severe depression, the "side effect" of sedation may be useful as long as it does not produce too much sedation, with the risk of falling. This is an important consideration especially in people who already have some impairment of thinking, increased confusion, disorientation, and agitation.[104]

Hypotensive effects: lowering of blood pressure to levels that are too low

Orthostatic (postural) hypotension, or the drop in blood pressure that occurs when someone stands up suddenly, is a common side effect of antidepressants, especially in older adults. It can be even more troublesome if the person is already at increased risk for this problem because he or she is taking other drugs to treat high blood pressure. As a result of such a drug-induced drop in blood pressure, falls that result in injury, heart attacks, and strokes can occur.[105] For this reason, before starting treatment with one of these antidepressants, blood pressure should be taken both in the lying position and after standing for two minutes.[106] This should be repeated after using the drug for several weeks.

Drug-induced parkinsonism

Like the antipsychotic drugs, many antidepressants can also cause drug-induced parkinsonism (see p. 212). Drug-induced parkinsonism involves the following symptoms: difficulty speaking or swallowing; loss of balance; mask-like face; muscle spasms; stiffness of arms or legs; trembling and shaking; unusual twisting movements of body.

Effects on heart rate and rhythm

These drugs can cause the heart to speed up. They can also cause a slowing down in the conduction of electricity through the heart, which is especially dangerous if someone already has heart block.[107] For this reason, a baseline electrocardiogram should be taken before starting any antidepressant therapy.

As can be seen from the chart below, the drugs with the fewest overall adverse effects in older adults are desipramine (Norpramin), which has a "mild" for all four kinds of adverse effects, and nortriptyline (Aventyl, Pamelor), which is "mild" for three of the four. Unfortunately, nortriptyline is not available generically as

Adverse Effects of Antidepressants in Older Adults				
Generic/ Brand Names	Anticholinergics*	Sedative	Hypotensive Effect	Heart Rate/ Rythm
fluoxetine/ Prozac**	none	none	none	none
bupropion/ Wellbutrin**	mild	none	none	none
desipramine/ Norpramin	mild	mild	mild	mild
nortriptyline/ Aventyl, Pamelor	moderate	mild	mild	mild
amoxapine/ Asendin	moderate	mild	moderate	moderate
maprotiline/ Ludiomil	moderate	moderate	moderate	mild
trazodone/ Desyrel	mild	moderate	moderate	moderate
imipramine/ Tofranil	moderate	moderate	moderate	moderate
doxepin/ Adapin, Sinequan	moderate	strong	moderate	moderate
amitriptyline/ Elavil	strong	strong	moderate	strong

mild = mild adverse effects
moderate = moderate adverse effects
strong = strong adverse effects

* see p. 218
** There is inadequate information for these drugs in older people to ensure that the risk of the adverse effects is as low as it appears; there is more information about nortriptyline and desipramine as far as their reduced amount of adverse effects on older adults in comparison with the drugs listed below them.

These listings are a composite of comparative ratings of eight of these drugs by four other researchers[108] and information from the references listed for fluoxetine and bupropion on the drug pages.

yet. Fluoxetine (Prozac) and bupropion (Wellbutrin) may have as few or fewer adverse effects as desipramine and nortriptyline but adequate comparative studies on older adults have not yet been published. The drug with the worst adverse effects profile in older adults is amitriptyline (Elavil), with "strong" adverse effects for three of the four categories. We list this drug as **Do Not Use.**

If the adverse effects of whichever drug is selected are too severe, or if the drug does not seem to be working, a discussion with your doctor about switching to a drug less likely to cause the troublesome effects is in order.

How To Reduce the Adverse Effects of Any of these Antidepressants

❑ Have a baseline electrocardiogram and blood pressure taken before starting.[109]
❑ Start with a dose of one-third to one-half the usual adult dose, meaning 15-25 milligrams a day, at bedtime. Increase the dose very slowly.[110] It may take 3 weeks to see an effect. A trial with one of these drugs should continue until it either works or causes persistent side effects.[111]
❑ Get a prescription for only 1 week's worth of pills since more pills increase the chance of a successful suicide attempt by people who are severely depressed.[112]
❑ Lower the dose gradually, as symptoms dictate, after successful treatment for several months.[113]

It is important to realize that long-term treatment with antidepressants is not always necessary even when the drug is being used to treat the kind of serious depression for which its use is proper. In one study, after patients had been successfully treated for four months with antidepressants, half were continued on their drugs and the other half were switched to a placebo. After an additional two months, most of the patients — either on the actual drug or the placebo — were still doing well, only about one-fourth, the same in both groups, had relapsed. [114]

Other recommendations for more effective and safer use of these drugs include:[115]

1. When starting a drug for a specific depressive illness, the doctor should monitor your response carefully to see if a different dose [or drug] should be used.
2. It should be made clear to you that depression can be an episodic illness, that recovery is expected and that the treatment will probably eventually be stopped.
3. If treatment with drugs is started as a trial in possible depression, you should be informed that it is a trial and that treatment will continue for a specified time, depending on the response of key symptoms.
4. The possibility of adverse effects should be evaluated carefully before these drugs are used primarily as sleeping pills or as an alternative to tranquilizers in the elderly.

LIMITED USE

Doxepin (*dox* e pin)
ADAPIN (Pennwalt)
SINEQUAN (Roerig)
Trazodone (*traz* oh done)
DESYREL (Mead Johnson)
Maprotiline (ma *proe* ti leen)
LUDIOMIL (CIBA)
Amoxapine (a *mox* a peen)
ASENDIN (Lederle)
Imipramine (im *ip* ra meen)
TOFRANIL (Geigy)

Generic: available

Family: Antidepressants (See p. 215 for discussion of depression.)

These five drugs are used to treat severe depression that is not caused by other drugs, by alcohol, or by emotional losses (such as a death in the family). You should *not* be taking them for anxiety or mild depression, or as a sleeping pill. Because these drugs have more harmful side effects (see chart, p. 219) than the two antidepressants desipramine and nortriptyline (see p. 232), we consider them to be of limited use to older adults.

If you are over 60, you will generally need to take one-third to one-half the dose used by younger adults. If the initial dose is not enough and needs to be increased, this should be done very slowly.

Trazodone can cause painful, prolonged penile erections (priapism) in men. If you suffer this reaction, stop taking the drug and notify your doctor. Amoxapine can cause tardive dyskinesia — uncontrolled movements of the jaws, tongue, and lips — an effect also seen with antipsychotic drugs

(see p. 211). Doxepin has especially strong sedative effects.

The length of time it takes an antidepressant to work can overlap with the time of spontaneous recovery especially if the depression is situational — caused by a death or other external circumstances. The majority of people lift themselves out of depression with friends or activities, such as exercise, work, reading, play, art, travel,

---

Warning: Special Mental and Physical Adverse Effects

Older adults are especially sensitive to the harmful anticholinergic effects of antidepressants such as these. Drugs in this family should not be used unless absolutely necessary.

Mental Effects: confusion, delirium, short-term memory problems, disorientation, and impaired attention.

Physical Effects: dry mouth, constipation, difficulty urinating (especially for a man with an enlarged prostate), blurred vision, decreased sweating with increased body temperature, sexual dysfunction, and worsening of glaucoma.

and spiritual resources. If depression is not overcome by these measures, seek help from mental health professionals, such as therapists or psychiatrists. Antidepressant drugs should be reserved for depression that is major and does not respond to psychotherapy alone.

Before You Use This Drug

Tell your doctor if you have or have had
- ❑ allergies to drugs
- ❑ alcohol dependence
- ❑ asthma*
- ❑ blood disorders*
- ❑ heart or blood vessel disease*
- ❑ stomach or intestinal disease*
- ❑ glaucoma*
- ❑ kidney or liver disease
- ❑ thyroid disease*
- ❑ manic-depressive illness, schizophrenia, or paranoia*
- ❑ retention of urine or enlarged prostate* *(for thazodone)*
- ❑ epilepsy or seizures, *not for maprotiline or doxepin*
- ❑ fever or sore throat, *for trazodone*
- ❑ blood in urine, *for trazodone*

Tell your doctor about any other drugs you take, including aspirin, herbs, vitamins, and other non-prescription products.
Ask your doctor to check your blood pressure, once while you are lying down and once after you have been standing up for at least 2 minutes, and to do an electrocardiogram.

When You Use This Drug

◆ Do not stop taking this drug suddenly. Your doctor must give you a schedule to lower your dose gradually, to prevent withdrawal symptoms such as headache, mood change, nausea, vomiting, diarrhea, or trouble sleeping and vivid dreams.

◆ Until you know how you react to this drug, do not drive or perform other activities requiring alertness. These drugs may cause blurred vision and drowsiness.

◆ It may take several weeks before you can tell that these drugs are working. If the drug works, talk with your doctor about lowering the dose gradually.

◆ Do not smoke. Smoking may increase the drug's effects on your heart.

◆ Do not drink alcohol or use other drugs that can cause drowsiness.

◆ You may feel dizzy when rising from a lying or sitting position. When getting out of bed, hang your legs over the side of the bed for a few minutes, then get up slowly. When getting up from a chair, stay beside the chair until you are sure that you are not dizzy. (See p. 14.)

◆ Check with your doctor before taking any other drugs, prescription or nonprescription. These drugs frequently interact with other drugs.

◆ The effects of these drugs may last for up to a week after you stop taking them. Avoid alcohol and heed all other warnings for this time period.

◆ If you plan to have any surgery, including dental, tell your doctor that you take one of these drugs.

How To Use This Drug

◆ Take with food to reduce stomach upset. *For trazodone,* taking with food will also reduce dizziness and lightheadedness.

◆ If you are taking any other drugs, take them 1 to 2 hours before you take your antidepressant.

◆ Capsules may be opened and mixed with food or drink.

◆ Do not store in the bathroom. Do not expose to heat, moisture, or strong light.

◆ *If you miss a dose, use the following guidelines:*
- If you are taking more than one dose a day of one of these drugs other than trazodone, take the missed dose as soon as you remember, but skip it if it is almost time for the next dose.
- If you are taking more than one dose a day of trazodone, take the missed dose as soon as you remember, but

---

* *not for trazodone*

skip it if it is less than 4 hours until your next scheduled dose.

- If you are taking your drug only once a day at bedtime, and you go to sleep without taking that dose, do not take it in the morning. Instead, call your doctor.
- **Do not take double doses.**

Interactions With Other Drugs

The following drugs are listed in *Evaluations of Drug Interactions*, 1991 as causing "highly clinically significant" or "clinically significant" interactions when used together with these drugs. There may be other drugs, especially those in the families of drugs listed below, that also will react with these antidepressants to cause severe adverse effects. Make sure to ask your doctor for a complete listing of them and let her or him know if you are taking any of these interacting drugs:

ADRENALIN (also in bee sting kits); alcohol; cimetidine; CYTOMEL; epinephrine; guanethidine; ISMELIN; ISORDIL; liothyronine; MELLARIL; nitroglycerin (sublingual); NITROSTAT; PARNATE; PRIMATENE MIST; TAGAMET; thioridazine; tolazamide; TOLINASE; tranylcypromine.

Adverse Effects

Call your doctor immediately:

❑ **if you experience signs of overdose:** confusion; severe drowsiness; fever; hallucinations; restlessness and agitation; seizures; shortness of breath; trouble breathing; unusually fast, slow, or irregular heartbeat; unusual tiredness, weakness; vomiting
❑ blurred vision or eye pain
❑ confusion, delirium, or hallucinations
❑ constipation
❑ fainting
❑ irregular heartbeat or slow or fast pulse
❑ feeling nervous or restless

❑ impaired sexual function
❑ shakiness
❑ trouble sleeping
❑ trouble urinating
❑ sore throat and fever
❑ yellow eyes or skin

For trazodone only:

❑ confusion
❑ muscle tremors
❑ prolonged, painful, inappropriate penile erection
❑ skin rash, hives, or itching
❑ abnormally slow or fast heartbeat

For amoxapine only:

❑ **if you experience signs of tardive dyskinesia:** lip smacking; chewing movements; puffing of cheeks; rapid, darting tongue movements; uncontrolled movements of arms or legs

Call your doctor if these symptoms continue:

❑ dizziness
❑ drowsiness
❑ dry mouth
❑ headache
❑ nausea or vomiting
❑ increased appetite for sweets*
❑ unpleasant taste in mouth*
❑ weight gain*
❑ muscle aches or pains; unusual tiredness or weakness, *for trazodone*

Periodic Tests

Ask your doctor which of these tests should be done periodically while you are taking this drug:

❑ blood cell counts
❑ blood pressure*
❑ pulse*
❑ glaucoma tests*
❑ liver function tests*
❑ kidney function tests
❑ heart function tests such as electrocardiogram (EKG)
❑ dental exams (at least twice yearly)

---

*not for trazodone

LIMITED USE

Buspirone
BUSPAR (Bristol Myers Squibb)

Generic: not available

Family: Tranquilizers (see p. 198)

Buspirone (*bu* spire own) is a new antianxiety agent, which differs chemically from the benzodiazepine drugs (see p. 198) and appears to lack the potential for addiction common to this family of drugs, such as Xanax and Valium. While buspirone is less apt than the benzodiazepines to cause drowsiness, drowsiness remains a common side effect. Although buspirone is preferred for older adults, compared to other drugs available,[116] information about buspirone is limited, and much is still unknown including its long-term safety and effectiveness.[117,118] Side effects are often paradoxical (drowsiness or insomnia, anorexia or weight gain). While buspirone is used for short-term anxiety, it takes a few weeks to work. In some people buspirone may increase anxiety, rather than alleviate it.[119] A decision to use buspirone should be reviewed periodically.

Anxiety is a universal emotion closely allied with appropriate fears.[120] No drug is useful for the stress of everyday living. Try non-drug therapies for anxiety first. Explore preventable causes of anxiety, such as overuse of caffeine, as well as medical/ physical causes. Drugs may control but do not cure anxiety.

If you already take a benzodiazepine (see p. 198) or antidepressant (see p. 215), your doctor should taper you off those drugs before trying buspirone. However, if you have already taken a benzodiazepine, the buspirone is less likely to be effective.[121]

Before You Use This Drug
Tell your doctor if you have or have had
❑ allergies to drugs
❑ alcohol or drug dependence
❑ high blood pressure
❑ kidney or liver disease
❑ thyroid disease
Tell your doctor about any other drugs you take, including aspirin, herbs, vitamins, and other non-prescription products.

When You Use This Drug
◆ Do not drink alcohol or use other drugs that can cause drowsiness.
◆ Until you know how you react to this drug, do not drive or perform other activities that require alertness. Buspirone may cause blurred vision and drowsiness.
◆ If you plan to have any surgery, including dental, tell your doctor that you take this drug.
◆ Do not take other drugs without checking with your doctor first — especially non-prescription drugs for appetite control, colds, coughs, hay fever, sinus problems, or sleep.

How To Use This Drug
◆ Swallow drug whole, or break in half to ease swallowing.
◆ If you miss a dose, take it as soon as you remember, but skip it if it is almost time for the next dose. **Do not take double doses.**
◆ Do not store in the bathroom. Do not expose to heat, moisture or strong light.

Interactions With Other Drugs

The following drugs are listed in the *United States Pharmacopeia Drug Information,* 1992 as having interactions of major significance when used with this drug. There may be other drugs, especially those in the families of drugs listed below, that also will react with this drug to cause severe adverse effects. Make sure to ask your doctor for a complete listing of them and let her or him know if you are taking any of these interacting drugs:

Taking buspirone with any MAO (monoamine oxidase) inhibitors may increase your blood pressure. Do not try buspirone for at least 10 days after stopping any of these MAO inhibitors:

deprenyl; ELDEPRYL; EUTONYL; EUTRON; furazolidine; FUROXONE; isocarboxazid; MARPLAN; MATULANE; NARDIL; pargyline; PARNATE; phenelzine; procarbazine; selegiline; tranylcypromine.

Adverse Effects

Call your doctor immediately:
- [ ] **if you experience signs of overdose:** severe dizziness; severe drowsiness; dry mouth; severe nausea and vomiting; unusually small pupils

- [ ] chest pain
- [ ] confusion or mental depression
- [ ] fast or pounding heartbeat

Call your doctor if these symptoms continue:
- [ ] anger, hostility
- [ ] blurred vision
- [ ] dizziness, lightheadedness
- [ ] constipation or diarrhea
- [ ] sleep or dream disturbance[122]
- [ ] drowsiness
- [ ] headache
- [ ] dry mouth
- [ ] involuntary movements
- [ ] muscle pain
- [ ] nasal congestion
- [ ] numbness
- [ ] restlessness, insomnia
- [ ] ringing in ears
- [ ] sweating
- [ ] unusual weakness, tiredness
- [ ] upset stomach
- [ ] urinary problems

Periodic Tests

Ask your doctor which of these tests should be done periodically while you are taking this drug:
- [ ] kidney function tests
- [ ] liver function tests

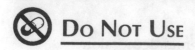 **DO NOT USE**

Alternative treatment: See Nondrug approaches, p. 204, Oxazepam, p. 237, and Buspirone, p. 224. See also Tranquilizers and Sleeping Pills, p. 198.

Butabarbital
BUTALAN (Lannett) BUTISOL (Wallace)
Pentobarbital
NEMBUTAL (Abbott)

Family: Barbiturates
Sleeping Pills

Butabarbital (byoo ta *bar* bi tal) and pentobarbital (pen toe *bar* bi tal) are used to promote sleep and to relieve tension and anxiety. **You should not use these drugs because they are addictive and cause serious side effects in people over 60.** The World Health Organization has designated them as drugs that older adults should not use.[123]

> One hazard of taking butabarbital or pentobarbital continuously for longer than several weeks is addiction. **Do not stop taking your drug suddenly.** With the help of your doctor, work out a schedule for slowly lowering the amount of the drug you take by about 5 to 10% each day. Keep a written record of the dosage reduction schedule with you. These steps will make it much easier to become drug free without developing distressing symptoms of drug withdrawal.

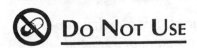 **DO NOT USE**

Alternative treatment: See Nortriptyline and Desipramine, p. 232.

Amitriptyline
ELAVIL (Merck)
ENDEP (Roche)

Family: Antidepressants (See p. 215 for discussion of depression.)

Amitriptyline (a mee *trip* ti leen) is used to treat depression, but we do not recommend its use because it has more harmful side effects than any other drug in its family (see chart, p. 219). If you need an antidepressant drug, either nortriptyline or desipramine is a better choice (see p. 232). The length of time it takes an antidepressant to work can overlap with the time of spontaneous recovery especially if the depression is situational — caused by a death or other external circumstances. The majority of people lift themselves out of depression with friends or activities, such as exercise, work, reading, play, art, travel, and spiritual resources. If depression is not overcome by these measures, seek help from mental health professionals, such as therapists or psychiatrists. Antidepressant drugs should be reserved for depression that is major and does not respond to psychotherapy alone.

Warning: Special Mental and Physical Adverse Effects

Older adults are especially sensitive to the harmful anticholinergic effects of antidepressants such as amitriptyline. Drugs in this family should not be used unless absolutely necessary.

Mental Effects: confusion, delirium, short-term memory problems, disorientation, and impaired attention.

Physical Effects: dry mouth, constipation, difficulty urinating (especially for a man with an enlarged prostate), blurred vision, decreased sweating with increased body temperature, sexual dysfunction, and worsening of glaucoma.

If you use amitripyline, ask your doctor about switching to another antidepressant. **Do not stop taking this drug suddenly.** Your doctor must give you a schedule to lower your dose *gradually,* to prevent withdrawal symptoms such as headache, mood change, nausea, vomiting, diarrhea, or trouble sleeping and vivid dreams.

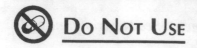 **Do Not Use**

Alternative treatment: See Nondrug approaches, p. 204, Oxazepam, p. 237, and Buspirone, p. 224. See also Tranquilizers and Sleeping Pills, p. 198.

Meprobamate
EQUANIL (Wyeth)
MILTOWN (Wallace)
SK-BAMATE (Smith Kline & French)

Family: Antianxiety Drugs

Meprobamate (me proe *ba* mate) is a tranquilizer. It is commonly misused to relieve occasional, short-term anxiety. **If you are suffering anxiety and tension from the stress of everyday life, you usually do not need an antianxiety drug.** There are safer ways to relieve such anxiety. If you do need a drug for anxiety, oxazepam (see p. 237) or buspirone (see p. 224) is a better choice than meprobamate.

Long-term treatment (longer than 4 months) of anxiety with meprobamate is rarely effective. It also puts you at risk of developing harmful side effects, such as drowsiness; dizziness; unsteady gait, with an increased risk of falls and hip fractures; impairment of thinking; memory loss; and addiction.

One hazard of taking meprobamate continuously for longer than several weeks is addiction. **Do not stop taking your drug suddenly.** With the help of your doctor, work out a schedule for slowly lowering the amount of the drug you take by about 5 to 10% each day. Keep a written record of the dosage reduction schedule with you. These steps will make it much easier to become drug free without developing distressing symptoms of drug withdrawal.

LIMITED USE

Lithium
ESKALITH (Smith Kline & French)
LITHOBID (Ciba)
LITHONATE (Reid-Rowell)

Generic: available

Family: Antimanic Drugs (See p. 215 for discussion of depression.)

Lithium (*lith* ee um) is used to treat manic episodes of manic depression, a condition in which a person's mood swings severely from normal to elated to depressed. It is also used to prevent or decrease the intensity of future manic episodes.

If you are over 60, you generally need to take less than the usual adult dose. Your doctor should frequently measure the levels of lithium in your blood.

Even when the amount of lithium in an older person's body is no more than is needed for it to work, the drug may cause harm to the central nervous system. Ideally, you should only use lithium if you have a normal salt (sodium) intake and normal heart and kidney function.[124]

Before You Use This Drug
Tell your doctor if you have or have had
❑ allergies to drugs
❑ heart or blood vessel disease
❑ Parkinson's disease
❑ epilepsy, seizures
❑ enlarged prostate or difficulty urinating
❑ kidney disease
❑ diabetes
❑ goiter, thyroid disease
❑ overactive parathyroid glands
❑ recent severe infection
❑ organic brain disease
❑ schizophrenia
❑ psoriasis
❑ a current low-salt diet

Tell your doctor about any other drugs you take, including aspirin, herbs, vitamins, and other non-prescription products.

When You Use This Drug
◆ It may take 1 to 3 weeks before you can tell that this drug is working.
◆ **Do not stop taking this drug suddenly. Your doctor must give you a schedule to lower your dose gradually, to prevent withdrawal symptoms.**
◆ See your doctor regularly to make sure that the drug is working and that you are not developing side effects. Your doctor should regularly measure the amount of drug in your body.
◆ Follow diet recommended by your doctor to avoid weight gain.
◆ Until you know how you react to this drug, do not drive or perform other activities requiring alertness. Lithium may cause blurred vision, drowsiness,

---

Heat Stress Alert

This drug can affect your body's ability to adjust to heat, putting you at risk of "heat stress." If you live alone, ask a friend to check you several times during the day. Early signs of heat stress are dizziness, lightheadedness, faintness, and slightly high temperature. Call your doctor if you have these signs.

Drink more fluids (water, fruit and vegetable juices) than usual, even if you're not thirsty, unless your doctor has told you otherwise. Do not drink alcohol.

fainting, or slow your reaction time.

◆ If you plan to have any surgery, including dental, tell your doctor that you take this drug.

How to Use This Drug

◆ Swallow extended-release tablets whole.

◆ Do not store in the bathroom. Do not expose to heat, moisture, or strong light. Do not let the liquid form freeze.

◆ If you miss a dose, take it as soon as you remember, but skip it if it is less than 2 hours until your next scheduled dose. If you are taking extended-release tablets, skip the missed dose if it is less than 6 hours until your next scheduled dose. **Do not take double doses.**

Interactions With Other Drugs

The following drugs are listed in *Evaluations of Drug Interactions*, 1991 as causing "highly clinically significant" or "clinically significant" interactions when used together with this drug. There may be other drugs, especially those in the families of drugs listed below, that also will react with this drug to cause severe adverse effects. Make sure to ask your doctor for a complete listing of them and let her or him know if you are taking any of these interacting drugs:

acetazolamide; ACHROMYCIN; ADVIL; ALDOMET; BRONKODYL; caffeine; CALAN; carbamazepine; chlorothiazide; chlorpromazine; CONSTANT-T; DIAMOX; DIURIL; ELIXOPHYLLIN; enalapril; FLAGYL; fluoxetine; HALDOL; haloperidol; ibuprofen; imipramine; INDOCIN; indomethacin; LOPRESSOR; MAZANOR; mazindol; methyldopa; metronidazole; MOTRIN; NAPROSYN; naproxen; NUPRIN; PANMYCIN; potassium iodide; PROZAC; QUIBRON-T-SR; SANOREX; SLO-BID; SLO-PHYLLIN; SOMOPHYLLIN; SUSTAIRE; TEGRETOL; tetracycline; THEO-24; THEOLAIR; theophylline; thioridazine; THORAZINE; TOFRANIL; VASOTEC; verapamil.

Adverse Effects

Call your doctor immediately:

❑ **if you experience signs of overdose:** *early signs* are diarrhea; drowsiness; loss of appetite; muscle weakness; nausea or vomiting; slurred speech; *late signs* are blurred vision; clumsiness; confusion; dizziness; seizures; trembling; increased amount of urine

❑ **if you have signs of parkinsonism:** difficulty speaking or swallowing; loss of balance; mask-like face; muscle spasms; stiffness of arms or legs; trembling and shaking; unusual twisting movements of body

❑ **if you experience signs of low thyroid hormone levels:** dry, rough skin; hair loss; hoarseness; swelling of feet or lower legs; swelling of neck (goitre); increased sensitivity to cold, fatigue

❑ fainting

❑ trouble breathing

❑ fast heartbeat, irregular pulse

❑ unusual weight gain

❑ blue color and pain in fingers or toes

❑ cold limbs

❑ headache

❑ eye pain, visual problems

❑ nausea, vomiting

Call your doctor if these symptoms continue:

❑ increased amount of urine

❑ increased thirst

❑ mild nausea

❑ trembling

❑ skin rash, acne

❑ bloated feeling

❑ fatigue

Periodic Tests

Ask your doctor which of these tests should be done periodically while you are taking this drug:

❑ white blood cell counts

❑ blood levels of lithium (more often if taking other drugs)

❏ blood levels of calcium
❏ electrocardiogram
❏ kidney function tests
❏ thyroid function tests

❏ weight evaluation
❏ Parathyroid hormone and calcium levels may rise above normal after long-term lithium therapy.

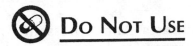 **Do Not Use**

Alternative treatment: For depression, see Nortriptyline and Desipramine, p. 232.

Amitriptyline and Chlordiazepoxide (combined)
LIMBITROL (Roche)

Family: Antidepressants (see p. 215)
Antianxiety Drugs

The brand-name drug Limbitrol contains a fixed combination of an antidepressant, amitriptyline (see p. 227), and a benzodiazepine (tranquilizer or antianxiety drug), chlordiazepoxide (see p. 246). It is used to treat moderate to severe depression associated with moderate to severe anxiety. We do not recommend that you use it, for several reasons.

First, combining an antidepressant with a benzodiazepine has not been shown to produce a more effective drug.[125] Second, taking these two drugs together raises the risk of harmful side effects. Chlordiazepoxide might increase the harmful anticholinergic effects of amitriptyline (see box below), and amitriptyline could increase the drowsiness caused by chlordiazepoxide.[126] Third, the antidepressant in this combination, amitriptyline, has more side effects than any other drug in its family (see chart, p. 219) and should not be used by older adults, either alone or in a combination such as this one.

If you use Limbitrol, ask your doctor if your treatment can be changed. Do not stop taking this drug suddenly. Your doctor may want to reduce your dose gradually over 1 or 2 months before you completely stop taking Limbitrol.

The length of time it takes an antidepressant to work can overlap with the time of spontaneous recovery especially if the depression is situational — caused by a death or other external circumstances. The majority of people lift themselves out of depression with friends or activities, such as exercise, work, reading, play, art, travel, and spiritual resources. If depression is not overcome by these measures, seek help from mental health professionals, such as therapists or psychiatrists. Antidepressant drugs should be reserved for depression that is major and does not respond to psychotherapy alone.

Warning: Special Mental and Physical Adverse Effects

Older adults are especially sensitive to the harmful anticholinergic effects of tricyclic antidepressants such as amitriptyline. Drugs in this family should not be used unless absolutely necessary.

Mental Effects: confusion, delirium, short-term memory problems, disorientation, and impaired attention.

Physical Effects: dry mouth, constipation, difficulty urinating (especially for a man with an enlarged prostate), blurred vision, decreased sweating with increased body temperature, sexual dysfunction, and worsening of glaucoma.

Desipramine
NORPRAMIN (Merrell Dow) PERTOFRANE (Rorer)
Nortriptyline
AVENTYL (Lilly) PAMELOR (Sandoz)

Generic: not available for nortriptyline

Family: Antidepressants (See p. 215 for discussion of depression.)

Desipramine (dess *ip* ra meen) and nortriptyline (nor *trip* ti leen) are used to treat severe depression that is not caused by other drugs, by alcohol, or by emotional losses (such as a death in the family). These two drugs produce fewer sedative effects and fewer harmful anticholinergic side effects (see box below) than some other antidepressants, and some clinicians suggest trying one of these two drugs before other drugs in their family (see p. 219 for comparison with other antidepressants). You should *not* be taking these drugs for mild depression or anxiety, or as a sleeping pill.

If you are over 60, you will generally need to take one-third to one-half the dose used for younger adults. If the initial dose is not enough and must be increased, this should be done very slowly under the guidance of your doctor. Your doctor should monitor the level of the drug in your bloodstream, because there is a point at which a higher drug level produces less benefit.

The length of time it takes an antidepressant to work can overlap with the time of spontaneous recovery especially if the depression is situational — caused by a death or other external circumstances. The majority of people lift themselves out of depression with friends or activities, such as exercise, work, reading, play, art, travel, and spiritual resources. If depression is not overcome by these measures, seek help from mental health professionals, such as therapists or psychiatrists. Antidepressant drugs should be reserved for depression that is major and does not respond to psychotherapy alone.

> *Warning: Special Mental and Physical Adverse Effects*
> Older adults are especially sensitive to the harmful anticholinergic effects of tricyclic antidepressants such as desipramine and nortriptyline. Drugs in this family should not be used unless absolutely necessary.
> *Mental Effects:* confusion, delirium, short-term memory problems, disorientation, and impaired attention.
> *Physical Effects:* dry mouth, constipation, difficulty urinating (especially for a man with an enlarged prostate), blurred vision, decreased sweating with increased body temperature, sexual dysfunction, and worsening of glaucoma.

Before You Use This Drug
Tell your doctor if you have or have had
- allergies to drugs
- alcohol dependence
- asthma
- blood disorders
- heart or blood vessel disease
- epilepsy, seizures
- stomach or intestinal disease
- glaucoma
- kidney, liver, or thyroid disease
- manic-depressive illness, schizophrenia, or paranoia
- retention of urine or enlarged prostate

Tell your doctor about any other drugs you take, including aspirin, herbs, vitamins, and other non-prescription products.

Ask your doctor to check your blood pressure, once while you are lying down and once after you have been standing up for at least 2 minutes, and to do an electrocardiogram.

When You Use This Drug

◆ **Do not stop taking your drug suddenly. Your doctor must give you a schedule to lower your dose gradually, to prevent withdrawal symptoms** such as headache, mood change, nausea, vomiting, diarrhea, or trouble sleeping and vivid dreams.

◆ Do not smoke. Smoking may increase the drug's effects on your heart.

◆ Until you know how you react to this drug, do not drive or perform other activities requiring alertness. These drugs may cause blurred vision and drowsiness.

◆ It may take several weeks before you can tell that these drugs are working. If the drug works, talk with your doctor about lowering the dose gradually.

◆ Do not drink alcohol or use other drugs that can cause drowsiness.

◆ You may feel dizzy when rising from a lying or sitting position. When getting out of bed, hang your legs over the side of the bed for a few minutes, then get up slowly. When getting up from a chair, stay by the chair until you are sure that you are not dizzy. (See p. 14.)

◆ Check with your doctor before taking any other drugs, prescription or nonprescription. These drugs frequently interact with other drugs.

◆ The effects of these drugs may last for up to a week after you stop taking them. Avoid alcohol and heed all other warnings for this time period.

◆ If you plan to have any surgery, including dental, tell your doctor that you take this drug.

How To Use This Drug

◆ Take with food to reduce stomach upset.

◆ If you are taking other drugs, take them 1 to 2 hours before taking your antidepressant.

◆ Capsules may be opened and mixed with food or drink.

◆ Do not store in the bathroom. Do not expose to heat, moisture, or strong light.

◆ *If you miss a dose, use the following guidelines:*
  - If you are taking your drug more than once a day, take the missed dose as soon as you remember, but skip it if it is almost time for your next scheduled dose.
  - If you are taking your drug only once a day at bedtime and you go to sleep without taking that dose, do not take it in the morning. Instead, call your doctor.
  - **Do not take double doses.**

Interactions With Other Drugs

The following drugs are listed in *Evaluations of Drug Interactions*, 1991 as causing "highly clinically significant" or "clinically significant" interactions when used together with desipramine. They may also interact with nortriptyline. There may be other drugs, especially those in the families of drugs listed below, that also will react with these antidepressants to cause severe adverse effects. Make sure to ask your doctor for a complete listing of them and let her or him know if you are taking any of these interacting drugs:

ADRENALIN (also in bee sting kits); cimetidine; CYTOMEL; epinephrine; ESIMIL; guanethidine; INDERAL; ISMELIN; ISORDIL; liothyronine; MELLARIL; nitroglycerin (sublingual); NITROSTAT; PARNATE; PRIMATENE; propranolol; TAGAMET; thioridazine; tolazamide; TOLINASE; tranylcypromine.

Adverse Effects

Call your doctor immediately:

❑ **if you experience signs of overdose:** confusion; severe drowsiness; fever; hallucinations; restlessness and agitation; seizures; shortness of breath; trouble breathing; unusually fast, slow,

or irregular heartbeat; unusual tiredness, weakness; vomiting
- ❑ **if you experience signs of parkinsonism:** difficulty speaking or swallowing; loss of balance; mask-like face; muscle spasms; stiffness of arms or legs; trembling and shaking; unusual twisting movements of body
- ❑ blurred vision or eye pain
- ❑ confusion, delirium, or hallucinations
- ❑ constipation
- ❑ fainting
- ❑ irregular heartbeat or slow or fast pulse
- ❑ feeling nervous or restless
- ❑ impaired sexual function
- ❑ shakiness
- ❑ trouble sleeping
- ❑ trouble urinating
- ❑ sore throat and fever
- ❑ yellow eyes or skin

Call your doctor if these symptoms continue:
- ❑ dizziness
- ❑ drowsiness
- ❑ dry mouth
- ❑ headache
- ❑ increased appetite for sweets
- ❑ nausea or vomiting
- ❑ unpleasant taste in mouth
- ❑ weight gain

Periodic Tests

Ask your doctor which of these tests should be done periodically while you are taking this drug:
- ❑ blood cell counts
- ❑ pulse
- ❑ blood pressure
- ❑ glaucoma tests
- ❑ desipramine blood levels
- ❑ liver function tests
- ❑ kidney function tests
- ❑ heart function tests such as electrocardiogram (EKG)
- ❑ dental exams, at least twice yearly

Fluoxetine
PROZAC (Lilly)

Generic: not available

Family: Antidepressants

Fluoxetine (flu *ox* eh teen) is used to treat severe depression that is not caused by other drugs, by alcohol, or by emotional losses (such as a death in the family). It is an effective medication in many patients including some whose depression has not improved on other drugs. Fluoxetine appears to be most appropriate for patients who are at special risk from the fatigue, low blood pressure, dry mouth, and constipation caused by other antidepressants. It is safer in overdoses than some other antidepressants. However, limited data on its safety and efficacy in older adults are available.

Fluoxetine may reduce the risk of suicide in depressed patients. However, there have been a few reports that fluoxetine may actually induce suicidal thoughts in selected patients, although this has not been confirmed.[127] You should *not* take this drug for mild depression or anxiety, or as a sleeping pill.

When you take this medicine you may experience some adverse effects. The most frequently reported adverse effects include nausea, anxiety, headache, and insomnia. These adverse effects tend to be worst at the start of treatment, and improve over a few weeks. Akathisia, or symptoms of restlessness, constant pacing, and purposeless movements of the feet and legs, may also occur. Dry mouth, sweating, diarrhea, tremor, loss of appetite, and dizziness are also common side effects.

Elderly patients, and those who experience troublesome agitation, anxiety, or insomnia at the recommended daily dose of 20 mg should start at lower doses (e.g. 5 mg) Many consultants to *The Medical Letter* think that the manufacturer's dosage recommendations are too high.[128] A liquid form of the medicine is now available for lower doses.

The length of time it takes an antidepressant to work can overlap with the time of spontaneous recovery especially if the depression is situational — caused by a death or other external circumstances. The majority of people lift themselves out of depression with friends or activities, such as exercise, work, reading, play, art, travel, and spiritual resources. If depression is not overcome by these measures, seek help from mental health professionals, such as therapists or psychiatrists. Antidepressant drugs should be reserved for depression that is major and does not respond to psychotherapy alone.

Warning

A small number of people taking fluoxetine have experienced intense, violent, suicidal thoughts, agitation, and impulsivity. Whether their symptoms were induced by fluoxetine or were related to their underlying psychological problems is unclear. As with any other antidepressant, fluoxetine should only be used under close medical supervision. Patients are advised to consider telling relatives and friends about their use of this drug and the risk of suicidal obsession and self-injurious behavior.

Do not take fluoxetine with monoamine oxidase (MAO) inhibitors (see Interactions With Other Drugs) because the combinations may produce a syndrome of rising temperature, tremor, and seizures.

Before You Use This Drug

Tell your doctor if you have or have had
❑ allergies to drugs
❑ suicidal thoughts or actions
❑ kidney or liver disease
❑ diabetes
❑ epilepsy or seizures

Tell your doctor about any other drugs you take, including aspirin, herbs, vitamins, and other non-prescription products.

When You Use This Drug

◆ Until you know how you react to this drug, do not drive or perform other activities requiring alertness. This drug may cause drowsiness.

◆ Do not drink alcohol or take other drugs that can cause drowsiness.

◆ You may feel dizzy when rising from a lying or sitting position. When getting out of bed, hang your legs over the side of the bed for a few minutes, then get up slowly. When getting up from a chair, stay by the chair until you are sure that you are not dizzy. (See p. 14.)

◆ Stop taking this drug and check with your doctor as soon as possible if you develop skin rash or hives.

◆ If you develop dryness of the mouth, take sips of water. If dry mouth persists for more than 2 weeks, check with your doctor.

◆ Check with your doctor before you take any other drugs, prescription or non-prescription. This drug frequently interacts with other drugs.

◆ The effects of this drug may last for several weeks after you stop taking it. Avoid alcohol and heed all other warnings for this time period.

How To Use This Drug

◆ Measure liquid with a calibrated teaspoon.

◆ Capsules may be opened and mixed with food or drink. Food does not affect the extent of absorption, although rate may be slightly decreased.

◆ If you are taking other drugs, take them 1 to 2 hours before taking fluoxetine.

◆ If you miss a dose, skip the missed dose, and continue with your next scheduled dose. **Do not take double doses**.
◆ Store both forms at room temperature with cap on tightly.
◆ Do not store in the bathroom. Do not expose to heat, moisture or strong light.

Interactions With Other Drugs

The following drugs are listed in *Evaluations of Drug Interactions*, 1991 as causing "highly clinically significant" or "clinically significant" interactions when used together with this drug. There may be other drugs, especially those in the families of drugs listed below, that also will react with this drug to cause severe adverse effects. Make sure to ask your doctor for a complete listing of them and let her or him know if you are taking any of these interacting drugs:

DESYREL; ESKALITH; lithium; LITHOBID; marijuana; trazodone.

At least two weeks should elapse between stopping a monoamine oxidase (MAO) inhibitor and starting fluoxetine. You should wait at least 5 weeks after stopping fluoxetine and starting one of these MAO inhibitors:

deprenyl; ELDEPRYL; EUTONYL; EUTRON; furazolidone; FUROXONE; isocarboxazid; MARPLAN; MATULANE; NARDIL; pargyline; PARNATE; phenelzine; procarbazine; selegiline; tranylcypromine.

Additionally, the *United States Pharmacopeia Drug Information*, 1992 lists these drugs as having interactions of major significance:

alcohol; COUMADIN; digoxin; LANOXIN; tryptophan; warfarin.

Any drug which affects the central nervous system, such as antihistamines or medication for hay fever, other allergies, or colds; sedatives, tranquilizers, or sleeping medicine; prescription pain medicine or narcotics; barbiturates; medicine for seizures; muscle relaxants; or anesthetics may also cause an increase in the frequency or intensity of adverse reactions. Fluoxetine can increase the blood levels of other antidepressants, potentially increasing adverse effects from those medications.

Adverse Effects

Call your doctor immediately:
❑ **if you experience signs of overdose:** agitation and restlessness, convulsions, seizures, unusual excitement, severe nausea and vomiting
❑ **if you experience signs of allergic reaction or serum sickness-like syndrome:** skin rash or hives associated with burning or tingling in fingers, hands, or arms; chills or fever; swollen glands; joint or muscle pain; swelling of feet or lower legs; or trouble breathing
❑ **if you experience signs of hypoglycemia:** anxiety; chills; cold sweats; confusion; cool, pale skin; difficulty in concentration; drowsiness; excessive hunger; fast heartbeat; headache; nervousness; shakiness; unsteady walk; unusual tiredness or weakness
❑ suicidal thoughts or behavior
❑ chills or fever
❑ joint or muscle pain
❑ skin rash, hives, or itching
❑ trouble breathing
❑ seizures
❑ unusual excitement
❑ swollen glands
❑ lack of energy

Call your doctor if these symptoms continue:
❑ anxiety and nervousness
❑ nausea, vomiting, or diarrhea
❑ stomach cramps, gas, or pain
❑ increased or decreased appetite or weight loss
❑ constipation
❑ frequent urination
❑ dry mouth
❑ change in taste
❑ drowsiness
❑ dizziness
❑ headache
❑ increased sweating

- ❑ insomnia
- ❑ disturbing dreams
- ❑ changes in vision
- ❑ chest pain
- ❑ irregular or fast heartbeat
- ❑ stuffy nose
- ❑ cough
- ❑ tiredness or weakness
- ❑ impaired concentration
- ❑ trembling or quivering
- ❑ impaired sexual function, or inability to achieve orgasm
- ❑ feeling of warmth or heat
- ❑ flushing or redness of skin, especially on face and neck

Periodic Tests
Ask your doctor which of these tests should be done periodically while you are taking this drug:
- ❑ blood pressure
- ❑ blood sugar test
- ❑ blood electrolytes, especially for sodium
- ❑ dental exam, at least twice yearly
- ❑ eye exam for glaucoma
- ❑ heart function tests, such as electrocardiogram (EKG)
- ❑ kidney function test
- ❑ liver function test
- ❑ pulse
- ❑ supervision of depression with suicidal tendencies

LIMITED USE

Oxazepam
SERAX (Wyeth)

Generic: available

Family: Benzodiazepine Sleeping Pills and Tranquilizers (see p. 198)

Oxazepam (ox *az* e pam) **is used to treat anxiety and is the only sleeping pill or tranquilizer in its family that we recommend for older adults.** Because oxazepam, like all the drugs in its family, is addictive, you should not be taking it to relieve the stress of daily life (see information in the box below). There are safer ways to deal with occasional and short-term tension, nervousness, and sleeplessness (see p. 204). Only in a very limited number of circumstances is a sleeping pill or tranquilizer really necessary.

Oxazepam, like Valium, Dalmane and Librium (see p. 246), belongs to a family of drugs called benzodiazepines (ben zoe dye *az* e peens). It is safer than these other drugs, and may be the safest benzodiazepine for older adults, because it is short-acting rather than long-acting, meaning that it is eliminated more quickly from your body. This reduces the risk that it will accumulate in your bloodstream and reach dangerously high levels, causing harmful

One hazard of taking oxazepam continuously for longer than several weeks is addiction. **Do not stop taking your drug suddenly.** With the help of your doctor, work out a schedule for slowly lowering the amount of the drug you take by about 5 to 10% each day. Keep a written record of the dosage reduction schedule with you. These steps will make it much easier to become drug free without developing distressing symptoms of drug withdrawal.

side effects. Another reason that oxazepam is safer than other drugs in its family is that your body does not convert it into chemicals called active metabolites that can produce adverse effects.[129]

Studies show that there is much less potential for abusing oxazepam than for abusing diazepam (Valium).[130,131] Oxazepam also may have a lower risk of addiction than benzodiazepines that act over a shorter period of time, such as lorazepam (Ativan), alprazolam (Xanax), and triazolam (Halcion).[132]

Oxazepam can cause side effects common to all benzodiazepines, and older adults are more likely to experience certain ones: confusion, drowsiness, and incoordination that can result in falls and hip fractures. Oxazepam causes no less memory impairment than any benzodiazepine, other than chlorazepate, a long-acting drug.[133]

Before You Use The Drug
Tell your doctor if you have or have had
❑ allergies to drugs
❑ liver problems

Rules For Safer Use Of Oxazepam

1. Use a low dose. The dose should be one-third to one-half the dose used for younger people. This means that the highest starting dose for older adults should be 7.5 milligrams 1 to 3 times a day, if used as a tranquilizer, or 7.5 milligrams at bedtime, if used as a sleeping pill. The generic tablet form of oxazepam is only available in a 15 milligram tablet, which should be broken in half to get a 7.5 milligram dose. This is one-half of a 15 milligram tablet, available generically,

2. Ask your doctor to limit the amount of your prescription to 7 days' worth of pills.

3. Ask your doctor to write *NO REFILL* on your prescription, so that you will not be inclined (because of the "good chemical feelings" these pills may provide) to refill the prescription 5 times without seeing the doctor again. This dangerously lax refill policy is perfectly legal because oxazepam and other similar drugs are not very carefully controlled by the government.

   By urging your doctor to write *NO REFILL* you are making sure that he or she will reevaluate your condition after you use oxazepam for a short time. You want to dicuss how you are doing with your anxiety or sleeping problem, rather than continuing to take the drug without a reevaluation. Continuing to take oxazepam without talking to your doctor could be the first step to addiction or other drug-induced problems.

4. At the end of the first day and every day that you use oxazepam, evaluate what you have done, on your own or by talking to others, to learn what makes you anxious. Evaluate what you have done to change the internal or external circumstances causing your anxiety. Keep a record of these evaluations. Talk to your doctor about reducing the dose of oxazepam as soon as a reduction seems appropriate. Since you only have enough medication for 1 week, it is unlikely that you will have become addicted this quickly.

5. Do not drive a car or operate dangerous machinery while using oxazepam.

6. Do not drink alcohol. Combining oxazepam and alcohol dangerously increases the effects of both. An overdose of oxazepam in combination with alcohol can be fatal.

7. Before using oxazepam, tell your doctor if you are taking other drugs with a sedative or "downer" effect, such as antidepressants, antipsychotics, antihistamines, narcotic painkillers, epilepsy medications, barbiturates, or other sleeping medications. Combining oxazepam with other drugs that have sedative effects dangerously increases the risks of both drugs.

❑ kidney problems
❑ brief periods of not breathing during sleep (sleep apnea)
❑ lung disease or breathing problems
❑ alcohol or drug dependence
❑ mental illness, depression
❑ myasthenia gravis
❑ glaucoma
❑ epilepsy, seizures

Tell your doctor about any other drugs you take, including aspirin, herbs, vitamins, and other non-prescription products.

When You Use This Drug

◆ Do not take more than prescribed. Oxazepam is addictive.
◆ Do not drink alcohol.
◆ Until you know how you react to this drug, do not drive or perform other activities requiring alertness. Oxazepam may cause drowsiness. **People who take drugs in this family may be more likely to have traffic accidents.**
◆ If you plan to have any surgery, including dental, tell your doctor that you take this drug.

How To Use This Drug

◆ Crush tablet and mix with food or water, or swallow whole. Take with food.
◆ If you miss a dose, take it if you remember within 1 hour of the time you were supposed to take it. Skip it if more than an hour has passed. **Do not take double doses.**

Interactions With Other Drugs

The following drugs are listed in *Evaluations of Drug Interactions,* 1991 as causing "highly clinically significant" or "clinically significant" interactions when used together with this drug. There may be other drugs, especially those in the families of drugs listed below, that also will react with this drug to cause severe adverse effects. Make sure to ask your doctor for a complete listing of them and let her or him know if you are taking any of these interacting drugs:

alcohol; BENADRYL; digoxin; diphenhydramine; KETALAR; ketamine; LANOXIN.

Adverse Effects

Call your doctor immediately:
❑ **if you experience signs of overdose:** prolonged confusion; severe drowsiness; slurred speech; shakiness; staggering; slow heartbeat; shortness of breath; trouble breathing; extreme weakness
❑ confusion, hallucinations
❑ trouble sleeping
❑ unusual excitement, irritability
❑ mental depression
❑ skin rash, itching
❑ sore throat and fever
❑ yellow eyes or skin
❑ sores in mouth or throat that last
❑ unusual bleeding or bruising
❑ clumsiness, unsteadiness, or falling

Call your doctor if these symptoms continue:
❑ clumsiness
❑ blurred vision or vision change
❑ dizziness, lightheadedness
❑ constipation or diarrhea
❑ drowsiness
❑ loss of bladder control
❑ headache
❑ dry mouth, increased thirst, or unusual mouth watering
❑ nausea or vomiting
❑ slurred speech
❑ tiredness, weakness
❑ joint or chest pain
❑ fast heartbeat
❑ nasal congestion

LIMITED USE

Chlorpromazine (klor *proe* ma zeen)
THORAZINE (Smith Kline & French)
Thioridazine (thye oh *rid* a zeen)
MELLARIL (Sandoz)
Trifluoperazine (trye floo oh *pair* a zeen)
STELAZINE (Smith Kline & French)
Fluphenazine (floo *fen* a zeen)
PROLIXIN (Squibb)
Haloperidol (ha loe *per* i dole)
HALDOL (McNeil Pharmaceutical)
Thiothixene (thye oh *thix* een)
NAVANE (Roerig)

Generic: available

Family: Antipsychotics (see p. 208)

All of these drugs are effective for treating mental illnesses called psychoses, including schizophrenia. They should not be used to treat anxiety; to treat the loss of mental abilities, for example due to Alzheimer's disease, in nonpsychotic people; to sedate; or to control restless behavior or other problems in nonpsychotic people. They should also be used sparingly, if at all, for treating depression in older people since the incidence of tardive dyskinesia, an often disabling adverse effect of these drugs, is 60% in older adults with depression who are given antipsychotic drugs.[134]

These antipsychotics can cause serious side effects, including tardive dyskinesia (involuntary movements of parts of the body), drug-induced parkinsonism (see p. 212), the "jitters," and weakness and muscle fatigue (see Adverse Effects).

The chart on p. 213 shows the major differences among these drugs. If your doctor has prescribed one of these drugs and it is causing an unwanted side effect, an alternative drug can be chosen by using this chart to find the drugs that cause less of that particular effect.

Whichever of these drugs you use, you should be taking between one-tenth and one-fifth of the dose used for younger adults.

Warning: Special Mental and Physical Adverse Effects

Older adults are especially sensitive to the harmful anticholinergic effects of antipsychotic drugs such as these. Drugs in this family should not be used unless absolutely necessary.

Mental Effects: confusion, delirium, short-term memory problems, disorientation, and impaired attention.

Physical Effects: dry mouth, constipation, difficulty urinating (especially for a man with an enlarged prostate), blurred vision, decreased sweating with increased body temperature, sexual dysfunction, and worsening of glaucoma.

Before You Use This Drug

Tell your doctor if you have or have had
- [ ] allergies to drugs
- [ ] heart or blood vessel disease
- [ ] Parkinson's disease
- [ ] epilepsy, seizures
- [ ] enlarged prostate or difficulty urinating
- [ ] glaucoma
- [ ] liver disease
- [ ] alcohol dependence
- [ ] lung disease or breathing problems
- [ ] breast cancer, *not for haloperidol*
- [ ] stomach ulcer, *not for haloperidol*
- [ ] bone marrow depression, *not for haloperidol*
- [ ] diabetes, *not for thiothixene*

Tell your doctor about any other drugs you take, including aspirin, herbs, vitamins, and other non-prescription products.

When You Use This Drug

- ◆ It may take 2 to 3 weeks before you can tell that your drug is working.
- ◆ **Do not stop taking your drug suddenly.** Your doctor must give you a schedule to lower your dose gradually, to prevent withdrawal symptoms such as nausea, vomiting, and stomach upset.
- ◆ Until you know how you react to this drug, do not drive or perform other activities requiring alertness. These drugs may cause blurred vision, drowsiness, and fainting.
- ◆ Do not drink alcohol or use other drugs that can cause drowsiness.
- ◆ You may feel dizzy when rising from a lying or sitting position. When getting out of bed, hang your feet over the side of the bed for a few minutes, then get up slowly. When getting out of a chair, stay by the chair until you are sure that you are not dizzy. (See p. 14.)
- ◆ If you plan to have any surgery, including dental, tell your doctor that you take this drug.

How To Use This Drug

- ◆ Take with food or **a full glass (8 ounces) of milk or water** to prevent stomach upset.

- ◆ Do not store in the bathroom. Do not expose to heat, moisture, or strong light. Do not let the liquid form freeze.
- ◆ If you take antacids or diarrhea drugs, take them at least 2 hours apart from taking your antipsychotic drug. This does not apply to haloperidol.
- ◆ Swallow extended-release chlorpromazine capsules whole.
- ◆ If you miss a dose, take it as soon as you remember, but skip it if it is almost time for the next dose. **Do not take double doses.**

Interactions With Other Drugs

The following drugs are listed in *Evaluations of Drug Interactions,* 1991 as causing "highly clinically significant" or "clinically significant" interactions when used together with one or more of these drugs. They may interact with all drugs in this family. There may be other drugs, especially those in the families of drugs listed below, that also will react with these antipsychotics to cause severe adverse effects. Make sure to ask your doctor for a complete listing of them and let her or him know if you are taking any of these interacting drugs:

AEROSPORIN; alcohol, ethyl; amphetamine; ANECTINE; benztropine; bromocriptine; CAPOTEN; captopril; carbamazepine; cimetidine; COGENTIN; DEMEROL; desipramine; diazoxide; ESIMIL; ESKALITH; guanethidine; INDERAL; ISMELIN; lithium carbonate; LITHOBID; LITHONATE; meperidine; NORPRAMIN; OBETROL; PARLODEL; PERTOFRANE; polymyxin B; propranolol; succinylcholine; TAGAMET; TEGRETOL.

Adverse Effects

Call your doctor immediately:
- [ ] **if you have signs of tardive dyskinesia:** lip smacking; chewing movements; puffing of cheeks; rapid, darting tongue movements; uncontrolled movements of arms or legs

❑ **if you have signs of parkinsonism:** difficulty speaking or swallowing; loss of balance; mask-like face; muscle spasms; stiffness of arms or legs; trembling and shaking; unusual twisting movements of body

❑ **if you have signs of restless leg (akathisia):** restless pacing, a feeling of the "jitters"

❑ **if you have signs of akinesia:** weakness, muscular fatigue, listlessness, depression. Although often confused with true depression, akinesia is actually the most common of a group of side effects called extrapyramidal effects (see p. 211).

❑ change or blurred vision

❑ difficulty urinating

❑ **if you have signs of nueroloptic malignant syndrome:** troubled or fast breathing; high or low blood pressure; increased sweating; loss of bladder control; muscle stiffness; seizures; unusual tiredness, weakness; fast heartbeat; irregular pulse; pale skin

❑ fever and sore throat

❑ yellow eyes or skin

❑ skin rash

❑ fainting

❑ abnormal bleeding or bruising, *not for haloperidol*

❑ sore mouth or gums, *not for haloperidol or thiothixene*

❑ nightmares, *not for haloperidol or thiothixene*

❑ hives or itching, *for haloperidol*

❑ hallucinations, *for haloperidol*

❑ restlessness and the need to keep moving, *for haloperidol*

❑ **if you experience signs of overdose of** *haloperidol*: severe breathing problems; dizziness; severe drowsiness; muscle stiffness or jerking; unusual tiredness or weakness

❑ **if you experience signs of overdose of** *thiothixene*: severe breathing problems; severe dizziness; severe drowsiness; fever; muscle stiffness or jerking; seizures; unusual excitement; unusually fast heartbeat; tiny pupils

Call your doctor if these symptoms continue:

❑ constipation

❑ decreased sexual ability

❑ decreased sweating

❑ dry mouth

❑ increased skin sensitivity to sun

❑ swelling or pain in breasts

❑ milk from breasts

❑ dizziness, lightheadedness, *not for haloperidol*

❑ drowsiness, *not for haloperidol*

❑ nasal congestion, *not for haloperidol*

❑ increased appetite and weight, *for thiothixene*

Periodic Tests

Ask your doctor which of these tests should be periodically done while you are taking this drug:

❑ blood cell counts

❑ glaucoma tests

❑ liver function tests

❑ observation for early signs of tardive dyskinesia

❑ reevaluation of need for the drug

❑ urine tests for bile and bilirubin, *not for haloperidol*

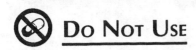 **DO NOT USE**

Alternative treatment: For depression, see *Nortriptyline and Desipramine, p. 232.*

Amitriptyline and Perphenazine (combined)
TRIAVIL (Merck)

Family: Antidepressants (see p. 215 for discussion of depression)
Antipsychotics (see p. 208)

The brand-name product Triavil contains a fixed combination of an antidepressant, amitriptyline (see p. 227), and an antipsychotic, perphenazine. It is used to treat moderate to severe anxiety, agitation, and depression. We do not recommend that you use it, for several reasons.

First, although Triavil is available in different strengths, the dose of each of its two ingredients is fixed and may not exactly fit your needs. **Second, combining an antipsychotic with an antidepressant has not been shown to produce a more effective drug.**[135] Third, using this combination raises the risk of harmful side effects, since it may cause any of the side effects of either of its ingredients, including severe drowsiness and other anticholinergic effects (see box below).[136] And fourth, the antidepressant ingredient in this combination, amitriptyline, has more side effects than any other drug in its family (see chart, p. 219) and should not be used by older adults either alone or in combinations such as this one.

The length of time it takes an antidepressant to work can overlap with the time of spontaneous recovery especially if the depression is situational — caused by a death or other external circumstances. The majority of people lift themselves out of depression with friends or activities, such as exercise, work, reading, play, art, travel, and spiritual resources. If depression is not overcome by these measures, seek help from mental health professionals, such as therapists or psychiatrists. Antidepressant drugs should be reserved for depression that is major and does not respond to psychotherapy alone.

If you use Triavil, talk to your doctor about changing your treatment. **Do not stop taking this drug suddenly.** Your doctor may want to give you a schedule to lower your dose *gradually* to prevent withdrawal symptoms, such as headache, mood change, nausea, vomiting, diarrhea, or trouble sleeping and vivid dreams.

Warning: Special Mental and Physical Adverse Effects

Older adults are especially sensitive to the harmful anticholinergic effects of tricyclic antidepressants such as amitriptyline. Drugs in this family should not be used unless absolutely necessary.

Mental Effects: confusion, delirium, short-term memory problems, disorientation, and impaired attention.

Physical Effects: dry mouth, constipation, difficulty urinating (especially for a man with an enlarged prostate), blurred vision, decreased sweating with increased body temperature, sexual dysfunction, and worsening of glaucoma.

LIMITED USE

Bupropion
WELLBUTRIN (Burroughs-Wellcome)

Generic: not available

Family: Antidepressants (see p. 215 for a discussion of depression)

Bupropion (byu *pro* pee on) is used to treat severe depression that is not caused by other drugs, alcohol, or emotional losses (such as death in the family). It can take four weeks to be effective. Bupropion controls, but does not cure depression. Although it has been used for several years in some people,[137] the manufacturer does not recommend use beyond six weeks. Bupropion is related to amphetamines and diethylpropion (Tenuate), but purportedly is not habit-forming. Although bupropion is preferred for the elderly by some doctors,[138] it has not been studied much in older people.

Weight loss is a common side effect. A number of people become restless when taking bupropion.

Higher doses increase likelihood of harmful effects. With doses more than 450 milligrams per day the risk of seizures increases tenfold and no one should take more than 450 mg per day.[139] Bupropion was temporarily banned in the United States for that reason. People age 60 and over are more likely to experience adverse effects, such as heart complications. Due to age-related decrease in kidney and liver function, the lowest effective dose should be used.

The length of time it takes an antidepressant to work can overlap with the time of spontaneous recovery especially if the depression is situational — caused by a death or other external circumstances. The majority of people lift themselves out of depression with friends or activities, such as exercise, work, reading, play, art, travel,

and spiritual resources. If depression is not overcome by these measures, seek help from mental health professionals, such as therapists or psychiatrists. Antidepressant drugs should be reserved for depression that is major and does not respond to psychotherapy alone.

Warning: Special Mental and Physical Adverse Effects

Older adults are especially sensitive to the harmful anticholinergic effects of antidepressants such as such as bupropion. Drugs in this family should not be used unless absolutely necessary.

Mental Effects: confusion, delirium, short-term memory problems, disorientation, and impaired attention.

Physical Effects: dry mouth, constipation, difficulty urinating (especially for a man with an enlarged prostate), blurred vision, decreased sweating with increased body temperature, sexual dysfunction, and worsening of glaucoma.

Before You Use This Drug
Do not use if you have or have had
- [ ] eating disorders, such as anorexia or bulimia
- [ ] seizures

Tell your doctor if you have or have had
- [ ] allergies to drugs
- [ ] bipolar disorder (manic depression)
- [ ] drug abuse
- [ ] electroshock therapy[140]
- [ ] head injury
- [ ] heart, kidney or liver problems
- [ ] myocardial infarction
- [ ] psychosis
- [ ] tumor of the central nervous system

Tell your doctor about any other drugs you take, including aspirin, herbs, vitamins, and other non-prescription products.

When You Use This Drug

◆ Until you know how you react to this drug, do not drive or perform other activities requiring alertness.
◆ Avoid using alcohol.

How To Use This Drug

◆ Swallow tablet whole. Take with food to lessen stomach upset.
◆ Space doses evenly apart during the day, but avoid taking at bedtime.
◆ If you miss a dose, take it as soon as you remember, but skip it if it is almost time for the next dose. **Do not take double doses.**
◆ Store tablets at room temperature with lid on firmly. Do not expose to high heat.

Interactions With Other Drugs

The following drugs are listed in the *United States Pharmacopeia Drug Information,* 1992 as having interactions of major significance when used with this drug. There may be other drugs, especially those in the families of drugs listed below, that also will react with this drug to cause severe adverse effects. Make sure to ask your doctor for a complete listing of them and let her or him know if you are taking any of these interacting drugs.

At least two weeks should elapse after you stop taking a monoamine oxidase (MAO) inhibitor and start taking bupropion. The same is true if you stop taking bupropion and then start one of these MAO inhibitors:

deprenyl; ELDEPRYL; EUTONYL; EUTRON; furazolidine; FUROXONE; isocarboxazid; MARPLAN; MATULANE; NARDIL; pargyline; PARNATE; phenelzine; procarbazine; selegiline; tranylcypromine.

Taking bupropion with other drugs that also affect the central nervous system adds to adverse effects, including risk of seizures:

alcohol; amitriptyline; chlorpromazine; clozapine; CLOZARIL; DESYREL; ELAVIL; ESKALITH; fluoxetine; HALDOL; haloperidol; lithium; LITHOBID; loxapine; LOXITANE; LUDIOMIL; maprotiline; MOBAN; molidone; NAVANE; PROZAC; thiothixene; THORAZINE; trazodone.

Adverse Effects

Call your doctor immediately:
❏ agitation, anxiety
❏ confusion
❏ convulsions
❏ fainting
❏ hallucinations
❏ severe headache
❏ irregular or fast heartbeat
❏ insomnia, restlessness
❏ skin rash, itching

Call your doctor if these symptoms continue:
❏ anger
❏ blood pressure becomes low or high
❏ constipation, diarrhea
❏ dizziness
❏ drowsiness
❏ dry mouth or increased saliva
❏ fever, chills
❏ impotence
❏ uncoordination
❏ inflammation of the mouth
❏ loss of appetite
❏ muscle spasms, tremor, twitching
❏ nausea or vomiting
❏ tinnitus, ringing in ears[141]
❏ increased sweating
❏ undesired weight change
❏ unusual tiredness
❏ increase in frequency of urination, especially at night, or difficult urination
❏ blurred vision

Periodic Tests

Ask your doctor which of these tests should be done periodically while you are taking this drug:
❏ kidney function tests
❏ liver function tests
❏ supervision for suicidal tendencies

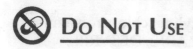 **DO NOT USE**

Alternative treatment: See nondrug approaches, p. 204, Buspirone, p. 224, and Oxazepam, p. 237.

Alprazolam (al *praz* oh lam)
XANAX (Upjohn)
Chlordiazepoxide (klor dye az e *pox* ide)
LIBRIUM (Roche)
Clorazepate (klor *az* e pate)
TRANXENE (Abbott)
Diazepam (dye *az* e pam)
VALIUM (Roche)
Estazolam (est *as* oh lamb)
PROSOM (Abbott)
Flurazepam (flure *az* e pam)
DALMANE (Roche)
Halazepam (hal *az* e pam)
PAXIPAM (Schering)
Lorazepam (lor *az* e pam)
ATIVAN (Wyeth)
Prazepam (*praz* e pam)
CENTRAX (Parke-Davis)
Quazepam (*kwayz* e pam)
DORAL (Wallace)
Temazepam (tem *az* e pam)
RESTORIL (Sandoz)
Triazolam (trye *ay* zoe lam)
HALCION (Upjohn)

Family: Benzodiazepine Sleeping Pills and Tranquilizers (see p. 198)

These twelve sleeping pills and tranquilizers all belong to the benzodiazepine (ben zoe dye *az* e peen) family. Although they are widely used for older adults, they present significantly higher risks to people over 60 and lack proven long-term benefits. These drugs can cause unsteady gait; dizziness; falling, with an increased risk of hip fractures; injurious automobile accidents; impairment of thinking and memory loss; and addiction. While some of these sleeping pills stay in the body so long you can still be sedated during the daytime, other drugs in this family stay in the body such a short time you can get rebound insomnia and become confused the following day.

Many older people who use these drugs should not be taking them. They have significant risks and are often prescribed unnecessarily.

Based on our review of the benzodiazepine drugs, which are all effective but differ in their degree of safety, we recommend (for limited use only) *oxazepam* (see p. 237) as the safest drug in this family for older adults who truly need a tranquilizer or sleeping pill. The non-benzodiazepine, buspirone (BuSpar), see p. 224, is also suggest for limited use.

These 13 benzodiazepine drugs (oxazepam and the 12 listed above) are different from each other, and the difference has to do with the different ways in which they are dangerous for older adults.

WHO specifically recommends that older adults should not use the most widely prescribed sleeping pill, Dalmane (flurazepam), "owing to a high incidence of adverse effects."[142] Seven other benzodiazepines are also more slowly cleared out of the body, especially in older adults, and can therefore accumulate, leading to increased risks. These drugs, which also should be avoided by older adults, include Valium (diazepam), Librium (chlordiazepoxide), Tranxene (chlorazepate), Centrax (prazepam), Paxipam (halazepam) Doral (quazepam) and Prosom (estazolam).

Another widely used sleeping pill, Halcion (triazolam),should also be avoided by older adults because it is so short-acting that it can cause rebound insomnia (increased sleeping problems when the drug effect has worn off), anxiety, serious amnesia (forgetfulness or memory loss) and violent, aggressive behavior. In 1992, Public Citizen's Health Research Group petitioned the Food and Drug Administration to ban Halcion. The new sleeping pill Prosom (estazolam) is in the same chemical sub-class as Halcion and, according to *The Medical Letter*, there is no reason to use it.[143] It also has the disadvantage of slow clearance from the body.

In a discussion of which of these drugs are best for older adults, it was stated that Serax (oxazepam) and Restoril (temazepam) were the drugs of choice.[144] But it has also been stated that "oxazepam (Serax) may be the safest benzodiazepine for the older patient" because **"oxazepam may offer the advantages of a short half-life and the absence of active metabolites"** (that is, chemicals into which the body converts the drug which can also have adverse effects).[145] In addition, recent studies have shown that oxazepam has much less of a "street" drug abuse potential than, for example, diazepam (Valium).[146,147]

If you are taking a tranquilizer or sleeping pill other than buspirone or oxazepam, ask your doctor to reevaluate your need for this drug. If you do need such a drug, you should be taking one of these two.

See pp. 198–207 for more discussion of the alternatives to sleeping pills and tranquilizers, the proper use of these drugs, and their safety problems.

One hazard of taking benzodiazepines continuously for longer than several weeks is addiction. **Do not stop taking your drug suddenly.** With the help of your doctor, work out a schedule for slowly lowering the amount of the drug you take by about 5 to 10% each day. Keep a written record of the dosage reduction schedule with you. These steps will make it much easier to become drug free without developing distressing symptoms of drug withdrawal.

Notes for Mind Drugs: Tranquilizers, Sleeping Pills, Antipsychotics, and Antidepressants

1. *National Prescription Audit*. I.M.S., Inc. Ambler, Pennsylvania, 1986.

2. *Drugs for the Elderly*. Denmark: World Health Organization, 1985.

3. Stewart RB, May FE, Hale WE, Marks RG. Psychotropic drug use in an ambulatory elderly population. *Gerontology* 1982; 28:328-35.

4. Ray WA. Prescribing patterns of drugs for the elderly. In *Pharmaceuticals for the Elderly*. Pharmaceutical Manufacturers Association, 1986.

5. Mellinger GD, Balter MB, and Uhlenhuth EH. Prevalence and correlates of the long-term regular use of anxiolytics. *Journal of the American Medical Association* 1984; 251:375-79. Of those people 65 and older who were using minor tranquilizers, 30.5% had been using them every day for at least 12 months.

6. *Statistical Abstracts of the United States*. U.S. Department of Commerce, 1987.

7. Mellinger, op. cit.

8. *National Prescription Audit*, op. cit.

9. *National Disease and Therapeutic Index*, I.M.S. Inc., Ambler, Pennsylvania., 1985.

10. Stewart, op. cit.

11. Ray, 1986, op. cit.

12. *Sleeping Pills, Insomnia, and Medical Practice*. Institute of Medicine, National Academy of Sciences, 1979.

13. Solomon F, White C, Arron D, Mendelson W. Sleeping pills, insomnia and medical practice. *New England Journal of Medicine* 1979; 300:803-8.

14. Ray, 1986, op. cit.

15. Ingman SR, Lawson IR, Pierpaoli PG, Blake P. A survey of the prescribing and administration of drugs in a long-term care institution for the elderly. *Journal of the American Geriatric Society* 1975; 23:309-16.

16. Perry SW, Wu A. Rationale for the use of hypnotic agents in a general hospital. *Annals of Internal Medicine* 1984; 100:441-6.

17. *Drug Utilization in the U.S*. Department of Health and Human Services, Food and Drug Administration, December 1986.

18. Hoffman-LaRoche mailing to physicians: "The later years...an optimistic outlook", 1979.

19. *Drug Utilization in the U.S.*, op. cit.

20. The fact that there are 2 million daily users 60 and over who use these drugs for a year or more is calculated as follows: 5.2% of people use minor tranquilizers daily for one year or more (Mellinger, op. cit.) and the 1985 U.S. population of people 60 and over was 39.53 million people (*Statistical Abstracts*, op. cit.). 5.2% of 39.53 is 2.06 million.

21. *Drugs for the Elderly*, op. cit.

22. Catalan J, Gath D, Edmonds G, Ennis J. The effects of non-prescribing of anxiolytics in general practice—I: controlled evaluation of psychiatric and social outcome. *British Journal of Psychiatry* 1984; 144:593-602.

23. Zung WK, Daniel JT, King RE, Moore DT. A comparison of prazepam, diazepam, lorazepam and placebo in anxious outpatients in non-psychiatric private practices. *Journal of Clinical Psychiatry* 1981; 42:280-1.

24. *Sleeping Pills, Insomnia, and Medical Practice*, op. cit.

25. Kolata G. Elderly become addicts to drug-induced sleep. *The New York Times*, February 1, 1992, p. 5.

26. Ray WA, Griffin MR, Schaffner W, Baugh DK, Melton J. Psychotropic drug use and the risk of hip fracture. *New England Journal of Medicine* 1987; 316:363-9.

27. Riggs BL, Melton LJ III. Involutional osteoporosis. *New England Journal of Medicine* 1986; 314:1676-86.

28. Buchner DM, Larson DB. Falls and fractures in patients with Alzheimer-type dementia. *Journal of the American Medical Association* 1987; 257:1492-5.

29. Ray WA, Fought RL, Decker MD. Psychoactive drugs and the risk of injurious motor vehicle crashes in elderly drivers. *American Journal of Epidemiology* 1992; 136:873-83.

30. *Statistical Abstracts of the United States*, op. cit.

31. Beck JC, Benson DF, Scheibel AB, Spar JE, Rubenstein LZ. Dementia in the elderly: The silent epidemic. *Annals of Internal Medicine* 1982; 97:231-41.

32. Larson EB, Kukull WA, Buchner D, Reifler BV. Adverse drug reactions associated with global cognitive impairment in elderly persons. *Annals of Internal Medicine* 1987; 107:169-73.

33. *Use and Misuse of Benzodiazepines*. Hearing before the Subcommittee on Health and Scientific Research of the Committee on Labor and Human Resources, United States Senate. September 10, 1979.

34. Busto U, Sellers EM, Naranjo CA, Cappell H, Sanchez-Craig M, Sykora K. Withdrawal reaction after long-term therapeutic use of benzodiazepines. *New England Journal of Medicine* 1986; 315:854-9.

35. Dement W. Presentation before the Health, Education and Welfare Joint Coordinating Council for Project Sleep. July 28, 1980.

36. Lakshminarayan S, Saohn SA, Hudson LD, Weil JV. Effect of diazepam on ventilatory response. *Clinical Pharmacology and Therapeutics* 1976; 20:178-83.

37. *The Medical Letter on Drugs and Therapeutics*. New York: The Medical Letter Inc., 1986; 28:99-106.

38. Lader M. Anxiety and its treatment. *Scrip Magazine* October 1992:46-8.

39. Catalan, op. cit.

40. Kolata, op. cit.

41. *Sleeping Pills, Insomnia, and Medical Practice*, op. cit.

42. *Physicians' Desk Reference*. 41st ed. Oradell, N.J.: Medical Economics Company, 1987. The FDA-approved labelling for all benzodiazepine tranquilizers states that there is no evidence of effectiveness for more than four months.

43. Vestal RE, ed. *Drug Treatment in the Elderly*. Sydney, Australia: ADIS Health Science Press, 1984:317-37.

44. *The Medical Letter on Drugs and Therapeutics*. New York: The Medical Letter Inc., 1981; 23:41-3.

45. *Drugs for the Elderly*, op. cit.

46. *The Medical Letter on Drugs and Therapeutics*. New York: The Medical Letter Inc., 1991; 33:91.

47. Avorn JL, Lamy PP, Vestal RE. Prescribing for the elderly—safely. *Patient Care* June 1982;14-62.

48. Vestal, op. cit.

49. Bergman U, Griffiths RR. Relative abuse of diazepam and oxazepam: Prescription forgeries and theft loss reports in Sweden. *Drug & Alcohol Dependence* 1986; 16:293-301.

50. Griffiths RR, McLeod DR, Bigelow GE, Liebson IA, Nowowieski P. Comparison of diazepam and oxazepam: preference, liking and extent of abuse. *Journal of Pharmaceutical and Experimental Therapeutics* 1984; 229:501-8.

51. Lamy PP. Pharmacological considerations in the treatment of Alzheimer's disease. *Geriatric Medicine Today* 1987; 6:29-53.

52. Vestal, op. cit.

53. National Institute of Mental Health, Epidemiological Catchment Area Data from 1981-1982.

54. *The Medical Letter on Drugs and Therapeutics* 1986, op. cit., p. 81-6.

55. *National Disease and Therapeutic Index*, I.M.S. Ambler Pennsylvania. Data is from 1984-1985.

56. Ray, 1986, op. cit.

57. Ray WA, Federspiel CF, Schaffner W. A study of antipsychotic drug use in nursing homes: Epidemiological evidence suggesting misuse. *American Journal of Public Health* 1980; 70:485-91.

58. Morgenstern H, Glazer WM, Niedzwiecki D, Nourjah P. The impact of neuroleptic medication on tardive dyskinesia. *American Journal of Public Health* 1987; 77:717-24. 22.9% of the estimated 1.3 million nursing home residents 65 and over 300,000 people, (*Statistical Abstracts of the United States*, 1986) are being given the antipsychotic drugs chronically.

59. Ibid.

60. The 450,000 estimate is based on the total U.S. non-institutionalized population 65 and over (27 million, *Statistical Abstracts of the United States*) multiplied by the estimates in Ray, 1986, op. cit., of community antipsychotic drug use-about 5% for all adults 65 and over multiplied by one-third because one-third of non-intitutionalized people using these drugs use them for three or four months or more (Morgenstern, op. cit.).

61. Estimate of total number of schizophrenics 65 years and over in the U.S. comes from multiplying the number of people 65 and over living in the community, 27 million, times 0.1%, the percentage of those 65 and over with active schizophrenia, to get 27,000 older non-institutionalized adults with schizophrenia. Then add the estimated number of nursing home residents 65 and over with schizophrenia (5% x 1.3 million = 65,000) for an estimated total of 92,000. All other psychotic disorders, such as the manic phase of manic depressive psychosis, which had a measured rate of 0.0 in people over 65 in the national survey of mental illness referred to at National Institute of Mental Health, op. cit, are not likely to add up to more than several thousand people 65 and over.

62. Again, using the estimates in Ray, 1986, op. cit., that for all people 65 and over in nursing homes, 39% get an antipsychotic drug and that 22.9% of all 65 and over nursing home residents, as in Morgenstern, op. cit., are chronic users, then 39% minus 22.9%, or 16.1%, are using these drugs for fewer than three or four months. Since there are 1.3 million residents 65 and over in nursing homes, multiplied by 16.1% gives a total of 209,000 non-chronic antipsychotic drug users in nursing homes. Similarly, using Ray, 1986, op. cit., finding that approximately 5% of all people 65 and over in the community are getting antipsychotic drugs and, from Morgenstern, op. cit., that 2/3 are non-chronic users, 900,000 non-institutionalized people 65 and over are also getting these drugs. 209,000 plus 900,000 equals 1,109,000 people.

63. Beers M, Avorn J, Soumerai SB, Everitt DE, Sherman DS, Salem S. Psychoactive medication use in intermediate-care facility residents. *Journal of the American Medical Association* 1988; 260:3016-20.

64. Ray, 1980, op. cit.

65. Barnes R, Veith R, Okinoto J, Raskind M, and Gumbrecht G. Efficacy of antipsychotic medicines in behaviorally disturbed dementia patients. *American Journal of Psychiatry* 1982; 139:1170-4.

66. Grimes JD. Drug-induced parkinsonism and tardive dyskinesia in non-psychiatric patients. *Canadian Medical Association Journal* 1982; 126:468.

67. Cooper JW, Francisco GE. Psychotropic drug usage in long term care facility geriatric patients, *Hospital Formulary* 1981; 16:407-13.

68. Ingman, op. cit.

69. Barton R and Hurst L. Unnecessary use of tranquilizers in elderly patients. *British Journal of Psychiatry* 1966; 112:989-90.

70. Shamoian CA. Psychogeriatrics. *Medical Clinics of North America* 1983; 67:361-78.

71. Reference 62, op. cit.

72. Evans LK. Sundown syndrome in institutionalized elderly. *Journal of the American Geriatrics Society* 1987; 35:101-8.

73. Peabody CE, Warner MD, Whiteford HA, and Hollister LE. Neuroleptics and the elderly. *Journal of the American Geriatrics Society* 1987; 35:233-8.

74. Yassa R, Nastase C, Dupont D, Thibeau M. Tardive dyskinesia in elderly psychiatric patients: a five-year study. *American Journal of Psychiatry* 1992; 149:1206-11.

75. Ray, 1987, op. cit.

76. *The Medical Letter on Drugs and Therapeutics*, 1986, op. cit., p. 104.

77. Evans, op. cit.

78. Barton, op. cit.

79. Yassa, op. cit.

80. Ray, 1980, op. cit.

81. *The Medical Letter on Drugs and Therapeutics*, 1986, op. cit., p. 81-6.

82. Stephen PJ, Williamson J. Drug-induced parkinsonism in the elderly. *The Lancet* 1984; ii:1082-3.

83. Grimes, op. cit.

84. Donlon PT, Stenson RL. Neuroleptic induced extrapyramidal symptoms. *Diseases of the Nervous System* 1976; 37:629-35.

85. Ibid.

86. Ayd FJ. A survey of drug-induced extrapyramidal reactions. *Journal of the American Medical Association* 1961; 175:102-8.

87. Mild, strong, and medium rankings of adverse effects are the averages of rankings from these three souces: Gilman AG, Goodman LS, Rall TW, Murad F, eds. *The Pharmacological Basis of Therapeutics*. 7th ed. New York: Macmillan, 1985.; Vestal, op. cit.; Everitt DE, Avorn J. Drug prescribing for the elderly. *Archives of Internal Medicine* 1986; 146:2393-6.

88. Ingman, op. cit.

89. Vestal, op. cit.

90. Salzman C. A primer on geriatric psychopharmacology. *American Journal of Psychiatry* 1982; 139:67-74.

91. *The Medical Letter on Drugs and Therapeutics*, 1986, op. cit., p. 81-5

92. Avorn, op. cit.

93. Thompson TL, Moran MG, Nies AS. Psychotropic drug use in the elderly. *New England Journal of Medicine* 1983; 308:194-8.

94. Thomas P. Primary care; Depressed elderly's best hope. *Medical World News* July 13, 1987:38-52.

95. Ibid.

96. Vestal, op. cit.

97. Salzman C. Clinical guidelines for the use of antidepressant drugs in geriatric patients. *Journal of Clinical Psychiatry* 1985; 46:38-44.

98. Shamoian, op. cit.

99. Duncan AJ, Campbell AJ. Antidepressant drugs in the elderly: are the indications as long term as the treatment? *British Medical Journal* 1988; 296:1230-2.

100. Shamoian, op. cit.

101. Ray, 1987, op. cit.

102. Riggs, op. cit.

103. Ray, 1992, op. cit.

104. Vestal, op. cit.

105. Thompson, op. cit.

106. Everitt, op. cit.

107. Vestal, op. cit.

108. Rankings of adverse effects are the averages of rankings from Vestal, op. cit; Thompson, op. cit; Salzman, op. cit; Everitt, op. cit.

109. Avorn, op. cit.

110. Ibid.

111. Thompson, op. cit.

112. Shamoian, op. cit.

113. Vestal, op. cit.

114. Georgotas A, McCue RE. Relapse of depressed patients after effective continuation therapy. *Journal of Affective Disorders* 1989; 17:159.

115. Duncan, op. cit.

116. *Drugs of Choice*. New Rochelle, NY: The Medical Letter,Inc., 1991:29-39.

117. *The Medical Letter on Drugs and Therapeutics*, 1986, op. cit., p. 117-8.

118. Buspirone — a radical advance in the treatment of anxiety? *The Lancet* 1988; 1:804-6.

119. American Society of Hospital Pharmacists. *American Hospital Formulary Service Drug Information*, Bethesda, MD, 1992:1355-61.

120. Gilman AG, Rall TW, Nies AS, Taylor P, eds. *The Pharmacological Basis of Therapeutics*. 8th ed. New York: Pergamon Press, 1990:428.

121. Dukes MNG, Beeley L. *Side Effects of Drugs Annual 12*, Amsterdam: Elsevier, 1988:45-6.

122. Manfredi RL, Kales A, Vgontzas AN, Bixler EO, Isaac MA, Falcone CM. Buspirone: sedative or stimulant effect? *American Journal of Psychiatry* 1991; 148:1213-7.

123. *Drugs for the Elderly,* op. cit., p. 27

124. Gilman, 1985, op. cit.

125. *Drug and Therapeutics Bulletin*, August 13, 1984, p. 62.

126. Shinn AF, Shrewsbury RP. *Evaluations of Drug Interactions*. 3rd ed. St. Louis, Toronto, Princeton: The C.V. Mosby Company, 1985:282.

127. Teicher MH, Glod C, Cole JO. Emergence of intense suicidal preoccupation during fluoxetine treatment. *American Journal of Psychiatry* 1990; 147:207-10.

128. *The Medical Letter on Drugs and Therapeutics*. New York: The Medical Letter Inc., 1990; 32:83-5.

129. Vestal, op. cit.

130. Bergman, op. cit.

131. Griffiths, op. cit.

132. Tyrer P, Murphy S. The place of benzodiazepines in psychiatric practice. *British Journal of Psychiatry* 1987; 151:719-23.

133. Lamy, op. cit.

134. Yassa, op. cit.

135. *Drug and Therapeutics Bulletin*, op. cit.

136. *USP DI, Drug Information for the Health Care Provider*. 6th ed. Rockville Md.: The United States Pharmacopeial Convention, Inc., 1986:240.

137. Harsch HH. Bupropion. *American Family Physician* 1991; 43:1789-90.

138. Gelenberg AJ. Imperfect drugs in an imperfect world. *Journal of Clinical Psychiatry* 1992; 53:39-40.

139. Davidson J. Seizures and bupropion: a review. *Journal of Clinical Psychiatry* 1989; 50:256-61.

140. Rudorfer MV, Manji HK, Potter WZ. Bupropion, ECT, and dopaminergic overdrive (letter). *American Journal of Psychiatry* 1991; 148:1101-2.

141. Settle EC. Tinnitus related to bupropion treatment. *Journal of Clinical Psychiatry* 1991; 52:352.

142. *Drugs for the Elderly*, op. cit.

143. *The Medical Letter on Drugs and Therapeutics*, 1991, op. cit.

144. Avorn, op. cit.

145. Vestal, op. cit.

146. Bergman, op. cit.

147. Griffiths, op. cit.

Painkillers and Arthritis Drugs

Non-narcotic Painkillers

Narcotic-containing Painkillers

Drugs for Arthritis and Gout

Immunosuppressants

Aspirin and Salicylates

The salicylates are used to relieve pain and to reduce fever and inflammation. Aspirin is the most well-known and frequently used salicylate. Other salicylates discussed in this book are salsalate and choline and magnesium salicylates.

Aspirin

Aspirin is the common name for a chemical called acetylsalicylic acid, or A.S.A. (as it is still known in Canada and some other countries). Aspirin, used as directed, is perhaps the most effective non-narcotic remedy, prescription or nonprescription, for pain, fever, and inflammation. Unfortunately, certain people should not use aspirin.

Aspirin Allergies

Some people are allergic to aspirin and may experience a wide variety of reactions, including hives, rash, swollen lymph nodes, generalized swelling, severe breathing difficulties, or a drop in blood pressure. Simple stomach discomfort following the use of aspirin or any other medication, however, does not indicate that you have an allergy.

Asthmatics seem to be particularly prone to aspirin allergies, as well as allergies to calcium carbaspirin, another member of the salicylate family.

If you have ever had an allergic reaction to aspirin or any other drug, be sure to tell your doctor. This kind of reaction can also occur in response to other related medications, which include prescription drugs containing salicylates or similar ingredients.

Aspirin and the Digestive Tract

Aspirin is a locally irritating, corrosive substance, which when used for a long time or in high doses can increase the likelihood of developing peptic ulcers[1] (in the lower part of the esophagus, the stomach, or the beginning of the small intestine). If you have ulcers, inflammation of the stomach (gastritis), or any form of stomach discomfort, you should not be taking even small quantities of aspirin, in any form.

Aspirin and Bleeding

Aspirin causes bleeding in the stomach; over time, it can weaken the ability to slow and contain bleeding throughout the body. Taking aspirin for a few days can increase the amount of bleeding during childbirth, after tooth extraction, and during surgery. Aspirin should not be taken for at least 5 days before surgery, even in small doses. Persons with serious liver disease, vitamin K deficiency or blood clotting disorders, or persons already taking blood thinners (anticoagulants, such as warfarin and heparin) or other drugs (see p. 268) should not take aspirin without strict supervision of a doctor or other health professional.

Aspirin should not be taken in very large doses (more than 12 regular-strength 325-milligram or 5-grain tablets per day) or for more than a few days without the supervision of a doctor. Even small doses used over a long period of time may leave certain predisposed individuals at an increased risk of serious bleeding after wounds or cuts.

Aspirin Preparations and Use

Aspirin is highly advertised, and there are many different brands from which to choose. **We recommend plain generic aspirin for intermittent use, such as for an occasional headache.**

Enteric-coated aspirin (coated so it does not dissolve in the stomach) causes much less blood loss than regular or buffered aspirin.[2] For this reason, **we recommend generic enteric-coated aspirin for everyone on long-term aspirin therapy, such as for arthritis.** Although a generic form of enteric-coated aspirin is available, it is more expensive than plain aspirin, but still less expensive than most other drugs for long-term treatment of arthritis. High-dose enteric-coated aspirin is now available (Easprin from Parke-Davis), but you pay for convenience.

National Institutes of Health arthritis expert Dr. Paul Plotz has said, referring to the treatment of arthritis when long-term use of aspirin is needed,

Enteric-coated aspirin is the best form of the drug. Indeed since the gastrointestinal side effects, the principal drawback of plain aspirin, are so much reduced and the drug is so well absorbed, enteric-coated aspirin is a close to perfect nonsteroidal inflammatory drug. It is available in several sizes and can be given twice a day with adequate serum [blood] levels.[3]

Enteric-coated aspirin should not be used for occasional problems, such as headaches, because it is absorbed more slowly than regular aspirin and takes more time to relieve pain.

Alka-Seltzer® contains aspirin and buffering agents and is much less irritating to the stomach than regular or buffered aspirin, but it is quite expensive and contains a great deal of salt (sodium).[4] If you have to restrict your intake of salt or take a salicylate for a long time, do not use Alka-Seltzer®. Since this drug contains aspirin, do not use it as an antacid.

Taking aspirin with food or after meals can decrease stomach upset. If you are on a high-dose salicylate treatment together with antacids, do not suddenly change (start or stop) the way that you take antacids without talking to your doctor first.

If you take aspirin or another salicylate regularly, the level of drug in your blood may have to be checked to make sure that you are taking the best dose. You should also have regular checkups and ask your doctor about the necessity of certain tests — hematocrit (a blood test), kidney and liver function tests, and hearing tests. Also ask if you should take vitamin C or vitamin K.

Salicylates should *not* be used by anyone with acute liver or kidney failure. They should be discontinued by anyone who has chronic liver or kidney disease if there is any sign of a worsening condition.[5] If you develop ringing in your ears or persistent stomach pain after using aspirin for a long time, call your doctor.

When you buy aspirin, make sure it is pure white and does not contain broken tablets. If it smells like vinegar, do not use it. Do not store your drug in the bathroom medicine cabinet because the heat or moisture might cause it to deteriorate and lose its effectiveness. Keep it away from heat and direct light.

Aspirin/Reye's Syndrome Alert
Do not use this product for treating chicken pox, flu, or flu-like illness. It will increase the risk of contracting Reye's syndrome, a rare but often fatal disease.

This warning appears in this book on the pages of drugs that contain aspirin and other salicylates. Although Reye's syndrome is not known to occur in adults over the age of 60, we want to alert *all* readers to the connection between these drugs and this disease. If members of your household and visitors who are under 40 need a drug to relieve pain or reduce fever, they should use acetaminophen (Tylenol, for example) rather than aspirin.

Narcotics

Narcotic drugs are prescribed to relieve pain and cough; to treat diarrhea not caused by poisoning; and to cause drowsiness before an operation. These drugs are addictive and have many side effects, and their use should be limited to the lowest dose for the shortest period of time except in the case of terminally ill people with extraordinary pain.

Use

Pain relief is the primary legitimate use of narcotics, which are effective for moderate to severe pain that has not responded to non-narcotic painkillers such as aspirin and other salicylates, acetaminophen, or nonsteroidal anti-inflammatory drugs (NSAIDs). Narcotics can be used alone or in combination with these drugs.

Most of the time when someone is able to swallow, they should first try a non-narcotic drug such as aspirin taken by mouth. If aspirin alone is not effective, it can be combined with a narcotic, such as codeine. These two drugs work in different ways and, when they are used together, they generally relieve pain that would otherwise require a higher dose of narcotic, while causing fewer side effects.[6] A sedative or antianxiety drug is just as effective as a narcotic, without causing vomiting like narcotics can.

Because narcotics are addictive and have many side effects, many doctors do not prescribe them freely. This reserve is not always appropriate. In the case of severe pain from late-stage cancer that has spread throughout the body, the pain is often undertreated as far as the use of narcotics is concerned. In an editorial in the *New England Journal of Medicine*, Dr. Marcia Angell wrote:

> *Pain is soul destroying. No patient should have to endure intense pain unnecessarily. The quality of mercy is essential to the practice of medicine; here, of all places, it should not be strained.*[7]

Wanted and Unwanted Effects of Narcotics

Narcotics affect the central nervous system, producing pain relief and drowsiness as well as less desirable effects. **Older adults may require less than the usual adult dose** to produce wanted effects because of their bodies' greater sensitivity to the drugs. Some of the adverse side effects seen more frequently in older adults are slow or troubled breathing (narcotics should never be given to anyone with depressed breathing); stimulation or confusion;[8] and hallucinations and unpleasant dreams, seen more in people using pentazocine.[9]

Other adverse effects are dizziness; drowsiness; feeling faint or lightheaded; nausea or vomiting (which might go away if you lie down for a while); blurry vision or change in vision (double vision); constipation (more often with long-term use and with codeine); difficult or painful urination or need to urinate often; general feeling of discomfort or illness; headache; dry mouth; loss of appetite; bad or unusual dreams; red or flushed face (more often with meperidine or methadone); redness, swelling, pain, or burning at place of injection; stomach pain or cramps; trouble sleeping; abnormal decrease in amount of urine; abnormal increase in sweating (more often with meperidine and methadone); abnormal nervousness, restlessness, tiredness, or weakness, and sexual problems.

Narcotics will add to the effects of alcohol and other drugs that slow down the nervous system: antihistamines (for hay fever or allergies); sedatives, tranquilizers, or sleeping pills; other narcotics; barbiturates (used to control seizures); certain antidepressants (tricyclic); and muscle relaxants. **Do not take any of these drugs or drink alcohol when you are taking a narcotic, unless your doctor has told you otherwise.**

One hazard of taking narcotics continuously for longer than several weeks is addiction. **Do not stop taking your drug suddenly.** With the help of your doctor, work out a schedule for slowly lowering the amount of the drug you take by about 5 to 10% each day. Keep a written record of the dosage reduction schedule with you. These steps will make it much easier to become drug free without developing distressing symptoms of drug withdrawal. Common withdrawal symptoms are body aches, diarrhea, goosebumps, loss of appetite, nausea or vomiting, nervousness or restlessness, runny nose, shivering or trembling, sneezing, cramps, trouble sleeping, unexplained fever, abnormal increase in sweating or yawning, abnormal irritability, abnormally fast heartbeat or weakness.

Taking Narcotics

Taking narcotics by mouth is preferred and is usually effective unless the pain is very severe.[10] The drugs can also be given in injections into the muscle or under the skin; intravenously, into the bloodstream, alone or mixed with a solution; or into the spinal cord.

Morphine sulfate is available as extended-release tablets which must be swallowed whole, but tablets of the other narcotics can be crushed. Meperidine sulfate oral solution should be mixed with a half glass of water before you drink it to decrease possible numbness of your mouth and throat.

If you are on a regular dosing schedule and you miss a dose, take it as soon as possible. But if it is almost time for the next dose, skip the missed dose and go back to the regular schedule. Do not take double doses. Drink plenty of liquids, as this may help decrease constipation. Call your doctor if you do not have a bowel movement for several days and feel uncomfortable. If you have diarrhea, do not take a drug to stop it. Instead, ask your doctor what to do.

Arthritis and Inflammation

Arthritis literally means an inflammation of a joint and is a blanket term for a number of ailments with differing significance, various causes, and diverse symptoms. Such conditions are usually characterized by pain when moving or putting weight on the joint. Inflammation (pain, heat, redness, and swelling) may or may not be present.

Pain, stiffness, swelling, or tenderness in any joint, or in the neck or lower back, which lasts longer than 6 weeks, warrants a trip to the doctor to determine the cause of the problem. A long delay in seeking help may result in irreversible damage to joints.

You should seek medical attention for pain in a joint immediately if:
◆ Joint pain or swelling is very sudden

and intense;
◆ Joint pain follows an injury (you may have a fracture near the joint); or
◆ Joint problems are accompanied by a fever above 100°F (38°C).

At least 31.6 million Americans suffer from some form of arthritis. The three most common types are rheumatoid arthritis, osteoarthritis, and gout. Each has a different cause, treatment, and probable outcome.

Rheumatoid Arthritis

Rheumatoid arthritis is an inflammation of the joints caused by disturbances in the body's immune system (which defends it against disease) and can occur at any age. Its victims are more likely to be female and include infants, teenagers, and middle-aged and older adults. It is often characterized by morning stiffness, along with pain and swelling in the joints of fingers, ankles, knees, wrists, and elbows, which improves as the day goes on. The distribution of affected joints is usually symmetrical; that is, if your right wrist is afflicted, your left wrist will probably be afflicted as well.

Treatment

There is no cure for rheumatoid arthritis, but the inflammation may be controlled under medical supervision. Drug therapy draws from two broad categories: the anti-inflammatory drugs and the antirheumatic drugs.

Anti-inflammatory Drugs
1. Nonsteroids
    salicylates
       aspirin
    nonsalicylates
       diclofenac
       etodolac
       fenoprofen
       flurbiprofen
       ibuprofen
       indomethacin
       ketoprofen
       meclofenamate
       naproxen
       piroxicam
       sulindac
       tolmetin
2. Steroids
    prednisone
    cortisone

Antirheumatic Drugs
1. Gold salts
    aurothioglucose
    gold sodium thiomalate
    auranofin
2. Antimalarial drugs
    hydroxychloroquine
    chloroquine
3. Penicillamine
4. Cytotoxic drugs
    methotrexate
    azathioprine
    cyclophosphamide

Anti-inflammatory drugs

Anti-inflammatory drugs can be further divided into *nonsteroidal* and *steroidal* drugs. *Nonsteroidal anti-inflammatory drugs (NSAIDs)* work by inhibiting formation of chemicals in the body that cause pain, fever, and inflammation. NSAIDs can be either salicylate, such as aspirin, or nonsalicylate, such as ibuprofen (Motrin, Rufen, Advil, Nuprin, Mediprin).

For rheumatoid arthritis, aspirin is the medication that many doctors use as first choice. The amount of aspirin required to reduce the inflammation of arthritis, however, approaches levels at which a small proportion of people may experience undesirable side effects. (High-dose aspirin therapy should never be started without medical supervision to determine the correct dose and to achieve the most therapeutic effect with the fewest side effects.)

Aspirin works when it is present in the bloodstream at a certain level, which varies among users. Effective blood levels of aspirin range between 15 and 30 milligrams per deciliter (tenth of a liter of blood). To achieve this level, between 9 and 23 regular (325 milligrams) aspirin tablets must be taken daily (3.0 to 7.5 grams of aspirin).[11] If you are taking aspirin, the level of the drug in your blood should be monitored periodically to prevent toxicity (poisoning). Signs of aspirin toxicity include ringing in the ears, rapid breathing (hyperventilation), mental confusion, shortness of breath, swelling of feet or lower legs (edema), dizziness, headache, nausea or vomiting, sweating, and thirst. These symptoms should be reported to your doctor immediately.

For chronic use, such as treatment of rheumatoid arthritis, we strongly recommend generic enteric-coated aspirin (the brand name version, Ecotrin, is almost twice as expensive). Studies have shown that enteric-coated aspirin provides the same amount of aspirin in the body but sharply decreases the amount of bleeding in comparison with plain aspirin.[12]

In addition to being as effective as any other arthritis drug in its family (nonsteroidal anti-inflammatory drugs), generic enteric-coated aspirin is less than one-fifth as expensive as piroxicam (Pfizer's Feldene), another NSAID. We recommend that piroxicam should not be used for people over 60 because of its increased risk of often fatal ulcers, intestinal perforation, and bleeding.

An early 1993 sampling of retail prices for various aspirin and nonaspirin arthritis drugs in drugstores in Washington, D.C. showed extraordinary differences between aspirin and others, except for ibuprofen. The most expensive drug was piroxicam ($84 a month, or $1008 a year for one 20-mg pill per day). The least expensive was generic enteric-coated aspirin ($11 a month, or $132 a year for a dose of 3 grams a day). Generic ibuprofen, at a dose of one 400-milligram pill three times a day, costs $10.71 a month or $128 a year, about the same as enteric-coated aspirin. Naproxen (Syntex's Naprosyn) costs $66 a month or $792 a year for a dose of two 375-mg pills a day.

Drug	Annual Cost
piroxicam (Feldene)	$1008
piroxicam (generic)	$ 593
naproxen (Naprosyn)	$ 792
generic ibuprofen	$ 128
generic enteric-coated aspirin	$ 132

All prescription drugs for rheumatoid arthritis are much more expensive than aspirin, have significant side effects, and are no more effective than aspirin. Like aspirin, other NSAIDs may also cause gastrointestinal bleeding or impair kidney function. Unless you have an allergy to aspirin or have experienced gastrointestinal problems while taking aspirin, enteric-coated aspirin is the drug of choice for rheumatoid arthritis. If you have had an allergic reaction or stomach problems after taking aspirin, however, another NSAID may be better tolerated. Read the information on individual NSAIDs for recommendations and adverse effects. Then discuss these choices with your doctor.

Steroids, the other type of anti-inflammatory drugs, are very important hormones that have two functions: controlling inflammation and regulating vital body functions. They are not generally recommended first for treatment of rheumatoid arthritis. Steroids may be useful, however, for older adults who cannot take or do not respond to an NSAID. They can be locally injected into a joint if a specific joint is causing considerable pain. Whenever possible, steroids are to be avoided because they are associated with numerous side effects (see p. 609), including an increased risk of developing the bone-weakening disease, osteoporosis (which is more likely to affect thin, small-boned white women).

Antirheumatic drugs

In contrast with the *anti-inflammatory drugs* just described, the *antirheumatic drugs* not only relieve symptoms, but may also slow the rheumatic disease process itself. Antirheumatic drugs, such as gold salts, should be reserved for people who have active rheumatoid arthritis that does not respond to salicylates or other NSAIDs because some form of toxicity is seen in more than 50% of people taking antirheumatic drugs.

Regardless of the drug therapy chosen by you and your doctor, an exercise program and physical therapy should be designed within the limits of pain. This will help to strengthen muscular action and maintain or improve range of motion in the joints.

Inflammation also occurs in other rheumatologic diseases such as ankylosing spondylitis, scleroderma, temporal arteritis, and polymyalgia rheumatica. Therapy follows the same general anti-inflammatory guidelines that are used to treat rheumatoid arthritis.

Osteoarthritis

Osteoarthritis is the most common type of arthritis, and is usually related to the aging of the joint. Often a mild condition, it may cause no symptoms or only occasional joint pain and stiffness. Most of the time osteoarthritis is not crippling, although a few people experience considerable pain and disability. It occasionally progresses to a point at which walking is difficult. Osteoarthritis frequently occurs in the finger joints, where it causes knobby bumps, and the spine, where it induces bone-like growths. These, however, do not commonly cause serious problems. Osteoarthritis can often be treated without medical supervision.

Unlike rheumatoid arthritis, osteoarthritis is a degenerative joint disease that does not always have inflammation as a symptom. Obesity (being excessively overweight) aggravates the wear and tear on the inside surface of the joint. Not surprisingly, the most severe form of osteoarthritis is the type that affects the joints that bear the body's weight, such as the hips and the knees. A marked improvement is often seen after weight loss and an exercise program that helps to preserve full range of movement in the affected joints.

Treatment

Enteric-coated aspirin is the best and least expensive way to relieve the pain of osteoarthritis. Unlike rheumatoid arthritis, which requires high doses of aspirin to reduce inflammation, two 325-mg tablets four times a day is often sufficient to control osteoarthritic pain in adults. Other pain relievers, including acetaminophen, are recommended for the person who cannot take aspirin. Be aware that in contrast to aspirin, acetaminophen relieves pain, but it is not effective in reducing inflammation. Therefore, we do not recommend the use of acetaminophen for the treatment of arthritis

unless it is clear that you have osteoarthritis which does not have a significant amount of inflammation.

Topical (skin) preparations marketed for treating arthritis (external salicylate-containing painkillers, such as Aspercreme and Myoflex) have no place in arthritis treatment. Salicylates (including aspirin) exert their effect on joints by absorption into the bloodstream. This is best done by swallowing tablets, not by applying cream.

Exercise should put an affected joint through its full range of motion. Swimming and walking are particularly good for this. You can start immediately and gradually improve your strength and flexibility. Under medical supervision, severe osteoarthritis is sometimes treated with physical therapy, orthopedic devices and, in extreme cases, surgery.

Gout

Gout is related to the formation of uric acid crystals in the joints. White blood cells respond to the crystals by releasing certain enzymes into the joint space. The release of these enzymes causes the intense pain and inflammation of an acute attack of gout. The big toe is a common location of gouty pain. Medical treatment by a professional is required, and is usually sought, as the pain typically comes on suddenly and is often severe.

Treatment

Gout therapy can be divided into treatment of acute (sudden) attacks and prevention of uric acid crystal formation. Colchicine relieves an acute attack by inhibiting the white blood cell response. NSAIDs are also effective for treating an acute attack, but require 12 to 24 hours before their onset of action. If you suffer from frequent attacks, or if your uric acid blood levels remain high between attacks, your doctor may prescribe either allopurinol or probenecid to reduce the uric acid in your body. Allopurinol decreases the amount of uric acid produced by the body. Probenecid increases the amount of uric acid that is eliminated by the body.

People who have gout should not use aspirin and other salicylates. Be aware that over-the-counter (nonprescription) products that contain aspirin cause retention of uric acid, and may result in a worsening of gouty arthritis. Aspirin also reduces the effectiveness of several antigout medications, for example probenecid.

Infectious Arthritis

Infectious arthritis occurs when a joint is invaded by bacteria, causing it to become red, hot, and swollen. It may be difficult to distinguish this type of arthritis from other types, as it frequently occurs in patients with other kinds of arthritis.

Treatment

This type of infection is almost always accompanied by fever and requires antibiotics, as directed by a physician, as soon as possible; otherwise the joint may be destroyed by the infectious process. No nonprescription preparations are appropriate as the sole treatment for infectious arthritis.

Flurbiprofen
ANSAID oral tablets (UpJohn)
OCUFEN eye solution (Allergan)

Generic: not available

Family: Nonsteroidal Anti-inflammatory Drugs "NSAIDs"
Arthritis Drugs (see p. 261)

Flurbiprofen (fler bih *pro* fen) is used to treat mild to moderate symptoms of rheumatoid arthritis, osteoarthritis, and bursitis. Your doctor may prescribe other arthritis drugs as well. The drug is used in drop form to dilate the eyes during cataract surgery. **In general, if you are over 60, you should take less than the usual adult dose, especially if you have decreased kidney function.**

Flurbiprofen belongs to the family of drugs called nonsteroidal anti-inflammatory drugs, shortened to NSAIDs (*n* sayds), often used to treat arthritis in older adults. Aspirin is just as effective as all these drugs and less costly (see p. 268). All the NSAIDs can cause serious harm, even fatalities, from bleeding in the stomach or intestines. Bleeding can occur at any time and without warning and older people are more likely to experience adversity from bleeding.

Elderly people are also more likely to have reduced liver and kidney function. So, some doctors believe people over age 70 should be started with half the usual dose of drugs in this group.[13]

Although flurbiprofen relieves symptoms, it does not cure any condition, nor delay progress of disease and can mask symptoms of infection.

Flurbiprofen belongs to the same family as ibuprofen (see p. 298) and aspirin (see p. 268). *The Medical Letter* found flurbiprofen about as effective as these drugs but much more costly.

Some rheumatologists (arthritis specialists) prefer aspirin to other drugs in its family for treating rheumatoid arthritis.[14] Aspirin is the best drug to treat pain and inflammation in people who do not have ulcers, or an allergy to aspirin.

Before You Use This Drug
Do not use if you have or have had
❑ an allergic reaction to aspirin, any other NSAID or iodides[15]
❑ herpes simplex (for eye drops)[16]
❑ kidney failure
❑ peptic ulcer

❏ liver disease
❏ nasal polyps
Tell your doctor if you have or have had
❏ allergies to drugs
❏ heart or kidney disease
❏ problems stopping bleeding
❏ high blood pressure
❏ hemorrhoids
❏ anemia
❏ asthma
❏ diabetes
❏ tuberculosis[17]
❏ urinary problems
Tell your doctor about any other drugs you take, including aspirin, herbs, vitamins, and other non-prescription products.

When You Use This Drug

◆ Do not drink alcohol. It irritates the stomach lining and increases the risk of stomach bleeding.
◆ Call your doctor immediately if you have flu-like symptoms (chills, fever, muscle aches or pains) shortly before or with a skin rash. This may indicate a serious reaction to flurbiprofen.
◆ You may feel dizzy when rising from a lying or sitting position. If you are lying down, hang your legs over the side of the bed for a few minutes, then get up slowly. When getting up from a chair, stay by the chair until you are sure that you are not dizzy. (See p. 14.)
◆ Avoid driving or other activities that require alertness because this drug may make you drowsy, dizzy, or lightheaded.
◆ If you plan to have any surgery, including dental, tell your doctor that you take this drug.

How To Use This Drug

◆ Take with food to reduce stomach irritation.
◆ Take with **a full glass (8 ounces) of water.** Do not lie down for 30 minutes afterwards.
◆ If you miss a dose, take it as soon as possible, but skip it if you don't remember until the next day. **Do not take double doses.**

◆ Instill eye drops according to instructions of your surgeon. Your eyes may sting temporarily.
◆ Store both tablets and eye drops at room temperature with cap on firmly. Do not expose to heat or light.

Interactions With Other Drugs

The following drugs are listed in *Evaluations of Drug Interactions,* 1991 as causing "highly clinically significant" or "clinically significant" interactions when used together with this drug. There may be other drugs, especially those in the families of drugs listed below, that also will react with this drug to cause severe adverse effects. Make sure to ask your doctor for a complete listing of them and let her or him know if you are taking any of these interacting drugs:
  bendroflumethiazide; BENEMID; CAPOTEN; captopril; COLBENEMID; COUMADIN; cyclosporine; DEXATRIM; digoxin; DILANTIN; DYAZIDE; DYRENIUM; ESKALITH; GARA-MYCIN; gentamicin; gold salts; INDERAL; LANOXIN; lithium; LITHOBID; methotrexate; MINIPRESS; MYOCHRYSINE; NALDEXON-DX; NATURETIN; phenylpropanolamine; phenytoin; prazosin; probenecid; propranolol; SANDIMMUNE; triamterene; warfarin.

Additionally, the *United States Pharmacopeia Drug Information,* 1992 lists these drugs as having interactions of major significance:
  aspirin; BUFFERIN; CEFOBID; cefoperazone; ECOTRIN.

Adverse Effects

Call your doctor immediately:
❏ abdominal pain
❏ back pain[18]
❏ bloody or black, tarry stools
❏ problems stopping bleeding
❏ breathing difficulty
❏ dizziness
❏ fever, chills, muscle aches or pain before or with a skin rash

- ❏ hives, itching, rash, or yellowing of skin
- ❏ swelling of face, lips, legs, or feet
- ❏ tremor
- ❏ unusual tiredness
- ❏ urination decreases or increases in frequency
- ❏ vision is blurred or changed
- ❏ vomiting

Call your doctor if these symptoms continue:
- ❏ constipation
- ❏ diarrhea
- ❏ depression
- ❏ drowsiness
- ❏ eyes burning or stinging
- ❏ forgetfulness
- ❏ gas, heartburn, indigestion, nausea
- ❏ headache

- ❏ insomnia
- ❏ nasal congestion
- ❏ nervousness
- ❏ ringing in ears
- ❏ weight change

Periodic Tests
Ask your doctor which of these tests should be done periodically while you are taking this drug:
- ❏ kidney function tests
- ❏ liver function tests
- ❏ stool tests for possible blood loss
- ❏ hematocrit and/or hemoglobin test
- ❏ blood concentrations of creatinine, potassium, and urea nitrogen
- ❏ white blood cell counts

Acetaminophen and Hydrocodone (combined)
BANCAP-HC (Forest)
VICODIN (Knoll)

Generic: available

Family: Painkillers
Fever Reducers
Narcotics (see p. 260)

Acetaminophen (see p. 318) and hydrocodone (hye droe *koe* done) are painkillers. Acetaminophen also reduces fever, but it does not relieve the redness, stiffness, or swelling of rheumatoid arthritis or other conditions that cause inflammation. Hydrocodone acts similarly to the narcotic drug codeine.

Together, these two drugs produce a rational combination that relieves pain better than acetaminophen alone but has less risk of side effects than the larger dose of hydrocodone that would be needed if hydrocodone were used alone. This

combination is available in tablets and in capsules.

Although this drug is the best choice in some situations, it is overused. Many people who are prescribed this combi-

One hazard of taking hydrocodone continuously for longer than several weeks is addiction. **Do not stop taking your drug suddenly**. With the help of your doctor, work out a schedule for slowly lowering the amount of the drug you take by about 5 to 10% each day. Keep a written record of the dosage reduction schedule with you. These steps will make it much easier to become drug free without developing distressing symptoms of drug withdrawal.

nation would get pain relief from acetaminophen alone, and would avoid the danger of becoming addicted to hydrocodone. So before taking this drug, ask your doctor about trying plain acetaminophen first.

Warning

There have been a number of case reports of liver damage involving a possible drug interaction between isoniazid, a medication used to prevent and treat tuberculosis, and acetaminophen, an over-the-counter painkiller and the active ingredient in Tylenol. Each drug alone is known to cause liver damage. Isoniazid alone, especially as people get older, has been documented to cause liver damage. Acetaminophen, alone in large doses or probably in combination with alcohol, also increases the risk of liver damage. The combination of acetaminophen with isoniazid, according to the authors of these case reports, may also be dangerous.

If you are taking isoniazid for tuberculosis or have a positive TB skin test and are using the drug, consult your physician before using acetaminophen or any combination product containing acetaminophen. Discuss alternatives to acetaminophen with your physician.[19,20]

Aspirin/Acetylsalicylic Acid
Plain 325 mg: **GENUINE BAYER ASPIRIN** (Glenbrook)
EMPIRIN (Burroughs Wellcome)
Enteric-coated 325 mg and 500 mg: **ECOTRIN** (SmithKline Consumer Products)
975 mg: **EASPRIN** (Parke-Davis)

Generic: available (except 975 mg product)

Family: Painkillers
Nonsteroidal Anti-inflammatory Drugs "NSAIDs"
Salicylates (see p. 258)
Fever Reducers

Aspirin (*as* pir in) relieves mild to moderate pain and reduces fever and inflammation. When you take aspirin for pain or fever, you are only treating *symptoms* of an underlying problem such as an infection. You are *not* treating the underlying problem itself. **You should not take aspirin if you have ulcers, a severely irritated stomach, gout, severe anemia, hemophilia or other bleeding problems, if you take an anticoagulant drug such as heparin or warfarin, or if you are allergic to aspirin or similar painkillers.**

Aspirin belongs to the family of drugs called nonsteroidal anti-inflammatory drugs, shortened to NSAIDs (*n* sayds), often used to treat arthritis in older adults. All the NSAIDs can cause serious harm, even fatalities, from bleeding in the stomach or intestines. Bleeding can occur at any time and without warning and older people are more likely to experience adversity from bleeding. Elderly people are also more likely to have reduced liver and kidney function. So, some doctors believe people over age 70 should be started with half the usual dose of drugs in this group.[21]

There are several forms of aspirin for different situations. If you take aspirin only occasionally, plain, generic aspirin is best. For long-term use, we strongly recommend aspirin that is "enteric-coated" (coated so it does not dissolve in the stomach), since it helps prevent the stomach bleeding that aspirin can cause and it can be taken twice a day. We do not recommend buffered aspirin (see p. 272), since it is no better than plain aspirin and is more costly.

In general, you should not take aspirin to reduce a fever until the cause of the fever is known. It is rarely *necessary* to reduce a fever, but if a fever is having harmful effects or is making you extremely uncomfortable, it can be treated with aspirin.[22] When you are taking aspirin for a fever, you should take it regularly (every 3 to 4 hours), and stop taking it when the underlying problem goes away or is controlled through other treatment.

If you have arthritis, either plain or enteric-coated aspirin may be the first drug your doctor prescribes. As long as you can tolerate high doses of aspirin for a long time, it is the best treatment. It might take 2 to 3 weeks or longer before aspirin is maximally effective. If the dose you are taking at first is not high enough, it should be increased slowly — more slowly for older adults than it would be for younger people. **In general, people over 60 should take less than the usual adult dose because of the risk of harmful side effects, such as stomach and intestinal problems.**

If you have joint pain and think that you might have arthritis, **do not try to treat yourself.** See your doctor. There are several kinds of arthritis, and different types require different treatments (see p. 261). **High-dose aspirin therapy can be dangerous if it is not monitored by a doctor.**

Doctors sometimes prescribe aspirin as a preventive measure for illnesses such as heart disease. If you have had a heart attack or are at risk of having sudden chest pain (unstable angina pectoris), your doctor may prescribe low, daily doses of aspirin to help prevent heart attacks. Aspirin also reduces the risk of stroke and death for some men who have had decreased blood flow to the brain (this has not been proven for women). Do not take aspirin for this purpose unless your doctor has prescribed it for you.

Aspirin/Reye's Syndrome Alert
Do not use this product for treating chicken pox, flu, or flu-like illness. It will increase the risk of contracting Reye's syndrome, a rare but often fatal disease.

Before You Use This Drug

Tell your doctor if you have or have had
- allergies to drugs
- a reaction to aspirin, other salicylates, or nonsteroidal anti-inflammatory drugs such as ibuprofen or naproxen
- bleeding problems
- ulcer or other stomach problems
- kidney, liver, or heart disease
- asthma, allergies, or nasal polyps
- anemia
- glucose-6-phosphate dehydrogenase deficiency
- gout
- overactive thyroid

Tell your doctor about any other drugs you take, including aspirin, herbs, vitamins, and other non-prescription products.

When You Use This Drug
- Do not drink alcohol. This combination increases the risk of stomach or intestinal bleeding.
- Never take more than the amount prescribed by your doctor or recommended on the package label.
- **Caution diabetics: see p. 516.**

◆ If you are treating yourself, call your doctor if your symptoms do not improve or if you have a fever that lasts more than 3 days or returns.
Do not take aspirin for 5 days before any surgery, unless your doctor tells you otherwise. Aspirin interferes with your body's ability to stop bleeding.
If you are on long-term or high-dose treatment, you should have regular checkups.
◆ Never place aspirin directly on teeth or gums because it irritates these tissues.
◆ Do not chew aspirin within 1 week after you have had any type of surgery in your mouth.

How To Use This Drug

◆ Take tablets and capsules with **a full glass (8 ounces) of water**. Do not lie down for 30 minutes.
Take with food to decrease stomach upset.
If you miss a dose, take it as soon as you remember, but skip it if it is almost time for the next dose. **Do not take double doses.**

Interactions With Other Drugs

The following drugs are listed in *Evaluations of Drug Interactions*, 1991 as causing "highly clinically significant" or "clinically significant" interactions when used together with this drug. There may be other drugs, especially those in the families of drugs listed below, that also will react with this drug to cause severe adverse effects. Make sure to ask your doctor for a complete listing of them and let her or him know if you are taking any of these interacting drugs:

acetazolamide; alcohol, ethyl; aluminum hydroxide/magnesium hydroxide; ANTURANE; CAPOTEN; captopril; chlorpropamide; COUMADIN; DEPAKENE; DIABINESE; DIAMOX; FOLEX; GARAMYCIN; gentamicin; heparin; MAALOX; MAALOX TC; MEDROL; MEXATE; methotrexate; methylprednisolone; RIOPAN; sulfinpyrazone; valproic acid; warfarin.

Adverse Effects

Call your doctor immediately:
❑ **if you experience signs of overdose:** severe or continuing headache; ringing or buzzing in ears; loss of hearing; severe or continuing diarrhea; dizziness or lightheadedness; confusion; extreme drowsiness; nausea or vomiting; stomach pain; abnormal increase in sweating; abnormally fast or deep breathing; abnormal thirst; abnormal or uncontrolled flapping of hands; vision problems; bloody urine; seizures; hallucinations; nervousness or excitement; trouble breathing; unexplained fever
❑ vomiting material that looks bloody or like coffee grounds
❑ bloody or black, tarry stools
❑ wheezing, tightness in chest, or trouble breathing
❑ skin rash, hives, or itching
❑ fainting or dizzy spells
Call your doctor if these symptoms continue:
❑ heartburn, indigestion, nausea, or stomach pain
❑ abnormal weakness or fatigue
❑ decreased urination

LIMITED USE

Probenecid
BENEMID (Merck)
SK-PROBENECID (Smith Kline & French)

Generic: available
Family: Antigout Drugs (see p. 261)
Antibiotic Therapy Aid

Probenecid (proe *ben* e sid) helps to prevent gout attacks. Gout occurs in people who have high levels of uric acid in their body, and an attack occurs when crystals of uric acid form in your joints and your body releases chemicals in response to the crystals. This causes pain and inflammation. Probenecid works by causing more uric acid to leave your body through the kidneys, thereby lowering the level of uric acid in your blood.

Probenecid will not relieve a gout attack that has already started. If you are taking probenecid, keep taking it during an attack, even if another drug is prescribed to treat the attack.

After you start using probenecid, you may still have gout attacks for a while. Keep taking the drug. If you take it regularly, the attacks gradually will become less frequent and less painful, and they may stop completely after several months.

Probenecid can increase your risk of getting kidney stones. To help prevent kidney stones while using probenecid, drink at least 10 to 12 full glasses (8 ounces each) of fluid each day, unless your doctor tells you otherwise. Too much vitamin C (see p. 575) also increases your risk of kidney stones, so do not take vitamin C supplements while taking probenecid unless you have checked with your doctor.

Before You Use This Drug
Tell your doctor if you have or have had
❑ allergies to drugs
❑ kidney problems
❑ kidney stones
❑ blood disease
❑ stomach ulcer
Tell your doctor about any other drugs you take, including aspirin, herbs, vitamins, and other non-prescription products.

When You Use This Drug
◆ Do not take aspirin and other drugs in its family (salicylates, see p. 258) because they may make probenecid less effective.
◆ Do not drink alcohol. Because alcohol increases the amount of uric acid in your blood, it may make your gout attacks more frequent and more difficult to control. It also increases the likelihood of stomach problems.
◆ **Caution diabetics:** Probenecid may cause false results in copper sulfate urine sugar tests (Clinitest). It will not interfere with glucose enzymatic urine sugar tests (Clinistix).

How To Use This Drug
◆ Take with food to decrease stomach upset. If this does not work and your stomach continues to be upset, check with your doctor.
◆ Do not expose to heat, moisture, or strong light. Do not store in the bathroom.
◆ If you miss a dose, take it as soon as you remember, but skip it if you don't remember until the next day. **Do not take double doses.**

Interactions With Other Drugs
The following drugs are listed in *Evaluations of Drug Interactions*, 1991 as causing "highly clinically significant" or "clinically significant" interactions when used to-

gether with this drug. There may be other drugs, especially those in the families of drugs listed below, that also will react with this drug to cause severe adverse effects. Make sure to ask your doctor for a complete listing of them and let her or him know if you are taking any of these interacting drugs:

aspirin; cephalothin; DILOR; dyphylline; ECOTRIN; FOLEX; INDOCIN; indomethacin; KEFLIN; LUFYLLIN; methotrexate; MEXATE; RETROVIR; zidovudine.

Adverse Effects
Call your doctor immediately:
- ❏ **if you experience signs of overdose:** convulsions; severe vomiting
- ❏ skin rash, hives, itching
- ❏ bloody or cloudy urine
- ❏ difficult or painful urination
- ❏ back pain

- ❏ trouble breathing
- ❏ unusual weight gain
- ❏ swelling of feet, legs, or face
- ❏ sore throat and fever
- ❏ unusual bleeding or bruising
- ❏ unusual tiredness or weakness
- ❏ decrease in amount of urine
- ❏ yellow eyes or skin

Call your doctor if these symptoms continue:
- ❏ headache
- ❏ loss of appetite
- ❏ nausea or vomiting
- ❏ dizziness
- ❏ flushing or redness of face
- ❏ frequent urge to urinate
- ❏ sore gums

Periodic Tests
Ask your doctor which of these tests should be done periodically while you are taking this drug:
- ❏ blood levels of uric acid

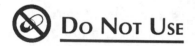 **DO NOT USE**

Alternative treatment: See Plain or Enteric-coated Aspirin, p. 258.

Buffered Aspirin
BUFFERIN (Bristol-Meyers)
ASCRIPTIN, ASCRIPTIN A/D (Rorer)

Family: Painkillers
Nonsteroidal Anti-inflammatory Drugs "NSAIDs"
Fever Reducers
Salicylates (see p. 258)

Buffered aspirin is aspirin with a "buffer" or "acid neutralizer" added. Advertisements for buffered aspirin claim that it relieves pain faster than plain aspirin because it is absorbed better, and also that it is less irritating to the stomach and intestines than plain aspirin. These claims cannot be justified.

The amount of buffer in buffered aspirin is very small, only a fraction of the amount found in even one teaspoon of many antacids. A Food and Drug Administration advisory committee found that although buffered aspirin may be absorbed more quickly than plain aspirin, it does *not* provide much faster pain relief. The committee also found *no* evidence that buffered aspirin is any gentler to the stomach than plain aspirin.[23] Alka-Seltzer®, a brand of buffered aspirin, should not be taken by anyone whose salt (sodium) intake has been limited.

If you take aspirin only occasionally, plain generic aspirin (see p. 268) is better than buffered, because it is much less expensive (about one-quarter of the price of Bufferin or Ascriptin) and relieves pain just as quickly. If you are taking aspirin for a long period of time, such as for arthritis, you should use generic enteric-coated aspirin, which actually does decrease the amount of irritation and bleeding in the stomach and which is also much less expensive than Bufferin or Ascriptin.

Aspirin/Reye's Syndrome Alert
Do not use this product for treating chicken pox, flu, or flu-like illness. It will increase the risk of contracting Reye's syndrome, a rare but often fatal disease.

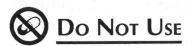 Do Not Use

Alternative treatment: See Enteric-coated Aspirin, p. 258.

Phenylbutazone
BUTAZOLIDIN (Geigy)
Oxyphenbutazone
TANDEARIL (Geigy)

Family: Nonsteroidal Anti-inflammatory Drugs "NSAIDs"
Arthritis Drugs (see p. 261)

Phenylbutazone (fen ill *byoo* ta zone) and oxyphenbutazone (ox ee fen *byoo* ta zone) relieve the pain and inflammation of rheumatoid arthritis and acute gout. **Do not use these drugs.** Oxyphenbutazone was taken off the market in 1986, but you or your friends or relatives may still have supplies of this drug and may be using it. Phenylbutazone is still being prescribed and sold but the World Health Organization has said that the drug should not be used by older people. [24] **Both drugs have caused numerous deaths and produce severe side effects.** They are toxic (poisonous) to bone marrow and can kill white blood cells.

These drugs belong to the family of drugs called nonsteroidal anti-inflammatory drugs, shortened to NSAIDs (*n* sayds), often used to treat arthritis in older adults. Aspirin is just as effective as all these drugs and less costly (see p. 268). All the NSAIDs can cause serious harm, even fatalities, from bleeding in the stomach or intestines. Bleeding can occur at any time and without warning and older people are more likely to experience adversity from bleeding. Elderly people are also more likely to have reduced liver and kidney function. So, some doctors believe people over age 70 should be started with half the usual dose of drugs in this group. [25]

Aspirin (see p. 268) is the drug of choice for treating pain, fever, and inflammation in people who do not have ulcers, gastritis (inflammation of the stomach), or an allergy to aspirin. Some rheumatologists (arthritis specialists) prefer aspirin to other drugs in this family for treating rheumatoid arthritis. [26]

If you are taking phenylbutazone or oxyphenbutazone, ask your doctor if you can switch to taking enteric-coated aspirin (aspirin coated so it won't dissolve in the stomach) twice a day. If you cannot take aspirin, ask about switching to another drug in this family such as ibuprofen (see p. 298). Each person responds differently to different NSAIDs.

LIMITED USE

Sulindac
CLINORIL (Merck)

Generic: available

Family: Nonsteroidal Anti-inflammatory
Drugs "NSAIDs"
Arthritis Drugs (see p. 261)

In older adults, sulindac (sul *in* dak) is used mainly to relieve the pain and inflammation of rheumatoid arthritis, osteoarthritis, and acute gout. **In general, if you are over 60, you should take less than the usual adult dose, especially if you have decreased kidney function.** Like indomethacin (see p. 291), to which it is chemically related, sulindac can cause headaches, drowsiness, and dizziness.

Sulindac belongs to the family of drugs called nonsteroidal anti-inflammatory drugs, shortened to NSAIDs (*n* sayds), often used to treat arthritis in older adults. Aspirin is just as effective as all these drugs and less costly (see p. 268). All the NSAIDs can cause serious harm, even fatalities, from bleeding in the stomach or intestines. Bleeding can occur at any time and without warning and older people are more likely to experience adversity from bleeding. Elderly people are also more likely to have reduced liver and kidney function. So, some doctors believe people over age 70 should be started with half the usual dose of drugs in this group.[27]

For most people, sulindac has no proven advantage over other drugs in this family. However, it may do less harm to the kidneys than other NSAIDs. Because of this, people with kidney disease may be able to take sulindac even if they can't take other drugs in its family, as long as they don't also have liver disease.[28]

Aspirin is the drug of choice for treating pain, fever, and inflammation in people who do not have ulcers, gastritis (inflammation of the stomach), or an allergy to aspirin. Some rheumatologists (arthritis experts) prefer aspirin to other drugs in its family for treating rheumatoid arthritis.[29]

If you are taking sulindac, ask your doctor if you can switch to taking enteric-coated aspirin (aspirin coated so it won't dissolve in the stomach) twice a day. If you can't take aspirin, ask about switching to another drug in this family such as ibuprofen (see p. 298). Each person responds differently to different NSAIDs.

Before You Use This Drug
Do not use if you have or have had
❑ an allergic reaction to aspirin, any other NSAID or iodides[30]
❑ kidney or heart failure
❑ peptic ulcers
❑ alcohol dependence
❑ cirrhosis of the liver
❑ nasal polyps or asthma
Tell your doctor if you have or have had
❑ allergies to drugs
❑ heart, kidney, or liver disease
❑ problems stopping bleeding
❑ high blood pressure
Tell your doctor about any other drugs you take, including aspirin, herbs, vitamins, and other non-prescription products.

When You Use This Drug
◆ Do not drink alcohol. It irritates the stomach lining and increases the risk of stomach bleeding.
◆ Call your doctor immediately if you have flu-like symptoms (chills, fever, muscle aches or pains) shortly before or with a skin rash. This may indicate a serious reaction to sulindac.

◆ You may feel dizzy when rising from a lying or sitting position. If you are lying down, hang your legs over the side of the bed for a few minutes, then get up slowly. When getting up from a chair, stay by the chair until you are sure that you are not dizzy. (See p. 14.)

◆ If you plan to have any surgery, including dental, tell your doctor that you take this drug.

How To Use This Drug

◆ Take with food to reduce stomach irritation.

◆ Take with **a full glass (8 ounces) of water.** Do not lie down for 30 minutes afterwards.

◆ If you miss a dose, take it as soon as possible, but skip it if you don't remember until the next day. **Do not take double doses.**

◆ Store at room temperature, with lid on tightly. Do not expose to moisture or heat. Do not store in the bathroom.

Interactions With Other Drugs

The following drugs are listed in *Evaluations of Drug Interactions*, 1991 as causing "highly clinically significant" or "clinically significant" interactions when used together with this drug. There may be other drugs, especially those in the families of drugs listed below, that also will react with this drug to cause severe adverse effects. Make sure to ask your doctor for a complete listing of them and let her or him know if you are taking any of these interacting drugs:

COUMADIN; cyclosporine; DILANTIN; labetalol; methotrexate; MINIPRESS; NORMODYNE; phenytoin; prazosin; SANDIMMUNE; TRANDATE; warfarin.

Adverse Effects

Call your doctor immediately:
❑ bloody or black, tarry stools
❑ confusion, forgetfulness
❑ mental depression, other mood or mental changes
❑ ringing or buzzing in ears
❑ swelling of feet or lower legs
❑ unusual weight gain
❑ abdominal/stomach pain or cramps
❑ vomiting blood or material that looks like coffee grounds
❑ bleeding sores on lips
❑ fainting
❑ fever, chills, muscle aches, or pain before or with a skin rash
❑ skin rash, itching, or peeling
❑ changes in vision or hearing
❑ unusual bleeding or bruising
❑ numbness or tingling in limbs
❑ sudden decrease in amount of urine

Call your doctor if these symptoms continue:
❑ dizziness or lightheadedness
❑ heartburn or indigestion
❑ nausea or vomiting
❑ constipation or diarrhea
❑ drowsiness

Periodic Tests

Ask your doctor which of these tests should be done periodically while you are taking this drug:
❑ kidney function tests
❑ liver function tests
❑ stool tests for possible blood loss
❑ hematocrit and/or hemoglobin test
❑ blood concentrations of creatinine, potassium, and urea nitrogen
❑ white blood cell counts

Codeine

Generic: available

Family: Narcotics (see p. 260)

Codeine (*koe* deen) relieves mild to moderate pain and also suppresses coughing. **Do not use codeine if you have a history of serious constipation.**

One hazard of taking codeine continuously for longer than several weeks is addiction. **Do not stop taking your drug suddenly.** With the help of your doctor, work out a schedule for slowly lowering the amount of the drug you take by about 5 to 10% each day. Keep a written record of the dosage reduction schedule with you. These steps will make it much easier to become drug free without developing distressing symptoms of drug withdrawal.

Before You Use This Drug
Tell your doctor if you have or have had
❑ allergies to drugs
❑ an unusual reaction to any narcotics
❑ brain disease or head injury
❑ colitis (inflammation of the colon)
❑ emphysema, asthma, or lung disease
❑ enlarged prostate or trouble urinating
❑ gallbladder disease or gallstones
❑ heart, kidney, or liver disease
❑ seizures
❑ underactive thyroid or adrenal gland
Tell your doctor about any other drugs you take, including aspirin, herbs, vitamins, and other non-prescription products.

When You Use This Drug
◆ Do not drink alcohol or take any drugs that make you drowsy unless you have checked with your doctor first. When codeine is combined with these substances, it will make you even more drowsy, which puts you at risk of having accidents.
◆ Do not drive or perform other activities that require alertness because this drug may make you drowsy, dizzy, or lightheaded.
◆ **This drug can increase the risk of hip fracture.**[31]
◆ If this drug seems less effective after a few weeks of use, **do not increase the dose.** Call your doctor instead.
◆ If you use this drug for a long time, have regular checkups.
◆ You may feel dizzy when rising from a lying or sitting position. If you are lying down, hang your legs over the side of the bed for a few minutes, then get up slowly. When getting up from a chair, stay by the chair until you are sure that you are not dizzy. (See p. 14.)
◆ If you plan to have any surgery, including dental, tell your doctor that you take this drug.

How To Use This Drug
◆ Do not store tablets in the bathroom.
◆ Protect liquid form from freezing.
◆ If you miss a dose, take it as soon as you remember, but skip it if it is almost time for the next dose. **Do not take double doses.**

Interactions With Other Drugs
The following drugs are listed in *Evaluations of Drug Interactions,* 1991 as causing "highly clinically significant" or "clinically significant" interactions when used together with this drug. There may be other drugs, especially those in the families of drugs listed below, that also will react with this drug to cause severe adverse effects. Make sure to ask your doctor for a complete listing of them and let her or him know if you are taking any of these interacting drugs:

carbamazepine; cimetidine;

chlorpromazine; COUMADIN; NARDIL; PENTOTHAL; phenelzine; TAGAMET; TEGRETOL; thiopental; THORAZINE; tubocurarine; warfarin.

Adverse Effects
Call your doctor immediately:
❑ **if you experience signs of overdose:** cold, clammy skin; convulsions; severe dizziness or drowsiness; nervousness or restlessness; confusion; small pupils; unconsciousness; abnormally low blood pressure; slow heartbeat; slow or troubled breathing; severe weakness
❑ feelings of unreality
❑ hallucinations (seeing, feeling, or hearing things that are not there)

❑ skin rash, hives, or itching
❑ depression
❑ ringing sound in ears
❑ slow, irregular, or troubled breathing
❑ swollen face
❑ trembling or uncontrolled muscle movements
❑ abnormal (slow, fast, or pounding) heartbeat
Call your doctor if these symptoms continue:
❑ dizziness
❑ drowsiness
❑ confusion
❑ feeling faint or lightheaded
❑ nausea or vomiting
❑ constipation
❑ sweating

LIMITED USE

Colchicine

Generic: available

Family: Antigout Drugs (see p. 261)

Colchicine (*kol* chi seen) prevents and treats gout attacks, and reduces inflammation and relieves pain from acute gouty arthritis.

Gout occurs in people who have high levels of uric acid in their body, and an attack occurs when crystals of uric acid form in the joints and the body responds by releasing harmful chemicals. This causes pain and inflammation.

Colchicine prevents and treats attacks by decreasing the amount of chemicals that your body releases into the joints. It does not lower the level of uric acid in your body, which is the root cause of the problem. Colchicine has several harmful side effects (see Adverse Effects) and you may be better off taking large doses of an anti-inflammatory drug such as naproxen (a nonsteroidal anti-inflammatory drug, see p.

302), which has fewer harmful effects. Stop taking colchicine and call your doctor immediately if you have diarrhea, nausea, vomiting, or stomach pain. **Older adults are more susceptible to colchicine's side effects. If you have decreased kidney function, you should be on a low dose of colchicine in order to reduce adverse effects such as muscle and nerve damage.**[32]

Before You Use This Drug
Tell your doctor if you have or have had
❑ allergies to drugs
❑ bone marrow depression or blood cell diseases
❑ heart, liver, or kidney disease
❑ severe intestinal disease
❑ ulcer or other stomach problem
Tell your doctor about any other drugs you take, including aspirin, herbs, vitamins, and other non-prescription products.

When You Use This Drug

◆ Do not take more than prescribed, even if the pain is not relieved or if you do not experience side effects.
◆ Do not drink alcohol. Because alcohol increases the amount of uric acid in your blood, it may make your gout attacks more frequent or more difficult to control. It also increases the likelihood of stomach problems.

How To Use This Drug

◆ If you take other drugs to prevent gout attacks and your doctor prescribes colchicine when you have an attack, keep taking the other drugs as directed by your doctor.
◆ *If you take colchicine only when you have an attack:* Take it at the first sign of attack. Stop taking it as soon as pain is relieved or if you experience nausea, vomiting, stomach pain, or diarrhea. Do not take it more often than every 3 days, unless your doctor tells you otherwise.
◆ *If you take colchicine regularly to prevent attacks:* Increase your dose, as directed by your doctor, at the first sign of an attack. Stop taking the larger dose as soon as pain is relieved or if you experience nausea, vomiting, stomach pain, or diarrhea. After the attack is over, return to your regular dose.
◆ Do not expose to heat, moisture, or strong light. Do not store in the bathroom.
◆ If you miss a dose, take it as soon as you remember, but skip it if it is almost time for the next dose. Do not take double doses.

Interactions With Other Drugs

Some other drugs that you may be taking (either over-the-counter or prescription drugs) can interact with this one, causing adverse effects. Find out from your doctor what these drugs are and let him or her know if you are taking any of them.

Adverse Effects

Call your doctor immediately:
❑ if you experience signs of overdose: bloody urine; burning feeling in stomach, throat, or skin; seizures; diarrhea; fever; mood or mental changes; severe muscle weakness; sudden decrease in amount of urine; difficulty breathing; severe vomiting
❑ numbness or tingling in hands or feet
❑ skin rash
❑ sore throat and fever
❑ unusual bleeding or bruising
❑ unusual tiredness or weakness
❑ redness or pain at injection site
Call your doctor if these symptoms continue:
❑ loss of appetite
❑ unusual hair loss

Periodic Tests

Ask your doctor which of these tests should be done periodically while you are taking this drug:
❑ complete blood counts

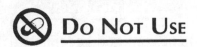 **DO NOT USE**

Alternative treatment: See Aspirin, p. 268, and Codeine, p. 276.

Propoxyphene
DARVON, DARVON-N (Lilly)

Propoxyphene and Acetaminophen (combined)
DARVOCET-N (Lilly) WYGESIC (Wyeth)

Propoxyphene, Aspirin, and Caffeine (combined)
DARVON COMPOUND, DARVON COMPOUND-65 (Lilly)

Family: Narcotics (see p. 260)

Propoxyphene (proe *pox* i feen) is a narcotic that relieves mild to moderate pain. **We recommend that you do not use it because it is no more effective than aspirin (see p. 268) or codeine (see p. 276) and it is much more dangerous than aspirin.** If you have taken aspirin for your pain and it has not worked, propoxyphene will probably not do any better.[33] In fact, some studies say that propoxyphene by itself is

> **These drugs can increase the risk of hip fracture.[37]**

no more effective than a sugar pill (placebo).[34] Most studies show that propoxyphene is less effective than aspirin **and that it has a potential for addiction and overdose.**[35]

Many people who have taken propoxyphene have become addicted to the

---

Warning

There have been a number of case reports of liver damage involving a possible drug interaction between isoniazid, a medication used to prevent and treat tuberculosis, and acetaminophen, an over-the-counter painkiller and the active ingredient in Tylenol. Each drug alone is known to cause liver damage. Isoniazid alone, especially as people get older, has been documented to cause liver damage. Acetaminophen, alone in large doses or probably in combination with alcohol, also increases the risk of liver damage. The combination of acetaminophen with isoniazid, according to the authors of these case reports, may also be dangerous.

If you are taking isoniazid for tuberculosis or have a positive TB skin test and are using the drug, consult your physician before using acetaminophen or any combination product containing acetaminophen. Discuss alternatives to acetaminophen with your physician.[38,39]

drug without knowing it. Thousands of these people have died, some through accidental overdoses. Several experts on drug prescribing for older adults have recommended that propoxyphene not be taken by this group.[36]

One hazard of taking propoxyphene continuously for longer than several weeks is addiction. **Do not stop taking your drug suddenly**. With the help of your doctor, work out a schedule for slowly lowering the amount of the drug you take by about 5 to 10% each day. Keep a written record of the dosage reduction schedule with you. These steps will make it much easier to become drug free without developing distressing symptoms of drug withdrawal.

Meperidine
DEMEROL (Winthrop-Breon)
Hydromorphone
DILAUDID (Knoll)

Generic: available

Family: Narcotics (see p. 260)

Meperidine (me *per* i deen) is a narcotic drug that relieves moderate to severe pain. Do not take this drug if you have taken antidepressant monoamine oxide inhibitors within the past 2 weeks (see Interactions With Other Drugs). **In general, if you are over 60, you should take less than the usual adult dose of meperidine, especially if you have kidney disease**.

Hydromorphone (hye droe *mor* fone), another narcotic, is related to morphine. Like morphine, it relieves severe pain that is not helped by non-narcotic drugs, such as pain from many kinds of cancer.

Before You Use This Drug
Tell your doctor if you have or have had
❑ allergies to drugs
❑ an unusual reaction to any narcotics
❑ brain disease or head injury
❑ colitis (inflammation of the colon)
❑ emphysema, asthma, or lung disease
❑ enlarged prostate or trouble urinating
❑ gallbladder disease or gallstones
❑ heart, kidney, or liver disease

❑ seizures
❑ underactive thyroid or adrenal gland
Tell your doctor about any other drugs you take, including aspirin, herbs, vitamins, and other non-prescription products.

When You Use This Drug
◆ Do not drink alcohol or take any drugs that make you drowsy without talking to your doctor. The narcotics will add to their effects, putting you at risk.
◆ Avoid driving or other activities that require alertness because these drugs may make you drowsy, dizzy, or lightheaded.

One hazard of taking meperidine or hydromorphone continuously for longer than several weeks is addiction. **Do not stop taking your drug suddenly**. With the help of your doctor, work out a schedule for slowly lowering the amount of the drug you take by about 5 to 10% each day. Keep a written record of the dosage reduction schedule with you. These steps will make it much easier to become drug free without developing distressing symptoms of drug withdrawal.

◆ If your drug seems less effective after a few weeks of use, **do not increase the dose**. Call your doctor instead.

◆ If you use a narcotic for a long time, have regular checkups.

◆ You may feel dizzy when rising from a lying or sitting position. If you are lying down, hang your legs over the side of the bed for a few minutes, then get up slowly. When rising from a chair, stay by the chair until you are sure that you are not dizzy. (See p. 14.)

◆ If you plan to have any surgery, including dental, tell your doctor that you take this drug.

How To Use This Drug

◆ *Liquid form of meperidine*: Mix with a half glass (4 ounces) of water and drink the mixture. The water will lessen the numbness that this drug can cause in your mouth and throat.

◆ *Suppository form of hydromorphone*: Remove wrapper, moisten suppository with water, lie on side, and insert into rectum.

◆ Do not store tablets in the bathroom. Heat and moisture can damage the drug.

◆ Store suppositories in the refrigerator.

◆ Prevent liquid form and suppositories from freezing.

◆ If you miss a dose, take it as soon as you remember, but skip it if it is almost time for the next dose. **Do not take double doses.**

Interactions With Other Drugs

The following drugs are listed in *Evaluations of Drug Interactions*, 1991 as causing "highly clinically significant" or "clinically significant" interactions when used together with this drug. There may be other drugs, especially those in the families of drugs listed below, that also will react with this drug to cause severe adverse effects. Make sure to ask your doctor for a complete listing of them and let her or him know if you are taking any of these interacting drugs:

carbamazepine; chlorpromazine; cimetidine; COUMADIN; NARDIL; PENTOTHAL; phenelzine; RIFADIN; rifampin; TAGAMET; TEGRETOL; thiopental; THORAZINE; tubocurarine; warfarin.

At least two weeks should elapse after you stop taking a monoamine oxidase (MAO) inhibitor and start taking demerol. The same is true if you stop taking bupropion and then start one of these MAO inhibitors:

deprenyl; ELDEPRYL; EUTONYL; EUTRON; furazolidine; FUROXONE; isocarboxizid; MARPLAN; MATULANE; NARDIL; pargyline; PARNATE; phenelzine; procarbazine; selegiline; tranylcypromine.

Adverse Effects

Call your doctor immediately:

❑ **if you experience signs of overdose:** cold, clammy skin; convulsions; severe dizziness or drowsiness; nervousness or restlessness; confusion; small pupils; unconsciousness; abnormally low blood pressure; slow heartbeat; slow or troubled breathing; severe weakness

❑ feelings of unreality

❑ hallucinations (seeing, feeling, or hearing things that are not there)

❑ skin rash, hives, or itching

❑ depression

❑ ringing sound in ears

❑ slow, irregular, or troubled breathing

❑ swollen face

❑ trembling or uncontrolled muscle movements

❑ abnormal (slow, fast, or pounding) heartbeat

Call your doctor if these symptoms continue:

❑ dizziness

❑ drowsiness

❑ confusion

❑ feeling faint or lightheaded

❑ nausea or vomiting

❑ constipation

❑ sweating

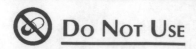 **DO NOT USE**

Alternative treatment: See Enteric-coated Aspirin, p. 268.

Salsalate
DISALCID (Riker)

Family: Salicylates (see p. 258)

Salsalate (*sal* sa late) belongs to the same family as aspirin and, like aspirin, relieves pain and reduces fever. Salsalate may cause fewer stomach problems than aspirin, but it may not be as effective and has the same potential side effects (see p. 258).[40] **It has no advantage over enteric-coated aspirin (see p. 268) and is more expensive.**[41] For the

vast majority of people, aspirin is the drug of choice and salsalate should not be used.

> ### Aspirin/Reye's Syndrome Alert
> Do not use this product for treating chicken pox, flu, or flu-like illness. It will increase the risk of contracting Reye's syndrome, a rare but often fatal disease.

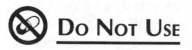 **DO NOT USE**

Alternative treatment: See Enteric-coated Aspirin, p. 268.

Diflunisal
DOLOBID (Merck)

Family: Nonsteroidal Anti-inflammatory Drugs "NSAIDs"
Arthritis Drugs (see p. 261)

Diflunisal (dye *floo* ni sal), like aspirin, relieves pain and inflammation. **It should not be used because it has no advantage over enteric-coated aspirin (see p. 268) and is much more expensive.**[42] Enteric-coated aspirin (aspirin coated so that it does not dissolve in the stomach) is the best drug for long-term treatment, such as for arthritis (see p. 261).

Diflunisal belongs to the family of drugs called nonsteroidal anti-inflammatory drugs, shortened to NSAIDs (*n* sayds), often used to treat arthritis in older adults. All the NSAIDs can cause serious harm, even fatalities, from bleeding in the stomach or intestines. Bleeding can occur at any time and without warning and older people are more likely to experience adversity from bleeding. Elderly people are also more likely to have reduced liver and kidney function. So, some doctors believe people over age 70 should be started with half the usual dose of drugs in this group.[43]

Aspirin with Codeine (combined)
EMPIRIN WITH CODEINE (Burroughs Wellcome)

Generic: available

Family: Painkillers
Fever Reducers
Nonsteroidal Anti-inflammatory
Drugs "NSAIDs"
Narcotics (see p. 260)

Aspirin (see p. 268) and codeine (see p. 276) are both effective painkillers. Together, they produce a rational combination drug that relieves pain better than aspirin alone but has less risk of side effects than the larger amount of codeine that would be needed if codeine were used alone. This combination is available in capsules and tablets.

Although this combination is the best drug for some situations, it is overused. Many people who are prescribed this combination would get pain relief from aspirin alone, and would avoid the harmful side effects codeine can have — addiction and constipation. So before taking this drug, ask your doctor about trying plain aspirin first.

Aspirin/Reye's Syndrome Alert
Do not use this product for treating chicken pox, flu, or flu-like illness. It will increase the risk of contracting Reye's syndrome, a rare but often fatal disease.

This drug can increase the risk of hip fracture.[46]

One hazard of taking codeine continuously for longer than several weeks is addiction. **Do not stop taking your drug suddenly.** With the help of your doctor, work out a schedule for slowly lowering the amount of the drug you take by about 5 to 10% each day. Keep a written record of the dosage reduction schedule with you. These steps will make it much easier to become drug free without developing distressing symptoms of drug withdrawal.

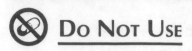 **DO NOT USE**

Alternative treatment: See Acetaminophen, p. 318.

Butalbital, Acetaminophen, and Caffeine (combined)
ESGIC (Forest)
FIORICET (Sandoz)

Family: Painkillers
Narcotics (see p. 260)

This combination of butalbital (byoo *tal* bi tal), acetaminophen (a *seat* am *in* o fen), and caffeine (ka *feen*) is marketed for tension headaches. When taking this product you are, in fact, taking three drugs, each with its own cautions, adverse effects, and drug interactions. Like other fixed-combination products, this combination curtails the ability to vary doses of each drug, irrationally combining in this case one effective painkiller (acetaminophen), one excessively dangerous drug (butalbital), and one ineffective drug (caffeine).

Caffeine has not proven effective in relieving pain. It can aggravate incontinence, produce insomnia, and lead to dependence-causing withdrawal headaches.

Butalbital is a barbiturate, and because of the serious side effects and addictive nature of all barbiturates, older adults should not use it and therefore should not take Esgic or Fioricet.

Acetaminophen is an effective painkiller, available separately without a prescription (see p. 318), as is aspirin (see p. 268). Either can relieve pain, but not the underlying condition. Regular use could mask the fever of a bacterial infection.

One hazard of taking butalbital continuously for longer than several weeks is addiction. **Do not stop taking your drug suddenly**. With the help of your doctor, work out a schedule for slowly lowering the amount of the drug you take by about 5 to 10% each day. Keep a written record of the dosage reduction schedule with you. These steps will make it much easier to become drug free without developing distressing symptoms of drug withdrawal.

Warning
There have been a number of case reports of liver damage involving a possible drug interaction between isoniazid, a medication used to prevent and treat tuberculosis, and acetaminophen, an over-the-counter painkiller and the active ingredient in Tylenol. Each drug alone is known to cause liver damage. Isoniazid alone, especially as people get older, has been documented to cause liver damage. Acetaminophen, alone in large doses or probably in combination with alcohol, also increases the risk of liver damage. The combination of acetaminophen with isoniazid, according to the authors of these case reports, may also be dangerous.

If you are taking isoniazid for tuberculosis or have a positive TB skin test and are using the drug, consult your physician before using acetaminophen or any combination product containing acetaminophen. Discuss alternatives to acetaminophen with your physician.[44,45]

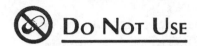 **DO NOT USE**

Alternative treatment: See Enteric-coated Aspirin, p. 268.

Piroxicam
FELDENE (Pfizer)

Family: Nonsteroidal Anti-inflammatory Drugs "NSAIDs"
Arthritis Drugs (see p. 261)

Piroxicam (peer *ox* i cam) relieves pain and inflammation caused by two kinds of arthritis, rheumatoid arthritis and osteoarthritis. **It has caused serious side effects and numerous deaths,** especially in older adults.[47,48] **People over 60 are more likely than other users of this drug to suffer stomach and intestinal bleeding, ulcers, and perforations.** These side effects have occurred *even* when patients were taking only the recommended dose. People in all age groups have had **serious skin reactions, some of which have been fatal,** while taking piroxicam.

Piroxicam belongs to the family of drugs called nonsteroidal anti-inflammatory drugs, shortened to NSAIDs (*n* sayds), often used to treat arthritis in older adults. Aspirin is just as effective as all these drugs and less costly (see p. 268). All the NSAIDs can cause serious harm, even fatalities, from bleeding in the stomach or intestines. Bleeding can occur at any time and without warning and older people are more likely to experience adversity from bleeding. Elderly people are also more likely to have reduced liver and kidney function. So, some doctors believe people over age 70 should be started with half the usual dose of drugs in this group.[49]

Although piroxicam is appealing because you only have to take it once a day, this "convenience" is *not* an advantage for older adults. Older adults eliminate drugs from their bodies more slowly than younger people, so a large once-a-day dose may not be eliminated as easily as smaller doses taken throughout the day. As a result, dangerous levels of the drug can accumulate in the bloodstream.

After receiving many reports of harmful reactions in older people taking piroxicam, the Canadian drug regulatory agency recommended that people over 65 start with a dose of 10 milligrams per day. This is half the U.S. recommended dose for adults.

Instead of piroxicam, we recommend equally effective and less dangerous drugs such as aspirin (see p. 268), which is also less expensive. Aspirin is the drug of choice for treating pain, fever, and inflammation in people who do not have ulcers, gastritis (inflammation of the stomach), or an allergy to aspirin. Some rheumatologists (arthritis specialists) still prefer aspirin to other drugs in its family (NSAIDs) for treating rheumatoid arthritis.[50]

If you are taking piroxicam, ask your doctor whether you can switch to taking enteric-coated aspirin (aspirin coated so it does not dissolve in the stomach) twice a day. If you cannot take aspirin, ask about switching to another, safer drug in this family such as ibuprofen (see p. 298). Each person may respond differently to different NSAIDs.

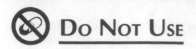 **DO NOT USE**

Alternative treatment: See Aspirin, p. 268, and Acetaminophen, p. 318.

Butalbital, Caffeine, and Aspirin (combined)
FIORINAL (Sandoz)

Butalbital, Caffeine, Aspirin, and Codeine (combined)
FIORINAL WITH CODEINE (Sandoz)

Family: Painkillers
Narcotics (see p. 260)

These are combination drugs composed of butalbital (*byoo* tal bi tal), caffeine (ka *feen*), aspirin (see p. 268), and (in the case of Fiorinal with Codeine) codeine (*koe* deen). Both of these combination drugs are used to relieve pain. They do contain two effective painkillers, aspirin and codeine, but they are *irrational* combinations because they also contain one ineffective drug (caffeine) and one excessively dangerous one (butalbital). We recommend that you do not use either of these drugs.

Caffeine has *not* been proven effective in relieving pain. Butalbital is a barbiturate, and because of the serious side effects and addictive nature of all barbiturates, older adults should not use Fiorinal or Fiorinal with Codeine.[51]

Aspirin and codeine, both effective painkillers, are available separately as well as combined with each other (see p. 283). There is no reason to take a product that combines these two useful painkillers with excessively dangerous butalbital and ineffective caffeine. It is much better to take plain aspirin (see p. 268) or acetaminophen (see p. 318), or, if necessary, aspirin or acetaminophen combined with codeine (see pp. 283, 319). Codeine can cause constipation and is addictive, so it should only be used if aspirin or acetaminophen alone does not work.

One hazard of taking butalbital or codeine continuously for longer than several weeks is addiction. **Do not stop taking your drug suddenly.** With the help of your doctor, work out a schedule for slowly lowering the amount of the drug you take by about 5 to 10% each day. Keep a written record of the dosage reduction schedule with you. These steps will make it much easier to become drug free without developing distressing symptoms of drug withdrawal.

Aspirin/Reye's Syndrome Alert
Do not use these products for treating chicken pox, flu, or flu-like illness. They will increase the risk of contacting Reye's syndrome, a rare but often fatal disease.

Fiorinal with Codeine can increase the risk of hip fracture.[52]

LIMITED USE

Methotrexate
FOLEX (Adria) MEXATE (Bristol)

Generic: available

Family: Antiarthritis Drugs (see p. 261)
 Anticancer Drugs

Methotrexate (meth o *trex* ate) is used to treat rheumatoid arthritis and a few types of cancer.

For rheumatoid arthritis, methotrexate should be used only for the most severe cases that have not responded to treatment with other drugs. Before prescribing methotrexate, your doctor should try anti-inflammatory drugs such as aspirin (see p. 268) or ibuprofen (see p. 298) and other antiarthritis drugs such as gold salts (see p. 311) or penicillamine. Only if these are not effective should you use methotrexate.

Methotrexate takes time to relieve the symptoms of arthritis, and you may not see improvement for weeks or months. Continue to take the drug as directed by your doctor, and also use a nonsteroidal anti-inflammatory drug other than aspirin until the methotrexate begins to work.

If you are using methotrexate for cancer, you may have to take it despite side effects such as sore mouth, stomach upset, nausea, vomiting, and loss of appetite. If a side effect is causing you problems, ask your doctor or other health professional to suggest ways to avoid or decrease the problem. Be aware, however, that some side effects are unavoidable. In fact, doctors use some side effects to tell whether the drug is working. Methotrexate can also cause liver and blood problems. For example, it can damage your bone marrow, disrupting the bone marrow's production of blood cells.

Drugs used to treat cancer often cause severe nausea and vomiting, either immediately after the drug is taken or several hours later. You can treat this kind of nausea and vomiting by changing your diet or by taking an antinausea drug. You should always try dietary changes first.[53]
❑ Eat small, frequent meals so your stomach is never empty.
❑ When you get up from sleeping or resting, eat some dry crackers or toast before you start being active.
❑ Drink carbonated drinks or other clear liquids such as soups and gelatin.
❑ Eat tart foods such as lemons and pickles.
❑ Do not eat foods with strong smells.

Before You Use This Drug
Do not use if you have or have had
❑ recent chicken pox exposure or infection
❑ shingles (herpes zoster)
Tell your doctor if you have or have had
❑ allergies to drugs
❑ alcohol dependence
❑ bone marrow depression
❑ gout
❑ kidney stones
❑ recent infection
❑ kidney or liver disease
❑ colitis
❑ stomach ulcers
❑ intestinal obstruction
❑ mouth sores or inflammation
Tell your doctor about any other drugs you take, including aspirin, herbs, vitamins, and other non-prescription products.

When You Use This Drug

◆ **Do not use more or less often or in a higher or lower dose than prescribed.** Check with your doctor before you stop using this drug.

◆ **Do not drink alcohol. It increases your chances of liver damage.**

◆ Try to stay out of the sun. Methotrexate makes your skin more sensitive to sunlight.

◆ **Do not get immunizations without your doctor's approval, and avoid exposure to people who have colds or other infections or who have recently been immunized.** Because methotrexate decreases the number of white blood cells, which fight infection, you are more likely to get an infection while you are taking it.

◆ Schedule regular visits with your doctor to check your blood counts, liver function, and progress on the drug.

◆ If you plan to have any surgery, including dental, tell your doctor that you take this drug.

How To Use This Drug

◆ Do not store in the bathroom. Do not expose to heat, strong light, or moisture.

◆ Call your doctor if you miss a dose or vomit shortly after taking the drug.

Interactions With Other Drugs

The following drugs are listed in *Evaluations of Drug Interactions*, 1991 as causing "highly clinically significant" or "clinically significant" interactions when used together with this drug. There may be other drugs, especially those in the families of drugs listed below, that also will react with this drug to cause severe adverse effects. Make sure to ask your doctor for a complete listing of them and let her or him know if you are taking any of these interacting drugs:

aspirin; BENEMID; cisplatin; CORTISPORIN; DILANTIN; EASPRIN; ECOTRIN; EMPIRIN; etretinate; ketoprofen; leucovorin; MATULANE; neomycin; ORUDIS; phenytoin; PLATINOL; probenecid; procarbazine; SEPTRA; SK-PROBENECID; TEGISON; trimethoprim/sulfamethoxazole; WELLCOVORIN.

Adverse Effects

Call your doctor immediately:
❏ black, tarry stools
❏ stomach pain
❏ diarrhea
❏ bloody vomit
❏ fever, chills, or sore throat
❏ unusual bleeding or bruising
❏ sores in mouth or on lips
❏ blood in urine
❏ swelling of feet or lower legs
❏ joint pain
❏ cough, shortness of breath
❏ dark urine, yellow eyes or skin

Call your doctor if these symptoms continue:
❏ nausea, vomiting, loss of appetite
❏ hair loss
❏ rash, hives, or itching
❏ acne or boils
❏ pale or reddened skin

Periodic Tests

Ask your doctor which of these tests should be done periodically while you are taking this drug:
❏ kidney function tests
❏ liver function tests, monthly
❏ blood levels of uric acid
❏ complete blood tests (including hematocrit, platelet count, white blood cell count), monthly
❏ examination for mouth ulcers

LIMITED USE

Azathioprine
IMURAN (Burroughs Wellcome)

Generic: unavailable in tablets

Family: Immunosuppressants

Azathioprine (aze *thy* o prin) is a potent drug reserved for severe conditions. It prevents rejection of transplanted organs, particularly kidneys, by suppressing the immune system. While azathioprine is also used in multiple sclerosis, severe skin diseases, and a number of other conditions, it is not yet approved for those conditions in the U.S. When all other treatments (rest, anti-inflammatory drugs, gold compounds) fail to relieve rheumatoid arthritis, azathioprine may slow damage to the joints and control symptoms but does not cure any condition. It is an alternative when surgery for some disabling arthritis cannot be done, and to lower the dose of steroids, often given along with azathioprine. It may take several weeks or even a few months for improvement to show.

Older people with age-related decrease in kidney function are more likely to need a low dose. In all ages, the lowest effective dose should be used.

During the first couple of weeks of therapy with azathioprine, nausea is common. Since azathioprine affects your immune system, you may get infections, which can be fatal, more easily. Azathioprine increases the risk of skin cancer, cervical cancer, Karposi's sarcoma, and leukemia.[54] These risks increase when the drug is used for transplants, and rises after the drug has been used for five years.[55] Azathioprine can also irritate your pancreas, damage your bone marrow, and harm your liver enough to be life-threatening. This liver damage is more apt to happen to men.[56] Lowering the dose may reverse some of these problems.

Before You Use This Drug

Because your risk of developing cancer would rise, discuss the benefit/risk balance of using azathioprine with your doctor if you are taking or have previously taken:
  ALKERAN; chlorambucil; cyclophosphamide; CYTOXAN; LEUKERAN; mephalan.

Tell your doctor if you have or have had
❑ allergies to drugs
❑ chicken pox presently or a recent exposure
❑ gout
❑ hepatitis
❑ herpes
❑ infection
❑ kidney or liver problems
❑ pancreatitis
❑ radiation therapy
❑ xanthine oxidase deficiency

Tell your doctor about any other drugs you take, including aspirin, herbs, vitamins, and other non-prescription products.

When You Use This Drug

◆ Keep your appointments for lab work. For the first two months blood tests should be done at least weekly, and at least monthly thereafter.

◆ Avoid places and people that expose you to bacterial or viral infections. During flu seasons avoid crowds. Report the first sign of any infection to your doctor: cough, hoarseness; fever, chills; lower back or side pain; or painful or difficult urination.

◆ Practice good hygiene. Wash your hands before touching your eyes or the inside of your nose.

◆ Check with your dentist about teeth cleaning methods suited to your condition. Check with your physician before having dental work done.

- Be cautious using knives, razors, nail clippers, and other sharp objects.
- Avoid engaging in contact sports, moving heavy objects, and activities where you might get bruised.
- Continue to rest, get physical therapy, and use anti-inflammatory drugs if you have rheumatoid arthritis.
- If you undergo emergency care, or surgery, including dental, tell your doctor that you take azathioprine.
- If you must take allopurinol, your dose of azathioprine should be reduced to one-fourth the usual dose.

How To Use This Drug

- Swallow tablet whole or break in half. If you take azathioprine once a day, take it at bedtime to reduce stomach upset. Otherwise, take it with food or after a meal.
- If your doctor prescribes a suspension, shake it well before measuring.
- *If you miss a dose, use the following guidelines:*
  - If you take the drug once a day, do not take the missed dose, nor double the next dose.
  - If you take the drug several times a day, then take it as soon as possible, or double the next dose only. Check with your doctor if you miss more than one dose.
- Store tablets at room temperature with lid on firmly. Do not expose to light and heat. Store other forms according to the prescription label.

Interactions With Other Drugs

The following drugs are listed in *Evaluations of Drug Interactions*, 1991 as causing "highly clinically significant" or "clinically significant" interactions when used together with this drug. There may be other drugs, especially those in the families of drugs listed below, that also will react with this drug to cause severe adverse effects. Make sure to ask your doctor for a complete listing of them and let her or him know if you are taking this interacting drug:

COUMADIN; warfarin. (Do not suddenly stop taking azathioprine or warfarin. Check with your doctor.)

Additionally, the *United States Pharmacopeia Drug Information*, 1992 lists these drugs as having interactions of major significance:

allopurinol; cyclosporine; live virus vaccines; LOPURIN; SABIN VACCINE; SANDIMMUNE; ZYLOPRIM.

(Avoid live virus vaccines, such as polio vaccines, for at least three months after stopping azathioprine. Not only might the vaccine not work, but you may be more apt to have adverse reactions to the vaccine. It is very important that you not come in close contact with anyone else, such as your grandchildren, getting live virus vaccines. If you must come in contact, wear a mask over your mouth and nose. Let someone else change and dispose of their diapers.)

Adverse Effects

Call your doctor immediately:
- bloody or black, tarry or pale stools
- bleeding or bruising
- breathing difficulty
- chills
- cough, hoarseness
- severe diarrhea
- dizziness
- fever
- rapid heartbeat
- severe nausea or vomiting
- pain in lower back, muscles, joints, side, or stomach
- pinpoint red spots, redness, blisters on skin
- sores in mouth or lips
- swelling of feet or legs
- unusual tiredness or weakness
- painful or difficult urination
- dark or bloody urine
- yellowing of eyes or skin

Call your doctor if these symptoms continue:
- abdominal pain
- constipation

- ❑ depression[57]
- ❑ hair loss
- ❑ headache
- ❑ heartburn
- ❑ loss of appetite
- ❑ low blood pressure
- ❑ nausea and vomiting
- ❑ skin rash, itching
- ❑ unusually deep suntan[58]

- ❑ blurred vision[59]

Adverse effects may persist after azathioprine is stopped.

Periodic Tests

Ask your doctor which of these tests should be done periodically while you are taking this drug:
- ❑ complete blood count (CBC)

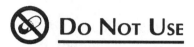 Do Not Use

Alternative treatment: See Enteric-coated Aspirin, p. 268.

Indomethacin
INDOCIN (Merck)

Family: Nonsteroidal Anti-inflammatory
Drugs "NSAIDs"
Arthritis Drugs (see p. 261)

Indomethacin (in doe *meth* a sin) relieves the pain and inflammation of rheumatoid arthritis and acute gout and reduces fever. **This drug is not recommended for older adults.**[60] It can cause depression, mood changes, and confusion. Indomethacin may also make epilepsy or Parkinson's disease worse, cause more stomach and intestinal bleeding than aspirin, and hide the signs of any infection you might have.[61,62,63]

Indomethacin belongs to the family of drugs called nonsteroidal anti-inflammatory drugs, shortened to NSAIDs (*n* sayds), often used to treat arthritis in older adults. Aspirin is just as effective as all these drugs and less costly (see p. 268). All the NSAIDs can cause serious harm, even fatalities, from bleeding in the stomach or intestines. Bleeding can occur at any time and without

warning and older people are more likely to experience adversity from bleeding. Elderly people are also more likely to have reduced liver and kidney function. So, some doctors believe people over age 70 should be started with half the usual dose of drugs in this group.[64]

Aspirin is the drug of choice for treating pain, fever, and inflammation in people who do not have ulcers, gastritis (inflammation of the stomach), or an allergy to aspirin. Some rheumatologists (arthritis specialists) prefer aspirin to other drugs in this family for treating rheumatoid arthritis.[65]

If you are taking indomethacin, ask your doctor whether you can switch to taking enteric-coated aspirin (aspirin coated so it does not dissolve in the stomach) twice a day. If you can't take aspirin, ask about switching to another, safer drug in this family such as ibuprofen (see p. 298). Each person responds differently to different NSAIDs.

LIMITED USE

Etodolac
LODINE (Wyeth-Ayerst)

Generic: not available

Family: Nonsteroidal Anti-inflammatory
Drugs "NSAIDs"
Arthritis Drugs (see p. 261)

Etodolac (et *o* dole ac) is used to treat mild
to moderate pain and symptoms of
osteoarthritis. In the United States etodolac
is not approved for the treatment of rheumatoid arthritis. **In general, if you are over
60, you should take less than the usual
adult dose, especially if you have decreased kidney function.** It takes about half
an hour for the drug to begin working.

Etodolac belongs to the family of drugs
called nonsteroidal anti-inflammatory
drugs, shortened to NSAIDs (*n* sayds),
often used to treat arthritis in older adults.
Aspirin is just as effective as all these drugs
and less costly (see p. 268). All the NSAIDs
can cause serious harm, even fatalities,
from bleeding in the stomach or intestines.
Bleeding can occur at any time and without
warning and older people are more likely
to experience adversity from bleeding.
Elderly people are also more likely to have
reduced liver and kidney function. So,
some doctors believe people over age 70
should be started with half the usual dose
of drugs in this group.[66]

Etodolac is comparable in effectiveness to
other NSAIDs, such as aspirin and several
prescription drugs. Like other NSAIDs,
etodolac relieves symptoms, but does not
cure any condition. Because NSAIDs relieve
pain and inflammation and reduce fever,
these drugs can mask signs of infection.
When taking etodolac, older people tend to
get more indigestion.[67]

Compared to other new drugs, etodolac
received a higher rate of adverse drug reports
in Britain, including deaths.[68] Etodolac can
impair liver function, may prolong bleeding
time, and damage bone marrow. Etodolac can
cause severe damage to the kidneys, even
kidney failure. This is more likely in the
elderly.[69]

Enteric-coated aspirin is the best and
least expensive way to relieve the pain of
osteoarthritis. Unlike the treatment of
rheumatoid arthritis, which requires high
doses of aspirin to reduce inflammation,
two 325-mg aspirin tablets four times a day
is often sufficient to control osteoarthritic
pain in adults. Other pain relievers, including acetaminophen, are recommended for
the person who cannot take aspirin.

For the treatment of osteoarthritis *The
Medical Letter* states that etodolac may offer
no advantage over the painkiller acetaminophen (Tylenol), which does not cause
gastrointestinal ulcers or bleeding and costs
less.[70]

Be aware that in contrast to aspirin,
acetaminophen relieves pain, but is not
effective in reducing inflammation. Therefore, we do not recommend the use of
acetaminophen for the treatment of arthritis
unless it is clear that you have osteoarthritis
which does not have a significant amount
of inflammation.

Before You Use This Drug
Do not use if you have or have had
❑ an allergic reaction to aspirin, any other
NSAID or iodides[71]
❑ bleeding ulcers
Tell your doctor if you have or have had
❑ allergies to drugs
❑ kidney or liver problems
❑ congestive heart failure
❑ hepatitis
❑ smoked

❑ stomach problems
Tell your doctor about any other drugs you take, including aspirin, herbs, vitamins, and other non-prescription products.

When You Use This Drug

◆ If you smoke, try to quit, since adverse effects of etodolac occur more often in smokers.[72]
◆ Do not drink alcohol. It irritates the stomach lining and increases the risk of stomach bleeding.
◆ Call your doctor immediately if you have flu-like symptoms (chills, fever, muscle aches or pains) shortly before or with a skin rash. This may indicate a serious reaction to etodolac.
◆ You may feel dizzy when rising from a lying or sitting position. If you are lying down, hang your legs over the side of the bed for a few minutes, then get up slowly. When getting up from a chair, stay by the chair until you are sure that you are not dizzy. (See p. 14.)
◆ Do not drive or perform other activities that require alertness because this drug may make you drowsy, dizzy, or lightheaded.
◆ If you plan to have any surgery, including dental, tell your doctor that you take this drug.

How To Use This Drug

◆ Take with food to reduce stomach irritation.
◆ Take with **a full glass (8 ounces) of water.** Do not lie down for 30 minutes afterwards.
◆ If you miss a dose, take it as soon as possible, but skip it if you don't remember until the next day. **Do not take double doses.**
◆ Store at room temperature with lid on firmly. Do not expose to moisture. Do not store in the bathroom.

Interactions With Other Drugs

The following drugs are listed in *Evaluations of Drug Interactions,* 1991 as causing "highly clinically significant" or "clinically significant" interactions when used together with this drug. There may be other drugs, especially those in the families of drugs listed below, that also will react with this drug to cause severe adverse effects. Make sure to ask your doctor for a complete listing of them and let her or him know if you are taking this interacting drug:

COUMADIN; warfarin.

Additionally, the *United States Pharmacopeia Drug Information,* 1992 lists these drugs as having interactions of major significance:

ASA; aspirin; BENEMID; CEFOBID; cefoperazone; COLBENEMID; DYAZIDE; DYRENIUM; ECOTRIN; ESKALITH; INDOCIN; indomethacin; lithium; LITHOBID; MEASURIN; methotrexate; probenecid; triamterene.

Adverse Effects

Call your doctor immediately:
❑ bloody or black, tarry stools
❑ bleeding or bruising, including bleeding of gums
❑ breathing difficulties
❑ fever, chills, muscle aches or pains with or before a rash
❑ dizziness
❑ skin rash, reddening or yellowing of skin
❑ swelling of legs, ankles, or feet
❑ blurred vision
❑ vomiting of blood or material that looks like coffee grounds

Call your doctor if these symptoms continue:
❑ abdominal cramps or pain
❑ constipation
❑ diarrhea
❑ depression
❑ headache
❑ gas, heartburn, indigestion
❑ itching
❑ nausea and vomiting
❑ nervousness
❑ ringing in the ears
❑ tiredness, weakness
❑ urination is frequent, difficult, or painful

❏ weight gain

Periodic Tests
Ask your doctor which of these tests should be done periodically while you are taking this drug:
❏ kidney function tests
❏ liver function tests

❏ stool tests for possible blood loss
❏ hematocrit and/or hemoglobin test
❏ blood concentrations of creatinine, potassium, urea nitrogen levels
❏ white blood cell counts

LIMITED USE

Allopurinol
LOPURIN (Boots)
ZYLOPRIM (Burroughs Wellcome)

Generic: available

Family: Antigout Drugs (see p. 261)

Allopurinol (al oh *pure* i nole) helps to prevent gout attacks. Gout occurs in people who have high levels of uric acid in their body, and an attack occurs when crystals of uric acid form in your joints and your body releases chemicals in response to the crystals. This causes pain and inflammation. Allopurinol works by decreasing your body's production of uric acid and thereby lowering the level of uric acid in your blood.

Allopurinol will not relieve a gout attack that has already started. If you are taking allopurinol, keep taking it during an attack, even if another drug is prescribed to treat the attack.

After you start using allopurinol, your gout attacks may become more frequent for a while. Keep taking the drug. If you take it regularly, the attacks gradually will become less frequent and less painful, and they may stop completely after several months.

Allopurinol can cause skin rashes, allergic reactions and kidney stones. **Stop taking allopurinol and call your doctor at the first sign of skin rash or allergic reaction.**

To help prevent kidney stones while taking allopurinol, drink at least 10 to 12 full glasses (8 ounces each) of fluid each day, unless your doctor tells you otherwise. Too much vitamin C (see p. 575) also increases your risk of forming kidney stones, so do not take vitamin C supplements while you are taking allopurinol unless you have checked with your doctor first.

Before You Use This Drug
Tell your doctor if you have or have had
❏ allergies to drugs
❏ kidney function impairment
Tell your doctor about any other drugs you take, including aspirin, herbs, vitamins, and other non-prescription products.

When You Use This Drug
◆ Do not drink alcohol. Because alcohol increases the amount of uric acid in your blood, it may make your gout attacks more frequent and more difficult to control. It also increases your risk of stomach problems.
◆ Until you know how you react to this drug, do not drive or perform other activities requiring alertness. Allopurinol can cause drowsiness.

How To Use This Drug

◆ Take with food to decrease stomach upset. If this does not work and your stomach continues to be upset, check with your doctor.

◆ Do not expose to heat, moisture, or strong light. Do not store in the bathroom.

◆ If you miss a dose, take it as soon as you remember, but skip it if you don't remember until the next day. **Do not take double doses.**

Interactions With Other Drugs

The following drugs are listed in *Evaluations of Drug Interactions*, 1991 as causing "highly clinically significant" or "clinically significant" interactions when used together with this drug. There may be other drugs, especially those in the families of drugs listed below, that also will react with this drug to cause severe adverse effects. Make sure to ask your doctor for a complete listing of them and let her or him know if you are taking any of these interacting drugs:

BRONKODYL; CONSTANT-T; cyclo-phosphamide; CYTOXAN; dicumarol; ELIXOPHYLLIN; mercaptopurine; NEOSAR; PURINETHOL; QUIBRON-T-SR; SLO-BID; SLOPHYLLIN; SOMOPHYLLIN; SUSTAIRE; THEO-24; THEOLAIR; theophylline; vidarabine.

Adverse Effects
Call your doctor immediately:
❑ skin rash, hives, itching
❑ bloody or cloudy urine
❑ difficult or painful urination
❑ lower back pain
❑ chills, fever, or muscle aches
❑ nausea or vomiting along with chills or fever
❑ numbness or tingling of hands or feet
❑ red, thick, or scaly skin
❑ sore throat and fever
❑ unusual bleeding or bruising
❑ unusual tiredness or weakness
❑ decrease in amount of urine
❑ yellow eyes or skin
Call your doctor if these symptoms continue:
❑ diarrhea
❑ drowsiness
❑ nausea, vomiting, or stomach pain

Periodic Tests
Ask your doctor which of these tests should be done periodically while you are taking this drug:
❑ complete blood counts
❑ liver function tests
❑ kidney function tests
❑ blood levels of uric acid

LIMITED USE

Meclofenamate
MECLOMEN (Parke-Davis)

Generic: available

Family: Nonsteroidal Anti-inflammatory Drugs "NSAIDs"
Arthritis Drugs (see p. 261)

In older adults, meclofenamate (me kloe *fen* am ate) is used mainly to relieve the pain and inflammation of two kinds of arthritis, rheumatoid arthritis and osteoarthritis. **In general, if you are over 60, you should take less than the usual adult dose, especially if you have decreased kidney function.**

Meclofenamate belongs to the family of drugs called nonsteroidal anti-inflamma-tory drugs, shortened to NSAIDs (*n* sayds), often used to treat arthritis in older adults. Aspirin is just as effective as all these drugs and less costly (see p. 268). All the NSAIDs can cause serious harm, even fatalities, from bleeding in the stomach or intestines. Bleeding can occur at any time and without warning and older people are more likely to experience adversity from bleeding. Elderly people are also more likely to have reduced liver and kidney function. So, some doctors believe people over age 70 should be started with half the usual dose of drugs in this group.[73]

Meclofenamate can cause stomach and intestinal problems, such as severe diarrhea.[74] It has also been linked with a few cases of serious blood cell abnormalities.[75] These blood cell abnormalities can occasionally be cured if they are caught early, so if you are taking meclofenamate, watch for the warning signs: fever and sore throat, ulcers (sores) in the mouth, easy bruising, and skin rashes. If you have any of these symptoms while taking this drug, call your doctor immediately. Stop taking meclofenamate immediately if you have a rash.

Aspirin is the drug of choice for treating pain, fever, and inflammation in people who do not have ulcers, gastritis (inflammation of the stomach), or an allergy to aspirin. Some rheumatologists (arthritis specialists) prefer aspirin to other drugs in its family for treating rheumatoid arthritis.[76] Meclofenamate should be used only if enteric-coated aspirin (see p. 268) and safer drugs in the NSAID family, such as ibuprofen and naproxen (see pp. 298, 302), do not provide relief.[77]

If you are taking meclofenamate, ask your doctor if you can switch to taking enteric-coated aspirin (aspirin coated so it will not dissolve in the stomach) twice a day. If you cannot take aspirin and are having trouble with side effects on meclofenamate, ask if you can switch to another drug in this family such as ibuprofen (see pg. 298). Each person responds differently to different NSAIDs.

Before You Use This Drug

Do not use if you have or have had
- ❑ an allergic reaction to aspirin, any other NSAID or iodides[78]
- ❑ kidney or heart failure
- ❑ peptic ulcers
- ❑ alcohol dependence
- ❑ cirrhosis of the liver
- ❑ nasal polyps or asthma

Tell your doctor if you have or have had
- ❑ allergies to drugs
- ❑ heart, kidney, or liver disease
- ❑ problems stopping bleeding
- ❑ high blood pressure
- ❑ epilepsy (seizures)
- ❑ mental depression or other psychiatric conditions
- ❑ Parkinson's disease
- ❑ lupus erythematosus

Tell your doctor about any other drugs you take, including aspirin, herbs, vitamins, and other non-prescription products.

When You Use This Drug

- ◆ Do not drink alcohol. It irritates the stomach lining and increases the risk of stomach bleeding.
- ◆ Call your doctor immediately if you have flu-like symptoms (chills, fever, muscle aches or pains) shortly before or with a skin rash. This may be a sign of a serious reaction to meclofenamate.
- ◆ You may feel dizzy when rising from a lying or sitting position. If you are lying down, hang your legs over the side of the bed for a few minutes, then get up slowly. When getting up from a chair, stay by the chair until you are sure that you are not dizzy. (See p. 14.)
- ◆ If you plan to have any surgery, including dental, tell your doctor that you take this drug.

How To Use This Drug

- ◆ Take with food to reduce stomach irritation.
- ◆ Take with **a full glass (8 ounces) of water**. Do not lie down for 30 minutes afterwards.

◆ If you miss a dose, take it as soon as possible, but skip it if you don't remember until the next day. **Do not take double doses.**

◆ Store at room temperature, with lid on tightly. Do not expose to moisture or heat. Do not store in the bathroom.

Interactions With Other Drugs

The following drugs are listed in *Evaluations of Drug Interactions*, 1991 as causing "highly clinically significant" or "clinically significant" interactions when used together with this drug. There may be other drugs, especially those in the families of drugs listed below, that also will react with this drug to cause severe adverse effects. Make sure to ask your doctor for a complete listing of them and let her or him know if you are taking any of these interacting drugs:

bendroflumethiazide; CAPOTEN; captopril; COUMADIN; cyclosporine; digoxin; DILANTIN; ESKALITH; FOLEX; GARAMYCIN; gentamicin; gold sodium thiomalate; INDERAL; LANOXIN; lithium; methotrexate; MINIPRESS; MYOCHRYSINE; NATURETIN; ORINASE; phenytoin; prazosin; propranolol; SANDIMMUNE; tolbutamide; warfarin.

Adverse Effects

Call your doctor immediately:

❑ **if you have signs of blood cell abnormalities:** fever and sore throat; ulcers in the mouth; easy bruising; skin rash

❑ bloody or black, tarry stools
❑ confusion, forgetfulness
❑ mental depression, other mood or mental changes
❑ ringing or buzzing in ears
❑ swelling of feet or lower legs
❑ unusual weight gain
❑ abdominal/stomach pain or cramps
❑ vomiting blood or material that looks like coffee grounds
❑ bleeding sores on lips
❑ fainting
❑ chills, fever, muscle aches or pain with or before a rash
❑ skin rash, itching, or peeling
❑ diarrhea
❑ changes in vision or hearing
❑ unusual bleeding or bruising
❑ numbness or tingling in limbs
❑ decrease in amount of urine

Call your doctor if these symptoms continue:
❑ dizziness or lightheadedness
❑ heartburn or indigestion
❑ nausea or vomiting
❑ constipation

Periodic Tests

Ask your doctor which of these tests should be done periodically while you are taking this drug:
❑ kidney function tests
❑ liver function tests
❑ stool tests for possible blood loss
❑ hematocrit and/or hemoglobin test
❑ blood concentrations of creatinine, potassium, and urea nitrogen
❑ white blood cell counts

Ibuprofen
Prescription: **MOTRIN** (Upjohn)
RUFEN (Boots)
Nonprescription: **ADVIL** (Whitehall)
NUPRIN (Bristol-Myers)
MEDIPREN (McNeil Consumer Products)

Generic: available

Family: Nonsteroidal Anti-inflammatory
Drugs "NSAIDs"
Arthritis Drugs (see p. 261)

Ibuprofen (eye byoo *proe* fen) is used to treat fever and pain, including pain caused by two kinds of arthritis, osteoarthritis and rheumatoid arthritis. **In general, if you are over 60, you should take less than the usual adult dose, especially if you have decreased kidney function.**

Ibuprofen belongs to the family of drugs called nonsteroidal anti-inflammatory drugs, shortened to NSAIDs (*n* sayds), often used to treat arthritis in older adults. Aspirin is just as effective as all these drugs and less costly (see p. 268). All the NSAIDs can cause serious harm, even fatalities, from bleeding in the stomach or intestines. Bleeding can occur at any time and without warning and older people are more likely to experience adversity from bleeding. Elderly people are also more likely to have reduced liver and kidney function. So, some doctors believe people over age 70 should be started with half the usual dose of drugs in this group.[79]

Some rheumatologists (arthritis specialists) prefer aspirin to other drugs in this family for treating rheumatoid arthritis. Aspirin is the best drug for treating pain, fever, and inflammation in people who do not have ulcers, gastritis (inflammation of the stomach), or an allergy to aspirin.

If you cannot use enteric-coated aspirin (aspirin coated so that it does not dissolve in the stomach), ibuprofen is generally the best second-choice drug because it has been studied longer than other drugs in this family and appears to have a good safety record. If you cannot take enteric-coated aspirin and are also bothered by side effects when taking ibuprofen, talk to your doctor about switching to another drug in this family. Each person responds differently to different NSAIDs.

Before You Use This Drug
Do not use if you have or have had
❑ an allergic reaction to aspirin, any other NSAID or iodides[80]
❑ kidney failure
❑ heart failure
❑ peptic ulcers
❑ alcohol dependence
❑ cirrhosis of the liver
❑ nasal polyps or asthma
Tell your doctor if you have or have had
❑ allergies to drugs
❑ heart, kidney, or liver disease
❑ problems stopping bleeding
❑ high blood pressure
Tell your doctor about any other drugs you take, including aspirin, herbs, vitamins, and other non-prescription products.

When You Use This Drug
◆ Do not drink alcohol. It irritates the stomach lining and increases the risk of stomach bleeding.
◆ Call your doctor immediately if you have flu-like symptoms (chills, fever, muscle aches or pains) shortly before or at the same time as a skin rash. This may be a sign of a serious reaction to ibuprofen.

- You may feel dizzy when rising from a lying or sitting position. If you are lying down, hang your legs over the side of the bed for a few minutes, then get up slowly. When getting up from a chair, stay by the chair until you are sure that you are not dizzy. (See p. 14.)
- If you plan to have any surgery, including dental, tell your doctor that you take this drug.

How To Use This Drug

- Take with food to reduce stomach irritation.
- Take with **a full glass (8 ounces) of water**. Do not lie down for 30 minutes afterwards.
- If you miss a dose, take it as soon as possible, but skip it if you don't remember it until the next day. **Do not take double doses.**
- Store at room temperature, with lid on tightly. Do not expose to moisture or heat. Do not store in the bathroom.

Interactions With Other Drugs

The following drugs are listed in *Evaluations of Drug Interactions*, 1991 as causing "highly clinically significant" or "clinically significant" interactions when used together with this drug. There may be other drugs, especially those in the families of drugs listed below, that also will react with this drug to cause severe adverse effects. Make sure to ask your doctor for a complete listing of them and let her or him know if you are taking any of these interacting drugs:

bendroflumethiazide; BENEMID; CAPOTEN; captopril; COUMADIN; cyclosporine; digoxin; DILANTIN; ESKALITH; FOLEX; GARAMYCIN; gentamicin; INDERAL; labetalol; LANOXICAPS; LANOXIN; lithium; methotrexate; MINIPRESS; NATURETIN; NORMODYNE; phenytoin; prazosin; probenecid; propranolol; SANDIMMUNE; TRANDATE; warfarin.

Adverse Effects

Call your doctor immediately:
- ❏ bloody or black, tarry stools
- ❏ mental depression, other mood or mental changes
- ❏ ringing or buzzing in ears
- ❏ swelling of feet or lower legs
- ❏ unusual weight gain
- ❏ abdominal/stomach pain or cramps
- ❏ vomiting blood or material that looks like coffee grounds
- ❏ bleeding sores on lips
- ❏ fainting
- ❏ chills, fever, muscle aches or pain with or before a rash
- ❏ skin rash, itching, or peeling
- ❏ changes in vision or hearing
- ❏ nose bleeds or any unusual bleeding or bruising
- ❏ numbness or tingling in limbs
- ❏ sudden decrease in amount of urine

Call your doctor if these symptoms continue:
- ❏ dizziness or lightheadedness
- ❏ heartburn or indigestion
- ❏ nausea or vomiting
- ❏ constipation or diarrhea
- ❏ drowsiness
- ❏ confusion, forgetfulness

Periodic Tests

Ask your doctor which of these tests should be done periodically while you are taking this drug:
- ❏ kidney function tests
- ❏ liver function tests
- ❏ stool tests for possible blood loss
- ❏ hematocrit and/or hemoglobin test
- ❏ blood concentrations of creatinine, potassium, and urea nitrogen
- ❏ white blood cell counts

LIMITED USE

Fenoprofen
NALFON (Dista)

Generic: not available

Family: Nonsteroidal Anti-inflammatory
Drugs "NSAIDs"
Arthritis Drugs (see p. 261)

In older adults, fenoprofen (fen oh *proe* fen)
is used mainly to relieve the pain and
inflammation of two kinds of arthritis,
rheumatoid arthritis and osteoarthritis, but
it is not the best drug for this purpose. **In
general, if you are over 60, you should
take less than the usual adult dose of
this drug.**

Fenoprofen belongs to the family of
drugs called nonsteroidal anti-inflammatory drugs, shortened to NSAIDs (*n* sayds),
often used to treat arthritis in older adults.
Aspirin is just as effective as all these drugs
and less costly (see p. 268). All the NSAIDs
can cause serious harm, even fatalities,
from bleeding in the stomach or intestines.
Bleeding can occur at any time and without
warning and older people are more likely
to experience adversity from bleeding.
Elderly people are also more likely to have
reduced liver and kidney function. So,
some doctors believe people over age 70
should be started with half the usual dose
of drugs in this group.[81]

Fenoprofen causes kidney disease in a
large percentage of people who take it,
compared with other drugs in its family
(NSAIDs),[82] so you should not take it if you
have impaired kidney function.[83] If you
have impaired hearing and take this drug
for a long time, you should have periodic
hearing tests.[84]

Aspirin (see pg. 268) is the drug of choice
for treating pain, fever, and inflammation
in people who do not have ulcers, gastritis
(inflammation of the stomach), or an allergy
to aspirin. Some rheumatologists (arthritis
specialists) prefer aspirin to other drugs in
this family for treating rheumatoid arthritis.[85] Fenoprofen should be used only if
enteric-coated aspirin (see p. 268) and other
safe drugs in this family, such as ibuprofen
and naproxen (see pp. 298, 302), do not
work.

If you are taking fenoprofen, ask
your doctor whether you can switch to
taking enteric-coated aspirin (aspirin
coated so it won't dissolve in the stomach)
twice a day. If you can't take aspirin and
are having trouble with side effects on
fenoprofen, ask if you can switch to another
drug in this family such as ibuprofen. Each
person responds differently to
different NSAIDs.

Before You Use This Drug
Do not use if you have or have had
❑ an allergic reaction to aspirin, any other
  NSAID or iodides[86]
❑ kidney or heart failure
❑ peptic ulcers
❑ alcohol dependence
❑ cirrhosis of the liver
❑ nasal polyps or asthma
Tell your doctor if you have or have had
❑ allergies to drugs
❑ heart, kidney, or liver disease
❑ problems stopping bleeding
❑ high blood pressure
*Tell your doctor about any other drugs you
take,* including aspirin, herbs, vitamins,
and other non-prescription products.

When You Use This Drug
◆ Do not drink alcohol. It irritates the
  stomach lining and increases the risk

of stomach bleeding.

◆ Call your doctor immediately if you have flu-like symptoms (chills, fever, muscle aches or pains) shortly before or with a skin rash. This may be a sign of a serious reaction to fenoprofen.

◆ You may feel dizzy when rising from a lying or sitting position. If you are lying down, hang your legs over the side of the bed for a few minutes, then get up slowly. When getting up from a chair, stay by the chair until you are sure that you are not dizzy. (See p. 14.)

◆ If you plan to have any surgery, including dental, tell your doctor that you take this drug.

How To Use This Drug

◆ Taking with food may reduce stomach irritation, but it will also decrease the drug's effectiveness.

◆ Take with **a full glass (8 ounces) of water**. Do not lie down for 30 minutes afterward.

◆ If you miss a dose, take it as soon as possible, but skip it if you don't remember until the next day. **Do not take double doses.**

◆ Store at room temperature, with lid on tightly. Do not expose to moisture or heat. Do not store in the bathroom.

Interactions With Other Drugs

The following drugs are listed in *Evaluations of Drug Interactions*, 1991 as causing "highly clinically significant" or "clinically significant" interactions when used together with this drug. There may be other drugs, especially those in the families of drugs listed below, that also will react with this drug to cause severe adverse effects. Make sure to ask your doctor for a complete listing of them and let her or him know if you are taking any of these interacting drugs:

bendroflumethiazide; BENEMID; CAPOTEN; captopril; COUMADIN; cyclosporine; digoxin; DILANTIN; ESKALITH; FOLEX; GARAMYCIN; gentamicin; gold sodium thiomalate; INDERAL; LANOXIN; lithium; methotrexate; MINIPRESS; MYOCHRYSINE; NATURETIN; phenytoin; prazosin; propranolol; probenecid; SANDIMMUNE; warfarin.

Adverse Effects

Call your doctor immediately:
❑ persistent headache
❑ bloody or black, tarry stools
❑ confusion, forgetfulness
❑ mental depression, other mood or mental changes
❑ ringing or buzzing in ears
❑ swelling of feet or lower legs
❑ unusual weight gain
❑ abdominal/stomach pain or cramps
❑ vomiting blood or material that looks like coffee grounds
❑ bleeding sores on lips
❑ fainting
❑ chills, fever, muscle aches or pain with or before a rash
❑ skin rash, itching, or peeling
❑ changes in vision or hearing
❑ nosebleeds or any unusual bleeding or bruising
❑ numbness or tingling in limbs
❑ sudden decrease in amount of urine
Call your doctor if these symptoms continue:
❑ dizziness or lightheadedness
❑ heartburn or indigestion
❑ nausea or vomiting
❑ constipation
❑ diarrhea
❑ drowsiness

Periodic Tests

Ask your doctor which of these tests should be done periodically while you are taking this drug:
❑ kidney function tests
❑ liver function tests
❑ stool tests for possible blood loss
❑ hematocrit and/or hemoglobin test
❑ blood concentrations of creatinine, potassium, and urea nitrogen
❑ white blood cell counts
❑ hearing tests, for prolonged use

Naproxen
NAPROSYN, ANAPROX (Syntex)

Generic: not available

Family: Nonsteroidal Anti-inflammatory
Drugs "NSAIDs"
Arthritis Drugs (see p. 261)

Naproxen (na *prox* en) relieves mild to
moderate pain and symptoms of
osteoarthritis, rheumatoid arthritis,
ankylosing spondylitis, tendonitis, bursitis,
and sudden gout attacks. **In general, if you
are over 60, you should take less than the
usual adult dose, especially if you have
decreased kidney function.**

Naproxen belongs to the family of drugs
called nonsteroidal anti-inflammatory
drugs, shortened to NSAIDs (*n* sayds),
often used to treat arthritis in older adults.
Aspirin is just as effective as all these
drugs and less costly (see p. 268). All
the NSAIDs can cause serious harm,
even fatalities, from bleeding in the stomach or intestines. Bleeding can occur at
any time and without warning and older
people are more likely to experience
adversity from bleeding. Elderly people
are also more likely to have reduced liver
and kidney function. So, some doctors
believe people over age 70 should be
started with half the usual dose of drugs
in this group.[87]

Some rheumatologists (arthritis specialists) prefer aspirin to other drugs in this
family for treating rheumatoid arthritis.[88]
Aspirin is the best drug for treating
pain, fever, and inflammation in people
who do not have ulcers, gastritis (inflammation of the stomach), or an allergy
to aspirin.

If you cannot take twice-a-day enteric-
coated aspirin (aspirin coated so it will not
dissolve in the stomach), naproxen may be
a good alternative. If you cannot take enteric-coated aspirin and are also bothered
by side effects when taking naproxen, talk
to your doctor about switching to another
drug in this family such as ibuprofen (see
p. 298). Each person responds differently to
different NSAIDs.

Before You Use This Drug
Do not use if you have or have had
❑ an allergic reaction to aspirin, any other
NSAID or iodides[89]
❑ kidney or heart failure
❑ peptic ulcers
❑ alcohol dependence
❑ cirrhosis of the liver
❑ nasal polyps or asthma
Tell your doctor if you have or have had
❑ allergies to drugs
❑ heart, kidney, or liver disease
❑ problems stopping bleeding
❑ high blood pressure
*Tell your doctor about any other drugs you
take,* including aspirin, herbs, vitamins,
and other non-prescription products.

When You Use This Drug
◆ Do not drink alcohol. It irritates the
stomach lining and increases the risk
of stomach bleeding.
◆ Call your doctor immediately if you
have flu-like symptoms (chills, fever,
muscle aches or pains) shortly before or
with a skin rash. This may indicate a
serious reaction to naproxen.
◆ You may feel dizzy when rising from a
lying or sitting position. If you are lying
down, hang your legs over the side of
the bed for a few minutes, then get up
slowly. When getting up from a chair,
stay by the chair until you are sure that
you are not dizzy. (See p. 14.)
◆ If you plan to have any surgery, including dental, tell your doctor that you take
this drug.

How To Use This Drug

◆ Take with food to reduce stomach irritation.

◆ Take with **a full glass (8 ounces) of water**. Do not lie down for 30 minutes afterwards.

◆ If you miss a dose, take it as soon as possible, but skip it if you don't remember until the next day. **Do not take double doses.**

◆ Store at room temperature, with lid on tightly. Do not expose to moisture or heat. Do not store in the bathroom.

Interactions With Other Drugs

The following drugs are listed in *Evaluations of Drug Interactions*, 1991 as causing "highly clinically significant" or "clinically significant" interactions when used together with this drug. There may be other drugs, especially those in the families of drugs listed below, that also will react with this drug to cause severe adverse effects. Make sure to ask your doctor for a complete listing of them and let her or him know if you are taking any of these interacting drugs:

bendroflumethazide; BENEMID; CAPOTEN; captopril; COLBENEMID; COUMADIN; cyclosporine; digoxin; DILANTIN; ESKALITH; FOLEX; GARAMYCIN; gentamicin; gold sodium thiomalate; INDERAL; INDOCIN; indomethacin; LANOXIN; lithium; methotrexate; MINIPRESS; MYOCHRYSINE; NATURETIN; phenytoin; prazosin; probenecid; propranolol; SANDIMMUNE; timolol; TIMOPTIC; warfarin.

Adverse Effects

Call your doctor immediately:

❑ bloody or black, tarry stools

❑ mental depression, other mood or mental changes

❑ ringing or buzzing in ears

❑ swelling of feet or lower legs

❑ unusual weight gain

❑ abdominal/stomach pain or cramps

❑ vomiting blood or material that looks like coffee grounds

❑ bleeding sores on lips

❑ fainting

❑ chills, fever, muscle aches or pain with or before a rash

❑ skin rash, itching, or peeling

❑ changes in vision or hearing

❑ nosebleeds or any unusual bleeding or bruising

❑ numbness or tingling in limbs

❑ sudden decrease in amount of urine

Call your doctor if these symptoms continue:

❑ dizziness or lightheadedness

❑ heartburn or indigestion

❑ nausea or vomiting

❑ constipation

❑ diarrhea

❑ drowsiness

❑ confusion, forgetfulness

Periodic Tests

Ask your doctor which of these tests should be done periodically while you are taking this drug:

❑ kidney function tests

❑ liver function tests

❑ stool tests for possible blood loss

❑ hematocrit and/or hemoglobin test

❑ blood concentrations of creatinine, potassium, and urea nitrogen

❑ white blood cell counts

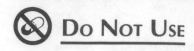 **DO NOT USE**

Alternative treatment: Rest, exercise, physical therapy, and an anti-inflammatory drug such as aspirin.

Orphenadrine, Aspirin, and Caffeine (combined)
NORGESIC FORTE (Riker)

Family: Muscle Relaxants
Painkillers

This combination of orphenadrine (or *fen* a dreen), aspirin, and caffeine is promoted to relieve the pain of muscle disorders. However, neither orphenadrine nor caffeine is effective for these conditions. Aspirin by itself may be helpful along with rest, exercise, physical therapy, or other treatment recommended by your doctor. When taking this product, you are, in fact, taking three drugs, each with its own cautions, adverse effects, and drug interactions. Like other fixed-combination products, this combination curtails the ability to vary doses of each drug.

Orphenadrine has not been shown to be any more effective than painkillers or anti-inflammatory drugs, such as aspirin by itself, for relieving the pain of local muscle spasm. It has a higher risk of side effects than these painkillers. Since orphenadrine is similar to a family of drugs called antihistamines, which are used to relieve symptoms of hay fever and other allergies (see p. 383), it may cause some of the same side effects and dangerous drug interactions as antihistamines. Some people taking orphenadrine experience blurred vision, dry mouth, mild excitement, temporary dizziness, and lightheadedness. Many of these effects occur more often in older adults. Orphenadrine is particularly dangerous for people who have glaucoma, myasthenia gravis, heart problems, or an enlarged prostate.

Aspirin relieves mild to moderate pain, but does not treat the underlying problem (see p. 268). Regular use could mask a fever due to bacterial infection. You should not take aspirin if you have ulcers, a severely irritated stomach, gout, severe anemia, hemophilia or other bleeding problems, if you take an anticoagulant drug such as heparin or warfarin, or if you are allergic to aspirin or similar painkillers.

Caffeine has not proven effective in relieving pain. It can aggravate incontinence, produce insomnia, and lead to dependence, causing withdrawal headaches. It can also irritate the stomach, so people with ulcers should avoid it.

Warning: Special Mental and Physical Adverse Effects

Older adults are especially sensitive to the harmful anticholinergic effects of orphenadrine because of its similarity to the antihistamines.

Mental Effects: confusion, delirium, short-term memory problems, disorientation, and impaired attention.

Physical Effects: dry mouth, constipation, difficulty urinating (especially for a man with an enlarged prostate), blurred vision, decreased sweating with increased body temperature, sexual dysfunction, and worsening of glaucoma.

Aspirin/Reye's Syndrome Alert

Do not use this product for treating chicken pox, flu, or flu-like illness. It will increase the risk of contracting Reye's syndrome, a rare but often fatal disease.

Ketoprofen
ORUDIS (Wyeth-Ayerst)

Generic: not available

Family: Nonsteroidal Anti-inflammatory
Drugs "NSAIDs"
Arthritis Drugs (see p. 261)

Ketoprofen (keat oh *pro* fen) relieves inflammation and pain. It is used to treat mild to moderate pain and symptoms of rheumatoid arthritis, osteoarthritis, and pain due to disease or injury. Improvement starts within a couple of weeks, while maximum improvement takes several weeks. **In general, if you are over 60, you should take less than the usual adult dose, especially if you have decreased kidney function.**

Ketoprofen belongs to the family of drugs called nonsteroidal anti-inflammatory drugs, shortened to NSAIDs (*n* sayds), often used to treat arthritis in older adults. Aspirin is just as effective as all these drugs and less costly (see p. 268). All the NSAIDs can cause serious harm, even fatalities, from bleeding in the stomach or intestines. Bleeding can occur at any time and without warning and older people are more likely to experience adversity from bleeding. Elderly people are also more likely to have reduced liver and kidney function. So, some doctors believe people over age 70 should be started with half the usual dose of drugs in this group.[90] Those underweight should also start with a low dose of ketoprofen.[91]

Also, women appear to be more susceptible to the adverse effects of ketoprofen.[92]

All NSAIDs relieve symptoms, but do not cure any condition, nor delay progress of disease and can mask symptoms of infection. Your doctor may also prescribe additional arthritis drugs for you.

Some rheumatologists (arthritis specialists) prefer aspirin to other drugs in this family for rheumatoid arthritis. Aspirin is the best drug to treat pain and inflammation in people who do not have ulcers, or an allergy to aspirin.

Before You Use This Drug
Do not use if you have or have had
❑ an allergic reaction to aspirin, any other NSAID or iodides[93]
❑ kidney disease
❑ peptic ulcers
Tell your doctor if you have or have had
❑ allergies to drugs
❑ kidney problems
❑ heart problems
❑ liver problems, such as cirrhosis, hepatitis, jaundice
❑ problems stopping bleeding
❑ high blood pressure
❑ anemia
❑ asthma[94]
❑ diabetes
❑ edema or swelling of legs
❑ hemorrhoids
❑ nasal polyps
❑ tuberculosis[95]
❑ urinary infections or other problems
Tell your doctor about any other drugs you take, including aspirin, herbs, vitamins, and other non-prescription products.

When You Use This Drug
◆ Do not drink alcohol. It irritates the stomach lining and increases the risk of stomach bleeding.
◆ Call your doctor immediately if you have flu-like symptoms (chills, fever, muscle aches or pains) shortly before or with a skin rash. This may indicate a serious reaction to ketoprofen.
◆ You may feel dizzy when rising from a lying or sitting position. If you are lying down, hang your legs over the

side of the bed for a few minutes, then get up slowly. When getting up from a chair, stay by the chair until you are sure that that you are not dizzy. (See p. 14.)

♦ Avoid driving or other activities that require alertness because this drug may make you drowsy, dizzy, or lightheaded.

♦ If you plan to have any surgery, including dental, tell your doctor that you take this drug.

How To Use This Drug

♦ Take with food, milk or an antacid to reduce stomach irritation. The antacid may delay time the drug takes to work.[96]

♦ Take with **a full glass (8 ounces) of water.** Do not lie down for 30 minutes afterwards.

♦ If you miss a dose, take it as soon as possible, but skip it if you don't remember until the next day. **Do not take double doses.**

♦ Store capsules at room temperature with cap on tightly. Do not expose to heat.

Interactions With Other Drugs

The following drugs are listed in *Evaluations of Drug Interactions*, 1991 as causing "highly clinically significant" or "clinically significant" interactions when used together with this drug. There may be other drugs, especially those in the families of drugs listed below, that also will react with this drug to cause severe adverse effects. Make sure to ask your doctor for a complete listing of them and let her or him know if you are taking any of these interacting drugs:

bendroflumethiazide; BENEMID; CAPOTEN; captopril; COLBENEMID; COUMADIN; cyclosporine; DEXATRIM; digoxin; DILANTIN; DYAZIDE; DYRENIUM; ESKALITH; GARAMYCIN; gentamicin; gold salts; INDERAL; LANOXIN; lithium; LITHOBID; methotrexate; MINIPRESS; MYOCHRYSINE; NALDECON-DX; NATURETIN; phenylpropanolamine; phenytoin; prazosin; probenecid; propranolol; SANDIMMUNE; triamterene; warfarin.

Additionally, the *United States Pharmacopeia Drug Information*, 1992 lists these drugs as having interactions of major significance:

aspirin; BUFFERIN; CEFOBID; cefoperazone; ECOTRIN.

Adverse Effects

Call your doctor immmediately:

❑ bloody or black, tarry stools
❑ problems stopping bleeding
❑ difficulty breathing
❑ chest pain or irregular heartbeat
❑ dizziness
❑ fever or chills
❑ hives, itching, skin rash, or yellowing of skin
❑ pain in joint or abdomen
❑ swelling of face, glands, lips, mouth, legs, or feet
❑ unusual tiredness
❑ urination decreases or increases in frequency
❑ vision becomes blurred or changed
❑ vomiting

Call your doctor if these symptoms continue:

❑ anxiety, nervousness
❑ constipation
❑ diarrhea
❑ depression
❑ difficulty concentrating
❑ drowsiness
❑ headache
❑ gas, indigestion, heartburn, nausea
❑ insomnia, nightmares
❑ irritability
❑ lack of appetite, undesired change in weight
❑ ringing in ears

Periodic Tests

Ask your doctor which of these tests should be done periodically while you are taking this drug:

❏ kidney function tests

❏ liver function tests
❏ stool tests for possible blood loss
❏ hematocrit and/or hemoglobin test
❏ blood concentrations of creatinine, potassium, and urea nitrogen
❏ white blood cell counts

Aspirin and Oxycodone (combined)
PERCODAN, PERCODAN-DEMI (Du Pont)

Generic: available

Family: Painkillers
Fever Reducers
Narcotics (see p. 260)

Aspirin (see p. 268) and oxycodone (ox i *koe* done) are painkillers. Oxycodone works similarly to narcotic drugs like morphine and has similar painkilling and addictive effects. Together, aspirin and oxycodone produce a rational combination drug that relieves pain better than aspirin alone but has less risk of side effects than the larger dose of oxycodone that would be needed if oxycodone were used alone.

Although this combination is the best choice in some situations, it is overused. Many people who are prescribed this combination would get pain relief from aspirin alone and would avoid the danger of becoming addicted to oxycodone. So before taking this drug, ask your doctor about trying plain aspirin first.

One hazard of taking oxycodone continuously for longer than several weeks is addiction. **Do not stop taking your drug suddenly.** With the help of your doctor, work out a schedule for slowly lowering the amount of the drug you take by about 5 to 10% each day. Keep a written record of the dosage reduction schedule with you. These steps will make it much easier to become drug free without developing distressing symptoms of drug withdrawal.

Aspirin/Reye's Syndrome Alert
Do not use this product for treating chicken pox, flu, or flu-like illness. It will increase the risk of contracting Reye's syndrome, a rare but often fatal disease.

Acetaminophen and Oxycodone (combined)
PERCOCET (Du Pont)
TYLOX (McNeil Pharmaceutical)

Generic: available

Family: Painkillers
Fever Reducers
Narcotics (see p. 260)

Acetaminophen (see p. 318) and oxycodone (oxi *koe* done) are both painkillers. Acetaminophen also reduces fever, but it does not relieve the redness, stiffness, or swelling of rheumatoid arthritis or other conditions that cause inflammation. Oxycodone works similarly to narcotic drugs like morphine and has similar painkilling and addictive effects.

Together, these two drugs produce a rational combination that relieves pain better than acetaminophen alone but has less risk of side effects than the larger dose of oxycodone that would be needed if oxycodone were used alone. This combination is available in tablets and capsules.

Although this combination is the best choice in some situations, it is overused. Many people who are prescribed this combination would get pain relief from acetaminophen alone, and would avoid the danger of becoming addicted to oxycodone. So before taking this drug, ask your doctor about trying plain acetaminophen first.

One hazard of taking oxycodone continuously for longer than several weeks is addiction. **Do not stop taking your drug suddenly.** With the help of your doctor, work out a schedule for slowly lowering the amount of the drug you take by about 5 to 10% each day. Keep a written record of the dosage reduction schedule with you. These steps will make it much easier to become drug free without developing distressing symptoms of drug withdrawal.

Warning
There have been a number of case reports of liver damage involving a possible drug interaction between isoniazid, a medication used to prevent and treat tuberculosis, and acetaminophen, an over-the-counter painkiller and the active ingredient in Tylenol. Each drug alone is known to cause liver damage. Isoniazid alone, especially as people get older, has been documented to cause liver damage. Acetaminophen, alone in large doses or probably in combination with alcohol, also increases the risk of liver damage. The combination of acetaminophen with isoniazid, according to the authors of these case reports, may also be dangerous.

If you are taking isoniazid for tuberculosis or have a positive TB skin test and are using the drug, consult your physician before using acetaminophen or any combination product containing acetaminophen. Discuss alternatives to acetaminophen with your physician.[97,98]

LIMITED USE

Hydroxychloroquine
PLAQUENIL (Winthrop-Breon)

Generic: not available

Family: Antiarthritis Drugs (see p. 261)

Hydroxychloroquine (hye drox ee *klor* oh kwin) is used to treat malaria, rheumatoid arthritis, and lupus erythematosus. Like other antiarthritis drugs, it reduces symptoms caused by inflammation. Because hydroxychloroquine has serious side effects, you should not be taking it for rheumatoid arthritis unless you have already tried other drugs that reduce inflammation and they have not worked.

Hydroxychloroquine takes time to produce results, and you may not notice improvement in your condition for weeks or months. Continue to take the drug as directed by your doctor, and use a nonsteroidal anti-inflammatory drug such as aspirin at the same time to relieve your symptoms until the hydroxychloroquine works. If the drug doesn't begin to work after 6 months, it should be discontinued.

Hydroxychloroquine can cause serious side effects, some of which may occur months after you have stopped using it. The drug can collect in your eyes and cause vision problems, so an eye specialist should check your eyes before and during your treatment with hydroxychloroquine. If you develop blurred vision, difficulty reading, or any other change in your vision, stop taking the drug and call your doctor. Hydroxychloroquine has also caused some cases of rash, hearing loss, muscle weakness, and blood disorders. You should not take a dose greater than 400 milligrams per day, since taking such a large dose for a long time increases your risk of side effects.

Keep this drug out of the reach of children. Children are especially sensitive to the effects of hydroxychloroquine, and some have died after taking as few as three or four tablets.

Before You Use This Drug
Tell your doctor if you have or have had
❑ allergies to drugs
❑ alcohol dependence
❑ liver problems
❑ severe blood disorders
❑ gastrointestinal disease
❑ glucose-6-phosphate dehydrogenase deficiency
❑ disorders of the nervous system or seizures
❑ psoriasis
❑ eye disease
Tell your doctor about any other drugs you take, including aspirin, herbs, vitamins, and other non-prescription products.

When You Use This Drug
◆ Do not drink alcohol.
◆ Until you know how you react to this drug, do not drive or perform other activities requiring alertness. Hydroxychloroquine causes lightheadedness and drowsiness.

How To Use This Drug
◆ Take with meals to reduce stomach upset.
◆ Do not expose to heat or direct light. Do not store in the bathroom.
◆ *If you miss a dose, use the following guidelines:*
  - If you take the drug once a week, take the missed dose as soon as you remember and resume your regular schedule.

- If you take the drug once a day, take the missed dose as soon as you remember, but skip it if you don't remember until the next day. **Do not take double doses.**
- If you take the drug more than once a day, take the missed dose if you remember less than an hour after you were supposed to take it. If more than an hour has passed since you were supposed to take it, skip it. Continue to follow your regular schedule. **Do not take double doses.**

Interactions With Other Drugs

The following drugs are listed in *Evaluations of Drug Interactions*, 1991 as causing "highly clinically significant" or "clinically significant" interactions when used together with this drug. There may be other drugs, especially those in the families of drugs listed below, that also will react with this drug to cause severe adverse effects. Make sure to ask your doctor for a complete listing of them and let her or him know if you are taking any of these interacting drugs:

digoxin; FLAGYL; LANOXICAPS; LANOXIN; metronidazole.

Adverse Effects
Call your doctor immediately:
❑ if you experience signs of overdose: difficulty breathing; drowsiness; fainting
❑ changes in vision
❑ seizures
❑ mood or mental changes
❑ hearing loss, ringing in ears
❑ unusual bleeding or bruising
❑ unusual muscle weakness

Call your doctor if these symptoms continue:
❑ diarrhea
❑ headache
❑ nausea, vomiting
❑ stomach cramps or pain
❑ bleaching of hair or hair loss
❑ dark discoloration of skin, nails, or inside of mouth
❑ skin rash or itching
❑ dizziness or lightheadedness
❑ nervousness or restlessness

Periodic Tests
Ask your doctor which of these tests should be done periodically while you are taking this drug:
❑ eye exams (before use, and at least annually during long-term use)

LIMITED USE

Aurothioglucose
SOLGANAL (Schering)

Gold Sodium Thiomalate
MYOCHRYSINE (Merck)

Generic: available for gold sodium thiomolate

Family: Gold Compound
Arthritis Drugs (see p. 261)

Aurothioglucose (aur oh thye oh *gloo* kose) and gold sodium thiomalate (thye oh *mah* late) are gold salts used to treat rheumatoid arthritis. These drugs have severe side effects. A large proportion of users show signs of toxicity from these drugs, and some side effects may occur many months after you stop taking the drug (see Adverse Effects). Because of the danger of side effects, you should only be taking gold salts for rheumatoid arthritis if you have already tried anti-inflammatory drugs without success.

Aurothioglucose and gold sodium thiomalate are injected into the muscle, and you may have joint pain for 1 or 2 days afterward.

These drugs cause gradual improvement, and you may not notice the improvement until you have been injected with a total of approximately 1,000 milligrams. Until the gold therapy begins to work, you should take a nonsteroidal anti-inflammatory drug such as aspirin at the same time to relieve your arthritis symptoms. If the cumulative dose of gold salts reaches 1,000 milligrams and you still do not notice any improvement, the drug should be discontinued.[99]

If you cannot tolerate the side effects of the injections, you may better tolerate auranofin, a recently approved gold salt that can be taken by mouth. It appears to have effects comparable to those of the gold injections. It is almost as effective and less toxic, although it commonly causes diarrhea.

Before You Use This Drug
Do not use if you have or have had
❑ severe side effects from previous gold treatments (bone marrow disease, low blood platelet count, severe skin rashes or intestinal diseases, formation of fibrous tissue in the lungs, protein in the urine)
Tell your doctor if you have or have had
❑ allergies to drugs
❑ bone marrow depression or blood cell diseases
❑ decreased circulation to the heart or brain
❑ extreme weakness
❑ kidney disease
❑ skin rash, hives, or eczema
❑ lupus erythematosus
❑ Sjogren's syndrome, *for aurothioglucose*
Tell your doctor about any other drugs you take, including aspirin, herbs, vitamins, and other non-prescription products.

When You Use This Drug
◆ You may lose consciousness and/or suffer allergic shock after an injection.

Interactions With Other Drugs
The following drugs are listed in *Evaluations of Drug Interactions*, 1991 as causing "highly clinically significant" or "clinically significant" interactions when used together with this drug. There may be other drugs, especially those in the families of drugs listed below, that also will react with this drug to cause severe

adverse effects. Make sure to ask your doctor for a complete listing of them and let her or him know if you are taking this interacting drug:

NAPROSYN; naproxen.

Adverse Effects

Call your doctor immediately, even if these occur many months after you stop taking the drug:
❑ skin rash or itching
❑ bloody or cloudy urine
❑ coughing or shortness of breath
❑ diarrhea or stomach pain
❑ swelling (edema)
❑ irritation or soreness of tongue or gums
❑ numbness or tingling in hands or feet
❑ metallic taste in mouth
❑ sore throat and fever
❑ sores or white spots in mouth or throat
❑ unusual bleeding or bruising
❑ unusual tiredness or weakness
❑ yellow eyes or skin

Call your doctor if these symptoms continue:
❑ dizziness, faintness
❑ flushing or redness of face
❑ nausea, vomiting
❑ gas, bloated feeling
❑ abdominal cramps or pain
❑ loss of appetite

Periodic Tests

Ask your doctor which of these tests should be done periodically while you are taking this drug:
❑ white blood cell counts*
❑ platelet counts*
❑ hemoglobin or hematocrit*
❑ liver function tests
❑ kidney function tests
❑ urinary protein (before each injection)

---

* Before each injection for the first 6 months, then less often as dosage decreases.

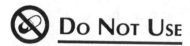 **Do Not Use**

Alternative treatment: See Aspirin, p. 268, and Aspirin and Codeine, p. 283.

Dihydrocodeine, Aspirin, and Caffeine (combined)
SYNALGOS-DC (Wyeth)

Family: Painkillers
Fever Reducers
Narcotics (see p. 260)

This is a combination drug composed of aspirin (see p. 268), caffeine (ka *feen*) and dihydrocodeine (dye hye droe *koe* deen). However, it is an *irrational* combination because it includes caffeine. There is no acceptable scientific evidence that caffeine helps to relieve pain. Another problem with this combination is that it includes

dihydrocodeine, which is related to codeine (see p. 276) and is addictive. Rather than taking this drug, ask your doctor about taking plain aspirin (see p. 268) or, if necessary, aspirin with codeine (see p. 283).

Aspirin/Reyes Syndrome
Do not use this product for treating chicken pox, flu, or flu-like illness. It will increase the risk of contracting Reye's syndrome, a rare but often fatal disease.

One hazard of taking dihydrocodeine continuously for longer than several weeks is addiction. **Do not stop taking your drug suddenly.** With the help of your doctor, work out a schedule for slowly lowering the amount of the drug you take by about 5 to 10% each day. Keep a written record of the dosage reduction schedule with you. These steps will make it much easier to become drug free without developing distressing symptoms of drug withdrawal.

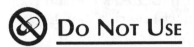 **DO NOT USE**

Alternative treatment: See Aspirin, p. 268, and Aspirin and Codeine, p. 283.

Pentazocine
TALWIN (Winthrop-Breon)

Pentazocine and Naloxone (combined)
TALWIN-NX (Winthrop-Breon)

Family: Narcotics (see p. 260)

Pentazocine (pen *taz* oh seen) relieves moderate to severe pain. **Older adults should not use this drug, either alone or in combination with naloxone, because of the high risk of side effects, especially confusion.** The risk is so high that the World Health Organization recommends that this drug not be used if possible.[100] Pentazocine is also addictive.

One hazard of taking pentazocine continuously for longer than several weeks is addiction. **Do not stop taking your drug suddenly.** With the help of your doctor, work out a schedule for slowly lowering the amount of the drug you take by about 5 to 10% each day. Keep a written record of the dosage reduction schedule with you. These steps will make it much easier to become drug free without developing distressing symptoms of drug withdrawal.

LIMITED USE

Tolmetin
TOLECTIN (McNeil Pharmaceutical)

Generic: available

Family: Nonsteroidal Anti-inflammatory
Drugs "NSAIDs"
Arthritis Drugs (see p. 261)

In older adults, tolmetin (*tole* met in) is used mainly to relieve the pain and inflammation of two kinds of arthritis, rheumatoid arthritis and osteoarthritis. **In general, if you are over 60, you should take less than the usual adult dose, especially if you have decreased kidney function.** Tolmetin has been reported to cause severe allergic reactions.[101] **You should never use tolmetin intermittently (on-and-off) because this greatly increases the risk of allergic reactions, which can be fatal.**

Tolmetin belongs to the family of drugs called nonsteroidal anti-inflammatory drugs, shortened to NSAIDs (*n* sayds), often used to treat arthritis in older adults. Aspirin is just as effective as all these drugs and less costly (see p. 268). All the NSAIDs can cause serious harm, even fatalities, from bleeding in the stomach or intestines. Bleeding can occur at any time and without warning and older people are more likely to experience adversity from bleeding. Elderly people are also more likely to have reduced liver and kidney function. So, some doctors believe people over age 70 should be started with half the usual dose of drugs in this group.[102]

Aspirin is the drug of choice for treating pain, fever, and inflammation in people who do not have ulcers, gastritis (inflammation of the stomach), or an allergy to aspirin. Some rheumatologists (arthritis specialists) prefer aspirin to other drugs in this family for treating rheumatoid arthritis.[103]

If you are taking tolmetin, ask your doctor if you can switch to taking enteric-coated aspirin (aspirin coated so it won't dissolve in the stomach) twice a day. If you cannot take aspirin and are having trouble with side effects on tolmetin, ask about switching to another NSAID such as ibuprofen or naproxen. Each person responds differently to different NSAIDs.

Before You Use This Drug
Do not use if you have or have had
❑ an allergic reaction to aspirin, any other NSAID or iodides[104]
❑ kidney or heart failure
❑ peptic ulcers
❑ alcohol dependence
❑ cirrhosis of the liver
❑ nasal polyps or asthma
Tell your doctor if you have or have had
❑ allergies to drugs
❑ heart, kidney, or liver disease
❑ problems stopping bleeding
❑ high blood pressure
❑ epilepsy (seizures)
❑ mental depression or other psychiatric conditions
❑ Parkinson's disease
❑ lupus erythematosus
Tell your doctor about any other drugs you take, including aspirin, herbs, vitamins, and other non-prescription products.

When You Use This Drug
◆ Do not drink alcohol. It irritates the stomach lining and increases the risk of stomach bleeding.
◆ Call your doctor immediately if you have flu-like symptoms (chills, fever, muscle aches or pains) shortly before or with a skin rash. This may indicate a serious reaction to tolmetin.

◆ You may feel dizzy when rising from a lying or sitting position. If you are lying down, hang your legs over the side of the bed for a few minutes, then get up slowly. When getting up from a chair, stay by the chair until you are sure that you are not dizzy. (See p. 14.)

◆ If you plan to have any surgery, including dental, tell your doctor that you take this drug.

How To Use This Drug

◆ Take with food to reduce stomach irritation.

◆ Take with **a full glass (8 ounces) of water**. Do not lie down within 30 minutes afterward.

◆ If you miss a dose, take it as soon as possible, but skip it if you don't remember it until the next day. **Do not take double doses.**

◆ Store at room temperature, with lid on tightly. Do not expose to moisture or heat. Do not store in the bathroom.

Interactions With Other Drugs

The following drugs are listed in *Evaluations of Drug Interactions*, 1991 as causing "highly clinically significant" or "clinically significant" interactions when used together with this drug. There may be other drugs, especially those in the families of drugs listed below, that also will react with this drug to cause severe adverse effects. Make sure to ask your doctor for a complete listing of them and let her or him know if you are taking any of these interacting drugs:

bendroflumethiazide; BENEMID; CAPOTEN; captopril; COUMADIN; cyclosporine; digoxin; DILANTIN; ESKALITH; FOLEX; GARAMYCIN; gentamicin; gold sodium thiomalate; INDERAL; LANOXIN; lithium; methotrexate; MINIPRESS; MYOCHRYSINE; NATURETIN; phenytoin; prazosin; probenecid; propranolol; SANDIMMUNE; warfarin.

Adverse Effects

Call your doctor immediately:

❏ bloody or black, tarry stools
❏ confusion, forgetfulness
❏ mental depression, other mood or mental changes
❏ ringing or buzzing in ears
❏ swelling of feet or lower legs
❏ unusual weight gain
❏ abdominal/stomach pain or cramps
❏ vomiting blood or material that looks like coffee grounds
❏ bleeding sores on lips
❏ fainting
❏ chills, fever, muscle aches or pain with or before a rash
❏ skin rash, itching, or peeling
❏ changes in vision or hearing
❏ unusual bleeding or bruising
❏ decrease in amount of urine

Call your doctor if these symptoms continue:

❏ dizziness or lightheadedness
❏ heartburn or indigestion
❏ nausea or vomiting
❏ constipation or diarrhea
❏ drowsiness

Periodic Tests

Ask your doctor which of these tests should be done periodically while you are taking this drug:

❏ kidney function tests
❏ liver function tests
❏ stool tests for possible blood loss
❏ hematocrit and/or hemoglobin test
❏ blood concentrations of creatinine, potassium, and urea nitrogen
❏ white blood cell counts

LIMITED USE

Choline and Magnesium Salicylates
TRILISATE (Purdue Frederick)

Choline Salicylate
ARTHROPAN (Purdue Frederick)

Magnesium Salicylate
DOAN'S PILLS (Jeffrey Martin)

Generic: available

Family: Salicylates (see p. 258)

Choline (*koe* leen) and magnesium salicy-lates (mag *nee* zee um sa *li* si lates), alone or combined, relieve pain and reduce fever. They offer few advantages over aspirin (see p. 268). If you are allergic to aspirin, you may be able to use choline and magnesium salicylates. These drugs may cause fewer stomach problems than plain aspirin but are more expensive, may not be as effective, and have the same potential side effects.[105] For the vast majority of people, aspirin is the drug of choice. For long-term use, enteric-coated aspirin is best because it helps prevent stomach bleeding.

If you are taking choline or magnesium salicylates and you are over 60 years old, you should probably take less than the usual adult dose because of the risk of harmful side effects.

Aspirin/Reye's Syndrome Alert
Do not use this product for treating chicken pox, flu, or flu-like illness. It will increase the risk of contracting Reye's syndrome, a rare but often fatal disease.

Before You Use This Drug
Tell your doctor if you have or have had
❏ allergies to drugs
❏ a reaction to aspirin, other salicylates, or nonsteroidal anti-inflammatory drugs such as ibuprofen or naproxen
❏ bleeding problems
❏ ulcer or other stomach problems
❏ anemia
❏ heart or liver disease
❏ gout
❏ overactive thyroid
Tell your doctor about any other drugs you take, including aspirin, herbs, vitamins, and other non-prescription products.

When You Use This Drug
◆ Do not drink alcohol. This combination increases the risk of stomach or intestinal bleeding.
◆ Never take more than the amount pre-scribed by your doctor or recommended on the package label.
◆ **Caution diabetics:** see p. 516.
◆ Do not take for 5 days before any sur-gery, unless your doctor or dentist tells you otherwise. These drugs interfere with your body's ability to stop bleeding.
◆ If you are on long-term or high-dose treatment, you should have regular checkups.
◆ Never place this drug directly on teeth or

gums because it is irritating to these tissues.

◆ Do not chew this drug within 1 week after you have any type of mouth surgery.

How To Use This Drug

◆ Take tablets and capsules with **a full glass (8 ounces) of water**. Oral solutions may be mixed with fruit juice just before taking. Take after meals or with food to help protect your stomach. Do not lie down for 30 minutes.

◆ Do not store in the bathroom. Do not expose to heat, moisture, or strong light.

◆ If you miss a dose, take it as soon as you remember, but skip it if it is almost time for the next dose. **Do not take double doses.**

Interactions With Other Drugs

The following drugs are listed in *Evaluations of Drug Interactions*, 1991 as causing "highly clinically significant" or "clinically significant" interactions when used together with this drug. There may be other drugs, especially those in the families of drugs listed below, that also will react with this drug to cause severe adverse effects. Make sure to ask your doctor for a complete listing of them and let her or him know if you are taking any of these interacting drugs:

acetazolamide; aluminum hydroxide; AMPHOJEL; ANTURANE; CAPOTEN; captopril; chlorpropamide; COUMADIN; DEPAKENE; DIABINESE; DIAMOX; FOLEX; MAALOX; magnesium hydroxide; MEDROL; methotrexate; methylprednisolone; sulfinpyrazone; valproic acid; warfarin.

Adverse Effects

Call your doctor immediately:

❏ **if you experience signs of overdose:** mild to severe or persistent headache; ringing or buzzing in ears; loss of hearing; severe or continuing diarrhea; dizziness or lightheadedness; extreme drowsiness; confusion; nausea or vomiting; stomach pain; abnormal increase in sweating; abnormally fast or deep breathing; abnormal thirst; abnormal or uncontrolled flapping of the hands; vision problems; bloody urine; seizures; hallucinations; nervousness or excitement; trouble breathing; unexplained fever

❏ vomiting material that looks bloody or like coffee grounds

❏ bloody or black, tarry stools

❏ wheezing, tightness in chest, or trouble breathing

❏ skin rash, hives, or itching

❏ fainting or dizzy spells

Call your doctor if these symptoms continue:

❏ heartburn or indigestion

❏ abnormal tiredness or weakness

Acetaminophen
TYLENOL (McNeil Consumer Products)

Generic: available

Family: Painkillers
Fever Reducers

Acetaminophen (a seat a *mee* noe fen), like aspirin, kills pain and reduces fever, but unlike aspirin does *not* help the redness, stiffness, or swelling of inflammation. Because of this, aspirin (see p. 268) is much more effective for treating the inflammation of arthritis.[106]

In general, you should not take anything to reduce a fever until the cause of the fever is known. It is rarely *necessary* to treat a fever. However, if a fever is having damaging effects or is making you extremely uncomfortable, it can be reduced with acetaminophen. When you are taking acetaminophen to reduce a fever, you should take it regularly every 3 or 4 hours, and stop taking it when the underlying problem is gone or has been controlled through other treatment.

One advantage of acetaminophen over aspirin is that acetaminophen does not cause the stomach bleeding that aspirin can cause. For this reason, doctors often prescribe or recommend acetaminophen to people who are likely to suffer from bleeding when they take aspirin. This includes people taking blood-thinning drugs like warfarin or heparin and people who have ulcers, gout, or bleeding problems such as hemophilia. Also, people who are allergic to aspirin can often take acetaminophen.

On the other hand, for most people, aspirin is not likely to cause harmful stomach effects if taken in small amounts for a short time.[107] And acetaminophen has its own harmful effects — it can cause liver damage, especially in older adults, if you take more than the recommended dose or if you take it continuously for more than 10 days.[108]

Warning
There have been a number of case reports of liver damage involving a possible drug interaction between isoniazid, a medication used to prevent and treat tuberculosis, and acetaminophen, an over-the-counter painkiller and the active ingredient in Tylenol. Each drug alone is known to cause liver damage. Isoniazid alone, especially as people get older, has been documented to cause liver damage. Acetaminophen, alone in large doses or probably in combination with alcohol, also increases the risk of liver damage. The combination of acetaminophen with isoniazid, according to the authors of these case reports, may also be dangerous.

If you are taking isoniazid for tuberculosis or have a positive TB skin test and are using the drug, consult your physician before using acetaminophen or any combination product containing acetaminophen. Discuss alternatives to acetaminophen with your physician.[109,110]

Before You Use This Drug
Tell your doctor if you have or have had
❑ allergies to drugs
❑ a reaction to acetaminophen
❑ alcohol dependence
❑ a viral infection
❑ kidney or liver disease
Tell your doctor about any other drugs you

take, including aspirin, herbs, vitamins, and other non-prescription products.

When You Use This Drug

If you are treating yourself with acetaminophen, call your doctor if you have a fever that lasts for more than 3 days or if your symptoms do not improve.
Do not take more than is recommended on the package or prescribed by your doctor.
Do not take for more than 10 days.
Do not drink alcohol. This combination increases the risk of liver damage.
Acetaminophen may affect the results of lab tests for blood sugar or uric acid.

How To Use This Drug

Do not store in the bathroom. Do not expose to heat, moisture, or strong light.
◆ Tablets may be crushed.
Avoid buffered (sodium-containing) acetaminophen and acetaminophen products that include other ingredients such as caffeine. They increase the likelihood of harmful drug interactions and side effects.

Interactions With Other Drugs

See Warning Box, p. 318
INH; isoniazid

Adverse Effects

Call your doctor immediately:
❏ if you experience signs of overdose: diarrhea; loss of appetite; nausea or vomiting; pain or cramps in stomach; sore or swollen upper abdomen; abnormal increase in sweating
❏ yellow eyes or skin
❏ bloody or cloudy urine
❏ trouble urinating, painful urination, or sudden decrease in amount of urine
❏ skin rash, hives, or itching
❏ unexplained fever or sore throat
❏ abnormal bleeding or bruising
❏ abnormal tiredness or weakness

Periodic Tests

Ask your doctor which of these tests should be done periodically while you are taking this drug:
❏ liver function tests, for long-term or high-dose therapy

Acetaminophen and Codeine (combined)
TYLENOL 3 (McNeil Pharmaceutical)

Generic: available

Family: Painkillers
Fever Reducers
Narcotics (see p. 260)

Acetaminophen (see p. 318) and codeine (see p. 276) are both effective painkillers. Together, they produce a rational combination drug that relieves pain better than acetaminophen alone but has less risk of side ef-

One hazard of taking codeine continuously for longer than several weeks is addiction. **Do not stop taking your drug suddenly.** With the help of your doctor, work out a schedule for slowly lowering the amount of the drug you take by about 5 to 10% each day. Keep a written record of the dosage reduction schedule with you. These steps will make it much easier to become drug free without developing distressing symptoms of drug withdrawal.

fects than the larger amount of codeine that would be needed if codeine were used alone. This combination is similar in effect to aspirin and codeine (see p. 283), except that acetaminophen, unlike aspirin, will not help the redness, stiffness, or swelling caused by rheumatoid arthritis or other types of inflammation. This combination is available in capsules and tablets and as a liquid.

Although this drug is the best choice in some situations, it is overused. Many people who are prescribed this combina- tion would get pain relief from acetaminophen alone, and would avoid the harmful side effects that codeine can cause — addiction and constipation. So before taking this drug, ask your doctor about trying plain acetaminophen first.

This drug can increase the risk of hip fracture.[111]

Warning

There have been a number of case reports of liver damage involving a possible drug interaction between isoniazid, a medication used to prevent and treat tuberculosis, and acetaminophen, an over-the-counter painkiller and the active ingredient in Tylenol. Each drug alone is known to cause liver damage. Isoniazid alone, especially as people get older, has been documented to cause liver damage. Acetaminophen, alone in large doses or probably in combination with alcohol, also increases the risk of liver damage. The combination of acetaminophen with isoniazid, according to the authors of these case reports, may also be dangerous.

If you are taking isoniazid for tuberculosis or have a positive TB skin test and are using the drug, consult your physician before using acetaminophen or any combination product containing acetaminophen. Discuss alternatives to acetaminophen with your physician.[112,113]

LIMITED USE

Diclofenac
VOLTAREN (Geigy)

Generic: not available

Family: Nonsteroidal Anti-inflammatory
Drugs "NSAIDs"
Arthritis Drugs (see p. 261)

Diclofenac (dick *low* fen ak) is used to treat mild to moderate pain and symptoms of rheumatoid arthritis, osteoarthritis, and spondylitis. **In general, if you are over 60, you should take less than the usual adult dose, especially if you have decreased kidney function.**

Diclofenac belongs to the family of drugs called nonsteroidal anti-inflammatory drugs, shortened to NSAIDs (*n* sayds), often used to treat arthritis in older adults. Aspirin is just as effective as all these drugs and less costly (see p. 268). All the NSAIDs can cause serious harm, even fatalities, from bleeding in the stomach or intestines. Bleeding can occur at any time and without warning and older people are more likely to experience adversity from bleeding. Elderly people are also more likely to have reduced liver and kidney function. So, some doctors believe people over age 70 should be started with half the usual dose of drugs in this group.[114] Like other NSAIDs, diclofenac relieves symptoms but does not cure any condition.

According to the International Agranulocytosis and Aplastic Anemia Study of 1986, toxic effects to the bone marrow and killing of white blood cells happen with diclofenac at a rate as high as with phenylbutazone[115] (see pg. 273). There have also been a number of cases of severe hepatitis in patients using diclofenac.[116]

Some rheumatologists (arthritis specialists) prefer aspirin to other drugs in its family (NSAIDs) for treating rheumatoid arthritis.[117] Aspirin is the best drug to treat pain and inflammation in people who do not have ulcers, or an allergy to aspirin. Another treatment is physiotherapy which can be used as an adjunct to drug therapies.[118]

Before You Use This Drug

Do not use if you have or have had

- ❑ an allergic reaction to aspirin, any other NSAID or iodides.[119]
- ❑ asthma
- ❑ kidney or heart failure
- ❑ peptic ulcers
- ❑ alcohol dependence
- ❑ cirrhosis of the liver
- ❑ nasal polyps or asthma
- ❑ hepatitis
- ❑ jaundice

Tell your doctor if you have or have had

- ❑ allergies to drugs
- ❑ heart, kidney or liver disease
- ❑ problems stopping bleeding
- ❑ high blood pressure

- ❑ blood transfusion[120]
- ❑ hemorrhoids[121]
- ❑ hepatitis
- ❑ occupational exposure to chemicals[122]
- ❑ psoriasis[123]
- ❑ salt-restricted diet[124]
- ❑ seizures[125]

Tell your doctor about any other drugs you take, including aspirin, herbs, vitamins, and other non-prescription products.

When You Use This Drug

- ◆ Do not drink alcohol. It irritates the stomach lining and increases the risk of stomach bleeding.
- ◆ Call your doctor immediately if you have flu-like symptoms (chills, fever, muscle aches or pains) shortly before or with a skin rash. This may indicate a serious reaction to diclofenac.
- ◆ You may feel dizzy when rising from a lying or sitting position. If you are lying down, hang your legs over the side of the bed for a few minutes, then get up slowly. When getting up from a chair, stay by the chair until you are sure that you are not dizzy. (See p. 14.)
- ◆ Do not drive or perform other activities that require alertness because this drug may make you drowsy, dizzy, or lightheaded.
- ◆ If you plan to have any surgery, including dental, tell your doctor that you take this drug.

How To Use This Drug

- ◆ Take with food to reduce stomach irritation.
- ◆ Take with **a full glass (8 ounces) of water.** Do not lie down for 30 minutes afterwards.
- ◆ If you miss a dose, take it as soon as possible, but skip it if you don't remember until the next day. **Do not take double doses.**
- ◆ Store at room temperature, with lid on tightly. Do not expose to moisture or heat. Do not store in the bathroom.

Interactions With Other Drugs

The following drugs are listed in *Evaluations of Drug Interactions*, 1991 as causing "highly clinically significant" or "clinically significant" interactions when used together with this drug. There may be other drugs, especially those in the families of drugs listed below, that also will react with this drug to cause severe adverse effects. Make sure to ask your doctor for a complete listing of them and let her or him know if you are taking any of these interacting drugs:

bendroflumethiazide; CAPOTEN; captopril; COUMADIN; cyclosporine; DEXATRIM; digoxin; DILANTIN; DYAZIDE; DYRENIUM; ESKALITH; GARAMYCIN; gentamicin; gold salts; INDERAL; LANOXIN; lithium; LITHOBID; methotrexate; MINIPRESS; MYOCHRYSINE; NALDECON-DX; NATURETIN; phenylpropanolamine; phenytoin; prazosin; propranolol; SANDIMMUNE; triamterene; warfarin.

Additionally, the *United States Pharmacopeia Drug Information*, 1992 lists these drugs as having interactions of major significance:

aspirin; BUFFERIN; CEFOBID; cefoperaxone; ECOTRIN.

Adverse Effects

Call you doctor immediately:
❏ bloody or black, tarry stools
❏ bleeding or bruising
❏ breathing difficulty
❏ changes in vision or hearing
❏ chest pain, or tightness in chest
❏ fainting
❏ flu-like symptoms
❏ numbness
❏ skin rash, itching, peeling
❏ ringing or buzzing in the ears
❏ seizures
❏ abdominal/stomach pain or cramps
❏ swelling of eyelids, lips, throat, legs or feet
❏ red urine,[126] or sudden decrease in amount of urine
❏ vomiting blood, or material that looks like coffee grounds
❏ sudden weight change

Call your doctor if these symptoms continue:
❏ loss of appetite
❏ confusion, forgetfulness
❏ constipation
❏ diarrhea
❏ dizziness
❏ drowsiness, fatigue
❏ gas, heartburn, indigestion
❏ hair loss, or changes in nails[127]
❏ headache
❏ nausea or vomiting

Periodic Tests

Ask your doctor which of these tests should be done periodically while you are taking this drug:
❏ kidney function tests
❏ liver function tests
❏ stool tests for possible blood loss
❏ hematocrit and/or hemoglobin test
❏ blood concentrations of creatinine, potassium, and urea nitrogen
❏ white blood cell counts

Lidocaine
XYLOCAINE (Astra)

Generic: available

Family: Anesthetics
Antiarrhythmics

Lidocaine (*lye* doe kane) is used to treat disturbances in heartbeats (arrhythmias) and as a local anesthetic. This page does not discuss its use for irregular heartbeats, since this use occurs mostly in the hospital. As a local anesthetic, a lidocaine injection or ointment is used for minor surgical procedures and for pain relief.

Before You Use This Drug
Do not use if you have or have had
❑ Adams-Stokes syndrome (fainting episodes due to brief failure of the heart to pump)
❑ complete heart block
❑ allergies to novocain
Tell your doctor if you have or have had
❑ allergies to drugs
❑ any heart problems
❑ congestive heart failure
❑ kidney or liver disease
❑ low blood pressure or shock due to fluid loss
Tell your doctor about any other drugs you take, including aspirin, herbs, vitamins, and other non-prescription products.

When You Use This Drug
◆ The ointment form of this drug (used as an anesthetic) should not be used for a long time.

How To Use This Drug
◆ Do not apply ointment to large areas of your body. Use the smallest amount that is effective, to avoid absorbing large amounts of the drug into your bloodstream.
◆ If you use this drug in your mouth or throat, do not eat or chew gum for 1 hour afterward. The drug's anesthetic effect may make it hard for you to swallow and increase your risk of badly biting your tongue or cheek.

Interactions With Other Drugs
The following drugs are listed in *Evaluations of Drug Interactions*, 1991 as causing "highly clinically significant" or "clinically significant" interactions when used together with this drug. There may be other drugs, especially those in the families of drugs listed below, that also will react with this drug to cause severe adverse effects. Make sure to ask your doctor for a complete listing of them and let her or him know if you are taking any of these interacting drugs:
amiodarone; cimetidine; CORDARONE; INDERAL; propranolol; ritodrine; succinylcholine; TAGAMET; YUTOPAR.

Adverse Effects
Call your doctor immediately:
❑ **if you experience signs of overdose:** blurred or double vision; nausea or vomiting; ringing in ears; tremors or twitching; convulsions; difficulty breathing; dizziness or fainting; unusually slow heartbeat
❑ itching or skin rash
❑ unusual swelling of skin (allergic reaction)
Call your doctor if these symptoms continue:
❑ pain at the site of injection
❑ anxiety, nervousness
❑ drowsiness
❑ feelings of coldness, heat, or numbness

Periodic Tests
Ask your doctor which of these tests should be done periodically while you are taking this drug:
❑ heart function tests, such as electrocardiogram (EKG)
❑ blood pressure
❑ blood levels of lidocaine and electrolytes

Notes for Painkillers and Arthritis Drugs

1. 42 *Federal Register* 35390. July 8, 1977.

2. *The Medical Letter on Drugs and Therapeutics.* New York: The Medical Letter Inc. 1991; 33:66.

3. Plotz P. Aspirin and Salicylates. In *Textbook of Rheumatology*, W. Kelley, ed., Philadelphia: Saunders, 1985.

4. *The Medical Letter on Drugs and Therapeutics.* New York: The Medical Letter Inc., 1976; 18:119.

5. Orland MJ, Saltman RJ, eds. *Manual of Medical Therapeutics.* 25th ed. Boston: Little, Brown and Company, 1986:373.

6. Gilman AG, Goodman LS, Rall TW, Murad F, eds. *The Pharmacological Basis of Therapeutics.* 7th ed. New York: Macmillan, 1985.

7. Angell M. The quality of mercy. *New England Journal of Medicine* 1982; 306:98-9.

8. Simonson W. *Medications and the Elderly.* Rockville, Maryland; Aspen Systems Corporation, 1984:116.

9. *The Medical Letter on Drugs and Therapeutics.* New York: The Medical Letter Inc., 1982; 24:96.

10. AMA Department of Drugs. *AMA Drug Evaluations.* 5th ed. Chicago: American Medical Association, 1983:70.

11. Vestal RE, ed. *Drug Treatment in the Elderly.* Sydney, Australia: ADIS Health Science Press, 1984:179.

12. Plotz, op. cit.

13. *USP DI, Drug Information for the Health Care Professional.* 12th ed. Rockville MD: The United States Pharmacopeial Convention, Inc., 1992:460-70.

14. *The Medical Letter on Drugs and Therapeutics.* New York: The Medical Letter Inc., 1980; 22:29-31.

15. Olin BR, ed. *Facts and Comparisons.* St. Louis: J.B. Lippincott Co., September 1992:251b.

16. American Society of Hospital Pharmacists. *American Hospital Formulary Service Drug Information*, Bethesda, MD, 1992:1698-9.

17. *USP DI*, 1992, op. cit.

18. Kaufhold J, Wilkowski M, McCabe K. Flurbiprofen-associated acute tubulointerstitial nephritis. *American Journal of Nephrology* 1991; 11:144-6.

19. Murphy R, Swartz R, Watkins PB. Severe acetaminophen toxicity in a patient receiving isoniazid. *Annals of Internal Medicine* 1990; 113:799-800.

20. Moulding TS, Redeker AG, Konel GC. Acetaminophen, isoniazid, and hepatic toxicity. *Annals of Internal Medicine*, 1991; 114:431.

21. *USP DI*, 1992, op. cit.

22. Orland, op. cit., p. 2.

23. 42 *Federal Register* 35480, July 8, 1977.

24. *Drugs for the Elderly.* Denmark: World Health Organization, 1985:27

25. *USP DI*, 1992, op. cit.

26. *The Medical Letter on Drugs and Therapeutics*, 1980, op. cit.

27. *USP DI*, 1992, op. cit.

28. Patrono C, Dunn MJ. The clinical significance of inhibition of renal prostaglandin synthesis. *Kidney International* 1987; 32:42.

29. *The Medical Letter on Drugs and Therapeutics,* 1980, op. cit.

30. Olin, op. cit.

31. Shorr RI. Opioid analgesics and the risk of hip fracture in the elderly: codeine and propoxyphene. *Journal of Gerontology* 1992; 47:M111-5.

32. Wallace SL, Singer JZ, Duncan GJ, Wigley FM, Kuncl RW. Renal function predicts colchicine toxicity: guidelines for the prophylactic use of colchicine in gout. *Journal of Rheumatology* 1991; 18:264-9.

33. Miller RR, et al. Propoxyphene hydrochloride: a critical review. *Journal of the American Medical Association* 1972; 213:996.

34. Moertel CG, et al. A comparative evaluation of marketed analgesic drugs. *New England Journal of Medicine* 1972; 286:813.

35. Avorn JL, Lamy PP, Vestal RE. Prescribing for the elderly—safely. *Patient Care* 1982; 16:14-62.

36. Ibid.

37. Shorr, op. cit.

38. Murphy, op. cit.

39. Moulding, op. cit.

40. Orland, op. cit., p. 373.

41. Plotz, op. cit.

42. Ibid.

43. *USP DI,* 1992, op. cit

44. Murphy, op. cit.

45. Moulding, op. cit.

46. Shorr, op. cit.

47. Wolfe S. The safety of piroxicam. *The Lancet* 1986; 2:808-9.

48. Armstrong CP, Blower AL. Ulcerogenicity of piroxicam. *British Medical Journal* 1987; 294:772.

49. *USP DI,* 1992, op. cit.

50. *The Medical Letter on Drugs and Therapeutics,* 1980, op. cit., p. 29-31.

51. *Drugs for the Elderly,* op. cit.

52. Shorr, op. cit.

53. Fong NL. Chemotherapy and Nutritional Management. In *Nutritional Management of the Cancer Patient,* edited by Walford. New York: Raven Press, 1979.

54. Younger IR, Harris DWS, Colver GB. Azathioprine in dermatology. *Journal of the American Academy of Dermatology* 1991; 25:281-6.

55. Yudkin PL, Ellison GW, Ghezzi A, Goodkin DE, Hughes RAC, McPherson K, Mertin J, Milanese C. Overview of azathioprine treatment in multiple sclerosis. *The Lancet* 1991; 338:1051-5.

56. American Society of Hospital Pharmacists, op. cit., p. 2252-5.

57. Singh G, Fries JF, Williams CA, Zatarain E, Spitz P, Block DA. Toxicity profiles of disease modifying antirheumatic drugs in rheumatoid arthritis. *The Journal of Rheumatology* 1991; 18:188-94.

58. Callen JP, Spencer LV, Burruss JB, Holtman J. Azathioprine: an effective, corticosteroid-sparing therapy for patients with recalcitrant cutaneous lupus erythematosus or with recalcitrant cutaneous leukocytoclastic vasculitis. *Archives of Dermatology* 1991; 127:515-22.

59. Singh, op. cit.

60. Orland, op. cit, p. 373.

61. *Physicians' Desk Reference.* 40th ed. Oradell, N.J.: Medical Economics Company, 1986:1187.

62. *USP DI, Drug Information for the Health Care Provider.* 6th ed. Rockville Md.: The United States Pharmacopeial Convention, Inc., 1986:871.

63. Kastrup EK, ed. *Facts and Comparisons.* St. Louis: J.B. Lippincott Co., July 1987:732b.

64. *USP DI*, 1992, op. cit.

65. *The Medical Letter on Drugs and Therapeutics*, 1980, op. cit.

66. *USP DI*, 1992, op. cit.

67. Balfour JA, Buckley MMT. Etodolac a reappraisal of its pharmacology and therapeutic use in rheumatic diseases and pain states. *Drugs* 1991; 42(2):274-99.

68. Bem JL, Breckenridge AM, Mann RD, Rawlins MD. Review of yellow cards (1986): report to the Committee on the Safety of Medicines. *British Journal of Clinical Pharmacology* 1988; 26:679-89.

69. Hughes G. Therapeutic choices for rheumatic disorders. *Gerontology* 1988; 34 (Suppl. 1):27-32.

70. *The Medical Letter on Drugs and Therapeutics.*, 1991, op. cit., p. 79-80.

71. Olin, op. cit.

72. Taha AS, McLaughlin S, Sturrock RD, Russell RI. Evaluation of the efficacy and comparative effects on gastric and duodenal mucosa of etodolac and naproxen in patients with rheumatoid arthritis using endoscopy. *British Journal of Rheumatology* 1989; 28:329-32.

73. *USP DI*, 1992, op. cit.

74. Gilman, op. cit., p. 698-9.

75. Ibid.

76. *The Medical Letter on Drugs and Therapeutics*, 1980, op. cit.

77. AMA, 1983, op. cit., p. 123.

78. Olin, op. cit.

79. *USP DI*, 1992, op. cit.

80. Olin, op. cit.

81. *USP DI*, 1992, op. cit.

82. George Washington University. *Drug Information Bulletin*, January/February 1987; 12(1).

83. Kastrup, op. cit., p. 251a-c.

84. Ibid.

85. *The Medical Letter on Drugs and Therapeutics*, 1980, op. cit.

86. Olin, op. cit.

87. *USP DI*, 1992, op. cit.

88. *The Medical Letter on Drugs and Therapeutics*, 1980, op cit.

89. Olin, op. cit.

90. *USP DI*, 1992, op. cit.

91. Veys EM. 20 years' experience with ketoprofen. *Scandanavian Journal of Rheumatology* 1991; Suppl. 90:3-44.

92. Ibid.

93. Olin, op. cit.

94. Dukes MNG, Beeley L. *Side Effects of Drugs Annual* 15, Amsterdam: Elsevier, 1991:101.

95. *USP DI*, 1992, op. cit.

96. Neuvonen PJ. The effect of magnesium hydroxide on the oral absorption of ibuprofen, ketoprofen and diclofenac. *British Journal of Clinical Pharmacology* 1991; 31:263-6.

97. Murphy, op. cit.

98. Moulding, op. cit.

99. Orland, op. cit., p. 375

100. *Drugs for the Elderly*, op. cit.

101. Kastrup, op. cit., p. 251a-c.

102. *USP DI*, 1992, op. cit.

103. *The Medical Letter on Drugs and Therapeutics*, 1980, op. cit.

104. Olin, op. cit.

105. Orland, op. cit., p. 373.

106. *The Medical Letter on Drugs and Therapeutics*, 1976, op. cit., p. 73.

107. Orland, op. cit., p. 2.

108. 42 *Federal Register*, 35480, July 8, 1977.

109. Murphy, op. cit.

110. Moulding, op. cit.

111. Shorr, op. cit.

112. Murphy, op. cit.

113. Moulding, op. cit.

114. *USP DI*, 1992, op. cit.

115. AMA Department of Drugs. *AMA Drug Evaluations*. 8th ed. Chicago: American Medical Association, 1991:1706-7.

116. Helfgott SM, Sandberg-Cook J, Zakim D, Nestler J. Diclofenac-associated hepatotoxicity. *Journal of the American Medical Association* 1990; 264:2660-2.

117. *The Medical Letter on Drugs and Therapeutics*, 1980, op. cit.

118. El-Hadidi T, El-Garf A. Double-blind study comparing the use of Voltaren EmulgelR versus regular gel during ultrasonic sessions in the treatment of localized traumatic and rheumatic painful conditions. *The Journal of International Medical Research* 1991; 19:219-27.

119. Olin, op. cit.

120. Gay GR. Another side effect of NSAIDs. *Journal of the American Medical Association* 1990; 264:2677-8.

121. Stadler P, Armstrong D, Margalith D, Saraga E, Stolte M, Lualdi P, Mautone G, Blum AL. Diclofenac delays healing of gastroduodenal mucosal lesions. *Digestive Diseases and Sciences* 1991; 36:594-600.

122. Gay, op. cit.

123. Dukes MNG, Beeley L. *Side Effects of Drugs Annual 13*, Amsterdam: Elsevier, 1989:80.

124. *USP DI*, 1992, op. cit.

125. Heim M, Nadvorna H, Azaria M. Grand mal seizures following treatment with diclofenac and pentazocine. *South African Medical Journal* 1990; 78:700-1.

126. Salama A, Gottsche B, Mueller-Eckhardt C. Autoantibodies and drug- or metabolite-dependent antibodies in patients with diclofenac-induced immune haemolysis. *British Journal of Haematology* 1991; 77:546-9.

127. Dukes, 1989, op. cit, p. 74.

Gastrointestinal Drugs

Diarrhea

Diarrhea is a change in the frequency and consistency of bowel movements, characterized by abnormally frequent passage of loose or watery stools. Diarrhea is common in older people and can be associated with underlying disease, complications of therapy (see **Common Causes of Acute Simple Diarrhea** below) or can be infectious in origin, usually due to a virus in the intestinal tract. Acute or sudden simple diarrhea lasts only a few days and typically improves with or without medication.

When older adults get diarrhea, they have a greater risk than younger adults of complications from the loss of fluid, sodium and potassium chloride and other electrolytes.

According to a recent study by the federal Centers for Disease Control, there were 28,538 Americans who died during a 9-year period for whom diarrhea was listed as an immediate or underlying cause of death. A disproportionate fraction of these deaths (51%) were in people older than 74, with a diarrhea death rate 10 times that of the total population. People 55 to 74 made up an additional 27% of diarrheal deaths so that 78% of deaths caused by diarrhea were in people 55 or older[1] even though this group makes up only 21% of the population.

Despite the heavy promotion and frequent use of ineffective and/or dangerous prescription or over-the-counter drugs, the world standard for hydrating patients with diarrhea is oral rehydration therapy. Many of the deaths in older adults described above might have been prevented if the patients had been given oral rehydration solution (ORS) (see box below).

Common Causes of Acute Simple Diarrhea

Acute diarrhea is often caused by a viral infection in the intestinal tract, food poisoning, anxiety, or a reaction to medication, food, or alcohol. Some drugs that commonly cause diarrhea include the following:

❑ Antibiotics taken for infections
❑ Antacids containing magnesium, such as Maalox and Mylanta
❑ Dietary supplements with magnesium[2]
❑ Drugs for high blood pressure
❑ All laxatives except the bulk-forming variety (those that contain psyllium, for example)
❑ Drugs for irregular heartbeat, such as quinidine (Duraquin; Quinaglute Dura-Tabs)

See Chapter 2, p. 45, for a longer list of drugs that can cause diarrhea.

How to Treat Acute Simple Diarrhea

❑ Do not eat or drink milk and dairy products, fresh fruits and vegetables, coffee, spicy foods, and other food you do not tolerate well.
❑ Do not consume drinks with a high sugar content like grape or apple juice, soft drinks including cola, ginger ale and sports drinks or eat highly sweetened foods such as candy, ice cream or Jello because they have too much sugar which can make the diarrhea worse.[3]
❑ Drink plenty of Oral Rehydration Solution (ORS)—the formula for which is shown in the box below. Once you have noticed watery diarrhea in the toilet bowl, you are probably already a liter (slightly more than a quart) dehydrated. This means you should, over the next several hours after first noticing the watery diarrhea, try to catch up with the fluids you have already lost by drinking 3 to 4 eight ounce glasses. Once you have caught up — this will be apparent because you will be well enough hydrated to pass urine — you should drink at least 4 additional 8 ounce glasses of ORS

every 12 hours until the diarrhea stops. Patients on a fluid or salt restricted diet should consult their physicians concerning the use of ORS.
❏ Do not eat salty foods like salty soup, potato chips or peanuts.
❏ Do not take medication not prescribed or directed by your doctor or other health professional.
❏ Take your temperature once a day.

When to Seek Help from a Health Professional

Get assistance when:
❏ severe diarrhea occurs in an older adult, particularly one who is very weak.
❏ fever is above 101°F (38.3°C).
❏ there is evidence of blood in the stools or black, tarry stools.
❏ diarrhea persists for more than three days.
❏ you suspect that a drug taken under the

direction of a doctor may be the cause of the diarrhea.
❏ diarrhea is accompanied by severe, incapacitating abdominal pain.
❏ diarrhea results in a severe loss of water (dehydration) characterized by dizziness while standing, confusion, or unresponsiveness.

How to Make Oral Rehydration Solution[4]
To 1 liter (slightly more than a quart) of clean water add:
❏ one-half of a level teaspoon of *salt*
❏ 8 level teaspoons of *sugar* (Caution: Before adding the sugar, taste the drink and be sure it is less salty than tears.)
❏ If it is available, you can add a mashed ripe banana which also provides potassium.

Constipation

For a discussion of ways to avoid, and if necessary, treat constipation, see Psyllium (p. 356). Also see a list of drugs (p. 42) which can cause constipation.

LIMITED USE

Aluminum Hydroxide
AMPHOJEL (Wyeth) ALAGEL (Century)
ALTERNAGEL (Stuart)

Generic: available

Family: Antacids

Aluminum hydroxide (a *loo* mi num hye *drox* ide) is used to treat ulcers and stomach upset caused by stomach acid, and to prevent a certain type of kidney stones. Older adults with metabolic bone diseases should not take aluminum antacids,[5] and those with kidney disease should not use them for a long time.[6]

The aluminum in this drug can cause constipation. If you become constipated while using aluminum hydroxide, ask your doctor about switching to a product that contains both aluminum and magnesium hydroxide (see p. 355).

The liquid form of this drug is better than tablets because it is more effective and costs less. If you use tablets, chew them thoroughly. If you take large doses of this drug or take it for a long time, see your doctor for regular checkups. If you are treating yourself with this drug, do not take it for longer than 2 weeks unless you check with your doctor.

Before You Use This Drug
Tell your doctor if you have or have had
❑ allergies to drugs
❑ severe abdominal pain
❑ blood in stools
❑ constipation
❑ prolonged diarrhea
❑ hemorrhoids
❑ intestinal blockage
❑ kidney disease
❑ metabolic bone disease
Tell your doctor about any other drugs you take, including aspirin, herbs, vitamins, and other non-prescription products.

When You Use This Drug
◆ **Call your doctor immediately if you have black, tarry stools or you vomit material that looks like coffee grounds. These are signs of a bleeding ulcer.**
◆ If you are on a low-salt (low-sodium) diet, ask your doctor or pharmacist to help you choose an antacid. Many antacids contain sodium.

How To Use This Drug
◆ Take 1 to 3 hours after meals and at bedtime for maximum effectiveness. Drink plenty of fluids.
◆ Do not take any other drugs by mouth for at least 1 or 2 hours after taking aluminum hydroxide.
◆ Do not expose to heat, moisture, or strong light. Do not store in the bathroom. Do not let the liquid form freeze.
◆ If you miss a dose, take it as soon as you remember, but skip it if it is almost time for the next dose. **Do not take double doses.**

Interactions With Other Drugs
The following drugs are listed in *Evaluations of Drug Interactions*, 1991 as causing "highly clinically significant" or "clinically significant" interactions when used together with this drug. There may be other drugs, especially those in the families of drugs listed below, that also will react with this drug to cause severe adverse effects. Make sure to ask your doctor for a complete listing of them and let her or him know if you are taking any of these interacting drugs:

ACHROMYCIN; aspirin; cholecalciferol; CIPRO; ciprofloxacin; DELTA-D; digoxin; ECOTRIN; KAYEXALATE; LANOXIN; PANMYCIN; sodium polystyrene sulfonate; tetracycline; vitamin D$_3$.

Adverse Effects
Call your doctor immediately:
❑ severe constipation
❑ bone pain, swelling of wrists
❑ loss of appetite, weight loss
❑ muscle weakness

Call your doctor if these symptoms continue:
❑ nausea, vomiting
❑ specked or whitish stools
❑ stomach cramps

Periodic Tests
Ask your doctor which of these tests should be done periodically while you are taking this drug:
❑ blood calcium, phosphate, and potassium levels

LIMITED USE

Meclizine
ANTIVERT (Roerig)

Generic: available

Family: Antinausea Drugs
Antihistamines (see p. 383)

Meclizine (*mek* li zeen) is used to prevent motion sickness. **It is also used to treat vertigo (dizziness), but it has not been proven effective for this purpose.**[7]

> ### Warning: Special Mental and Physical Adverse Effects
> Older adults are especially sensitive to the harmful anticholinergic effects of meclizine. Drugs in this family should not be used unless absolutely necessary.
> *Mental Effects:* confusion, delirium, short-term memory problems, disorientation, and impaired attention.
> *Physical Effects:* dry mouth, constipation, difficulty urinating (especially for a man with an enlarged prostate), blurred vision, decreased sweating with increased body temperature, sexual dysfunction, and worsening of glaucoma.

If you are taking meclizine to prevent motion sickness, take it at least 1 hour before traveling. Do not take more than is recommended.

If you have asthma, glaucoma, an obstructed intestine, or an enlarged prostate gland, meclizine can make your symptoms worse.[8] If you take meclizine regularly for some time and you are also taking high doses of aspirin or other drugs in the salicylate family, the meclizine may hide signs of an aspirin or salicylate overdose.[9]

Before You Use This Drug
Tell your doctor if you have or have had
❑ allergies to drugs
❑ problems with urination
❑ glaucoma
❑ peptic ulcer or intestinal obstruction
❑ enlarged prostate
Tell your doctor about any other drugs you take, including aspirin, herbs, vitamins, and other non-prescription products.

When You Use This Drug
◆ Do not drink alcohol or use drugs that cause drowsiness.

◆ Until you know how you react to this drug, do not drive or perform other activities requiring alertness.

How To Use This Drug

◆ Take with food or milk to decrease stomach upset.
◆ Do not expose to heat, moisture, or strong light. Do not store in the bathroom. Do not let the liquid form freeze.
◆ If you miss a dose, take it as soon as you remember, but skip it if it is almost time for the next dose. **Do not take double doses.**

Interactions With Other Drugs

The following drug is listed in *Evaluations of Drug Interactions*, 1991 as causing "highly clinically significant" or "clinically significant" interactions when used together with this drug. There may be other drugs that also will react with this drug to cause severe adverse effects. Make sure to ask your doctor for a complete listing of them and let her or him know if you are taking this interacting drug:

alcohol.

Adverse Effects

Call your doctor if these symptoms continue:
❑ drowsiness
❑ blurred vision
❑ dry mouth, nose, or throat
❑ difficulty urinating

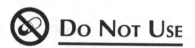 **Do Not Use**

Alternative treatment: For diarrhea, see Diarrhea, p. 332. For spastic colon, see Psyllium, p. 356.

Atropine

Family: Antispasmodics
Anticholinergics

Atropine (*a* tro peen) is used to relieve abdominal discomfort from cramping (spasms) and to control diarrhea. **It has such severe side effects that older adults should not use it.** Even if you are taking only the usual adult dose, you may suffer from excitement, restlessness, drowsiness, or confusion.[10] If you are taking atropine, ask your doctor to change your medication.

> **Warning: Special Mental and Physical Adverse Effects**
> Older adults are especially sensitive to the harmful anticholinergic effects of a family of drugs known as belladonna alkaloids. Atropine is in this family. Drugs in this family should not be used unless absolutely necessary.
> *Mental Effects*: confusion, delirium, short-term memory problems, disorientation, and impaired attention.
> *Physical Effects*: dry mouth, constipation, difficulty urinating (especially for a man with an enlarged prostate), blurred vision, decreased sweating with increased body temperature, sexual dysfunction, and worsening of glaucoma.

Nizatidine
AXID (Lilly)

Generic: not available

Family: Stomach Acid Blockers

Nizatidine (ni *zat* id dean) blocks release of stomach acid, especially at night. It is used to treat duodenal ulcers and gastric ulcers. Nizatidine can relieve symptoms such as ulcer pain and heartburn, and reduces or eliminates use of antacids. It is not for minor digestive complaints. Healing takes at least four weeks for duodenal ulcers, longer for gastric ulcers. Eight to twelve weeks is often recommended in the elderly.[11]

Nizatidine belongs to the same family as cimetidine (Tagamet), famotidine (Pepcid), and ranitidine (Zantac). At this time, nizatidine and famotidine have fewer reports of drug interactions, but their safety is otherwise similar to that of the other acid-blocking drugs and all are about equally effective.[12]

Long-term safety of nizatidine is still unknown.[13,14] Information about nizatidine's effect on heart rate in the elderly, and use with beta-blockers, or calcium channel blockers is limited.[15,16]

Ulcers often come back after a few months. So for frequent, severe recurrences, maintenance therapy is used. Confusion is a possible adverse effect, but this also occurs with other drugs in this family.[17] Elderly people are more apt to have reduced function of kidney and liver.[18,19] **If you have reduced kidney function, your doctor should start you on a low, or less frequent, dose.**

Cigarette smoking can delay healing of ulcers.[20] Some people find relief of reflux esophagitis by elevating the head of the bed. Liquid antacids of magnesium and aluminum in low doses are as effective at healing ulcers as stomach blockers, and less costly. However, long-term use of antacids has risks. Antacids with aluminum can cause bone damage, ones with magnesium can cause severe diarrhea. Too much calcium or sodium also can cause serious problems. If ulcer symptoms worsen or bleeding occurs medical help should be sought.

Before You Use This Drug
Tell your doctor if you have or have had
❑ allergies to drugs
❑ kidney or liver problems
Tell your doctor about any other drugs you take, including aspirin, herbs, vitamins, and other non-prescription products.

When You Use This Drug
◆ **Call your doctor immediately if you have black, tarry stools or if you vomit material that looks like coffee grounds. These are signs of a bleeding ulcer.**
◆ If you take an antacid take it at least 30 minutes apart from nizatidine. One source suggests taking stomach blockers 2 hours before antacids.[21]
◆ Do not drink alcohol or smoke.
◆ Avoid any food and drink that triggers your ulcer.
◆ Check with your doctor before taking any aspirin, ibuprofen or other NSAIDs. These drugs can cause or aggravate ulcers.

How To Use This Drug
◆ Swallow capsule whole. You may take with food, or mix contents of the capsule with 4 ounces of a compatible liquid, such as apple juice, cranberry juice, or Gatorade. Those mixtures can be referigerated up to 48 hours. If you use other liquids, do not store the mixture. Avoid vegetable juice or any liquid in which the powder does not dissolve.[22]

◆ Make sure that one of your doses is taken at bedtime.

◆ Take all the nizatidine your doctor prescribed even if you feel better.

◆ Do not expose to heat, moisture, or strong light. Do not store in the bathroom.

◆ If you miss a dose, take it as soon as you remember, but skip it if it is almost time for the next dose. **Do not take double doses.**

Interactions With Other Drugs

The following drugs are listed in *Evaluations of Drug Interactions*, 1991 as causing "highly clinically significant" or "clinically significant" interactions when used together with this drug. There may be other drugs, especially those in the families of drugs listed below, that also will react with this drug to cause severe adverse effects. Make sure to ask your doctor for a complete listing of them and let her or him know if you are taking any of these interacting drugs:

ANECTINE; BiCNU; bone marrow depressants; carbamazepine; clozapine; CLOZARIL; COUMADIN; DILANTIN; ELIXOPHYLLIN; imipramine; morphine; phenytoin;[23] succinylcholine;

TEGRETOL; THEO-DUR; theophylline; TOFRANIL; warfarin.[24]

Additionally, the *United States Pharmacopeia Drug Information*, 1992 lists this drug as having interactions of major significance:

ketoconazole; NIZORAL (if you must take this drug also, take your nizatidine 2 hours afterwards).

Adverse Effects

Call your doctor immediately:

❑ confusion

❑ hallucinations

❑ sore throat and fever

❑ slow, fast or irregular heartbeat

❑ skin rash or yellowing of skin or eyes

❑ difficulty breathing or speaking

Call your doctor if these symptoms continue:

❑ depression

❑ diarrhea

❑ drowsiness

❑ fatigue

❑ hair loss

❑ headache

❑ itching

❑ muscle cramps or pain

❑ nasal congestion[25]

❑ nausea

❑ increased sweating

Sulfasalazine
AZULFIDINE (Pharmacia)

Generic: available

Family: Gastrointestinal Drugs

Sulfasalazine (sul fa *sal* a zeen) is used to treat two diseases of the intestines: ulcerative colitis and Crohn's disease. The drug is usually taken for a long time. If your disease improves enough, you may be able to lower your dose to a maintenance level. If your condition continues to improve, you

may be able to stop using the drug for periods of time. Ask your doctor about this.

If you have impaired kidney function, you may need to take less than the usual adult dose.

Before You Use This Drug

Tell your doctor if you have or have had

❑ allergies to drugs

❑ an unusual reaction to sulfa drugs, furosemide, thiazide diuretics (water

pills), or diabetes or glaucoma drugs taken by mouth
- ❑ glucose-6-phosphate dehydrogenase deficiency
- ❑ kidney or liver disease
- ❑ porphyria
- ❑ stomach or intestinal blockage

Tell your doctor about any other drugs you take, including aspirin, herbs, vitamins, and other non-prescription products.

When You Use This Drug

- ◆ **Check with your doctor to make certain your fluid intake is adequate and appropriate.**
- ◆ Call your doctor if your symptoms (including diarrhea) do not improve in a month or so or if they get worse. Schedule regular visits to your doctor to check your progress.
- ◆ Your urine may turn orange-yellow in color. This is no cause for alarm.
- ◆ **Take all the sulfasalazine your doctor prescribed, even if you begin to feel better. If you stop too soon, your symptoms could come back.**
- ◆ Do not give this drug to anyone else. Throw away outdated drugs.
- ◆ **Caution diabetics:** see p. 516.
- ◆ Stay out of the sun as much as possible, and call your doctor if you get a rash, hives, or any other skin reaction. This drug makes you more sensitive to the sun.
- ◆ Ask your doctor about how to get more folic acid in your diet. You may need more folic acid than usual while taking sulfasalazine.
- ◆ If you plan to have any surgery, including dental, tell your doctor that you take this drug.

How To Use This Drug

- ◆ Take with **a full glass (8 ounces) of water** on an **empty stomach**, at least 1 hour before or 2 hours after meals. Shake liquid form before using. Swallow tablets whole.
- ◆ Do not store in the bathroom. Do not

expose to heat, moisture, or strong light. Do not let the liquid form freeze.
- ◆ If you miss a dose, take it as soon as you remember, but skip it if it is almost time for the next dose. **Do not take double doses.**

Interactions With Other Drugs

The following drugs are listed in *Evaluations of Drug Interactions,* 1991 as causing "highly clinically significant" or "clinically significant" interactions when used together with this drug. There may be other drugs, especially those in the families of drugs listed below, that also will react with this drug to cause severe adverse effects. Make sure to ask your doctor for a complete listing of them and let her or him know if you are taking any of these interacting drugs:

COUMADIN; digoxin; FOLEX; LANOXICAPS; LANOXIN; methotrexate; ORINASE; tolbutamide; warfarin.

Adverse Effects

Call your doctor immediately:
- ❑ itching or skin rash
- ❑ aching joints or muscles
- ❑ difficulty swallowing
- ❑ fever, pale skin, sore throat
- ❑ abnormal bleeding or bruising
- ❑ abnormal tiredness or weakness
- ❑ yellow eyes or skin

Call your doctor if these symptoms continue:
- ❑ diarrhea
- ❑ dizziness or headache
- ❑ loss of appetite
- ❑ nausea or vomiting

Periodic Tests

Ask your doctor which of these tests should be done periodically while you are taking this drug:
- ❑ complete blood counts
- ❑ proctoscopy, sigmoidoscopy
- ❑ urine tests
- ❑ liver and kidney function tests, if you take this drug for a long time

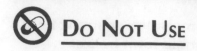 **DO NOT USE**

Alternative treatment: For diarrhea, see *Diarrhea,* p. 332. For spastic colon, see *Psyllium,* p. 356.

Dicyclomine
BENTYL (Lakeside/Merrell Dow)

Family: Antispasmodics
Anticholinergics

Dicyclomine (dye *sye* kloe meen) is used to relieve abdominal discomfort from cramping (spasms). **Although the effective and usual adult dose is 160 milligrams per day, older adults have an unacceptably high rate of side effects at this dose.** In addition to its anticholinergic effects (see box), dicyclomine may cause excitement or confusion.[26]

A respected drug reference book recommends that dicyclomine be discontinued if your condition does not improve after 2 weeks of treatment or if side effects force your doctor to lower your dose to below 80 milligrams per day. There are no documented data available on dicyclomine's safety at doses of 80 to 160 milligrams daily for periods longer than 2 weeks.[27]

We believe that older adults should not use dicyclomine because of the high rate of serious side effects. If you use it, ask your doctor to change your medication.

> ### Warning: Special Mental and Physical Adverse Effects
>
> Older adults are especially sensitive to the harmful anticholinergic effects of a family of drugs known as belladonna alkaloids. Dicyclomine is in this family. Drugs in this family should not be used unless absolutely necessary.
>
> *Mental Effects:* confusion, delirium, short-term memory problems, disorientation, and impaired attention.
>
> *Physical Effects:* dry mouth, constipation, difficulty urinating (especially for a man with an enlarged prostate), blurred vision, decreased sweating with increased body temperature, sexual dysfunction, and worsening of glaucoma.

Sucralfate
CARAFATE (Marion)

Generic: not available

Family: Antiulcer Drugs

Sucralfate (soo *kral* fate) is used to treat ulcers. After you take it, it forms a gummy substance that sticks to the part of your stomach where the ulcer is. This protects the ulcer from stomach acid and prevents further damage to the ulcer and the stomach lining.

You should not take sucralfate for minor digestive problems. Do not take sucralfate for more than 12 weeks unless your doctor tells you to.

Sucralfate can cause constipation.

Before You Use This Drug
Tell your doctor if you have or have had
❏ allergies to drugs
Tell your doctor about any other drugs you take, including aspirin, herbs, vitamins, and other non-prescription products.

When You Use This Drug
◆ **Call your doctor immediately if you have black, tarry stools or you vomit material that looks like coffee grounds. These are signs of a bleeding ulcer.**
◆ Take antacids for ulcer pain.

How To Use This Drug
◆ Do not chew tablets.
◆ Take on an empty stomach, at least 1 hour before or 2 hours after eating, and take a dose at bedtime.
◆ Do not expose to heat, moisture, or strong light. Do not store in the bathroom.

◆ If you miss a dose, take it as soon as you remember, but skip it if it is almost time for the next dose. **Do not take double doses.**

Interactions With Other Drugs
The following drugs are listed in *Evaluations of Drug Interactions,* 1991 as causing "highly clinically significant" or "clinically significant" interactions when used together with this drug. There may be other drugs, especially those in the families of drugs listed below, that also will react with this drug to cause severe adverse effects. Make sure to ask your doctor for a complete listing of them and let her or him know if you are taking any of these interacting drugs:

ACHROMYCIN; DILANTIN; norfloxacin; NOROXIN; phenytoin; tetracycline.

Adverse Effects
Call your doctor if these symptoms continue:
❏ constipation
❏ dizziness, lightheadedness
❏ backache
❏ drowsiness
❏ dry mouth
❏ indigestion, nausea
❏ stomach cramps or pain
❏ skin rash, hives, itching

Periodic Tests
Ask your doctor which of these tests should be done periodically while you are taking this drug:
❏ blood levels of phosphate

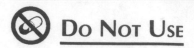 **DO NOT USE**

Alternative treatment: See Psyllium, p. 356.

Docusate
COLACE (Mead Johnson)
SURFAK (Hoechst-Roussel)

Family: Stool-softener Laxatives

Docusate (*dok* yoo sate) is a laxative that works by softening your stools. **You should not take it for simple constipation.** Docusate and other laxatives in its family can cause long-lasting damage to your intestine and can interfere with your body's use of nutrients. Docusate can also be dangerous if you are taking other drugs at the same time, since it can make your body absorb the other drugs at an increased rate. Since there are other laxatives that are safer than docusate, we do not recommend that you use it.

Many people take laxatives more often than they need to. This is dangerous for several reasons. First, some laxatives, such as docusate, can have harmful side effects. Second, all laxatives can be habit-forming. If you take them too often or for too long, your body will become less able to pass stools without them. This leads to a cycle of abuse in which you become dependent on laxatives and have to take them continuously. If you think you have become dependent on laxatives, talk to your doctor.

When do you really need to take a laxative? You should not take a laxative to "clean out your system" or to make your body act more "normally." Nor should you take a laxative just because you are having less than one bowel movement a day. It is untrue that everyone must have a bowel movement (stool) daily. Perfectly healthy people may have from two bowel movements per week to three bowel movements per day.

If the frequency of your bowel movements has decreased, if you are having bowel movements less than twice a week, or if you are having difficulty in passing stools, you are constipated, but this does not mean that you need a laxative. It is better to treat simple, occasional constipation without drugs, by eating a high-fiber diet that includes whole-grain breads and cereals, raw vegetables, raw and dried fruits, and beans, and by drinking plenty of nonalcoholic liquids (6 to 8 glasses per day). This type of diet will both prevent and treat constipation, and it is less costly than taking drugs. Regular exercise — at least 30 minutes per day of swimming, cycling, jogging, or brisk walking — will also help your body maintain regularity.

If you are constipated while traveling or at some other time when it is hard for you to eat properly, it may be appropriate to take a laxative for a short time. The only type of laxative you should use for self-medication is a bulk-forming laxative such as psyllium (see p. 356). This type usually takes effect in 12 hours to 3 days, compared with docusate which takes effect 1 or 2 days after the first dose, but may require 3 to 5 days of treatment. Even bulk-forming laxatives should only be used occasionally.

If you are on a special diet such as a low-salt or low-sugar diet, ask your doctor or pharmacist to help you choose a laxative without ingredients you are trying to avoid. Some laxatives contain sugar (up to half of the product), salt (up to 250 milligrams per dose), or the artificial sweetener NutraSweet®.

LIMITED USE

Prochlorperazine
COMPAZINE (Smith Kline & French)

Generic: available

Family: Antinausea Drugs
Antipsychotics (see p. 208)

Prochlorperazine (proe klor *pair* a zeen) is used to control nausea and vomiting, to treat serious mental illness (psychosis), and to manage behavior problems in mentally retarded people.

For severe nausea and vomiting, you should only be taking prochlorperazine if you have already tried making changes in your diet (see box below) and this has not worked. This drug has "questionable value" in treating psychosis[28] and has not been proven effective for managing behavior problems of mentally retarded people.

Prochlorperazine can cause serious side effects: drug-induced parkinsonism (see p. 212) and tardive dyskinesia (involuntary movements of parts of the body, which may last indefinitely). More information appears under Adverse Effects. **If you are over 60, you should generally be taking less than the usual adult dose.**

Before You Use This Drug
Tell your doctor if you have or have had
❑ allergies to drugs
❑ an unusual reaction to other antipsychotics (see p. 240 for examples)
❑ heart or blood vessel disease
❑ Parkinson's disease
❑ epilepsy, seizures
❑ enlarged prostate or difficulty urinating
❑ diabetes
❑ glaucoma
❑ liver disease
❑ bone marrow depression
❑ lung disease or breathing problems
❑ alcohol dependence

Warning: Special Mental and Physical Adverse Effects

Older adults are especially sensitive to the harmful anticholinergic effects of antipsychotic drugs such as prochlorperazine. Drugs in this family should not be used unless absolutely necessary.

Mental Effects: confusion, delirium, short-term memory problems, disorientation, and impaired attention.

Physical Effects: dry mouth, constipation, difficulty urinating (especially for a man with an enlarged prostate), blurred vision, decreased sweating with increased body temperature, sexual dysfunction, and worsening of glaucoma.

Drugs used to treat cancer often cause severe nausea and vomiting, either immediately after the drug is taken or several hours later. You can treat this kind of nausea and vomiting by changing your diet or by taking an anti-nausea drug. You should always try dietary changes first.[29]
❑ Eat small, frequent meals so your stomach is never empty.
❑ When you get up from sleeping or resting, eat some dry crackers or toast before you start being active.
❑ Drink carbonated drinks or other clear liquids such as soups and gelatin.
❑ Eat tart foods such as lemons and pickles.
❑ Do not eat foods with strong smells.

❑ breast cancer
❑ stomach ulcer
Tell your doctor about any other drugs you take, including aspirin, herbs, vitamins, and other non-prescription products.

When You Use This Drug

◆ **Do not stop taking this drug suddenly. Your doctor must give you a schedule to lower your dose gradually, to prevent withdrawal symptoms** such as nausea, vomiting, stomach upset, trembling, dizziness, and symptoms of Parkinson's disease.

It may take 2 or 3 weeks before you can tell that this drug is working.

Until you know how you react to this drug, do not drive or perform other activities requiring alertness. Prochlorperazine can cause blurred vision, drowsiness, and fainting.

Do not drink alcohol or use drugs that cause drowsiness.

You may feel dizzy when rising from a lying or sitting position. When getting out of bed, hang your legs over the side of the bed for a few minutes, then get up slowly. When getting up from a chair, stay by the chair until you are sure that you are not dizzy. (See p. 14.)

If you plan to have any surgery, including dental, tell your doctor that you take this drug.

How To Use This Drug

Take with food or **a full glass (8 ounces)** of milk or water to prevent stomach upset. Swallow extended-release capsules whole.

◆ If you take antacids or drugs for diarrhea, take them at least 2 hours apart from prochlorperazine.

◆ Do not store in the bathroom. Do not expose to heat, moisture, or strong light. Do not let the liquid form freeze.

◆ If you miss a dose, take it as soon as you remember, but skip it if it is almost time for the next dose. **Do not take double doses.**

Interactions With Other Drugs

The following drugs are listed in *Evaluations of Drug Interactions*, 1991 as causing "highly clinically significant" or "clinically significant" interactions when used together with this drug. There may be other drugs, especially those in the families of drugs listed below, that also will react with this drug to cause severe adverse effects. Make sure to ask your doctor for a complete listing of them and let her or him know if you are taking any of these interacting drugs:

AEROSPORIN; alcohol; amphetamines; ANECTINE; benztropine; bromocriptine; CAPOTEN; captopril; carbamazepine; COGENTIN; DEMEROL; desipramine; DEXEDRINE; diazoxide; ESKALITH; guanethidine; HYPERSTAT; INDERAL; ISMELIN; lithium; meperidine; NORPRAMIN; PARLODEL; PERTOFRANE; polymyxin B; propranolol; succinylcholine; TEGRETOL.

Adverse Effects

Call your doctor immediately:

❑ **if you experience signs of tardive dyskinesia:** lip smacking; chewing movements; puffing of cheeks; rapid, darting tongue movements; uncontrolled movements of arms or legs

❑ **if you experience signs of parkinsonism:** difficulty speaking or swallowing; loss of balance; mask-like face; muscle spasms; stiffness of arms or legs; trembling and shaking; unusual twisting movements of body

❑ change in vision, blurring

❑ difficulty urinating

❑ **if you experience signs of neuroleptic malignant syndrome:** troubled or fast breathing; fever; high or low blood pressure; increased sweating; loss of bladder control; muscle stiffness; seizures; unusual tiredness, weakness; fast heartbeat; irregular pulse; pale skin

❑ fever; sore mouth, gums, or throat

- ❏ abnormal bleeding or bruising
- ❏ nightmares
- ❏ fainting
- ❏ skin rash
- ❏ yellow eyes or skin

Call your doctor if these symptoms continue:
- ❏ constipation
- ❏ decreased sexual ability
- ❏ decreased sweating
- ❏ dizziness, lightheadedness
- ❏ drowsiness
- ❏ dry mouth
- ❏ increased skin sensitivity to sun
- ❏ nasal congestion

- ❏ swelling or pain in breasts
- ❏ milk from breasts

Periodic Tests
Ask your doctor which of these tests should be done periodically while you are taking this drug:
- ❏ blood cell counts
- ❏ glaucoma tests
- ❏ liver function tests
- ❏ urine tests for bile and bilirubin
- ❏ observation for early signs of tardive dyskinesia
- ❏ evaluation of continued need for prochlorperazine

LIMITED USE

Misoprostol
CYTOTEC (Searle)

Generic: not available

Family: Ulcer Drug

Misoprostol (mice o *prost* all) is used to prevent ulcers, specifically, gastric ulcers caused by aspirin, ibuprofen, and other nonsteroidal anti-inflammatory drugs (NSAIDs) commonly used to treat arthritis. NSAIDs can cause serious harm, even fatalities from bleeding in the stomach or intestines. Misoprostol is a synthetic prostaglandin drug which may protect the lining of the stomach and modestly decreases gastric acid.

People with high risk of ulcers from NSAIDs include the elderly, people with another debilitating disease, and those who had an ulcer previously. **Misoprostol should only be used by those who had an ulcer previously. However, arthritis in such people should be severe to warrant treatment with both an NSAID and misoprostol.** Healing of ulcers may be slower in people who smoke.

The elderly, the target group "at high risk from the complications of gastric ulcer," are also at high risk from the complications of misoprostol. Misoprostol has been shown to alter bone metabolism in animals, and to alter chemical markers of bone metabolism in humans. Though the drug is intended for life-long use by older people with arthritic conditions, a group known to be at risk for osteoporosis (thinning and weakening of the bones), little information has been gathered by its manufacturer on misoprostol's long-term effect on the human skeleton.

Diarrhea is a common adverse effect of misoprostol, ranging from minor to severe enough to be life-threatening.[30,31,32] In older people loss of fluids and minerals from diarrhea can in turn worsen blood pressure, or cause heart, kidney, and mental problems. Misoprostol predictably causes diarrhea in a significant number of patients who may tolerate it poorly. In clinical trials the incidence of loose stools ranged from 14 to 40%.

Since too many people receive NSAIDs for too long for no reason, approach taking one drug to treat the adverse effects of another drug with great caution. Many of these patients have conditions which can be treated with more conservative measures, or with generic acetaminophen (which does not induce stomach ulcers) for pain relief. Of patients chronically taking NSAIDs, 2 to 5% will develop a serious complication requiring hospitalization, but there is no evidence that misoprostol prevents the serious, life-threatening gastro-intestinal complications associated with NSAIDs.

Warning
Misoprostol is contraindicated, because of its abortifacient property, in women who are pregnant. Patients must be advised of the abortifacient property and warned not to give the drug to others.

Before deciding to take misoprostol along with an NSAID, ask your doctor why misoprostol was prescribed and how long you could expect to take it. Ask if a different arthritis drug with a lower incidence of side effects can be used. Also inquire if alternate therapy is possible.[33,34,35,36] If you develop a duodenal ulcer, instead of a gastric ulcer, one of the stomach blockers should be tried first.[37] Also, consider the expense, since the price of misoprostol in the United States usually exceeds the cost of the drug you are taking for arthritis.[38,39,40]

Before You Use This Drug
Do not take this drug if you have or have had[41]
❑ Crohn's disease
❑ inflammatory bowel disease
❑ ulcerative colitis
Tell your doctor if you have or have had
❑ allergies to drugs
❑ cerebral vascular disease
❑ coronary artery disease
❑ heart problems
❑ epilepsy
❑ kidney problems
❑ low blood pressure
❑ osteoporosis

When You Use This Drug
◆ Restrict your use of alcohol and cigarettes, which aggravate ulcers.
◆ Limit your intake of foods which you know bother your stomach, or cause diarrhea.
◆ Use antacids and laxatives which do not contain magnesium.
◆ Drink liquids to replace fluids lost by diarrhea.

How To Use This Drug
◆ Swallow tablets whole or break in half. Take with or after meals to lessen chance of diarrhea.
◆ If you miss a dose, take it as soon as you remember, but skip it if it is almost time for the next dose. **Do not take double doses.**
◆ Do not expose to heat, moisture, or strong light. Do not store in the bathroom.

Interactions With Other Drugs
Some other drugs that you may be taking (either over-the-counter or prescription drugs) can interact with this one, causing adverse effects. Find out from your doctor what these drugs are and let him or her know if you are taking any of them.

Adverse Effects
Call your doctor immediately:
❑ if you experience signs of overdose:[42] severe drowsiness; convulsions, muscle twitching; abdominal pain; fever; heartbeat slows or becomes more rapid; dizziness; shortness of breath
❑ severe diarrhea
Call your doctor if these symptoms continue:
❑ confusion[43]
❑ constipation or diarrhea

❑ cramps
❑ gas
❑ headache

❑ heartburn, indigestion
❑ nausea or vomiting
❑ urinary incontinence[44]

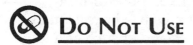 **DO NOT USE**

Alternative treatment: See Psyllium, p. 356.

Docusate and Casanthranol (combined)
DIALOSE PLUS (Stuart) PERI-COLACE (Mead Johnson)
Docusate and Danthron (combined)
DOXIDAN (Hoechst)*
MODANE PLUS (Adria)*

Family: Stool-softener Laxatives
Stimulant Laxatives

The combination of docusate (see p. 342) and casanthranol (ka *san* thra nole) and the combination of docusate and danthron (*dan* thron), are laxatives which combine two drugs, one that works by softening your stools and the other that works as a stimulant. All three of the ingredients in these two products can cause serious health problems. **You should not take these combinations to treat simple constipation.**

Danthron is a possible cancer-causing agent in humans. All danthron-containing products have been recalled in the United States. If you have such a product, take it back to your pharmacist for a refund.

Casanthranol is a stimulant laxative, a type that is not recommended to treat simple constipation. If you take this type of laxative for a long time, it gradually reduces your intestine's ability to work efficiently. This causes increasing constipation and a disease of the large intestine called cathartic colon, in which the intestine becomes enlarged and will not move without chemical stimulation. According to one

pharmacology textbook, "the medical importance of the stimulant laxatives stems more from their popularity and abuse than from their valid therapeutic applications."[45]

Docusate is a stool-softener laxative. This type of laxative can cause lasting damage to the intestine and can interfere with your body's absorption of nutrients. Docusate may also make your body absorb other drugs at an increased rate, so the combination of docusate with some other drugs may be dangerous.

Many people take laxatives more often than they need to. When do you really need them? You should not take a laxative to "clean out your system" or to make your body act more "normally." Nor should you take a laxative just because you are having less than one bowel movement a day. It is untrue that everyone must have a bowel movement (stool) daily. Perfectly healthy people may have from two bowel movements per week to three bowel movements per day.

If the frequency of your bowel movements has decreased, if you are having bowel movements less than twice a week, or if you are having difficulty in passing stools, you are constipated, but this does not mean that you need a laxative. It is better to treat simple, occasional

* Danthron-containing products are no longer available in the U.S. but may still be in people's medicine cabinets.

constipation without drugs, by eating a high-fiber diet that includes whole-grain breads and cereals, raw vegetables, raw and dried fruits, and beans, and by drinking plenty of nonalcoholic liquids (6 to 8 glasses per day). This type of diet will both prevent and treat constipation, and it is less costly than taking drugs. Regular exercise — at least 30 minutes per day of swimming, cycling, jogging, or brisk walking — will also help your body maintain regularity.

If you are constipated while traveling or at some other time when it is hard for you to eat properly, it may be appropriate to take a laxative for a short time. The only type of laxative you should use for self-medication is a bulk-forming laxative such as psyllium (see p. 356). This type usually takes effect in 12 hours to 3 days, compared with docusate which takes effect 1 or 2 days after the first dose, but may require 3 to 5 days. Even bulk-forming laxatives should only be used occasionally.

If you are on a special diet such as a low-salt or low-sugar diet, ask your doctor or pharmacist to help you choose a laxative without ingredients you are trying to avoid. Some laxatives contain sugar (up to half of the product), salt (up to 250 milligrams per dose), or the artificial sweetener NutraSweet®.

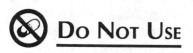 **DO NOT USE**

Alternative treatment: For spastic colon, see Psyllium, p. 356.

Atropine, Hyoscyamine, Scopolamine, and Phenobarbital (combined)
DONNATAL (Robins)

Family: Antispasmodics
Anticholinergics
Barbiturates

This combination of atropine (see p. 336), hyoscyamine (hye oh *sye* a meen), scopolamine (skoe *pol* a meen), and phenobarbital (see p. 544) is used to relieve abdominal discomfort from cramps (spasms) and to reduce the amount of acid produced in the stomach. **It is an irrational mixture of drugs[46] that is dangerous for older adults to use.**

Atropine, hyoscyamine, and scopolamine, three of the four ingredients in this combination, have severe side effects that make them too dangerous for older adults to use (see below). Even if you are taking only the usual adult dose, you may suffer from excitement, restlessness, drowsiness, or confusion.[47]

> *Warning: Special Mental and Physical Adverse Effects*
>
> Older adults are especially sensitive to the harmful anticholinergic effects of a family of drugs called belladonna alkaloids. Atropine, hyoscyamine and scopolamine are all in this family. Drugs in this family should not be used unless absolutely necessary.
>
> *Mental Effects*: confusion, delirium, short-term memory problems, disorientation, and impaired attention.
>
> *Physical Effects*: dry mouth, constipation, difficulty urinating (especially for a man with an enlarged prostate), blurred vision, decreased sweating with increased body temperature, sexual dysfunction, and worsening of glaucoma.

Phenobarbital, the fourth drug in this combination, causes problems so serious that the World Health Organization has said older adults should not use it.[48] Epilepsy is the only reason to take this drug. You can easily become addicted to phenobarbital. If you stop taking this drug suddenly, you will probably suffer withdrawal symptoms such as anxiety, restlessness, muscle twitching, trembling hands, weakness, dizziness, vision problems, nausea, vomiting, trouble sleeping, faintness, and lightheadedness. Later, you will suffer more serious symptoms such as convulsions, seizures, and hallucinations.

These may last for more than 2 weeks after you stop taking phenobarbital.

One hazard of taking Donnatal continuously for longer than several weeks is addiction. **Do not stop taking your drug suddenly.** With the help of your doctor, work out a schedule for slowly lowering the amount of the drug you take by about 5 to 10% each day. Keep a written record of the dosage reduction schedule with you. These steps will make it much easier to become drug free without developing distressing symptoms of drug withdrawal.

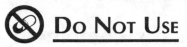 **Do Not Use**

Alternative treatment: See Psyllium, p. 356.

Bisacodyl
DULCOLAX (Boehringer Ingelheim)

Family: Stimulant Laxatives

Bisacodyl (bis a *koe* dill) is a stimulant laxative. **We do not recommend taking it to treat constipation.** If you take stimulant laxatives for a long time, they gradually reduce your intestine's ability to work efficiently. This causes increasing constipation and a disease of the large intestine called cathartic colon, in which the intestine becomes enlarged and will not move without chemical stimulation. According to one pharmacology textbook, "the medical importance of the stimulant laxatives stems more from their popularity and abuse than from their valid therapeutic applications."[49]

Many people take laxatives more often than they need to. This is dangerous for several reasons. First, some laxatives, such as bisacodyl, can have harmful side effects. Second, all laxatives can be habit-forming. If you take them too often or for too long, your body will become less able to pass

stools without them. This leads to a cycle of abuse in which you become dependent on laxatives and have to take them continuously. If you think you have become dependent on laxatives, talk to your doctor.

When do you need a laxative? You should not take a laxative to "clean out your system" or to make your body act more "normally." Nor should you take a laxative just because you are having less than one bowel movement a day. It is untrue that everyone must have a bowel movement (stool) daily. Perfectly healthy people may have from two bowel movements per week to three bowel movements per day.

If the frequency of your bowel movements has decreased, if you are having bowel movements less than twice a week, or if you are having difficulty in passing stools, you are constipated, but this does not mean that you need a laxative. It is better to treat simple, occasional constipation without drugs, by eating a high-fiber diet that includes whole-grain breads and cereals, raw vegetables, raw and dried fruits, and beans, and by drinking plenty of nonalcoholic liquids (6 to 8 glasses per day). This type of diet will both prevent and treat constipation, and it is less costly than taking drugs. Regular exercise — at least 30 minutes per day of swimming, cycling, jogging, or brisk walking — will also help your body maintain regularity.

If you are constipated while traveling or at some other time when it is hard for you to eat properly, it may be appropriate to take a laxative for a short time. The only type of laxative you should use for self-medication is a bulk-forming laxative such as psyllium (see p. 356). This type usually takes effect in 12 hours to 3 days, compared with docusate which takes effect 1 or 2 days after the first dose, but may require 3 to 5 days of treatment. Even bulk-forming laxatives should only be used occasionally.

If you are on a special diet such as a low-salt or low-sugar diet, ask your doctor or pharmacist to help you choose a laxative without ingredients you are trying to avoid. Some laxatives contain sugar (up to half of the product), salt (up to 250 milligrams per dose), or the artificial sweetener NutraSweet®.

Aluminum Hydroxide and Magnesium Trisilicate (combined) GAVISCON, GAVISCON-2 (Marion)

Generic: not available

Family: Reflux Esophagitis Drugs

This combination of aluminum hydroxide (see p. 334) and magnesium trisilicate (mag *nee* zee um tri *sill* i kate) is used to temporarily relieve heartburn caused by reflux esophagitis. In reflux esophagitis, acidic stomach contents flow backwards up into the esophagus (tube leading from the mouth to the stomach), causing a burning sensation under the breastbone.

You should not be taking Gaviscon and Gaviscon-2, two brand-name products which contain this combination of drugs, for ulcers or serious stomach upset due to stomach acid. They do not contain enough aluminum hydroxide and magnesium trisilicate to neutralize stomach acid. Instead, you should be taking a combination of aluminum hydroxide and magnesium hydroxide (see p. 355).

By combining aluminum with magnesium, this product reduces the problems that either substance alone can cause. Aluminum can cause constipation, and magnesium can cause diarrhea, but when the two are combined in one product, these effects are often balanced out. However, the combination may still cause either constipation or diarrhea.

Take each dose with **a full glass (8 ounces) of water.** The liquid form is better than tablets because it is more effective and costs less. If you use tablets, chew them thoroughly. If you take large doses of this drug or use it for a long time, see your doctor for regular checkups. If you are treating yourself with this drug, do not take it for more than 2 weeks unless you check with your doctor.

Older adults with metabolic bone diseases should not take aluminum antacids,[50] and those with kidney disease should not use them for a long time.[51] Taking magnesium trisilicate for a long time or in large doses may cause kidney stones.[52] Anyone with severe kidney disease should not use magnesium antacids.[53]

Before You Use This Drug

Do not use if you have or have had
❏ severely reduced kidney function
❏ metabolic bone disease
Tell your doctor if you have or have had
❏ allergies to drugs
❏ constipation
Tell your doctor about any other drugs you take, including aspirin, herbs, vitamins, and other non-prescription products.

When You Use This Drug

◆ Call your doctor immediately if you have black, tarry stools or you vomit material that looks like coffee grounds. These are signs of a bleeding ulcer.

How To Use This Drug

◆ Take immediately after meals and at bedtime for maximum effectiveness. Drink plenty of fluids.
◆ Do not take any other drugs by mouth for at least 1 or 2 hours after taking this drug.
◆ Do not expose to heat, moisture, or strong light. Do not store in the bathroom. Do not let the liquid form freeze.
◆ If you miss a dose, take it as soon as you remember, but skip it if it is almost time for the next dose. **Do not take double doses.**

Interactions With Other Drugs

The following drugs are listed in *Evaluations of Drug Interactions,* 1991 as causing "highly clinically significant" or "clinically significant" interactions when used together with this drug. There may be other drugs, especially those in the families of drugs listed below, that also will react with this drug to cause severe adverse effects. Make sure to ask your doctor for a complete listing of them and let her or him know if you are taking any of these interacting drugs:

ACHROMYCIN; aspirin; cholecalciferol; CIPRO; ciprofloxacin; DELTA-D; digoxin; ECOTRIN; KAYEXALATE; LANOXIN; sodium polystyrene sulfonate; tetracycline; vitamin D_3.

Adverse Effects

Call your doctor immediately:
❏ difficult or painful urination
❏ irregular heartbeat
❏ mood or mental changes
❏ unusual tiredness or weakness
❏ severe constipation
❏ swelling of feet or lower legs
❏ bone pain, swelling of wrists
❏ loss of appetite, weight loss
❏ muscle weakness
Call your doctor if these symptoms continue:
❏ nausea or vomiting
❏ specked or whitish stools
❏ stomach cramps
❏ diarrhea or laxative effect

Periodic Tests

Ask your doctor which of these tests should be done periodically while you are taking this drug:
❏ blood calcium, phosphate, and potassium levels
❏ kidney function tests

LIMITED USE

Alternative treatment: See Diarrhea, p. 332.

Loperamide
IMODIUM (Janssen)

Generic: available

Family: Antispasmodics
Anticholinergics

Loperamide (loe *per* a mide) is used to treat severe diarrhea. When older adults get diarrhea, they have a greater risk than younger people of complications from the loss of fluid, sodium and potassium chloride, and other electrolytes.[54] If you occasionally get short-term diarrhea, you can probably control it without using drugs (see p. 332). If non-drug treatments do not control your diarrhea, ask your doctor if loperamide is appropriate for you. The first-choice treatment for acute diarrhea is oral rehydration solution (ORS) (see p. 332).

If you use loperamide, do not take more than four 2-milligram capsules of loperamide per day (total of 8 milligrams).[55] An overdose can depress your breathing severely and can cause coma, permanent brain damage, and sometimes death.

If you still have diarrhea after using loperamide for 2 days, or if you develop a fever, stop taking the drug and call your doctor.[56]

Warning: Special Mental and Physical Adverse Effects

Older adults are especially sensitive to the harmful anticholinergic effects of loperamide. Drugs in this family should not be used unless absolutely necessary.

Mental Effects: confusion, delirium, short-term memory problems, disorientation, and impaired attention.

Physical Effects: dry mouth, constipation, difficulty urinating (especially for a man with an enlarged prostate), blurred vision, decreased sweating with increased body temperature, sexual dysfunction, and worsening of glaucoma.

Before You Use This Drug
Do not use if you have or have had
❑ severe inflammation of the colon
❑ diarrhea caused by antibiotics
Tell your doctor if you have or have had
❑ allergies to drugs
❑ a condition in which constipation must be avoided
❑ dehydration
❑ infectious diarrhea
❑ liver problems
Tell your doctor about any other drugs you take, including aspirin, herbs, vitamins, and other non-prescription products.

When You Use This Drug
◆ **Call your doctor immediately if diarrhea continues past 2 days or if you get a fever.**
◆ To prevent severe constipation, stop taking this drug once your diarrhea stops.
◆ Until you know how you react to this drug, do not drive or perform other activities requiring alertness. Loperamide may cause drowsiness.
◆ Have regular checkups if you use loperamide for a long time.

How To Use This Drug
◆ Do not take more than prescribed.
◆ Do not expose to heat or direct light. Do not store in the bathroom. Do not let the liquid form freeze.
◆ If you miss a dose, take it as soon as you remember, but skip it if it is almost

time for the next dose. **Do not take double doses.**

Interactions With Other Drugs

Some other drugs that you may be taking (either over-the-counter or prescription drugs) can interact with this one, causing adverse effects. Find out from your doctor what these drugs are and let him or her know if you are taking any of them.

Adverse Effects

Call your doctor if these symptoms continue:
- ❑ constipation
- ❑ skin rash
- ❑ dry mouth
- ❑ loss of appetite
- ❑ stomach pain
- ❑ drowsiness
- ❑ nausea or vomiting
- ❑ unexplained fever
- ❑ bloated feeling

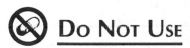 **Do Not Use**

Alternative treatment: For spastic colon, see Psyllium, p. 356.

Chlordiazepoxide and Clidinium (combined)
LIBRAX (Roche)

Family: Ulcer and Irritable Bowel Drugs

This combination of chlordiazepoxide (see p. 246) and clidinium (kli *di* nee um) is used to treat ulcers and colitis. It is said to relieve the abdominal discomfort from cramping (spasms), reduce the amount of stomach acid, and relax the digestive system. **However, it is an *irrational* and ineffective mixture of drugs**[57] which older adults should not use.

One of the ingredients in this combina-

tion, chlordiazepoxide, is a tranquilizer. **Because of this ingredient, this product is *addictive*.** Chlordiazepoxide (sold by itself as Librium) belongs to a family of drugs called benzodiazepines (see p. 198) that can cause confusion, muscle incoordination leading to falls and hip fractures, and drowsiness in older adults. We believe that

> *Warning: Special Mental and Physical Adverse Effects*
> Older adults are especially sensitive to the harmful anticholinergic effects of drugs such as clidinium. Drugs in this family should not be used unless absolutely necessary.
> *Mental Effects*: confusion, delirium, short-term memory problems, disorientation, and impaired attention.
> *Physical Effects*: dry mouth, constipation, difficulty urinating (especially for a man with an enlarged prostate), blurred vision, decreased sweating with increased body temperature, sexual dysfunction, and worsening of glaucoma.

> One hazard of taking chlordiazepoxide continuously for longer than several weeks is addiction. **Do not stop taking your drug suddenly.** With the help of your doctor, work out a schedule for slowly lowering the amount of the drug you take by about 5 to 10% each day. Keep a written record of the dosage reduction schedule with you. These steps will make it much easier to become drug free without developing distressing symptoms of drug withdrawal.

people 60 years of age and older should not use chlordiazepoxide. Other drugs in the benzodiazepine family are sometimes appropriate to treat anxiety or sleeping problems on a *short-term* basis, but because they are addictive, they should be used only as a last resort. They should not be used to treat digestive problems.

Clidinium has such severe side effects that older adults should not use it (see warning box). Even if you are taking only the usual adult dose, you may suffer excitement, restlessness, drowsiness, or confusion.[58] Clidinium can also reduce the amount of saliva. Since saliva fights bacteria in the mouth, a decrease in the amount of saliva leads to erosion of the gums and teeth, and later to dental or denture problems like tooth decay.

If you are taking this combination of chlordiazepoxide and clidinium, ask your doctor to prescribe another drug. If you have used the drug continuously for several weeks or longer, ask for a schedule that lowers your dose gradually.

The Food and Drug Administration concluded that this drug lacks evidence of effectiveness.

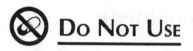 **Do Not Use**

Alternative treatment: See Diarrhea—treating without drugs, p. 332.

Diphenoxylate and Atropine (combined)
LOMOTIL (Searle)

Family: Antidiarrheals (see p. 332)

This combination of diphenoxylate (dye fen *ox* i late) and atropine (see p. 336) is used to treat severe diarrhea. Because of serious side effects, we recommend that older adults not use this product.

If you occasionally have short-term diarrhea, it is best to treat it without drugs using oral rehydration solution (ORS) (see p. 332). If nondrug treatments do not control your diarrhea, see your doctor. This combination of diphenoxylate and atropine should never be used to self-treat diarrhea. If you are using it, talk to your doctor about changing to a different drug.

Diphenoxylate can depress your breathing, causing severe shortness of breath or troubled breathing.[59] An overdose can cause severe respiratory depression and coma, possibly leading to permanent brain damage or death.[60]

Warning: Special Mental and Physical Adverse Effects

Older adults are especially sensitive to the harmful anticholinergic effects of a family of drugs called belladonna alkaloids. Atropine is in this family. Drugs in this family should not be used unless absolutely necessary.

Mental Effects: confusion, delirium, short-term memory problems, disorientation, and impaired attention.

Physical Effects: dry mouth, constipation, difficulty urinating (especially for a man with an enlarged prostate), blurred vision, decreased sweating with increased body temperature, sexual dysfunction, and worsening of glaucoma.

Aluminum Hydroxide and Magnesium Hydroxide (combined)
MAALOX, MAALOX TC (Rorer)
Magaldrate
RIOPAN (Ayerst)

Generic: available

Family: Antacids

The mixture of aluminum hydroxide (see p. 334) and magnesium hydroxide (see p. 363) neutralizes stomach acid and is used to treat ulcers and stomach upset caused by stomach acid. Magaldrate (*mag* al drate), a chemical combination of aluminum hydroxide and magnesium hydroxide, is used in the same way.

By combining aluminum with magnesium, these drugs reduce the problems that either substance alone can cause. Aluminum can cause constipation, and magnesium can cause diarrhea, but when the two are combined in one product, these effects are often balanced out. However, the combination may still cause either constipation or diarrhea.

Take each dose with **a full glass (8 ounces) of water.** The liquid form is better than tablets because it is more effective and costs less. If you use tablets, chew them thoroughly. If you take large doses of one of these drugs or use it for a long time, see your doctor for regular checkups. If you are treating yourself with this drug, do not take it for more than 2 weeks unless you check with your doctor.

Older adults with metabolic bone diseases should not take antacids that contain aluminum,[61] and those with kidney disease should not use them for a long time.[62] Anyone with severe kidney disease should not use magnesium antacids.[63]

Before You Use This Drug
Do not use if you have or have had
❑ severely reduced kidney function
❑ metabolic bone disease

Tell your doctor if you have or have had
❑ allergies to drugs
❑ severe abdominal pain
❑ blood in stools
❑ inflammation of the colon (colitis)
❑ diverticulitis
❑ prolonged diarrhea
❑ severe or prolonged constipation
❑ intestinal blockage
❑ kidney disease
Tell your doctor about any other drugs you take, including aspirin, herbs, vitamins, and other non-prescription products.

When You Use This Drug
◆ **Call your doctor immediately if you have black, tarry stools or you vomit material that looks like coffee grounds. These are signs of a bleeding ulcer.**
◆ If you are on a low-salt (low-sodium) or low-phosphate diet, ask your doctor or pharmacist to help you choose an antacid. Many brands contain one of these substances.

How To Use This Drug
◆ Take 1 to 3 hours after meals and at bedtime for maximum effectiveness. Drink plenty of fluids.
◆ Do not take any other drugs by mouth for at least 1 to 2 hours after taking this drug.
◆ Do not expose to heat, moisture, or strong light. Do not store in the bathroom. Do not let liquid form freeze.
◆ If you miss a dose, take it as soon as you remember, but skip it if it is almost time for the next dose. **Do not take double doses.**

Interactions With Other Drugs
The following drugs are listed in *Evaluations of Drug Interactions,* 1991 as causing

"highly clinically significant" or "clinically significant" interactions when used together with this drug. There may be other drugs, especially those in the families of drugs listed below, that also will react with this drug to cause severe adverse effects. Make sure to ask your doctor for a complete listing of them and let her or him know if you are taking any of these interacting drugs:

ACHROMYCIN; aspirin; cholecalciferol; CIPRO; ciprofloxacin; DELTA-D; digoxin; ECOTRIN; KAYEXALATE; LANOXIN; sodium polystyrene sulfonate; tetracycline; vitamin D$_3$.

Adverse Effects
Call your doctor if these symptoms continue:
❏ nausea or vomiting
❏ stomach cramps
❏ diarrhea or laxative effect

Periodic Tests
Ask your doctor which of these tests should be done periodically while you are taking this drug:
❏ blood calcium, phosphate, and potassium levels
❏ kidney function tests

Psyllium
METAMUCIL (Searle)
PERDIEM (Rorer)

Generic: available

Family: Bulk-forming Laxatives
Cholesterol-lowering Drugs (see p. 70)

Psyllium (*sill* i yum) is a laxative that works by absorbing water and softening the stools in your intestine. Fiber that you get from food works exactly the same way. **Since a diet high in fiber, combined with plenty of nonalcoholic liquids, has the same effect as psyllium, this drug is usually not necessary.** Eating high-fiber foods is preferable to taking psyllium because these foods give you essential nutrients in addition to fiber.

When do you really need to take a laxative? You should not take a laxative to "clean out your system" or to make your body act more "normally." Nor should you take a laxative just because you are having less than one bowel movement a day. It is untrue that everyone must have a bowel

movement (stool) daily. Perfectly healthy people may have from two bowel movements per week to three bowel movements per day.

If the frequency of your bowel movements has decreased, if you are having bowel movements less than twice a week, or if you are having difficulty in passing stools, you are constipated, but this does not mean that you need a laxative. It is better to treat simple, occasional constipation by eating a high-fiber diet — one that includes whole-grain breads and cereals, raw vegetables, raw and dried fruits, and beans — and by drinking plenty of nonalcoholic liquids (6 to 8 glasses per day). This type of diet will both prevent and treat constipation, and it is less costly than taking drugs. Regular exercise — at least 30 minutes per day of swimming, cycling, jogging, or brisk walking — will also help your body maintain regularity.

If you are constipated while you are traveling or at some other time when it is difficult for you to eat properly, using psyllium may be appropriate. Psyllium usually takes effect in 12 hours to 3 days.

If you are on a special diet such as a low-salt or low-sugar diet, ask your doctor or pharmacist to help you choose a laxative that does not contain ingredients you are trying to avoid. Some psyllium products contain sugar (up to half of the product) or salt (up to 250 milligrams per dose).

Before You Use This Drug

Tell your doctor if you have or have had
❏ allergies to drugs
❏ severe abdominal pain
❏ rectal bleeding
❏ impacted bowel movement
❏ occupational exposure to psyllium
❏ obstruction of the intestine
❏ problems with swallowing
Tell your doctor about any other drugs you take, including aspirin, herbs, vitamins, and other non-prescription products.

When You Use This Drug

◆ Check with your doctor to make certain your fluid intake is adequate and appropriate. If you do not get enough fluids, the laxative will not work properly and may dry and harden, clogging the intestine.
◆ Do not use for more than 1 week. If you have used psyllium for a week, stop taking it to see if a high-fiber diet and liquids alone will work. If your constipation continues for longer than a week, call your doctor.

How To Use This Drug

◆ Take each dose with a full glass of water or juice.
◆ If you take any other drugs, take them at least 2 hours before or after the time you take psyllium.
◆ Do not expose to heat, moisture, or strong light. Do not store in the bathroom.

Interactions With Other Drugs

Some other drugs that you may be taking (either over-the-counter or prescription drugs) can interact with this one, causing adverse effects. Find out from your doctor what these drugs are and let him or her know if you are taking any of them.

Adverse Effects

Call your doctor immediately:
❏ trouble swallowing
❏ intestinal obstruction (cramping, bloating, nausea)

Periodic Tests

Ask your doctor which of these tests should be done periodically while you are taking this drug:
❏ blood glucose and potassium levels, if used for a long time

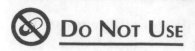 **DO NOT USE**

Alternative treatment: See Aluminum Hydroxide and Magnesium Hydroxide, p. 355.

Magnesium Hydroxide, Aluminum Hydroxide, and Simethicone (combined)
MYLANTA, MYLANTA-II (Stuart)

Family: Antiflatulents (Anti-gas)
Antacids

This combination of magnesium hydroxide (see p. 363), aluminum hydroxide (see p. 334), and simethicone (see p. 359) is used both as an antacid and as an antiflatulent (anti-gas) drug. As an antacid, it is used to treat ulcers and serious stomach upset caused by stomach acid and to relieve heartburn. As an antiflatulent, it is used to relieve "excess gas."

We do not recommend this widely used drug because it contains an ineffective and unnecessary ingredient, simethicone. There is no convincing evidence that simethicone, alone or in combination with other drugs, is effective in treating so-called excess gas.[64] Since this drug has no benefit, there is no reason to take it. If you need an antacid, use a combination of magnesium hydroxide and aluminum hydroxide (see p. 355). **Do not waste your money on products that contain simethicone.**

If you think that you suffer from "excess gas," it may be that you actually have a bloated feeling from overeating or discomfort from eating the wrong food. In this case, no anti-gas drug will help you because the problem has nothing to do with gas. If you do have excess gas in your stomach, the best way to treat it is to reduce the amount of air that you swallow. You can do this by cutting down on smoking, carbonated drinks, and gum-chewing, which make you swallow air. A dry mouth (which may be due to anxiety or a drug you are taking) and badly fitting dentures also make you swallow more air, so correcting these problems will help.

Most gas in the large intestine is created when bacteria come into contact with carbohydrates, especially those found in cabbage, broccoli, and beans.[65] This bacterial action is normal, as is the passing of gas (flatus). Different people pass different amounts of gas, and passing gas is no cause for medical concern.

Older adults with metabolic bone disease should not take antacids that contain aluminum,[66] and those with kidney disease should not use them for a long time.[67] Anyone with severe kidney disease should not use magnesium antacids.[68]

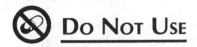 **DO NOT USE**

Alternative treatment: Reduce the causes of "excess gas" (see below).

Simethicone
MYLICON (Stuart)
PHAZYME (Reed & Carnrick)

Family: Antiflatulents (Anti-gas)

Simethicone (si *meth* i kone) is marketed as a drug to reduce the amount of "excess gas" and the discomfort that it causes. **There is no convincing evidence that this drug, alone or combined with others, is effective for this purpose.[69] Do not waste your money on products containing simethicone that claim to relieve "excess gas."**

If you think that you suffer from "excess gas," it may be that you actually have a bloated feeling from overeating or discomfort from eating the wrong food. In this case, no anti-gas drug will help you because the problem has nothing to do with gas. If you do have excess gas in your stomach, the best way to treat it is to reduce the amount of air that you swallow. You can do this by cutting down on smoking, carbonated drinks, and gum-chewing, which make you swallow air. A dry mouth (which may be due to anxiety or a drug you are taking) and badly fitting dentures also make you swallow more air, so correcting these problems will help.

Most gas in the large intestine is created when bacteria come into contact with carbohydrates, especially those found in cabbage, broccoli, and beans.[70] This bacterial action is normal, as is the passing of gas (flatus). Different people pass different amounts of gas, and passing gas is no cause for medical concern.

Famotidine
PEPCID (Merck)

Generic: not available

Family: Stomach Acid Blockers

Famotidine (fam *oat* id ine) blocks release of stomach acid. It is used to treat duodenal ulcers, gastric ulcers, and esophageal acid reflux. Famotidine can relieve symptoms of heartburn, and ulcer pain. It is not for minor digestive complaints. Over four weeks, famotidine can heal ulcers, and prevent the need for surgery. Famotidine belongs to the same family as cimetidine (Tagamet), ranitidine (Zantac) and nizatidine (Axid). At this time, nizatidine and famotidine have fewer reports of drug interactions, but their safety is otherwise similar to that of the other acid-blocking drugs and all are about equally effective.[71]

Ulcers often come back after a few months. So for frequent, severe recurrences, maintenance therapy is used. But long-term safety of famotidine is still unknown.[72] Confusion is a possible adverse effect, but this also occurs with other drugs in this family.[73] Elderly people are more apt to have reduced function of kidney and liver.[74,75] **If you have reduced kidney function, your doctor should start you on a low, or less frequent, dose.**

Cigarette smoking can delay healing.[76] Liquid antacids of magnesium and aluminum in low doses are as effective at healing ulcers as stomach blockers, and less costly.[77,78,79] However, long-term use of antacids has risks. Antacids with aluminum can cause bone damage, ones with magnesium can cause severe diarrhea. Too much calcium or sodium also cause serious problems. If ulcer symptoms worsen or bleeding occurs medical help should be sought.

Before You Use This Drug
Tell your doctor if you have or have had
❑ allergies to drugs
❑ kidney and liver problems
Tell your doctor about any other drugs you take, including aspirin, herbs, vitamins, and other non-prescription products.

When You Use This Drug
◆ **Call your doctor immediately if you have black, tarry stools or if you vomit material that looks like coffee grounds. These are signs of a bleeding ulcer.**
◆ If you take an antacid take it at least 30 minutes apart from famotidine. One source suggests taking stomach blockers 2 hours before antacids.[80]
◆ Do not drink alcohol or smoke.
◆ Avoid any food and drink that triggers your ulcer.
◆ Check with your doctor before taking any aspirin, ibuprofen or other NSAIDs. These drugs can cause or aggravate ulcers.

How To Use This Drug
◆ Swallow tablet whole. If you use the suspension shake it well before measuring.
◆ Take with meals. Make sure that one of your doses is taken at bedtime.
◆ Take all the famotidine your doctor prescribed even if you feel better.
◆ Do not expose to heat, moisture, or strong light. Do not store in the bathroom. The suspension may be refrigerated,[81] but avoid freezing. Discard the suspension after 30 days.
◆ If you miss a dose, take it as soon as you remember, but skip it if it is almost time for the next dose. **Do not take double doses.**

Interactions With Other Drugs
The following drugs are listed in *Evaluations of Drug Interactions*, 1991 as causing "highly clinically significant" or "clinically significant" interactions when used together with this drug. There may be other drugs, especially those in the families of drugs listed below, that also will react with this drug to cause severe adverse effects. Make sure to ask your doctor for a complete listing of them and let her or him know if you are taking any of these interacting drugs:

ANECTINE; BiCNU; bone marrow depressants; carbamazepine; clozapine; CLOZARIL; COUMADIN; DILANTIN; ELIXOPHYLLIN; imipramine; morphine; phenytoin;[82] succinylcholine; TEGRETOL; THEO-DUR; theophylline;[83] TOFRANIL; warfarin.[84]

Additionally, the *United States Pharmacopeia Drug Information*, 1992 lists this drug as having interactions of major significance:

ketoconazole; NIZORAL (if you also must take this drug, take your famotidine 2 hours after you take it).

Adverse Effects
Call your doctor immediately:
❑ confusion
❑ hallucinations
❑ fever
❑ chest pain, or slow, fast or irregular heartbeat[85,86]
❑ abdominal pain
❑ difficulty breathing
❑ dizziness
❑ eye sensitivity to light
❑ seizure
❑ skin rash

- swelling around eyes, face, lips,
- throbbing headache[87]

Call your doctor if these symptoms continue:
- constipation or diarrhea

- depression
- headache
- loss of appetite
- ringing in ears
- tiredness or weakness

LIMITED USE

Promethazine
PHENERGAN (Wyeth)

Generic: available

Family: Antinausea Drugs
Antipsychotics (see p. 208)
Antihistamines

Promethazine (proe *meth* a zeen) is most often used to treat severe nausea or vomiting, after the patient has already tried dietary changes without relief (see box below). It is also used to treat or prevent allergy symptoms and motion sickness and to promote sleep and sedation, but because of its serious side effects, it should *not* be used for these purposes.

Promethazine can cause serious side effects: drug-induced parkinsonism (see p. 212) and tardive dyskinesia (involuntary movements of parts of the body, which may last indefinitely). More information appears under Adverse Effects. Taking large doses of promethazine or taking it for a long time could increase your chance of experiencing these and other side effects. If you have used promethazine regularly for some time,

---

Warning: Special Mental and Physical Adverse Effects

Older adults are especially sensitive to the harmful anticholinergic effects of antipsychotics and antihistamines such as promethazine. Drugs in these families should not be used unless absolutely necessary.

Mental Effects: confusion, delirium, short-term memory problems, disorientation, and impaired attention.

Physical Effects: dry mouth, constipation, difficulty urinating (especially for a man with an enlarged prostate), blurred vision, decreased sweating with increased body temperature, sexual dysfunction, and worsening of glaucoma.

Drugs used to treat cancer often cause severe nausea and vomiting, either immediately after the drug is taken or several hours later. You can treat this kind of nausea and vomiting by changing your diet or by taking an antinausea drug. You should always try dietary changes first.[88]
- Eat small, frequent meals so your stomach is never empty.
- When you get up from sleeping or resting, eat some dry crackers or toast before you start being active.
- Drink carbonated drinks or other clear liquids such as soups and gelatin.
- Eat tart foods such as lemons and pickles.
- Do not eat foods with strong smells.

ask your doctor if your drug can be changed in order to avoid developing serious side effects.

If you are over 60, you should generally be taking less than the usual adult dose.

Before You Use This Drug

Tell your doctor if you have or have had
- allergies to drugs
- an unusual reaction to other antipsychotics (see p. 240 for examples)
- heart or blood vessel disease
- Parkinson's disease
- epilepsy, seizures
- enlarged prostate or difficulty urinating
- diabetes
- glaucoma
- liver disease
- bone marrow depression
- lung disease or breathing problems
- alcohol dependence
- breast cancer
- stomach ulcer

Tell your doctor about any other drugs you take, including aspirin, herbs, vitamins, and other non-prescription products.

When You Use This Drug
- **Do not stop taking this drug suddenly. The dosage must be gradually decreased by your doctor to prevent withdrawal symptoms** such as nausea, vomiting, stomach upset, trembling, dizziness, and symptoms of Parkinson's disease.
- It may take 2 or 3 weeks before you can tell that this drug is working.
- Until you know how you react to this drug, do not drive or perform other activities requiring alertness. Promethazine may cause blurred vision, drowsiness, and fainting.
- Do not drink alcohol or take drugs that cause drowsiness.
- You may feel dizzy when rising from a lying or sitting position. When getting out of bed, hang your legs over the side of the bed for a few minutes, then get up slowly. When getting up from a chair,

stay by the chair until you are sure that you are not dizzy. (See p. 14.)
- If you plan to have any surgery, including dental, tell your doctor that you take this drug.

How To Use This Drug
- Take with food or **a full glass (8 ounces) of milk or water** to prevent stomach upset.
- If you take antacids or drugs for diarrhea, take them at least 2 hours apart from promethazine.
- Do not store in the bathroom. Do not expose to heat, moisture, or strong light. Do not let the liquid form freeze.
- If you miss a dose, take it as soon as you remember, but skip it if it is almost time for the next dose. **Do not take double doses.**

Interactions With Other Drugs

The following drugs are listed in *Evaluations of Drug Interactions*, 1991 as causing "highly clinically significant" or "clinically significant" interactions when used together with this drug. There may be other drugs, especially those in the families of drugs listed below, that also will react with this drug to cause severe adverse effects. Make sure to ask your doctor for a complete listing of them and let her or him know if you are taking any of these interacting drugs:

AEROSPORIN; alcohol; benztropine; bromocriptine; CAPOTEN; captopril; COGENTIN; DEMEROL; desipramine; diazoxide; HYPERSTAT; INDERAL; meperidine; NORPRAMIN; PARLODEL; PERTOFRANE; polymyxin B; propranolol; succinylcholine.

Adverse Effects

Call your doctor immediately:
- **if you experience signs of tardive dyskinesia:** lip smacking; chewing movements; puffing of cheeks; rapid, darting tongue movements; uncontrolled movements of arms or legs

❏ **if you experience signs of parkinsonism:** difficulty speaking or swallowing; loss of balance; mask-like face; muscle spasms; stiffness of arms or legs; trembling and shaking; unusual twisting movements of body
❏ change in vision, blurring
❏ difficulty urinating
❏ **if you experience signs of neuroleptic malignant syndrome:** troubled or fast breathing; fever; high or low blood pressure; increased sweating; loss of bladder control; muscle stiffness; seizures; unusual tiredness, weakness; fast heartbeat; irregular pulse; pale skin
❏ fever, sore mouth, gums, or throat
❏ abnormal bleeding or bruising
❏ nightmares
❏ fainting
❏ skin rash
❏ yellow eyes or skin
Call your doctor if these symptoms continue:
❏ constipation

❏ decreased sexual ability
❏ decreased sweating
❏ dizziness, lightheadedness
❏ drowsiness
❏ dry mouth
❏ increased skin sensitivity to sun
❏ nasal congestion
❏ swelling or pain in breasts
❏ milk from breasts

Periodic Tests
Ask your doctor which of these tests should be done periodically while you are taking this drug:
❏ blood cell counts
❏ glaucoma test
❏ liver function tests
❏ urine tests for bile and bilirubin
❏ observation for tremors or jerking movements, early signs of tardive dyskinesia
❏ evaluation of continued need for promethazine

LIMITED USE

Magnesium Hydroxide
PHILLIPS' MILK OF MAGNESIA (Glenbrook)
M.O.M (Ulmer)

Generic: available

Family: Antacids
Laxatives

Magnesium hydroxide (mag *nee* zium hye *drox* ide) is both a laxative and an antacid. As a laxative, this drug may be used occasionally but should not be used regularly (see p. 356 for alternatives). As an antacid, this drug is stronger than aluminum hydroxide (see p. 334), but it tends to cause diarrhea. **Older adults who have severe kidney disease should not use magnesium antacids.**[89]

Take each dose of magnesium hydroxide with **a full glass (8 ounces) of water.** The liquid form is better than tablets because it is more effective and costs less. If you use tablets, chew them thoroughly. If you take large doses of magnesium hydroxide or use it for a long time, see your doctor for regular checkups. If you are treating yourself with this drug, do not take it for more than 2 weeks unless you check with your doctor.

Before You Use This Drug
Tell your doctor if you have or have had
❏ allergies to drugs

- ❏ abdominal pain
- ❏ blood in stools
- ❏ inflammation of the colon (colitis)
- ❏ diverticulitis
- ❏ prolonged diarrhea
- ❏ intestinal blockage
- ❏ kidney disease

Tell your doctor about any other drugs you take, including aspirin, herbs, vitamins, and other non-prescription products.

When You Use This Drug

◆ **Call your doctor immediately if you have black, tarry stools or you vomit material that looks like coffee grounds. These are signs of a bleeding ulcer.**

◆ If you are on a low-salt (low-sodium) diet, ask your doctor or pharmacist to help you choose an antacid or laxative. Many brands contain sodium.

How To Use This Drug

◆ If you are taking magnesium hydroxide as an antacid, take it 1 to 3 hours after meals and at bedtime for maximum effectiveness. Drink plenty of fluids.

◆ Do not take any other drugs by mouth for at least 1 or 2 hours after taking magnesium hydroxide.

◆ Do not expose to heat, moisture, or strong light. Do not store in the bathroom. Do not let the liquid form freeze.

◆ If you miss a dose, take it as soon as you remember, but skip it if it is almost time for the next dose. **Do not take double doses.**

Interactions With Other Drugs

The following drugs are listed in *Evaluations of Drug Interactions*, 1991 as causing "highly clinically significant" or "clinically significant" interactions when used together with this drug. There may be other drugs, especially those in the families of drugs listed below, that also will react with this drug to cause severe adverse effects. Make sure to ask your doctor for a complete listing of them and let her or him know if you are taking any of these interacting drugs:

ACHROMYCIN; aspirin; CIPRO; ciprofloxacin; digoxin; ECOTRIN; KAYEXALATE; LANOXIN; sodium polystyrene sulfonate; tetracycline.

Adverse Effects

Call your doctor immediately:
- ❏ difficult or painful urination
- ❏ dizziness, lightheadedness
- ❏ irregular heartbeat
- ❏ mood or mental changes
- ❏ unusual tiredness or weakness

Call your doctor if these symptoms continue:
- ❏ diarrhea or laxative effect
- ❏ nausea, vomiting
- ❏ stomach cramps

LIMITED USE

Omeprazole
PRILOSEC (Merck)

Generic: not available

Family: Ulcer Drugs

Omeprazole (o *mep* ra zole) is used short-term to treat gastroesophageal reflux as well as duodenal and gastric ulcers resistant to the usual treatment with acid blockers or antacids. It is the drug of choice for long-term treatment of Zollinger-Ellison syndrome, although it does not alter the course of the disease.

Warning
In long-term (2 year) studies in rats, omeprazole caused an increase in carcinoid tumors of the stomach. Although such tumors have not yet been demonstrated in humans, using the drug for long-term therapy is not advisable, except for the treatment of Zollinger-Ellison syndrome.

Omeprazole inhibits secretion of the gastric acid, whereas stomach acid blockers, such as cimetidine (Tagamet), prevent production of the acid. Compared to stomach acid blockers, omeprazole relieves pain more quickly during the first two weeks,[90] and generally has fewer adverse effects short-term. Preventing the need for surgery is especially desirable in the elderly.[91,92,93] For ulcers, treatment takes a few weeks; for Zollinger-Ellison syndrome, a few years. To maintain effectiveness in treating Zollinger-Ellison syndrome, the dose may need to be increased annually.[94] Individual response to omeprazole varies considerably. In older people, decreased liver function may affect the response. Relapse of acid reflux is common. Long-term suppression of acid can lead to intestinal infections.[95,96] It is uncertain whether long-term suppression of stomach acid may also cause stomach cancer.[97,98,99,100,101,102,103,104]

For now, omeprazole is recommended for short-term treatment of severe refractory reflux esophagitis or peptic ulcers only when other agents such as H$_2$ antagonists (stomach acid blockers, such as cimetidine (Tagamet)) or antacids do not work. Omeprazole is more costly than stomach acid blockers, but less costly than surgery. For all these conditions try to avoid foods which trigger your condition, and avoid alcohol and smoking. Also, avoid drugs known to aggravate ulcers, especially aspirin, ibuprofen, and other nonsteroidal anti-inflammatory drugs (NSAIDs) (see p. 262). Ask your doctor if acetaminophen could be substituted. If these practices are not enough, try liquid antacids next. Long-term use of antacids also has risks. Aluminum can cause bone damage, magnesium severe diarrhea. Too much calcium and sodium also causes problems.

If you have gastric reflux or Zollinger-Ellison syndrome, try raising the head of your bed six inches.[105] If you have reflux esophagitis try eating smaller, low-fat meals, more frequently, but do not eat for at least two hours before bedtime. Check with your doctor about other medications that aggravate the esophagus. If symptoms worsen or bleeding occurs, call your doctor.

Before You Use This Drug
Tell your doctor if you have or have had
❑ allergies to drugs
❑ heart problems[106]
❑ liver problems[107]
❑ pernicious anemia[108,109]

Tell your doctor about any other drugs you take, including aspirin, herbs, vitamins, and other non-prescription products.

When You Use This Drug

◆ Try to stop smoking, since smoking may delay healing, especially of large ulcers.[110,111]

◆ Follow a diet recommended by your doctor.

How To Use This Drug

◆ Swallow capsule whole. Do not crush, chew, or open the capsule.

◆ Take omeprazole about a half an hour before a meal. If you take it once a day, schedule it in the morning. You may take with or without antacids.

◆ Take for the full amount of time prescribed by your doctor, even if you are feeling better.

◆ Do not expose to heat, moisture, or strong light. Do not store in the bathroom. Do not let the liquid form freeze.

◆ If you miss a dose, take it as soon as you remember, but skip it if it is almost time for the next dose. **Do not take double doses.**

Interactions With Other Drugs

The following drugs are listed in *Evaluations of Drug Interactions,* 1991 as causing "highly clinically significant" or "clinically significant" interactions when used together with this drug. There may be other drugs, especially those in the families of drugs listed below, that also will react with this drug to cause severe adverse effects. Make sure to ask your doctor for a complete listing of them and let her or him know if you are taking this interacting drug:

cyclosporine; SANDIMMUNE.

Additionally, the *United States Pharmacopeia Drug Information,* 1992 and *Drug Interactions and Updates,* 1991 list these drugs as having interactions of major significance:

COUMADIN; diazepam; digoxin;[113,114] DILANTIN; LANOXIN; phenytoin;[112] VALIUM; warfarin.

Adverse Effects

Call your doctor immediately:

❑ bleeding or bruising
❑ breathing difficulty[115]
❑ fever
❑ mouth sores
❑ sore thoat
❑ unusual tiredness or weakness[116]
❑ cloudy or bloody urine

Call your doctor if these symptoms continue:

❑ abdominal pain
❑ anxiety[117]
❑ breast enlargement in men[118,119]
❑ chest pain
❑ constipation or diarrhea
❑ cough
❑ depression[120]
❑ dizziness
❑ drowsiness
❑ painful erections
❑ gas
❑ headache
❑ heartburn
❑ muscle or back pain
❑ nausea or vomiting
❑ numbness[121]
❑ skin rash or itching

LIMITED USE

Metoclopramide
REGLAN (Robins)

Generic: available

Family: Antinausea Drugs
Antipsychotics (see p. 208)

Metoclopramide (met oh *kloe* pra mide) has several uses. For people who have a condition in which the stomach takes too long to empty, it relieves symptoms such as nausea, vomiting, loss of appetite, heartburn, and a feeling of fullness. It also controls reflux esophagitis, a condition in which the stomach contents flow backwards into the esophagus (the tube connecting the mouth to the stomach), causing heartburn. It prevents nausea and vomiting caused by chemotherapy for cancer. This drug should not be used to treat motion sickness or vertigo (dizziness).[122]

If you are suffering nausea and vomiting

Drugs used to treat cancer often cause severe nausea and vomiting, either immediately after the drug is taken or several hours later. You can treat this kind of nausea and vomiting by changing your diet or by taking an antinausea drug. You should always try dietary changes first.[127]
- Eat small, frequent meals so your stomach is never empty.
- When you get up from sleeping or resting, eat some dry crackers or toast before you start being active.
- Drink carbonated drinks or other clear liquids such as soups and gelatin.
- Eat tart foods such as lemons and pickles.
- Do not eat foods with strong smells.

---

from cancer chemotherapy, you should try changing your diet to relieve these effects before taking a drug such as metoclopramide (see box below).

Metoclopramide can cause serious side effects: severe drowsiness,[123] drug-induced parkinsonism (see p. 212),[124] and tardive dyskinesia (involuntary movements of parts of the body, which may last indefinitely). The latter two conditions can occur when the drug is used over a long period of time,[125] especially in people with impaired kidney function.[126] More information appears under Adverse Effects.

If you are over 60, you should generally be taking less than the usual adult dose because older adults often do not tolerate metoclopramide well.

Before You Use This Drug
Do not use if you have or have had
- epilepsy
- bleeding, obstruction, or perforation of the stomach or intestine
Tell your doctor if you have or have had
- allergies to drugs
- liver disease
- Parkinson's disease
- kidney disease
Tell your doctor about any other drugs you take, including aspirin, herbs, vitamins, and other non-prescription products.

When You Use This Drug
- Do not drink alcohol or use drugs that cause drowsiness.
- Until you know how you react to this drug, do not drive or perform other activities requiring alertness. Metoclopramide can cause drowsiness.

How To Use This Drug

◆ Take 30 minutes before meals and at bedtime for maximum effectiveness. Do not take more than prescribed.

◆ Do not expose to heat, moisture, or strong light. Do not store in the bathroom. Do not let the liquid form freeze.

◆ If you miss a dose, take it as soon as you remember, but skip it if it is almost time for the next dose. **Do not take double doses.**

Interactions With Other Drugs

The following drugs are listed in *Evaluations of Drug Interactions*, 1991 as causing "highly clinically significant" or "clinically significant" interactions when used together with this drug. There may be other drugs, especially those in the families of drugs listed below, that also will react with this drug to cause severe adverse effects. Make sure to ask your doctor for a complete listing of them and let her or him know if you are taking any of these interacting drugs:

cyclosporine; digoxin; LANOXICAPS; LANOXIN; SANDIMMUNE.

Adverse Effects

Call your doctor immediately:

❑ **if you experience signs of overdose:** confusion; severe drowsiness; muscle spasms; shuffling walk; tic-like, jerky movements of head and face; shaking, trembling hands

❑ **if you experience signs of tardive dyskinesia:** lip smacking; chewing movements; puffing of cheeks; rapid, darting movements of tongue; uncontrolled movements of arms or legs

❑ **if you experience signs of parkinsonism:** difficulty speaking or swallowing; loss of balance; mask-like face; muscle spasms; stiffness of arms or legs; trembling and shaking; unusual twisting movements of body

Call your doctor if these symptoms continue:

❑ drowsiness
❑ restlessness, trouble sleeping
❑ unusual tiredness or weakness
❑ breast tenderness and swelling
❑ constipation or diarrhea
❑ depression, irritability
❑ dizziness
❑ headache
❑ nausea
❑ skin rash
❑ dry mouth

Periodic Tests

Ask your doctor which of these tests should be done periodically while you are taking this drug:

❑ clinical exams for tremors and jerky movements

Cimetidine
TAGAMET (Smith Kline & French)

Generic: available

Family: Stomach Acid Blockers

Cimetidine (sye *met* i deen) blocks the release of stomach acid and is used to treat ulcers and conditions caused by excess stomach acid. Similar drugs in this family include ranitidine (Zantac), nizatidine (Axid) and famotidine (Pepcid). You should not be taking cimetidine for minor digestive complaints such as occasional upset stomach, nausea, or heartburn, as there is no evidence that it is effective for treating these problems.

Ulcers often come back after a few months. So for frequent, severe recurrences, maintenance therapy is used. Confusion is a possible adverse effect, but this also occurs with other drugs in this family.[128] Elderly people, are more apt to have reduced function of kidney and liver.[129] **If you have reduced kidney function, your doctor should start you on a low or less frequent dose.**

If you are over 60, you should generally be taking less than the usual adult dose of cimetidine, especially if you have reduced kidney or liver function. Your body eliminates cimetidine more slowly than younger people's bodies.[130] This means that more of the drug stays in your body for a longer time, which puts you at a higher risk of side effects, particularly dizziness and confusion.[131] Rarely, people taking cimetidine have developed bone marrow depression, a serious side effect in which your bone marrow is unable to normally produce blood cells. Cimetidine has been shown to cause benign tumors in the testicles of rats,[132] and it can reduce men's sperm count (and therefore their ability to father children) if it is taken regularly for at least 9 weeks.[133]

Cigarette smoking can delay healing of ulcers.[134] Some people find relief of reflux esophagitis by elevating the head of the bed.

Liquid antacids of magnesium and aluminum in low doses are as effective at healing ulcers as stomach acid blockers, and less costly. However, long-term use of antacids has risks. Antacids with aluminum can cause bone damage, ones with magnesium can cause severe diarrhea. Too much calcium or sodium also causes serious problems. If ulcer symptoms worsen or bleeding occurs medical help should be sought.

Before You Use This Drug
Tell your doctor if you have or have had
❑ allergies to drugs
❑ kidney or liver disease
Tell your doctor about any other drugs you take, including aspirin, herbs, vitamins, and other non-prescription products.

When You Use This Drug
◆ Call your doctor immediately if you have black, tarry stools or if you vomit material that looks like coffee grounds. These are signs of a bleeding ulcer.
◆ If you take an antacid take it at least 30 minutes apart from cimetidine. One source suggests taking stomach acid blockers 2 hours before antacids.[135]
◆ Do not drink alcohol or smoke.
◆ Avoid any food and drink that triggers your ulcer.
◆ Check with your doctor before taking any aspirin, ibuprofen or other NSAIDs. These drugs can cause or aggravate ulcers.
◆ Do not expose yourself to organophosphate pesticides, such as Diazinon.[136]

How To Use This Drug
◆ Take with meals. Make sure that one of your doses is taken at bedtime.

◆ Tablets have an odor. This is normal and no cause for concern.

◆ Do not expose to heat, moisture, or strong light. Do not store in the bathroom. Do not let the liquid form freeze.

◆ If you miss a dose, take it as soon as you remember, but skip it if it is almost time for the next dose. **Do not take double doses.**

Interactions With Other Drugs

The following drugs are listed in *Evaluations of Drug Interactions*, 1991 as causing "highly clinically significant" or "clinically significant" interactions when used together with this drug. There may be other drugs, especially those in the families of drugs listed below, that also will react with this drug to cause severe adverse effects. Make sure to ask your doctor for a complete listing of them and let her or him know if you are taking any of these interacting drugs:

BiCNU; BRONKODYL; carbamazepine; carmustine; clozapine; CLOZARIL; CONSTANT-T; COUMADIN; diazepam; DILANTIN; ELIXOPHYLLIN; flecainide; glipizide; GLUCOTROL; imipramine; INDERAL; lidocaine; M S CONTIN; morphine; phenytoin; procainamide; PRONESTYL; propranolol; QUIBRON-T-SR; QUINIDEX; quinidine; ROXANOL; SLO-BID; SLO-PHYLLIN; SOMOPHYLLIN; succinylcholine; SUSTAIRE; TAMBOCOR; TEGRETOL; THEO-24; THEOLAIR; theophylline; TOFRANIL; VALIUM; warfarin; XYLOCAINE.

Additionally, the *United States Pharmacopeia Drug Information*, 1992 lists this drug as having interactions of major significance:

ketoconazole; NIZORAL.

Adverse Effects

Call your doctor immediately:
❏ confusion
❏ hallucinations
❏ sore throat and fever
❏ unusual bleeding or bruising
❏ slow, fast, or irregular heartbeat
❏ unusual tiredness or weakness

Call your doctor if these symptoms continue:
❏ decreased sexual ability
❏ diarrhea
❏ dizziness or headache
❏ muscle cramps or pain
❏ skin rash
❏ enlarged or sore breasts

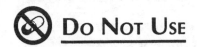 **Do Not Use**

Alternative treatment: Dietary modifications, see p. 343.

Trimethobenzamide
TIGAN (Beecham)

Family: Antinausea Drugs
Anticholinergics

Trimethobenzamide (trye meth oh *ben* za mide) is used to relieve nausea and vomiting, but **there is no convincing proof that it is effective.**[137] It has little or no value for preventing or treating vertigo (dizziness) or motion sickness.[138]

If you have been taking trimethobenzamide regularly for some time and you have also been taking high doses of aspirin or other similar drugs (salicylates), the trimethobenzamide can hide the signs of an aspirin or salicylate overdose.[139] Rarely, trimethobenzamide causes convulsions, and this is more common among older users of the drug.[140]

> *Warning: Special Mental and Physical Adverse Effects*
> Older adults are especially sensitive to the harmful anticholinergic effects of trimethobenzamide. Drugs in this family should not be used unless absolutely necessary.
> *Mental Effects*: confusion, delirium, short-term memory problems, disorientation, and impaired attention.
> *Physical Effects*: dry mouth, constipation, difficulty urinating (especially for a man with an enlarged prostate), blurred vision, decreased sweating with increased body temperature, sexual dysfunction, and worsening of glaucoma.

Ranitidine
ZANTAC (Glaxo)

Generic: not available

Family: Stomach Acid Blockers

Ranitidine (ra *nit* te deen) blocks the release of stomach acid and is used to treat ulcers and conditions caused by excess stomach acid. Similar drugs in this family include cimetidine (Tagamet), famotidine (Pepcid) and nizatidine (Axid). You should not be taking ranitidine for minor digestive complaints such as occasional upset stomach, nausea, or heartburn.

Ulcers often come back after a few months. So for frequent, severe recurrences, maintenance therapy is used. Confusion is a possible adverse effect, but this also occurs with other drugs in this family.[141] Elderly people are more apt to have reduced function of kidney and liver.[142,143] **If you have reduced kidney function, your doctor should start you on a low, or less frequent dose.**

If you are over 60, you should generally be taking less than the usual adult dose of ranitidine, especially if you have reduced kidney or liver function. Your body eliminates ranitidine more slowly than younger people's bodies.[144] This means that more of the drug stays in your body for a longer time, which puts you at a higher risk of side effects, especially confusion. Ranitidine is less likely than cimetidine to cause enlarged breasts, decreased sexual ability, dizziness and confusion.[145]

Cigarette smoking can delay healing of ulcers.[146] Some people find relief of reflux esophagitis by elevating the head of the bed.

Liquid antacids of magnesium and aluminum in low doses are as effective at healing ulcers as stomach acid blockers, and less costly. However, long-term use of antacids has risks. Antacids with aluminum can cause bone damage, ones with magnesium can cause severe diarrhea. Too much calcium or sodium also causes serious problems. If ulcer symptoms worsen or bleeding occurs medical help should be sought.

Before You Use This Drug
Tell your doctor if you have or have had
❑ allergies to drugs
❑ kidney or liver disease
Tell your doctor about any other drugs you take, including aspirin, herbs, vitamins, and other non-prescription products.

When You Use This Drug
◆ **Call your doctor immediately if you have black, tarry stools or if you vomit material that looks like coffee grounds. These are signs of a bleeding ulcer.**
◆ If you take an antacid take it at least 30 minutes apart from ranitidine. One source suggests taking stomach acid blockers 2 hours before antacids.[147]
◆ Avoid any food and drink that triggers your ulcer.
◆ Check with your doctor before taking any aspirin, ibuprofen or other NSAIDs. These

drugs can cause or aggravate ulcers.
◆ Do not drink alcohol or smoke.

How To Use This Drug
◆ Make sure that one of your doses is taken at bedtime.
◆ Do not expose to heat, moisture, or strong light. Do not store in the bathroom. Do not let the liquid form freeze.
◆ If you miss a dose, take it as soon as you remember, but skip it if it is almost time for the next dose. **Do not take double doses.**

Interactions With Other Drugs
The following drugs are listed in *Evaluations of Drug Interactions,* 1991 as causing "highly clinically significant" or "clinically significant" interactions when used together with this drug. There may be other drugs, especially those in the families of drugs listed below, that also will react with this drug to cause severe adverse effects. Make sure to ask your doctor for a complete listing of them and let her or him know if you are taking any of these interacting drugs:

COUMADIN; glipizide; GLUCOTROL; procainamide; PRONESTYL; QUINIDEX; quinidine; warfarin.

Adverse Effects
Call your doctor immediately:
❑ confusion
❑ hallucinations
❑ sore throat and fever
❑ unusual bleeding or bruising
❑ slow, fast, or irregular heartbeat
❑ unusual tiredness or weakness
Call your doctor if these symptoms continue:
❑ constipation, diarrhea
❑ dizziness or headache
❑ nausea
❑ skin rash
❑ stomach pain

Notes for Gastrointestinal Drugs

1. Lew JF, Glass RI, Gangarosa RE, Cohen IP, Bern C, Moe CL. Diarrheal deaths in the United States, 1979 through 1987: a special problem for the elderly. *Journal of the American Medical Association* 1991; 265:3280-4.

2. Fine KD, Santa Ana CA, Fordtran JS. Diagnosis of magnesium-induced diarrhea. *New England Journal of Medicine* 1991; 324:1012-7.

3. *Training Manual for Treatment and Prevention of Childhood Diarrhea with Oral Rehydration Therapy, Proper Nutrition and Hygiene* 1992. International Child Health Foundation, P.O. Box 1205, 10227 Wincopa Circle, Columbia Md 21044.

4. Recipe for Oral Rehydration Solution. From Werner D, Thuman C, Maxell J. *Where There Is No Doctor; A Village Health Care Handbook* 1992. The Hesperian Foundation, P.O. Box 1692, Palo Alto, CA 94302.

5. *USP DI, Drug Information for the Health Care Provider.* 6th ed. Rockville Md.: The United States Pharmacopeial Convention, Inc., 1986:190.

6. *The Medical Letter on Drugs and Therapeutics.* New York: The Medical Letter Inc., 1982; 24:61.

7. *Physicians' Desk Reference.* 40th ed. Oradell, N.J.: Medical Economics Company, 1986:1520.

8. Kastrup EK, ed. *Facts and Comparisons.* St. Louis: J.B. Lippincott Co., July 1987:258-2591.

9. *USP DI*, 1986, op. cit., p. 979.

10. *USP DI, Drug Information for the Health Care Provider.* 7th ed. Rockville Md.: The United States Pharmacopeial Convention, Inc., 1987:366.

11. Freston JWA. Overview of medical therapy of peptic ulcer disease. *Gastroenterology Clinics of North America* 1990; 19:121-40.

12. *The Medical Letter on Drugs and Therapeutics.* New York: The Medical Letter Inc., 1991; 33:111-4.

13. Lipsy RJ, Fennerty B, Faggan TC. Clinical review of histamine$_2$ receptor antagonists. *Archives of Internal Medicine* 1990; 150:745-51.

14. Sontag SJ. The medical management of reflux esophagitis; role of antacids and acid inhibition. *Gastroenterology Clinics of North America* 1990; 19:683-712.

15. Halabi A, Kirch W. Negative chronotropic effects of nizatidine. *Gut* 1991; 32:630-4.

16. Lipsy RJ, Fagan TC, Fennerty B. Histamine$_2$ receptor antagonists and cardiovascular drugs. *Archives of Internal Medicine* 1991; 151:814-5.

17. Karlstadt RG, Palmer RH. Unrecognized drug interactions with famotidine and nizatidine. *Archives of Internal Medicine* 1991; 151:810.

18. Gilman AG, Rall TW, Nies AS, Taylor P, eds. *The Pharmacological Basis of Therapeutics.* 8th ed. New York: Pergamon Press, 1990:899-902.

19. Dukes MNG, Beeley L. *Side Effects of Drugs Annual* 14, Amsterdam: Elsevier, 1990; 317.

20. Sontag, op. cit.

21. Lipsy, 1990, op. cit.

22. Lantz MD, Wozniak TJ. Stability of nizatidine in extemporaneous oral liquid preparations (abstract). *American Journal of Hospital Pharmacy* 1990; 47:2716.

23. Shinn AF. Unrecognized drug interactions with famotidine and nizatidine. *Archives of Internal Medicine* 1991; 151:814.

24. Karlstadt, op. cit.

25. Cloud ML, Offen WW, Robinson M. Nizatidine versus placebo in gastroesophageal reflux disease: a 12-week multicenter randomized, double-blind study. *The American Journal of Gastroenterology* 1991; 86:1735-42.

26. *USP DI*, 1987, op. cit., p. 766.

27. *Physicians' Desk Reference*. 41st ed. Oradell, N.J.: Medical Economics Company, 1987:1068.

28. Gilman AG, Goodman LS, Rall TW, Murad F, eds. *The Pharmacological Basis of Therapeutics*. 7th ed. New York: Macmillan, 1985:402.

29. Fong NL. Chemotherapy and Nutritional Management. In *Nutritional Management of the Cancer Patient*. New York: Raven Press, 1979.

30. Gabriel SE. Is misoprostol prophylaxis indicated for NSAID induced adverse gastrointestinal events? An epidemiologic opinion. *The Journal of Rheumatology* 1991; 18:958-60.

31. Koretz RL. Prevention of NSAID-induced gastric ulcer. *Annals of Internal Medicine* 1991; 115:911-2.

32. Kornbluth A, Gupta R, Gerson CD. Life-threatening diarrhea after short-term misoprostol use in a patient with Crohn ileocolitis. *Annals of Internal Medicine* 1990; 113: 474-5.

33. Clearfield HR. Management of NSAID-induced ulcer disease. *American Family Physician* 1992; 45:255-8.

34. Mazzuca SA, Brandt KD, Anderson SL, Musick BS, Katz BP. The therapeutic approaches of community based primary care practitioners to osteoarthritis of the hip in an elderly patient. *The Journal of Rheumatology* 1991; 18:1593-1600.

35. Rubin W. Medical treatment of peptic ulcer disease. *Medical Clinics of North America* 1991; 75:981-98.

36. Dukes, 1990, op. cit., p. 90-1.

37. Rubin, op. cit.

38. Gabriel, op. cit.

39. Renfrew RA. Prevention of NSAID-induced gastric ulcer (letter). *Annals of Internal Medicine* 1991; 115:912-3.

40. Mazzuca, op. cit.

41. Kornbluth, op. cit.

42 Graber DJ, Meier KH. Acute misoprostol toxicity. *Annals of Emergency Medicine* 1991; 20:549-51.

43. Morton MR, Robbins ME. Delirium in an elderly woman possibly associated with administration of misoprostol. *DICP, The Annals of Pharmacotherapy* 1991; 25:133-4.

44. Fossaluzza V, Di Benedetto P, Zampa A, De Vita S. Misoprostol-induced urinary incontinence. *Journal of Internal Medicine* 1991; 230:463-4.

45. Gilman, 1985, op. cit., p. 999.

46. AMA Department of Drugs. *AMA Drug Evaluations*. 1st ed. Chicago: American Medical Association, 1971:594.

47. *USP DI*, 1987, op. cit., p. 366.

48. *Drugs for the Elderly*. Denmark: World Health Organization, 1985:27.

49. Gilman, 1985, op. cit., p. 999.

50. *USP DI*, 1986, op. cit., p. 190.

51. *The Medical Letter on Drugs and Therapeutics*, 1982, op. cit.

52. *USP DI*, 1986, op. cit., p. 192.

53. *The Medical Letter on Drugs and Therapeutics*, 1982, op. cit.

54. *USP DI*, 1986, op. cit., p. 956.

55. Phone conversation with James Butt, M.D., Professor of Medicine, University of Missouri, School of Medicine, Columbia MO, January 5,1987.

56. Kastrup, op. cit., p. 324c.

57. AMA, 1971, op. cit.

58. *USP DI*, 1987, op. cit., p. 587.

59. *USP DI*, 1986, op. cit., p. 693.

60. *Physicians' Desk Reference*, 1986, op. cit., p. 1690.

61. *USP DI*, 1986, op. cit., p. 190.

62. *The Medical Letter on Drugs and Therapeutics*, 1982, op. cit.

63. Ibid.

64. *The Medical Letter on Drugs and Therapeutics*. New York: The Medical Letter Inc., 1975; 17:80.

65. Ibid.

66. *USP DI*, 1986, op. cit., p. 190.

67. *The Medical Letter on Drugs and Therapeutics*, 1982, op. cit.

68. Ibid.

69. *The Medical Letter on Drugs and Therapeutics*, 1975, op. cit.

70. Ibid.

71. *The Medical Letter on Drugs and Therapeutics*, 1991, op. cit.

72. Sontag, op. cit.

73. Karlstadt, op. cit.

74. Gilman, 1990, op. cit.

75. Dukes, 1990, op. cit., p. 317.

76. Sontag, op. cit.

77. Gilman, 1990, op. cit.

78. *The Medical Letter on Drugs and Therapeutics*, 1991, op. cit.

79. Sontag, op. cit.

80. Lipsy, 1990, op. cit.

81. American Society of Hospital Pharmacists. *American Hospital Formulary Service Drug Information*. Bethesda, MD, 1992:1759-63.

82. Ibid.

83. Ibid.

84. Shinn, op. cit.

85. Ahmad S. Famotidine and cardiac arrhythmia. *DICP, The Annals of Pharmacotherapy* 1991; 25:315.

86. Halabi, op. cit.

87. Dukes, 1990, op. cit., p. 317.

88. Fong, op. cit.

89. *The Medical Letter on Drugs and Therapeutics*, 1982, op. cit.

90. Lampkin TA, Ouellet D, Hak LJ, Dukes GE. Omeprazole: a novel antisecretory agent for the treatment of acid-peptic disorders. *DICP, The Annals of Pharmacotherapy* 1990; 24:393-402.

91. Langman M. Omeprazole. *British Medical Journal* 1991; 303:481-2.

92. Lind T, Cederberg C, Olausson M, Olbe L. Omeprazole in elderly duodenal ulcer patients: relationship between reduction in gastric acid secretion and fasting plasma gastrin. *European Journal of Clinical Pharmacology* 1991; 40:557-60.

93. Richter JE. Gastroesophageal reflux: diagnosis and management. *Hospital Practice* 1992; 27:59-66.

94. Maton PN, Vinayek R, Frucht H, McArthur KA, Miller LS, Saeed ZA, Gardner JD, Jensen RT. Long-term efficacy and safety of omeprazole in patients with Zollinger-Ellison syndrome: a prospective study. *Gastroenterology* 1989; 97:827-36.

95. Dukes MNG, Beeley L. *Side Effects of Drugs Annual* 15, Amsterdam: Elsevier, 1991: 397.

96. Sontag, op. cit.

97. Omeprazole (letters). *British Medical Journal* 1991; 303:1200-1.

98. Lampkin, op. cit.

99. Langman, op. cit.

100. Maton, op. cit.

101. Parkinson A, Hurwitz A. Omeprazole and the induction of human cytochrome P-450: a response to concerns about potential adverse effects. *Gastroenterology* 1991; 100:1157-64.

102. Misiewicz JJ. and Poynter D. Omeprazole and genotoxicity (letters). *The Lancet* 1990; 335:611.

103. Sachs G, Scott D, Reuben M. Omeprazole and the gastric mucosa (abstract). *Digestion* 1990; 47(Supp. 1):35.

104. Wright NA, Goodlad RA. and Diaz de Rojas F. Omeprazole and genotoxicity (letters). *The Lancet* 1990; 335:909-10.

105. Richter, op. cit.

106. Langman, op. cit.

107. Walker S, Klotz U, Sarem-Aslani A, Treiber G, Bode JC. Effect of omeprazole on nocturnal intragastric pH in cirrhotics with inadequate antisecretory response to ranitidine. *Digestion* 1991; 48:179-84.

108. Langman, op. cit.

109. Lind, op. cit.

110. Lysy J, Karmeli F, Wengrower D, Rachmilewitz D. Effect of duodenal ulcer healing by omeprazole and ranitidine on the generation of gastroduodenal eicosanoids, platelet-activating factor, pepsinogen A, and gastrin in duodenal ulcer patients. *Scandinavian Journal of Gastroenterology* 1992; 27:13-9.

111. McTavish D, Buckley MMT, Heel RC. Omeprazole: an updated review of its pharmacology and therapeutic use in acid-related disorders. *Drugs* 1991; 42(1):138-70.

112. Hansten and Horn; *Drug Interactions & Updates*, Lea Febiger, Malvern, PA, 1990, Updates of October, 1991.

113. Ibid.

114. Langman, op. cit.

115. Marks DR, Joy JV, Bonheim NA. Hemolytic anemia associated with the use of omeprazole. *The American Journal of Gastroenterology* 1991; 86:217-8.

116. Ibid.

117. Lampkin, op. cit.

118. Convens C, Verhelst J, Mahler C. Painful gynaecomastia during omeprazole therapy. *The Lancet* 1991; 338:1153.

119. Santucci L, Farroni F, Fiorucci S, Morelli A. Gynecomastia during omeprazole therapy. *New England Journal of Medicine* 1991; 324:635.

120. Lampkin, op. cit.

121. Sontag, op. cit.

122. Kastrup, op. cit, p. 258-259l.

123. AMA Department of Drugs. *AMA Drug Evaluations*. 5th ed. Chicago: American Medical Association, 1983:536-7.

124. Bateman DN, Rawlins MD, Simpson JM. Extrapyramidal reactions with metoclopramide. *British Medical Journal* 1985; 291:930-2.

125. *USP DI*, 1986, op. cit., p. 1025.

126. AMA, 1983, op. cit.

127. Fong, op. cit.

128. Karlstadt, op. cit.

129. Gilman, 1990, op. cit.

130. Vestal RE, ed. *Drug Treatment in the Elderly*. Sydney, Australia: ADIS Health Science Press, 1984:250.

131. *USP DI*, 1986, op. cit., p. 525.

132. Vestal, op. cit.

133. Van Thiel DH, Gavaler JS, Smith WI, Paul G. Hypothalmic-pituitary-gonadal dysfunction in men using cimetidine. *The New England Journal of Medicine* 1979; 300:1012.

134. Sontag, op. cit.

135. Lipsy, 1990, op. cit.

136. According to University of Texas (Dallas) expert on drug toxicity, Dr. Thomas L. Kurt, MD, MPH, cimetidine can interfere with the body's clearance of organophosphate pesticides, since it inhibits the liver enzyme which breaks them down. As a result, there can be increased levels of pesticides in the body and increased pesticide toxicity.

137. *The Medical Letter on Drugs and Therapeutics*. New York: The Medical Letter Inc., 1974; 16:48.

138. AMA, 1983, op. cit.

139. *USP DI*, 1986, op. cit., p. 1505.

140. AMA, 1983, op. cit.

141. Karlstadt, op. cit.

142. Gilman, 1990, op. cit.

143. Dukes, 1990, op. cit., p. 317.

144. Vestal, op. cit.

145. *USP DI*, 1986, op. cit., p. 1323.

146. Sontag, op. cit.

147. Lipsy, 1990, op. cit.

Cold, Cough, Allergy, and Asthma Drugs

Antihistamines and Decongestants

Cough and Cold Drugs

Asthma Drugs

Drugs to Treat Lung Disease

Cold, Cough, Allergy, and Hay Fever

Cold

The viral infection we call "the common cold" can usually be treated without any professional help by rest and plenty of liquids, occasionally aided by the use of simple over-the-counter (nonprescription) remedies for certain symptoms. *There are no drugs that can kill the viruses that cause colds.*

A cold cannot be "cured" except by time, but you are less likely to catch a cold if you do not smoke, since smoking paralyzes the hair-like cells that clean out the body's airways. Colds are usually spread by hand more often than they are spread through the air. It's a good idea to prevent the spread of viruses by trying not to touch your eyes, mouth, and nose, and by washing your hands frequently when you are ill or with an ill person.

Certain other illnesses appear similar to colds, but warrant medical advice. If you have a high fever (above 101°F or 38.3°C) accompanied by shaking chills and you are coughing up thick phlegm, or if coughing or breathing deeply causes sharp chest pain, you may have pneumonia. You should call your doctor for diagnosis and appropriate treatment.

The safest, best, and least expensive way to care for a cold is to not take anything at all and let the illness run its short, *usually self-limiting course.* If necessary, purchase single-ingredient products to treat the individual symptoms that you have.

What Is the Common Cold?

The common cold is a viral infection of the upper respiratory tract (nose, throat, and upper airways), resulting in inflammation of the mucous membrane lining of those areas. The most common symptoms are runny nose, sneezing, and a sore throat.

How to Treat a Cold
Nondrug measures

A cold is best treated without drugs by drinking plenty (at least 8 to 10 full (8 ounce) glasses per day) of nonalcoholic liquids (especially warm or hot liquids), getting enough rest, and not smoking.

Drugs to use

If symptoms do *not* respond to these nondrug measures and interfere with normal activities, the following products are safe and effective. Please note that all of the drug products we recommend for treating various cold symptoms — stuffy nose, fever, nonproductive cough — are available without a prescription (over-the-counter, OTC). **None of the prescription cough or cold drugs among the 364 most-prescribed drugs for older adults is recommended; 17 of the 18 drugs are classed as "Do Not Use."**

For a runny nose

No OTC or prescription drug is appropriate. A runny nose promotes drainage and should not be treated with medication. If it lasts longer than a week, call your doctor.

For a stuffy nose

If your nose is blocked, especially if you can't breathe through it, use nose drops or spray containing oxymetazoline hydrochloride (Afrin, for example), xylometazoline hydrochloride (4-Way Long Acting Nasal Spray, for example), or phenylephrine hydrochloride (Neo-Synephrine nose drops and nasal spray, for example). Buy a less expensive generic or store brand product if it is available. **Do not use these drugs for more than 3 days.**

For fever, headaches and body aches

Use aspirin or acetaminophen, if needed (see pp. 268 and 318). (Also see Reye's Syndrome Warning, p. 269.)

For a cough

A *productive cough* (when you are coughing something up) should not be treated. If you have an *unproductive (dry) cough* that keeps you from sleeping, use dextromethorphan, available in Hold, St. Joseph's Cough Syrup for Children, or Sucrets Cough Control Formula. Buy a less expensive generic or store brand dextromethorphan product if it is available.

Examples of cold remedies not to use
Oral nasal decongestants (pills or syrup)

We do not recommend the use of any nasal decongestants that are taken by mouth for treatment of a cold, although a Food and Drug Administration (FDA) panel has found three ingredients safe and effective. These include ingredients in the OTC drugs Afrinol, Actifed and Sudafed, and 12 of the 18 prescription cough and cold drugs presented in this book. The reason we do not recommend them is that they all contain large amounts of amphetamine-like drugs which can increase your heart rate and blood pressure. In addition, they can make you jittery and keep you awake. By using nose drops or spray, for 1 to 3 days (**No more**), you get less than 1/25th as much of these drugs just in your nose where needed, instead of all over your body as you do when you take these drugs by mouth.

Antihistamines

Although the FDA has tentatively approved these drugs, we do not recommend the use of the following drugs *for treatment of a cold*, largely because they are ineffective for this purpose: Chlor-Trimeton and Dimetane (OTC) nor any of the prescription antihistamines (see p. 379).

The most widely read book on drugs, a standard reference for doctors called *The Pharmacological Basis of Therapeutics*, says this about the use of antihistamines for treating the common cold: **"Despite early claims and persistent popular belief, histamine-blocking drugs [antihistamines] are without value in combating the common cold."** Antihistamines also have a sedative effect.

Another reason to avoid unnecessary use of antihistamines is that older adults are more sensitive to their adverse effects. (See Chapter 2: *Adverse Drug Reactions*, p. 9.)

Eight of the 18 prescription cough and cold drugs that are in this book contain an antihistamine and are therefore classed as "Do Not Use." They include Novafed A, Ornade, Trinalin, Actifed*, Dimetapp*, Tavist-D, Naldecon, and Tussionex. All of these 8 also contain an oral decongestant.

Commonly used oral OTC cold remedies that contain an antihistamine, a decongestant, or both and are also labeled "Do Not Use" include Alka-Seltzer Plus, Chlor-Trimeton Decongestant, Comtrex, Contac, Contac Severe Cold Formula, Coricidin, Coricidin-'D', CoTylenol, Dimetane Decongestant, Dristan Advanced Formula, Drixoral, Maximum Strength Tylenol Sinus Medication, Nyquil, Pyrroxate, Sinarest, Sine-Aid, Sine-Off, Sinutab, Sudafed Plus, Triaminic Syrup, Triaminicin Tablets, and Vicks Formula 44D.

Cough — A Necessary Evil

Your lungs clean themselves constantly in order to maintain efficient breathing. Mucus normally lines the walls of the lungs and captures foreign particles, such as inhaled smoke and infecting virus particles. Hair-like cells push this out of the lungs. Coughing adds an additional, rapid-fire means of removing unwanted material from the lungs.

A cough is beneficial as long as it is bringing up material, such as sputum (phlegm), from your airways and lungs. This is called a *productive cough* and is often seen with colds, bronchitis, and pneumonia. A dry, hacking, *nonproductive* cough, on the

---

* available OTC as well

other hand, can be irritating and keep you awake at night. Cough can also be part of a chronic condition, such as asthma or emphysema, or it may be caused by cigarette smoking.

Cough resulting from a chronic condition should be evaluated by your doctor. You should also seek medical advice if your sputum (phlegm) becomes greenish, yellowish, or foul smelling; if your cough is accompanied by a high fever lasting several days; if coughing or breathing deeply causes sharp chest pain; or if you develop shortness of breath—you may have pneumonia. Anyone who coughs up blood should call a doctor.

Types of Coughs

A *productive cough* is useful in helping you to recover from a cold or flu. You should do what you can to encourage the clearance of material from your lungs by "loosening up" the mucus. This is the purpose of an expectorant, which thins secretions so that they can be removed more easily by coughing (or "expectoration"). **The best expectorant is water**, especially in warm liquids such as soup, which thins the mucus and increases the amount of fluid in the respiratory tract. A moist environment also helps this effort. You should drink plenty of liquids and supplement this, if you can, by moistening the air with a humidifier or plain water steamed by a vaporizer. A pan of water on the radiator can help in the winter.

A *nonproductive cough* — a dry cough bringing up no mucus—may be treated with a cough suppressant, also called an antitussive. A cough that keeps you up at night or is extremely exhausting may also call for the use of one of these agents. Cough suppressants should be used in a single-ingredient product. Rest and plenty of fluids are also in order.

Cough Remedies (Not to Use)

As mentioned above, the only time a cough medicine should be used is to sup-

press a nonproductive cough preventing sleep or other activities. The only drug recommended is single-ingredient dextromethorphan. Codeine, present in many prescription cough medicines, is *not* recommended for coughs. It is addictive and likely to cause constipation, especially in older adults (see Tussi-Organidin and Tussionex).

Another ingredient in prescription (and OTC) cough products that we recommend against using is the expectorant guaifenesin (in all Robitussin products). We believe guaifenesin lacks evidence of effectiveness in loosening secretions (see Entex, Entex LA, and Robitussins).

Fever, Headache, and Muscle Aches

Fever, headache, and muscle aches are sometimes fellow travelers of the common cold. They are best treated without drugs—in other words, with rest and adequate fluids—or with plain aspirin or acetaminophen. (A generic or store brand is as effective as heavily advertised brand names like Bayer, Datril, and Tylenol and generally costs less.)

Never give aspirin, however, to a feverish person under 40 years old: he or she may have influenza rather than a cold. There is strong evidence that young people who take aspirin when they have flu (or chicken pox) have a greatly increased risk of later getting Reye's syndrome. This is a rather rare but potentially fatal disease that often leaves its victims impaired for life, if they survive.

In addition, a fever that climbs above 103°F (39.4°C) calls for calling a doctor, as does a fever at or above 100°F (38°C) that lasts for more than 4 days. Under either of these circumstances, the patient probably does not have a cold.

Seek medical help when any of the following occur:
❏ A fever greater than 101° F (38.3° C) accompanied by shaking chills and coughing up thick phlegm (especially if greenish or foul smelling)

❑ Sharp chest pain when you take a deep breath
❑ Cold-like symptoms that do not improve after 7 days
❑ Any fever greater than 103°F or 39.4°C
❑ Coughing up blood
❑ A painful throat with any of the following
  1) Pus (yellowish-white spots) on the tonsils or the throat
  2) Fever greater than 101° F (38.3° C)
  3) Swollen or tender glands or bumps in the front of the neck
  4) Exposure to someone who has a documented case of "strep" throat
  5) A rash that came during or after a sore throat
  6) A history of rheumatic fever, rheumatic heart disease, kidney disease, or chronic lung disease such as emphysema or chronic bronchitis

Allergy and Hay Fever

If you suffer from an itchy and runny nose, watery eyes, sneezing, and a tickle in the back of your throat, then you probably have an allergy. An allergy means a "hypersensitivity" to a particular substance called an "allergen."

Hypersensitivity means that the body's immune system, which defends against infection, disease, and foreign bodies, reacts inappropriately to the allergen. Examples of common allergens are pollen, mold, ragweed, dust, feathers, cat hair, makeup, walnuts, aspirin, shellfish, poison ivy, and chocolate.

There are four common types of allergic responses, although many substances can cause more than one type of response in a given person:
◆ Itchy and runny nose, watery eyes, sneezing, and a tickle in the back of your throat. This type of allergy is sometimes called *allergic rhinitis* and is commonly caused by exposure to allergens in the air, such as pollen, dust, and animal feathers or hair. It is called "hay fever" when it occurs seasonally, such as in

response to ragweed in the fall.
◆ Hives or other skin reactions. These commonly result from something you eat or from skin exposure to an allergenic substance, such as poison ivy or chemicals on the job or in your hobby shop. Allergic skin reactions may also follow insect bites or an emotional disturbance.
◆ Asthma (see p. 388).
◆ Sudden, generalized itching, rapidly followed by difficulty breathing, and possible shock (extremely low blood pressure) or death. This rare and serious allergic response, called *anaphylaxis*, usually occurs as a response to certain injections (including allergy shots), drugs (including antibiotics such as penicillin and many arthritis drugs especially Tolectin/tolmetin), and insect bites as from a bee or wasp. This reaction may become increasingly severe with repeated exposures. Anaphylaxis is a medical emergency requiring an *immediate* trip to an emergency room, clinic, or doctor's office. **If you are likely to have an anaphylactic response to an allergen, such as a bee sting, in a locale where medical attention may be out of reach, you should obtain a prescription from a doctor for an emergency kit containing injectable epinephrine to keep with you, and learn how to use it.**

How to Treat Allergic Symptoms
The best way to treat an allergy is to discover its cause and, if possible, to avoid the substance. Sometimes this is easy, but in many cases it is not. If, for example, your eyes swell, your nose runs, and you break out in hives each time you are around cats, avoid cats and you have solved your problem.

If, however, you sneeze during one particular season (typically, late spring, summer, or fall) each year or all year round, there is not too much you can do to avoid the pollens, dust or grass particles in the air. Some people find relief in an indoor retreat where it is cooler, closed, and less dusty, but this is not always possible.

If you can't seem to figure out the cause of your allergy, have tried eliminating most of the common allergens from your environment, and are still suffering significant discomfort, you may have to see your doctor or another health professional. It is possible that you may be an appropriate candidate for skin testing, and may be referred to a doctor specializing in allergies.

Beware of the allergist who sends you home with a long list of substances to avoid because they gave positive patch tests. Even if you avoid all of them, you may be left with your allergy if none of the ones on the list is the particular one responsible for your symptoms.

When identifying the cause of your allergy is not possible, then you may choose to treat the symptoms. Because allergy symptoms are caused primarily by the release of a chemical in your body called *histamine*, a class of drugs known as the *antihistamines* is the most effective initial treatment available. We recommend that you use antihistamines in a single-ingredient preparation to treat your symptoms.

Allergic rhinitis should not be treated with topical nasal decongestants (drops, sprays, and inhalers), that are recommended for treating the *temporary* stuffy nose of a cold. Allergies are long-term conditions, lasting for weeks, months, or years, and use of these topical decongestants for more than a few days can lead to rebound congestion (an increase in nasal stuffiness after the medication wears off) and sometimes permanent damage to the membranes lining the nose. If you think your congestion is caused by allergies, don't use an OTC nasal spray, or you may eventually find that you can't breathe through your nose without it.

Drugs for allergy
Antihistamines
Of the products sold for allergy, we recommend that you **use a single-ingredient product containing only an antihistamine.** Antihistamines are the most effective ingredients you can buy for treating an allergy, and you will minimize the side effects by buying the single-ingredient formulation.

A major side effect of antihistamines is drowsiness. If they make you drowsy, you should avoid driving a motor vehicle or operating heavy machinery while taking these drugs. Even if they don't make you drowsy, they may still slow your reaction time. Additionally, keep in mind that drowsiness is increased dramatically by adding other sedatives, including alcoholic beverages.

The amount of drowsiness produced by an antihistamine differs depending on the person who takes it and the antihistamine that is used. Of antihistamines classified by the FDA as safe and effective for OTC use, **those causing the least drowsiness are chlorpheniramine maleate, brompheniramine maleate, pheniramine maleate and clemastine.** For daytime use, we urge you to use one of these.

Other FDA-approved antihistamines, causing somewhat more sedation, are pyrilamine maleate and thonzylamine maleate. Those causing a great deal of drowsiness include diphenhydramine hydrochloride and doxylamine succinate, which are the ingredients in currently available OTC sleep aids.

The advent of the less-sedating but, as it turns out, potentially more dangerous prescription antihistamines such as astemizole and terfenadine has lessened the tendency of physicians and patients to use the lowest possible dose of the older, less expensive and safer antihistamines such as chlorpheniramine maleate, the active ingredient in Chlor-Trimeton and dozens of other prescription and over-the-counter allergy medicines. By trying a lower dose, you may find that you significantly reduce the sedating effects and avoid the possible danger and expense of astemizole and terfenadine

Another common side effect of antihistamines is dryness of the mouth, nose, and throat. Other less common side effects include blurred vision, dizziness, loss of appetite, nausea, upset stomach, low blood pressure, headache, and loss of coordination. Difficulty in urinating is often a problem in older men with enlarged prostate glands. Antihistamines occasionally cause nervousness, restlessness, or insomnia, especially in children.

For antihistamine treatment of allergies, your first choice should be a low dose of chlorpheniramine maleate or brompheniramine maleate, available in OTC single-ingredient products such as Chlor-Trimeton or Dimetane or generically. Check the label and be sure that nothing else is in the product. Chlor-Trimeton Decongestant or Dimetane Decongestant both contain additional ingredients which

Antihistamine Costs[1] for 14 Days Treatment

brompheniramine maleate	generic	$ 1.88
	Dimetane	$ 6.91
chlorpheniramine maleate	generic	$ 2.45
	Chlor-trimeton	$ 9.28
clemastine	Tavist	$25.38
diphenydramine	generic	$ 4.10
	Benadryl	$21.74
astemizole	Hismanal	$22.29
ciproheptadine	Periactin	$20.70
terfenadine	Seldane	$22.92

are not necessary for the treatment of allergy. Less-expensive store brand or generic equivalents are often available and should be purchased if possible. If you can't find them, ask the pharmacist; he or she should have them behind the counter if they are not on display.

You should not use antihistamines for self-medication if you have asthma, glaucoma, or difficulty urinating due to enlargement of the prostate gland.

Nasal decongestants
Many over-the-counter products sold for allergies contain amphetamine-like nasal

decongestants, such as pseudoephedrine hydrochloride or ingredients found in many oral cold preparations (see earlier discussion on oral decongestants for colds). Some of these side effects and adverse reactions (such as jitteriness, sleeplessness, and potential heart problems) occur even more frequently when they are used to treat allergies because allergy medication is usually taken for a longer period of time than a cold remedy is.

More to the point, nasal decongestants do not treat the symptoms most frequently experienced by allergy sufferers: the runny nose, itchy and watery eyes, sneezing, cough, and the tickle in the back of the throat. They treat only a stuffy nose—not the major problem for most allergy sufferers.

Examples of OTC nasal decongestants that are labeled to treat allergy symptoms "without drowsiness" (since they do not contain antihistamines) include Afrinol and Sudafed. We do not recommend the use of these products for allergies.

Combination allergy products
As usual in the OTC market (particularly in the cold and allergy area), most products available are fixed-combination products, using a "shotgun" approach to your ailment. The majority of allergy combination products contain *antihistamines and nasal decongestants*; some also contain pain relievers. We do *not* recommend any of these for self-treatment.

It is our opinion that nasal decongestants should not be used for allergy symptoms that are appropriate for self-treatment. The likelihood of side effects is increased by taking a combination product, and decongestants are seldom useful for allergy symptoms.

Examples of OTC combination drugs for allergy, which we *cannot* recommend, are

Actifed, A.R.M., Allerest, Chlor-Trimeton Decongestant, Dimetane Decongestant, Drixoral, and Sudafed Plus. Many of the combination cold products that we urge you not to use are also marketed for allergic symptoms and hay fever. We do not recommend using any of these products for allergies either.

Asthma, Chronic Bronchitis, and Emphysema

Asthma, chronic bronchitis, and emphysema all occur commonly, may occur together, and may have similar treatments.

Asthma is a disease in which the smaller air passages in the lungs are hyperirritable. Attacks, which may be initiated by various influences, lead to narrowing of the airways and difficulty with breathing. Most asthmatics have only occasional trouble breathing. When this occurs, wheezing, chest tightness, and an unproductive cough usually accompany the sensation of shortness of breath.

Chronic bronchitis is a disease in which the cells lining the lungs secrete excess mucus, leading to a chronic cough, usually accompanied by phlegm. **Emphysema** is due to destruction of the walls of lung air sacs, leading to shortness of breath, with or without a cough. There is a fair degree of overlap between these two diseases, and they are sometimes lumped together into "chronic obstructive pulmonary disease" or COPD. Wheezing may occur with chronic bronchitis or emphysema.

Bronchitis, asthma, or emphysema may be mild. For some people, however, these diseases can become life-threatening or can cause restriction in life-style. For all people afflicted with these problems, the types of drugs prescribed to treat or prevent the attacks are quite strong. If used incorrectly, they may be very dangerous—in an immediate way—to the health of the user. **For this reason, both the diagnosis and the treatment of these disorders should be supervised by a doctor.**

Asthma attacks are commonly caused by exposure to specific allergens, air pollutants, industrial chemicals, or infection; they can be caused by exercise (especially in cold air). Asthma can be worsened by emotional factors, and the disease often runs in families. Other ailments common to many asthma sufferers, or their family members, are hay fever and an allergic skin condition called eczema.

Chronic bronchitis or emphysema is most commonly the end result of many years of cigarette smoking. Other causes include occupational or environmental air pollution, chronic lung infections, and hereditary factors.

Asthma, chronic bronchitis, and emphysema may be occupational illnesses (a problem related to the workplace). Asthma frequently occurs among meat wrappers, bakers, woodworkers, and farmers, and among workers exposed to specific chemicals. Chronic bronchitis frequently is the result of exposure to dusts and noxious gases.

You cannot diagnose yourself. Asthma, chronic bronchitis, and emphysema must be diagnosed by a doctor or other health professional. These diseases may cause symptoms similar to congestive heart failure or pneumonia, two other common conditions that cause breathing difficulties. Both may be worsened by many of the kinds of drugs used to treat asthma or COPD. Therefore it is extremely important that you have your condition properly diagnosed before starting any medication.

Treatment

The treatment of asthma or COPD, like its diagnosis, should be determined by a doctor. Attacks can be very frightening, and sufferers often overtreat themselves, especially when the desired relief has not been provided by the recommended dosage. **Do not use more—or less—than the prescribed dose of any asthma or bronchitis medication without first consulting your doctor.**

All medications for the treatment of these disorders, including those available without a prescription, should be chosen by you and your doctor together. A doctor is likely to prescribe one or more prescription drugs for the asthmatic. The currently available nonprescription (over-the-counter) drugs are not the best drugs even for the treatment of minor or infrequent asthmatic episodes. The drug of choice for treatment of occasional acute symptoms of asthma is an inhaled beta$_2$-agonist, such as albuterol (Proventil; Ventolin), pirbuterol (Maxair) or terbutaline (Brethine; Bricanyl).[2] These drugs are also commonly used for chronic bronchitis or emphysema.

Corticosteroids such as oral prednisone, or inhaled beclomethasone (Beclovent; Vanceril), flunisolide (Aerobid), and triamcinolone (Azmacort) are commonly used when severe acute symptoms of asthma do not improve after treatment with inhaled albuterol or terbutaline.[3] These are not used in COPD unless there is a component of asthma on top of the COPD.

Theophylline and aminophylline are commonly used for suppressing the symptoms of chronic asthma, bronchitis, or emphysema. Aminophylline is identical to theophylline except that aminophylline contains a salt called ethylenediamine, which has caused rashes and hives in some people. Oxtryphylline (Choledyl) is not recommended because it is no more effective than theophylline, but costs more. These drugs must be taken *exactly* as prescribed, and the level of drug in the bloodstream must be monitored by a doctor. These measures will prevent adverse effects and ensure the optimal dose.

Proper Use Of Inhalers

To receive the most benefit from your inhaler, follow the directions below[4] even though they may not agree with the directions on the drug manufacturer's packaging. Always shake well before taking each dose. Remove the plastic cap that covers the mouthpiece. Hold the inhaler upright, approximately 1 to 1-1/2 inches from your lips. Open your mouth widely. Breathe out as fully as you comfortably can. Breathe in deeply as you press down on the can with your index finger. When you have finished breathing in, hold your breath as long as you comfortably can (try to hold it for 10 seconds). This allows time for the medication to treat your lungs before you breath it out. If you have difficulty with hand-breath coordination, as many people do, ask your doctor for an "add-on" device that attaches to your inhaler. It allows you to close your lips around the inhaler, yet still receive the full therapeutic benefit from that dose.

If your doctor has told you to take more than one puff at each treatment, wait one minute, shake the can again, and repeat. If you also take a bronchodilator, in addition to the corticosteroids, you should inhale the bronchodilator first. Wait *15 minutes* before inhaling the corticosteroids. This allows more corticosteroid to be absorbed in the lungs.

Your inhaler should be cleaned *every* day. To do this properly, remove the can from the plastic case. Under warm running water, rinse the plastic case and cap. Dry thoroughly. Using a gentle, twisting motion, replace the metal can into the case. Put the cap on the mouthpiece.

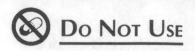 **DO NOT USE**

Alternative treatment: See Cold, Cough, Allergy, and Hay Fever, p. 382.

Triprolidine and Pseudoephedrine (combined)
ACTIFED (Burroughs Wellcome)

Family: Cold and Allergy Drugs (see p. 382)

This combination of triprolidine (trye *proe* li deen) and pseudoephedrine (soo doe e *fed* rin) is marketed as a drug that relieves congestion and other problems caused by allergies and the common cold. Actifed, a brand-name product, is advertised as a remedy for sneezing, runny nose, and other symptoms of nasal congestion. **You should not use it.** Fixed-combination products containing an antihistamine (triprolidine) and a decongestant (pseudoephedrine) exemplify the "shotgun" approach to treating cold and allergy symptoms, which are better treated with individual drugs for individual symptoms. **The combination lacks clinical evidence of effectiveness.**

If you want to treat congestion caused by an allergy, the best treatment is an antihistamine such as triprolidine. If you want to treat congestion caused by a cold, the best treatment is a decongestant nose spray or nose drops. There is no reason to combine an antihistamine and a decongestant in one product.

Triprolidine is an effective antihistamine for treating hay fever and other allergies. If you have congestion caused by an allergy, taking triprolidine or another antihistamine alone will help. There is no satisfactory evidence that allergy patients benefit from adding a decongestant such as pseudoephedrine to an antihistamine. Triprolidine can cause drowsiness, loss of coordination, mental inattention, and dizziness.[5]

If your congestion is caused by a cold rather than an allergy, you can use decongestant nasal sprays or drops such as phenylephrine, oxymetazoline, or xylometazoline, all available without a prescription. Any of these is a better choice than a drug like pseudoephedrine, which can have dangerous side effects because you take it by mouth and it affects your whole body. Do not use decongestant nasal sprays or drops longer than 3 days (see p. 382).

Warning
Pseudoephedrine can cause or worsen high blood pressure. It is especially dangerous for people who have high blood pressure, heart disease, diabetes, or thyroid disease. People over 60 are more likely than younger people to experience effects on the heart and blood pressure, restlessness, nervousness, and confusion. Do not use pseudoephedrine during or within 14 days following administration of monoamine oxidase (MAO) inhibitors.

Warning: Special Mental and Physical Adverse Effects
Older adults are especially sensitive to the harmful anticholinergic effects of antihistamines such as triprolidine. Drugs in this family should not be used unless absolutely necessary.

Mental Effects: confusion, delirium, short-term memory problems, disorientation, and impaired attention.

Physical Effects: dry mouth, constipation, difficulty urinating (especially for a man with an enlarged prostate), blurred vision, decreased sweating with increased body temperature, sexual dysfunction, and worsening of glaucoma.

Chlorpheniramine
ALERMINE (Reid-Rowell)
CHLOR-TRIMETON (Schering)

Generic: available

Family: Antihistamines (see p. 382)

Chlorpheniramine (klor fen *eer* a meen) relieves the symptoms of hay fever and other allergic reactions. **Do not use it to treat a cold.** Colds and allergies have different causes, and chlorpheniramine is not effective against either the cause of a cold or its symptoms. In fact, the drug can make a cold or cough worse by thickening nasal secretions and drying mucous membranes. It also causes drowsiness, which is a problem for anyone who must remain alert.

Chlorpheniramine can cause harmful side effects, and these are more common in people over 60 than in younger people. They include confusion; dizziness; fainting; difficult or painful urination; dry mouth, nose, or throat; nightmares; unusual excitement, nervousness, restlessness, or irritabil-

---

Warning: Special Mental and Physical Adverse Effects

Older adults are especially sensitive to the harmful anticholinergic effects of antihistamines such as chlorpheniramine. Drugs in this family should not be used unless absolutely necessary.

Mental Effects: confusion, delirium, short-term memory problems, disorientation, and impaired attention.

Physical Effects: dry mouth, constipation, difficulty urinating (especially for a man with an enlarged prostate), blurred vision, decreased sweating with increased body temperature, sexual dysfunction, and worsening of glaucoma.

---

ity. If you have any of these symptoms while taking chlorpheniramine, ask your doctor about changing or discontinuing this drug. **Since older people can be more sensitive to the usual adult dose, start with a low dose. This may decrease adverse effects.**

Avoid exposure to things which trigger your allergy, such as animals, bedding, chemicals, cosmetics, drugs, dust, foods, molds, pollens or smoke. Many people with mildly red, itching eyes require no treatment. Cold compresses to the eyes may prove helpful. Using eye drops with vasoconstrictors whitens eyes for awhile, but rebound redness can occur. Misuse of vasoconstrictors sets up a vicious cycle.

Before You Use This Drug
Tell your doctor if you have or have had
❑ allergies to drugs
❑ asthma
❑ problems with urination
❑ glaucoma
❑ enlarged prostate
Tell your doctor about any other drugs you take, including aspirin, herbs, vitamins, and other non-prescription products.

When You Use This Drug
◆ **Do not use more often or in a higher dose than prescribed. Overuse increases your risk of side effects.**
◆ Do not drink alcohol or use other drugs that can cause drowsiness.
◆ Until you know how you react to this drug, do not drive or perform other activities requiring alertness.
◆ If you plan to have any surgery, including dental, tell your doctor that you take this drug.

How To Use This Drug

◆ Do not expose to heat, moisture, or strong light. Do not store in the bathroom. Do not allow liquid form to freeze.
◆ Take with food, water, or milk to avoid stomach upset.
◆ Swallow extended-release forms whole.
◆ If you miss a dose, take it as soon as you remember, but skip it if it is almost time for the next dose. **Do not take double doses.**

Interactions With Other Drugs

The following drugs are listed in *Evaluations of Drug Interactions*, 1991 as causing "highly clinically significant" or "clinically significant" interactions when used together with this drug. There may be other drugs, especially those in the families of drugs listed below, that also will react with this drug to cause severe adverse effects. Make sure to ask your doctor for a complete listing of them and let her or him know if you are taking any of these interacting drugs:

alcohol; DILANTIN; phenytoin.

Adverse Effects

Call your doctor immediately:
❏ **if you experience signs of overdose:** clumsiness or unsteadiness; dry mouth, nose, or throat; flushed or red face; shortness of breath; trouble breathing; seizures; hallucinations; trouble sleeping; severe drowsiness; faintness or lightheadedness
❏ sore throat and fever
❏ unusual bleeding or bruising
❏ unusual tiredness or weakness
Call your doctor if these symptoms continue:
❏ thickening bronchial secretions
❏ change in vision
❏ confusion
❏ difficult or painful urination
❏ nightmares
❏ loss of appetite
❏ unusual excitement, nervousness, restlessness, or irritability
❏ ringing or buzzing in ears
❏ skin rash
❏ stomach upset or pain
❏ increased sweating
❏ unusually fast heartbeat
❏ increased sensitivity to sun (rash, hives, skin reactions)

Limited Use

Aminophylline
AMOLINE (Major)
SOMOPHYLLIN, SOMOPHYLLIN-DF (Fisons)

Generic: available

Family: Asthma Drugs (see p. 388)

Aminophylline (am in *off* i lin) is used to treat symptoms of *chronic* asthma, bronchitis, and emphysema, including trouble breathing, wheezing, chest tightness, or shortness of breath. It opens airways in the lungs and increases the flow of air through them, making breathing easier.

Aminophylline is identical to theophylline (see p. 401), except that aminophylline contains a salt called ethylenediamine, which has caused rashes and hives in some people.[6] For this reason, theophylline is preferable to aminophylline if you need to take a drug in this family by mouth.

(Both drugs are also available in an intravenous form for hospital use.)

You must take aminophylline *exactly* as prescribed. Because there is a narrow range between a helpful and harmful amount of this drug in your body, your doctor must monitor your dose and the level of the drug in your bloodstream. Too little aminophylline may bring on an asthma attack; too much can lead to an overdose. The more serious signs of an overdose include seizures, irregular heart rhythms, and pounding heartbeat. Less severe signs may or may not appear before the serious ones.[7]

The preferred forms of aminophylline are the liquid and the uncoated, plain tablets. These are absorbed best by the body. The enteric-coated tablets and some sustained-release forms are unreliable. The elixir form contains alcohol.

Avoid exposure to things which trigger your allergies or asthma, such as animals, bedding, chemicals, cosmetics, drugs, dust, mold, foods, pollens or smoke. Wearing a mask reduces inhalation of drugs, pollens and smoke. Aspirin can trigger asthma in people who are aspirin-allergic, as can beta-blockers. Infections aggravate lung problems.

During epidemics of respiratory illnesses, avoid crowded places, and wash your hands to help prevent getting infected. If you have asthma, get a flu vaccination.

Note: The information on this page addresses the care of asthma that is *not* serious enough to need emergency treatment.

Before You Use This Drug
Do not use if you have or have had
- ❑ an allergy to caffeine or any other xanthine, such as theobromine found in chocolate or theophylline

Tell your doctor if you have or have had
- ❑ allergies to drugs
- ❑ alcohol dependence
- ❑ irregular heartbeats
- ❑ heart disease
- ❑ diarrhea
- ❑ fibrocystic breast disease
- ❑ stomach inflammation
- ❑ ulcers
- ❑ prolonged fever
- ❑ respiratory infections
- ❑ liver disease
- ❑ thyroid disease
- ❑ a recent low-protein, high-carbohydrate or high-protein, low-carbohydrate diet
- ❑ regularly smoked marijuana or tobacco in the last two years

Tell your doctor about any other drugs you take, including aspirin, herbs, vitamins, and other non-prescription products.

When You Use This Drug
- ◆ **Do not use more often or in a higher dose than prescribed by your doctor.** Do not change brands or dosage forms without checking with your doctor or pharmacist first.
- ◆ Reduce your intake of charcoal-broiled foods and foods that contain caffeine, such as chocolate, cocoa, tea, coffee, and colas.

Extreme caution should be used when fluoroquinolones such as ciprofloxacin (Cipro), enoxacin (Penetrex), lomafloxacin (Maxaquin), norfloxacin (Chibroxin, Noroxin), and ofloxacin (Floxin) are to be prescribed in conjunction with aminophylline or theophylline, particularly in elderly patients. Prudence would suggest that aminophylline doses be adjusted, perhaps reduced by 30% to 50% at the initiation of fluoroquinolone therapy. The reduction in dose must be guided by the clinical conditions of the patient, the use of other concomitant medication, and the baseline value of the aminophylline serum concentration. In addition, serum aminophylline levels should be obtained following the initiation of a fluoroquinolone no later than 2 days into therapy.[8]

◆ Call your doctor immediately if you get a fever, diarrhea, or the flu while taking aminophylline, because these increase your chance of developing side effects from the drug.

◆ If you plan to have any surgery, including dental, tell your doctor that you take this drug.

How To Use This Drug

◆ Take on an empty stomach, at least 1 hour before or 2 hours after meals, to increase absorption. If the drug upsets your stomach, take with food instead.

◆ Do not expose to heat, moisture, or strong light. Do not store in the bathroom.

◆ If you miss a dose, take it as soon as you remember, but skip it if it is almost time for the next dose. **Do not take double doses.**

Interactions With Other Drugs

The following drugs are listed in *Evaluations of Drug Interactions*, 1991 as causing "highly clinically significant" or "clinically significant" interactions when used together with this drug. There may be other drugs, especially those in the families of drugs listed below, that also will react with this drug to cause severe adverse effects. Make sure to ask your doctor for a complete listing of them and let her or him know if you are taking any of these interacting drugs:

allopurinol; ANTABUSE; ANTIMINTH; CALAN; carbamazepine; CHIBROXIN; cimetidine; CIPRO; ciprofloxacin; DILANTIN; disulfuram; ERYTHROCIN; erythromycin; ESKALITH; FLOXIN; FLUOTHANE; halothane; INDERAL; LASIX; lithium; LUMINAL; mexiletine; MEXITIL; MINTEZOL; norfloxacin; NOROXIN; ofloxacin; pancuronium; PCE; phenobarbital; phenytoin; propranolol; pyrantelopamate; RIFADIN; rifampin; TAGAMET; TEGRETOL; thiabendazole; tobacco; verapamil; ZYLOPRIM.

Adverse Effects

Call your doctor immediately:

❑ **if you experience signs of overdose:** bloody or black, tarry stools; confusion or change in behavior; convulsions; diarrhea; dizziness or lightheadedness; flushed or red face; headache; increased urination; irritability; loss of appetite; muscle twitching; continued or severe nausea; stomach cramps or pain; trembling; trouble sleeping; unusually fast breathing; pounding or irregular heartbeat; abnormal tiredness or weakness; vomiting blood or material that looks like coffee grounds

❑ heartburn and/or vomiting

❑ skin rash or hives

❑ chest pain

❑ decrease in blood pressure

❑ chills or fever

Periodic Tests

Ask your doctor which of these tests should be done periodically while you are taking this drug:

❑ blood levels of aminophylline

❑ lung function tests

Hydroxyzine
ATARAX (Roerig)
HY-PAM (Lemmon)
VISTARIL (Pfizer)

Generic: available

Family: Antihistamines (see p. 382)

Hydroxyzine (hy *drox* i zeen) is used to treat itching and hives caused by allergic reactions and to relieve drug withdrawal symptoms, nausea, and anxiety. It also promotes sleep and is commonly found in nonprescription sleeping pills. If you need a sleeping pill, an antihistamine such as hydroxyzine is preferable to the overprescribed and addictive benzodiazepine sleeping pills and tranquilizers such as Valium, Librium, and Dalmane (see p. 198).

Do not use hydroxyzine to treat a cold. Colds and allergies have different causes, and hydroxyzine is not effective against either the cause of a cold or its symptoms. In fact, it can make a cold or cough worse by thickening nasal secretions and drying mucous membranes. It also causes drowsiness, which is a problem for anyone who must remain alert.

Hydroxyzine can cause harmful side effects, and these are more common in people over 60. They include confusion; dizziness; fainting; difficult or painful urination; dry mouth, nose, or throat; nightmares; unusual excitement, nervousness, restlessness, or irritability. If you have any of these while taking hydroxyzine, ask your doctor about changing or discontinuing this drug. **Since older people can be more sensitive to the usual adult dose, start with a low dose. This may decrease adverse effects.**

Avoid exposure to things which trigger your allergy, such as animals, bedding, chemicals, cosmetics, drugs, dust, foods, molds, pollens or smoke. Many people with mildly red, itching eyes require no treatment. Cold compresses to the eyes may prove helpful. Using eye drops with vasoconstrictors whitens eyes for awhile, but rebound redness can occur. Misuse of vasoconstrictors sets up a vicious cycle.

Warning: Special Mental and Physical Adverse Effects

Older adults are especially sensitive to the harmful anticholinergic effects of antihistamines such as hydroxyzine. Drugs in this family should not be used unless absolutely necessary.

Mental Effects: confusion, delirium, short-term memory problems, disorientation, and impaired attention.

Physical Effects: dry mouth, constipation, difficulty urinating (especially for a man with an enlarged prostate), blurred vision, decreased sweating with increased body temperature, sexual dysfunction, and worsening of glaucoma.

Before You Use This Drug
Tell your doctor if you have or have had
❏ allergies to drugs
❏ asthma
❏ problems with urination
❏ glaucoma
❏ enlarged prostate
Tell your doctor about any other drugs you take, including aspirin, herbs, vitamins, and other non-prescription products.

When You Use This Drug
◆ **Do not use more often or in a higher dose than prescribed. Overuse increases your risk of side effects.**

♦ Do not drink alcohol or use other drugs that can cause drowsiness.

♦ Until you know how you react to this drug, do not drive or perform other activities requiring alertness.

♦ If you plan to have any surgery, including dental, tell your doctor that you take this drug.

How To Use This Drug

♦ Do not expose to heat, moisture, or strong light. Do not store in the bathroom. Do not allow liquid form to freeze.

♦ Take with food, water, or milk to decrease stomach upset.

♦ If you miss a dose, take it as soon as you remember, but skip it if it is almost time for the next dose. **Do not take double doses.**

Interactions With Other Drugs

Some other drugs that you may be taking (either over-the-counter or prescription drugs) can interact with this one, causing adverse effects. Find out from your doctor what these drugs are and let him or her know if you are taking any of them.

Adverse Effects

Call your doctor immediately:

❑ **if you experience signs of overdose:** severe drowsiness, oversedation; faintness

❑ seizures

❑ trembling or shakiness

❑ skin rash

Call your doctor if these symptoms continue:

❑ drowsiness

❑ dry mouth

Ipratropium
ATROVENT (Boehringer Ingelheim)

Generic: not available

Family: Drugs to treat bronchitis and lung disease

Ipratropium (ip ra *trop* ee um) prevents and relieves difficult breathing, coughing, and wheezing from lung diseases, such as bronchitis and emphysema. It is not approved for the treatment of asthma. It is an anticholinergic drug in the same family as atropine. Ipratropium takes about 15 minutes to work and lasts about 3 to 6 hours. So while effective for maintenance therapy, it is not useful by itself to treat asthma attacks because of its delayed onset of action. However, ipratropium may be useful with other drugs. It offers an alternative to theophylline in people with chronic obstructive lung disease.

Ipratropium enlarges the bronchial tubes, but may also enlarge the intestines.[9] It does not control symptoms nor reduce inflammation, a drawback for treating asthma according to a recent report of the International Asthma Management Project.[10]

Warning: Special Mental and Physical Adverse Effects

Older adults are especially sensitive to the harmful anticholinergic effects of drugs such as ipratropium. Drugs in this family should not be used unless absolutely necessary.

Mental Effects: confusion, delirium, short-term memory problems, disorientation, and impaired attention.

Physical Effects: dry mouth, constipation, difficulty urinating (especially for a man with an enlarged prostate), blurred vision, decreased sweating with increased body temperature, sexual dysfunction, and worsening of glaucoma.

Ipratropium may thicken secretions in the lungs, cause retention of urine, and cause or worsen narrow angle glaucoma. It does not relieve nasal congestion or sneezing. While ipratropium is often preferred for use in people over age 60, it should be used cautiously in older men with prostate problems.[11]

Before You Use This Drug

Tell your doctor if you have or have had
❑ allergies to drugs
❑ glaucoma, narrow angle
❑ prostate problems
❑ difficult urination

Tell your doctor about any other drugs you take, including aspirin, herbs, vitamins, and other non-prescription products.

When You Use This Drug

◆ Check with your doctor if symptoms do not improve 30 minutes after using ipratropium.
◆ If you plan to have any surgery, including dental, tell your doctor that you take this drug.

How To Use This Drug

◆ If you also use a beta-agonist (Alupent, Brethaire, Brethine, Bricanyl, Bronkosol, Maxair, Metaprel, Proventil, Ventolin) use it 5 minutes before using ipratropium.
◆ If you also use a corticosteroid (Azmacort, Beclovent, Vanceril) or cromolyn (Intal) inhaler, use ipratropium 5 minutes before using those inhalers.
◆ Avoid getting ipratropium in your eyes. Use a well-fitting mask, goggles, T-piece extension, or at least close your eyes.[12,13,14]
◆ Shake canister well before using. Dilute solutions before using, according to instructions.
◆ Inhale through the mouth according to instructions for the inhaler. If you use more than one inhalation, wait one minute between inhalations. Do not use more than 12 inhalations in 24 hours.
◆ If you use a spacer device or nebulizer be sure you understand the instructions for use. Ask questions and practice until you are comfortable using the device. Ask your doctor if a paper bag can be substituted.[15]
◆ If you miss a dose, take it as soon as you remember, but skip it if it is almost time for the next dose. **Do not take double doses.**
◆ Do not expose to heat, moisture, or strong light. Do not store in the bathroom. Store metered dose inhaler at room temperature. Store solutions according to instructions on the label.
◆ Discard solutions of ipratropium without a preservative within 24 hours at room temperature, or 48 hours of refrigeration.
◆ Discard solutions with preservative stored at room temperature after 7 days.
◆ Discard mixtures of ipratropium and albuterol or metaproterenol, with a preservative, after 7 days at room temperature.
◆ Discard cannisters with fluorocarbon propellants according to local waste disposal laws.

Interactions With Other Drugs

The following drugs are listed in *Evaluations of Drug Interactions*, 1991 as causing "highly clinically significant" or "clinically significant" interactions when used together with this drug. There may be other drugs, especially those in the families of drugs listed below, that also will react with this drug to cause severe adverse effects. Make sure to ask your doctor for a complete listing of them and let her or him know if you are taking this interacting drug:

cromolyn solution (If mixed with ipratropium a cloudy sludge will form. Do not use such mixtures.); INTAL; NASALCROM.

Adverse Effects

Call your doctor immediately:
❑ dizziness
❑ unusually fast heartbeat

- ❏ skin rash or hives
- ❏ large pupils
- ❏ sores or ulcers on lips or in mouth
- ❏ tremor

Call your doctor if these symptoms continue:
- ❏ constipation
- ❏ cough
- ❏ dry mouth, hoarseness

- ❏ headache
- ❏ nausea
- ❏ nasal congestion
- ❏ nervousness
- ❏ metallic taste
- ❏ unusual tiredness or weakness
- ❏ difficult urination
- ❏ blurred vision, eye pain

Diphenhydramine
BENADRYL (Parke-Davis)
SOMINEX FORMULA (Beecham Products)

Generic: available

Family: Antihistamines (see p. 382)

Diphenhydramine (di fen *hye* dra meen) is used to treat allergic reactions, coughing, insomnia, motion sickness, and Parkinson's disease. **Do not use it to treat a cold.** Colds and allergies have different causes, and diphenhydramine is not effective against either the cause of a cold or its symptoms. In fact, it can make a cold worse by thickening nasal secretions and drying mucous membranes. It also causes drowsiness, which is a problem for anyone who must remain alert.

Diphenhydramine can cause harmful side effects. These are more common in people over 60 than in younger people. They include confusion; dizziness; fainting; difficult or painful urination; dry mouth, nose, or throat; nightmares; unusual excitement, nervousness, restlessness, or irritability. If you have any of these symptoms while taking diphenhydramine, ask your doctor about changing or discontinuing this drug. **Since older people can be more sensitive to the usual adult dose, start with a low dose. This may decrease adverse effects.**

Avoid exposure to things which trigger your allergy, such as animals, bedding, chemicals, cosmetics, drugs, dust, foods, molds, pollens or smoke. Many people with mildly red, itching eyes require no treatment. Cold compresses to the eyes may prove helpful. Using eye drops with vasoconstrictors whitens eyes for awhile, but rebound redness can occur. Misuse of vasoconstrictors sets up a vicious cycle.

Warning: Special Mental and Physical Adverse Effects

Older adults are especially sensitive to the harmful anticholinergic effects of antihistamines such as diphenhydramine. Drugs in this family should not be used unless absolutely necessary.

Mental Effects: confusion, delirium, short-term memory problems, disorientation, and impaired attention.

Physical Effects: dry mouth, constipation, difficulty urinating (especially for a man with an enlarged prostate), blurred vision, decreased sweating with increased body temperature, sexual dysfunction, and worsening of glaucoma.

Before You Use This Drug

Tell your doctor if you have or have had
❑ allergies to drugs
❑ asthma
❑ problems with urination
❑ glaucoma
❑ enlarged prostate
Tell your doctor about any other drugs you take, including aspirin, herbs, vitamins, and other non-prescription products.

When You Use This Drug

◆ **Do not use more often or in a higher dose than prescribed. This will increase the risk of side effects and will not increase the effectiveness of the drug.**
◆ Do not drink alcohol or use other drugs that can cause drowsiness.
◆ Until you know how you react to this drug, do not drive or perform other activities requiring alertness.
◆ If you plan to have any surgery, including dental, tell your doctor that you take this drug.

How To Use This Drug

◆ Do not expose to heat, moisture, or strong light. Do not store in the bathroom. Do not allow liquid form to freeze.
◆ Take with food, water, or milk to decrease stomach irritation.
◆ Swallow extended-release forms whole.
◆ If you miss a dose, take it as soon as you remember, but skip it if it is almost time for the next dose. **Do not take double doses.**

Interactions With Other Drugs

The following drugs are listed in *Evaluations of Drug Interactions,* 1991 as causing "highly clinically significant" or "clinically significant" interactions when used together with this drug. There may be other drugs, especially those in the families of drugs listed below, that also will react with this drug to cause severe adverse effects. Make sure to ask your doctor for a complete listing of them and let her or him know if you are taking any of these interacting drugs:

alcohol, ethyl; DILANTIN; phenytoin; RESTORIL; temazepam.

Adverse Effects

Call your doctor immediately:
❑ if you experience signs of overdose: clumsiness or unsteadiness; dry mouth, nose, or throat; flushed or red face; shortness of breath; trouble breathing; seizures; hallucinations; trouble sleeping; severe drowsiness; faintness or lightheadedness
❑ sore throat and fever
❑ unusual bleeding or bruising
❑ unusual tiredness or weakness
Call your doctor if these symptoms continue:
❑ thickening bronchial secretions
❑ change in vision
❑ confusion
❑ difficult or painful urination
❑ nightmares
❑ loss of appetite
❑ unusual excitement, nervousness, restlessness, or irritability
❑ ringing or buzzing in ears
❑ skin rash
❑ stomach upset or pain
❑ increased sweating
❑ unusually fast heartbeat
❑ increased sensitivity to sun (rash, hives, skin reactions)

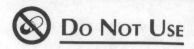 **DO NOT USE**

Alternative treatment: See Albuterol and Terbutaline, p. 422.

Isoetharine
BETA-2 (Nephron)
BRONKOSOL, BRONKOMETER (Winthrop-Breon)

Family: Asthma Drugs (see p. 388)

Isoetharine (eye soe *eth* a reen) is used to treat mild asthma, chronic bronchitis, emphysema, or occasional spasms of the airways called bronchospasm. If you have any of these conditions, the best drug to use is either albuterol or terbutaline (see p. 422), rather than isoetharine.

Isoetharine is an older inhaled drug that lasts for a shorter time than albuterol (see p. 422).[16] It is more likely to cause high blood pressure and an increase in your heart rate than the similar drugs albuterol, metaproterenol, and terbutaline.[17] If you are using isoetharine and have side effects, ask your doctor to change your inhalant to albuterol or terbutaline.

Whichever drug you take, use only the inhaled forms. Do not use the tablets, capsules, or liquids. Because these forms are swallowed, the drug is distributed throughout the body, increasing the risk of side effects. An inhaler deposits most of the drug in the lungs, where it is needed.

Theophylline
BRONKODYL (Winthrop-Breon)
SUSTAIRE (Pfizer)
SLO-BID (Rorer)
THEOLAIR (Riker)
THEO-24 (Searle)
CONSTANT-T (Geigy)
ELIXOPHYLLIN (Forest)
QUIBRON-T-SR (Bristol)
SLO-PHYLLIN (Rorer)
SOMOPHYLLIN-CRT (Fisons)
SOMOPHYLLIN-T (Fisons)

Generic: available

Family: Asthma Drugs (see p. 388)

Theophylline (thee *off* i lin) is used to treat symptoms of *chronic* asthma, bronchitis, and emphysema, including trouble breathing, wheezing, chest tightness, or shortness of breath. The drug opens airways in the lungs and increases the flow of air through them, making breathing easier. **If you are over 60, you will generally need to take less than the usual adult dose.**

Theophylline does not take effect right away, so a faster-acting drug must be used in situations where immediate action is necessary. In these situations, such as for occasional acute asthma, the best drug to use is inhaled albuterol or terbutaline (see p. 422).

You must take theophylline *exactly* as prescribed. Because there is a narrow range between a helpful and harmful amount of this drug in your body, your doctor must monitor your dose and the level of this drug in your bloodstream. Too little theophylline may bring on an asthma attack; too much can lead to an overdose. The more serious signs of an overdose are seizures, irregular heart rhythms, and pounding heartbeat. Less severe signs may or may not appear before the serious ones.[18]

The preferred forms of theophylline are the liquid and the plain, uncoated tablets. These forms are absorbed best by the body. The sustained-release forms that you take once a day are unreliable. The elixir form

Extreme caution should be used when fluoroquinolones such as ciprofloxacin (Cipro), enoxacin (Penetrex), lomafloxacin (Maxaquin), norfloxacin (Chibroxin, Noroxin), and ofloxacin (Floxin) are to be prescribed in conjunction with aminophylline or theophylline, particularly in elderly patients. Prudence would suggest that amino-phylline doses be adjusted, perhaps reduced by 30% to 50% at the initiation of fluoroquinolone therapy. The reduction in dose must be guided by the clinical conditions of the patient, the use of other concomitant medication, and the baseline value of the theophylline serum concentration. In addition, serum theophylline levels should be obtained following the initiation of a fluoroquinolone no later than 2 days into therapy.[19]

contains alcohol. The suppository form is absorbed erratically by your body and should not be used.

Avoid exposure to things which trigger your allergies or asthma, such as animals, bedding, chemicals, cosmetics, drugs, dust, mold, foods, pollens or smoke. Wearing a mask reduces inhalation of drugs, pollens and smoke. Aspirin can trigger asthma in people who are aspirin-allergic, as can beta-blockers. Infections aggravate lung problems.

During epidemics of respiratory illnesses, avoid crowded places, and wash your hands to help prevent getting infected. If you have asthma, get a flu vaccination.

Note: The information on this page addresses the care of asthma that is *not* serious enough to need emergency treatment.

Before You Use This Drug
Do not use if you have or have had
❑ an allergy to caffeine or another xanthine, such as theobromine found in chocolate
Tell your doctor if you have or have had
❑ allergies to drugs
❑ alcohol dependence
❑ irregular heartbeats
❑ heart disease
❑ diarrhea
❑ fibrocystic breast disease
❑ stomach inflammation
❑ ulcers
❑ prolonged fever
❑ respiratory infections
❑ liver disease
❑ thyroid disease
❑ a recent low-protein, high-carbohydrate or high-protein, low-carbohydrate diet
❑ regularly smoked marijuana or tobacco in the last two years
Tell your doctor about any other drugs you take, including aspirin, herbs, vitamins, and other non-prescription products.

When You Use This Drug
◆ **Do not use more often or in a higher dose than prescribed by your doctor.** Do not change brands or dosage forms without checking with your doctor or pharmacist first.
◆ Reduce your intake of charcoal-broiled foods and foods that contain caffeine, such as chocolate, cocoa, tea, coffee, and colas.
◆ Call your doctor immediately if you get a fever, diarrhea, or the flu while taking theophylline, because these increase your chance of developing side effects from the drug.
◆ If you plan to have any surgery, including dental, tell your doctor that you take this drug.

How To Use This Drug
◆ Swallow the coated or sustained-release tablets whole. Do not crush, break, or chew them.
◆ Take on an empty stomach, (at least 1 hour before or 2 hours after meals) with **a full glass (8 ounces) of water.** Take your last dose of the day with a full glass of water at least an hour before bedtime to improve your body's absorption of the drug. If the drug upsets your stomach, take with food instead.
◆ Do not expose to heat, moisture, or strong light. Do not store in the bathroom.
◆ If you miss a dose, take it as soon as you remember, but skip it if it is almost time for the next dose. **Do not take double doses.**

Interactions With Other Drugs
The following drugs are listed in *Evaluations of Drug Interactions*, 1991 as causing "highly clinically significant" or "clinically significant" interactions when used together with this drug. There may be other drugs, especially those in the families of drugs listed below, that also will react with this drug to cause severe adverse effects. Make sure to ask your doctor for a complete listing of them and let her or him know if you are taking any of these interacting drugs:

allopurinol; ANTABUSE; ANTIMINTH; ARM A CHAR;

CALAN; carbamazepine; charcoal; CHIBROXIN; cimetidine; CIPRO; ciprofloxacin; DILANTIN; disulfuram; EES; E-MYCIN; ERYTHROCIN; erythromycin; ESKALITH; FLOXIN; flu vaccine; furosemide; ILOSONE; INDERAL; interferon; LASIX; lithium carbonate; LITHOBID; LITHONATE; LOPURIN; LUMINAL; mexiletine; MEXITIL; norfloxacin; NOROXIN; ofloxacin; PBR/12; phenobarbital; phenytoin; propranolol; pyrantel pamoate; rifampin; RIFADIN; ROFERON; TAGAMET; TEGRETOL; tobacco; verapamil; ZYLOPRIM.

Adverse Effects
Call your doctor immediately:
❑ **if you experience signs of overdose:** bloody or black, tarry stools; confusion or change in behavior; seizures; diarrhea; dizziness or lightheadedness; flushed or red face; headache; increased urination; irritability; loss of appetite; muscle twitching; continued or severe nausea; stomach cramps or pain; trembling; trouble sleeping; unusually fast breathing; pounding or irregular heartbeat; abnormal tiredness or weakness; vomiting blood or material that looks like coffee grounds
❑ heartburn and/or vomiting
❑ skin rash or hives
❑ chest pain
❑ decrease in blood pressure
❑ chills or fever

Periodic Tests
Ask your doctor which of these tests should be done periodically while you are taking this drug:
❑ blood levels of theophylline
❑ lung function tests

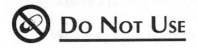 **Do Not Use**

Alternative treatment: See Theophylline, p. 401.

Oxtriphylline
CHOLEDYL (Parke-Davis)

Family: Asthma Drugs (see p. 388)

Oxtriphylline (ox *trye* fi lin) is used to treat symptoms of *chronic* asthma, bronchitis, and emphysema. It opens airways in the lungs and increases the flow of air through them, making breathing easier. Oxtriphylline is identical to theophylline, except that it contains a salt not found in theophylline. **It is no more effective than theophylline (see p. 401), yet it costs more.**[20] If you take oxtriphylline, ask your doctor to change your prescription to theophylline.

If you continue to use oxtriphylline, take it *exactly* as prescribed. Because there is a narrow range between a helpful and a harmful amount of this drug in your body, your doctor should monitor your dose and the level of the drug in your bloodstream. Too little oxtriphylline may bring on an asthma attack; too much can lead to an overdose. The more serious signs of an overdose include seizures, irregular heart rhythms, and pounding heartbeat. Less severe signs may or may not appear before the serious ones.[21]

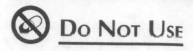 **DO NOT USE**

Alternative treatment: See Cold, Cough, Allergy, and Hay Fever, p. 382.

Brompheniramine and Phenylpropanolamine (combined)
DIMETAPP (Robins)

Family: Cold and Allergy Drugs (see p. 382)

This combination of brompheniramine (brome fen *eer* a meen) and phenylpropanolamine (fen ill proe pa *nole* a meen) is marketed as a drug that relieves congestion and other problems caused by allergies and the common cold. Dimetapp, a brand-name product, is advertised as a remedy for sneezing, runny nose, and other symptoms of nasal congestion. You should not use it, for two reasons.

First, the long-lasting tablet form of this drug is unacceptable because your body does not absorb it gradually at an even rate. This means that levels of the drug in your body may vary significantly over time rather than staying constant. Second, fixed-combination products containing an antihistamine (brompheniramine) and a decongestant (phenylpropanolamine) exemplify the "shotgun" approach to treating cold and allergy symptoms, which are better treated with individual drugs for individual symptoms. **The combination lacks clinical evidence of effectiveness.**

If you want to treat congestion caused by an allergy, the best treatment is an antihistamine such as brompheniramine. If you

want to treat congestion caused by a cold, the best treatment is a decongestant nose spray or nose drops. There is no reason to combine an antihistamine and a decongestant in one product.

Brompheniramine is an effective antihistamine for treating hay fever and other allergies. If you have congestion caused by an allergy, taking brompheniramine or another antihistamine alone will help. There is no satisfactory evidence that allergy patients benefit from adding a decongestant such as phenylpropanolamine to an antihistamine. Brompheniramine can cause drowsiness, loss of coordination, mental inattention, and dizziness.

If your congestion is caused by a cold rather than an allergy, you can use decongestant nasal sprays or drops such as phenylephrine, oxymetazoline, or xylometazoline, all available without a

> ### Warning
> Phenylpropanolamine (PPA) can cause or worsen high blood pressure. It is especially dangerous for people who have high blood pressure, heart disease, diabetes, or thyroid disease. People over 60 are more likely than younger people to experience effects on the heart and blood pressure, restlessness, nervousness, and confusion.

> ### Warning: Special Mental and Physical Adverse Effects
> Older adults are especially sensitive to the harmful anticholinergic effects of antihistamines such as brompheniramine. Drugs in this family should not be used unless absolutely necessary.
> *Mental Effects*: confusion, delirium, short-term memory problems, disorientation, and impaired attention.
> *Physical Effects*: dry mouth, constipation, difficulty urinating (especially for a man with an enlarged prostate), blurred vision, decreased sweating with increased body temperature, sexual dysfunction, and worsening of glaucoma.

prescription. Any of these is a better choice than a drug like phenylpropanolamine, which can have dangerous side effects because you take it by mouth and it affects

your whole body. Do not use decongestant nasal sprays or drops longer than 3 days (see p. 382).

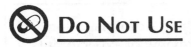 **Do Not Use**

Alternative treatment: See Cold, Cough, Allergy, and Hay Fever, p. 382.

Guaifenesin, Phenylpropanolamine, and Phenylephrine (combined)
ENTEX (Norwich Eaton)

Family: Cold and Allergy Drugs (see p. 382)

This combination of guaifenesin (gwye *fen* e sin) (see p. 425), phenylpropanolamine (fen ill proe pa *nole* a meen), and phenylephrine (fen ill *ef* rin) is marketed as a drug that relieves the symptoms of nasal and airway congestion. It contains two decongestants (phenylpropanolamine and phenylephrine) and a drug that is supposed to work as an expectorant, thinning mucus in the airways so that it can be coughed up more easily (guaifenesin). Entex, a brand-name product, is prescribed for sneezing, runny nose, and other symptoms of nasal congestion. You should not use it, for several reasons.

First, guaifenesin, the most widely used expectorant, has not been proven effective. No well-designed study has shown that it works, despite the efforts of drug manufacturers to convince people that it does.

Second, fixed-combination products containing an expectorant and decongestants exemplify the "shotgun" approach to treating cold symptoms, which are better treated with individual drugs for individual symptoms. **The combination lacks clinical evidence of effectiveness.**

Third, this product contains duplicates from a class of drugs. There is no reason to believe that two nasal decongestants in a

product make it any more effective than an adequate amount of one. Increasing the number of drugs raises the risk of unwanted side effects without increasing the benefits.

Fourth, phenylpropanolamine, one of the decongestants in this product, may have major harmful effects on blood pressure and the heart (see box below).

If you want to treat a stuffy nose caused by a cold (not an allergy), you can use decongestant nasal sprays or drops such as phenylephrine, oxymetazoline, or xylometazoline, all available without a prescription. Any of these is a better choice than a drug like phenylpropanolamine, which can have dangerous side effects because you take it by mouth and it affects your whole body. Do not use decongestant nasal sprays or drops longer than 3 days (see p. 382).

> *Warning*
> Phenylpropanolamine (PPA) can cause or worsen high blood pressure. It is especially dangerous for people who have high blood pressure, heart disease, diabetes, or thyroid disease. People over 60 are more likely than younger people to experience effects on the heart and blood pressure, restlessness, nervousness, and confusion.

If you have a cough, it is not necessarily a good idea to take a cough suppressant. Coughing clears mucous plugs and thick secretions from your airways and opens collapsed segments of your lungs. Drinking lots of liquids, especially soup and other hot drinks, and inhaling steam from hot showers and warm baths will help to loosen secretions and clean and soothe mucous membranes.

If you have a dry, irritating cough that is not producing mucus and that interferes with your sleep, you may benefit from a cough suppressant. The best non-narcotic treatment is generic dextromethorphan, which you can get without a prescription. **If your cough persists, you should see a doctor or other health professional, especially if you are a smoker.**

> A Food and Drug Administration advisory panel review of expectorants found that all nonprescription expectorants on the market lack evidence of effectiveness.

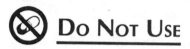 **DO NOT USE**

Alternative treatment: See Cold, Cough, Allergy, and Hay Fever, p. 382.

Guaifenesin and Phenylpropanolamine (combined)
ENTEX LA (Norwich Eaton)

Family: Cold and Allergy Drugs (see p. 382)

This combination of guaifenesin (gwye *fen* e sin) (see p. 425) and phenylpropanolamine (fen ill proe pa *nole* a meen) is marketed as a drug that relieves symptoms of nasal and airway congestion. It contains a decongestant (phenylpropanolamine) and a drug that is supposed to work as an expectorant, thinning mucus in the airways so that is can be coughed up more easily (guaifenesin). Entex LA, a brand-name product, is prescribed for sneezing, runny nose, and other symptoms of nasal congestion. You should not use it, for several reasons.

First, guaifenesin, the most widely used expectorant, has not been proven effective. No well-designed study has shown that it works, despite the efforts of drug manufacturers to convince people that it does.

Second, fixed-combination products containing an expectorant and a decongestant exemplify the "shotgun" approach to treating cold symptoms, which are better treated with individual drugs for individual symptoms. **The combination lacks clinical evidence of effectiveness.**

Third, phenylpropanolamine may have major effects on blood pressure and the heart (see below). And fourth, the long-lasting tablet form of this product is unacceptable because your body does not absorb it gradually at an even rate. This means that levels of the drug in your body may vary significantly over time rather than staying constant.

If you want to treat a stuffy nose caused by a cold (not an allergy), you can use decongestant nasal sprays or drops such as phenylephrine, oxymetazoline, or xylometazoline, all available without a prescription. Any of these is a better choice than a drug like phenylpropanolamine, which can have dangerous side effects because you take it by mouth and it affects your whole body. Do not use decongestant nasal sprays or drops longer than 3 days (see p. 382).

If you have a cough, it is not necessarily a good idea to take a cough suppressant.

Coughing clears mucous plugs and thick secretions from your airways and opens collapsed segments of your lungs. Drinking lots of liquids, especially soup and other hot drinks, and inhaling steam from hot showers and warm baths will help to loosen secretions and clean and soothe mucous membranes.

If you have a dry, irritating cough that is not producing mucus and that interferes with your sleep, you may benefit from a cough suppressant. The best non-narcotic treatment is generic dextromethorphan, which you can get without a prescription. **If your cough persists, you should see a doctor or other health professional, especially if you are a smoker.**

> ### Warning
> Phenylpropanolamine (PPA) can cause or worsen high blood pressure. It is especially dangerous for people who have high blood pressure, heart disease, diabetes, or thyroid disease. People over 60 are more likely than younger people to experience effects on the heart and blood pressure, restlessness, nervousness, and confusion.

> A Food and Drug Administration advisory panel review of expectorants found that all nonprescription expectorants on the market lack evidence of effectiveness.

Cromolyn
GASTROCOM Capsules (Fisons)
INTAL Capsules/Inhaler (Fisons)
NASALCROM Nasal Solution (Fisons)

Generic: available

Family: Allergy and Asthma Drugs (see p. 382)

Cromolyn (*chrome* o lynn) is used by inhalation to reduce the frequency and severity of bronchial asthma and bronchospasm. It is of no value in treating an asthma attack or in *status asthmaticus*. Cromolyn is also used nasally to prevent severe symptoms of allergies. It is effective for nasal congestion only when congestion is due to an allergy.[22] Use of cromolyn often reduces or eliminates the use of antihistamines, decongestants, or steroids. The International Asthma Management Project recently released a report urging the treatment of inflammation in asthma with cromolyn or corticosteroids.[23] Concerns about systemic steroid use include suppressing the adrenals, and causing glaucoma and cataracts.[24,25,26]

While cromolyn is relatively safe,[27,28,29,30,31] **older people are more likely to have reduced kidney and liver function, so a lower dose of cromolyn may be required.** Response to the cromolyn is unpredictable and it may take a month for benefits to be noticeable.

Oral cromolyn is also used to relieve symptoms of mastocytosis (abdominal pain, diarrhea, headache, itching). An eyedrop form of cromolyn (Opticrom) has been off the U.S. market for more than a year, and no date to manufacture it again has been set yet.

Avoid exposure to things which trigger your allergies or asthma, such as animals, bedding, chemicals, cosmetics, drugs, dust, mold, foods, pollens or smoke. Wearing a mask reduces inhalation of dusts, pollens and smoke. Aspirin can trigger asthma in people who are aspirin-allergic, as can beta-blockers. Infections aggravate lung problems.

During epidemics of respiratory illnesses, avoid crowded places, and wash your hands to help prevent getting infected. If you have asthma, get a flu vaccination.

Before You Use This Drug

Tell your doctor if you have or have had
- allergies to drugs
- glaucoma
- heart, kidney or liver problems
- high blood pressure
- severe or constant coughing or wheezing[32]

Tell your doctor about any other drugs you take, including aspirin, herbs, vitamins, and other non-prescription products.

When You Use This Drug

- Do not use cromolyn during an asthma attack. It may worsen the attack.
- Rinsing the mouth and gargling with water before and/or after your treatment may prevent irritation of the mouth, nose, and throat, and prevent hoarseness.
- If you also take steroid drugs, your doctor may gradually reduce your dose after you are taking cromolyn.
- Avoid drugs that may trigger asthma. Check with your doctor about using aspirin. If you use beta-blockers orally or in the eye, or ACE inhibitors check with your doctor about changing drugs, or reviewing your dose.[33,34]
- If you plan to have any surgery, including dental, tell your doctor that you take this drug.

How To Use This Drug

Ask for a demonstration of any device you are expected to use. Do not hesitate to ask or repeat questions until you feel comfortable using any inhaler device. When used for seasonal allergy begin at least one week before the season. For exercise or environmentally induced asthma, start no more than one hour before anticipated exercise or exposure.

For the aerosol for oral inhalation:
- Invert the can, then shake well.
- Exhale as completely as possible.
- Place mouthpiece into the mouth. Close lips loosely around it. Tilt inhaler upward and head backward, then inhale deeply while actuating the inhaler. (Some physicians recommend placing inhaler about 2 inches from the front of the open mouth.) Remove inhaler from mouth. Hold breath a few seconds, then exhale slowly.
- Avoid contact with the eyes.
- Clean the inhaler and plastic mouthpiece with warm water.
- Do not puncture, burn, or incinerate the container. It contains fluorocarbons.

For the capsules for oral inhalation:
- Do not swallow the capsules
- Load capsule in the Spinhaler according to instructions.
- Exhale as completely as possible, then place mouthpiece between the lips, tilt inhaler upward, head backward, and inhale deeply and rapidly with an even breath. Remove inhaler for a few seconds, then exhale. Repeat the process until all the powder is inhaled. A light dusting of powder remaining in the capsule is normal.
- Do not exhale into the device, since moisture from breath interferes with the operation.
- Be aware of adverse effects due to lactose in the Spinhaler powder (cough, wheezing, bronchospasm, irritation of the throat and lungs).
- Dismantle Spinhaler weekly and clean in warm water. Dry thoroughly.
- To improve distribution of cromolyn in the lungs, a bronchodilator is sometimes used 5 minutes prior to the cromolyn.[35,36]

For the solution for oral inhalation:
- If specified, mix with other drug solutions no more than 90 minutes before

use. If mixture changes color, or contains particles, do not use it.[37]

◆ Use with power-operated nebulizer with a flow rate of 6 to 8 liters per minute, and equipped with face mask or mouthpiece. Do not use hand-operated nebulizers, which deliver too small a volume.

For the solution for nasal inhalation:

◆ Clear your nasal passages first.

◆ Prime metered spray device prior to initial use.

◆ Spray in each nostril, while inhaling.

◆ Replace spray device every six months. Do not clean it.

For the oral capsules for dilution to swallow:

◆ Do not use these capsules in Spinhaler.

◆ Capsules are intentionally oversized to prevent spilling powder when capsule is opened.

◆ A half hour before meals, open the capsule(s) and stir in 4 ounces of hot water until dissolved, then add 4 ounces of cold water. Do not mix with fruit juice, milk, or foods. Drink the entire 8 ounces.

For all forms:

◆ Read instructions for using the devices carefully. An instruction sheet should come with each package.

◆ Check with your doctor if there is no improvement.

◆ Do not stop taking because of an attack, but do not take during an attack.

◆ To be effective cromolyn must be taken regularly. If you miss a dose, take it as soon as you remember, then space remaining doses for the day at regular intervals. **Do not take more often than prescribed.**

◆ Do not expose to heat, moisture, or strong light. Do not store in the bathroom.

Interactions With Other Drugs

Some other drugs that you may be taking (either over-the-counter or prescription drugs) can interact with this one, causing adverse effects. Find out from your doctor what these drugs are and let him or her know if you are taking any of them.

Adverse Effects

Call your doctor immediately:

❑ difficulty breathing or swallowing
❑ chest pain
❑ chills
❑ dizziness
❑ severe headache
❑ muscle pain
❑ nausea or vomiting
❑ skin rash or hives
❑ increased sweating
❑ swelling of face, lips, eyes, mouth, joints, hands, feet
❑ urge to urinate frequently, or pain on urination
❑ severe wheezing

Call your doctor if these symptoms continue:

❑ cough
❑ diarrhea
❑ drowsiness
❑ dryness or irritation of mouth or throat
❑ headache
❑ hoarseness
❑ nosebleed, or severe nasal congestion
❑ sneezing
❑ unpleasant taste
❑ watering eyes

LIMITED USE

Astemizole
HISMANAL (Janssen)

Generic: not available

Family: Antihistamines (see p. 382)

Astemizole (ast *m* is ol), a newer antihistamine, relieves symptoms of hay fever and allergies. It has not been shown to be more effective than older antihistamines, such as chlorpheniramine, and is 20 times more expensive.[38]

The advent of these less-sedating but, as it turns out, potentially more dangerous antihistamines has lessened the tendency of physicians and patients to use the lowest possible dose of the older, less expensive and safer antihistamines such as chlorpheniramine maleate, the active ingredient in Chlor-Trimeton and dozens of other prescription and over-the-counter allergy medicines. By trying a lower dose, you may find that you significantly reduce the sedating effects and avoid the possible danger and expense of astemizole.

Do not use astemizole to treat a cold. In fact, the drug can make a cold or cough worse by thickening nasal secretions and drying mucous membranes.

Compared to older antihistamines, onset of action of astemizole is slow, sometimes taking a few days.[39] Astemizole is less apt to cause drowsiness and anticholinergic effects.[40,41] However, if drowsiness or other adverse effects do occur, these may persist several weeks after the drug is stopped.[42]

Astemizole can cause harmful side effects, and these are more common in people over 60. These include headache, fatigue, weight gain, nervousness, dizziness, nau-

> *Warning: Do Not Exceed the Recommended Dose of 10 mg (One Tablet Daily)*
>
> Rare cases of serious cardiovascular adverse events including death, cardiac arrest, QT prolongation, torsades de pointes, and other ventricular arrhythmias have been observed in patients exceeding recommended doses of astemizole. While the majority of such events have occurred following substantial overdoses of astemizole, torsades de pointes (arrhythmias) have very rarely occurred at reported doses as low as 20-30 mg daily (2-3 times the recommended daily dose). Data suggest that these events are associated with elevation of astemizole and/or astemizole metabolite levels, resulting in the electrocardiographic QT prolongation. In view of the potential for cardiac arrhythmias, adherence to the recommended dose should be emphasized.
>
> Some patients appear to increase the dose of astemizole in an attempt to accelerate the onset of action. Patients should be advised not to do this and not to use astemizole on an as needed basis for immediate relief of symptoms.
>
> Since astemizole is extensively metabolized by the liver, its use in patients with significant liver dysfunction should generally be avoided.
>
> In some cases, severe arrhythmias have been preceded by episodes of fainting. **Fainting in patients receiving astemizole should lead to discontinuation of treatment and appropriate clinical evaluation, including electrocardiographic testing** (looking for QT prolongation and ventricular arrhythmia).

sea, diarrhea, abdominal pain, dry mouth, inflammed throat and eyes, nosebleed, painful joints, and sunburn.[43,44] If you have any of these symptoms ask your doctor about changing or discontinuing this drug.

Since older people can be more sensitive to the usual adult dose, start with a low dose. This may decrease adverse effects.

Avoid exposure to things which trigger your allergy, such as animals, bedding, chemicals, cosmetics, drugs, dust, foods, molds, pollens or smoke. Many people with mildly red, itching eyes require no treatment. Cold compresses to the eyes may prove helpful. Using eye drops with vasoconstrictors whitens eyes for awhile, but rebound redness can occur. Misuse of vasoconstrictors sets up a vicious cycle.

Warning: Special Mental and Physical Adverse Effects

Older adults are especially sensitive to the harmful anticholinergic effects of antihistamines such as astemizole. Drugs in this family should not be used unless absolutely necessary.

Mental Effects: confusion, delirium, short-term memory problems, disorientation, and impaired attention.

Physical Effects: dry mouth, constipation, difficulty urinating (especially for a man with an enlarged prostate), blurred vision, decreased sweating with increased body temperature, sexual dysfunction, and worsening of glaucoma.

Before You Use This Drug

Tell your doctor if you have or have had
- allergies to drugs
- asthma
- problems with urination
- glaucoma
- heart problems
- liver disease
- enlarged prostate

Tell your doctor about any other drugs you take, including aspirin, herbs, vitamins, and other non-prescription products.

When You Use This Drug
- ◆ **Do not use more often or in a higher dose than prescribed. Overuse increases your risk of side effects.**
- ◆ Do not drink alcohol or use other drugs that can cause drowsiness.
- ◆ Until you know how you react to this drug, do not drive or perform other activities requiring alertness.
- ◆ If you plan to have any surgery, including dental, tell your doctor that you take this drug.
- ◆ Protect yourself from sunburn.

How To Use This Drug
- ◆ Do not expose to heat, moisture, or strong light. Do not store in the bathroom.
- ◆ Swallow tablet whole, or break tablets in half to ease swallowing.
- ◆ Take once a day, preferably at bedtime. Abstain from food two hours before and one hour after taking astemizole.
- ◆ If you miss a dose at bedtime, you may take it soon after awakening, but be wary of drowsiness. Skip it if it is almost time for the next dose. **Do not take double doses.**

Interactions With Other Drugs

The following drugs are listed in *Evaluations of Drug Interactions*, 1991 as causing "highly clinically significant" or "clinically significant" interactions when used together with this drug. There may be other drugs, especially those in the families of drugs listed below, that also will react with this drug to cause severe adverse effects. Make sure to ask your doctor for a complete listing of them and let her or him know if you are taking this interacting drug:

ketoconazole; NIZORAL.

Adverse Effects

Call your doctor immediately:
- if you experience signs of overdose: clumsiness or unsteadiness; dry mouth, nose, or throat; flushed or red face;

shortness of breath, trouble breathing; seizures; hallucinations; trouble sleeping; severe drowsiness; faintness or lightheadedness.
- ❏ numbness in arms or legs[45]
- ❏ sore throat or fever
- ❏ unusual bleeding or bruising
- ❏ unusual tiredness or weakness

Call your doctor if these symptoms continue:
- ❏ thickening bronchial secretions

- ❏ change in vision
- ❏ confusion
- ❏ difficult or painful urination
- ❏ nightmares
- ❏ undesired weight gain
- ❏ skin rash
- ❏ headaches
- ❏ unusually fast heartbeat
- ❏ drowsiness
- ❏ swelling of tissue

Pirbuterol
MAXAIR (3M Riker)

Generic: not available

Family: Asthma Drugs

Pirbuterol (per *butte* er all) is used to prevent and treat asthma, as well as to treat bronchitis and emphysema. Within 5 minutes it begins to subdue wheezing and improve breathing. Pirbuterol controls symptoms, but does not cure any condition. It belongs to the same family as albuterol (Proventil) and terbutaline (Brethaire). According to Goodman and Gilman's *The Pharmacological Basis of Therapeutics*, there is little basis to choose one of this drug family over another.[46] As with all bronchodilators, it should be used cautiously by the elderly.[47] **If you are over 60, you will generally need to take less than the usual adult dose of this drug, especially if you have heart disease.**

Whichever of these drugs you take, use only the inhaled form. Do not take the tablets, capsules, or liquids. Because these forms are swallowed, the drug is distributed throughout your body, increasing the risk of side effects. An inhaler deposits most of the drug in the lungs, where it is needed.

Sometimes tolerance to pirbuterol develops. It can produce changes in your blood pressure, heart rate, pulse, and impede the flow of bile.[48] Fatal, paradoxical bronchospasms can occur. In fact related drugs caused epidemics of asthma deaths in other countries several years ago.[49]

Since pirbuterol does not relieve inflammation of the lungs, The International Asthma Management Project recommends the use of bronchodilators, such as pirbuterol, be kept to a mininum in the treatment of asthma.[50] Sometimes pirbuterol is used along with corticosteroids or theophylline.

Avoid exposure to things which trigger your allergies or asthma, such as animals, bedding, chemicals, cosmetics, drugs, dust, mold, foods, pollens or smoke. Wearing a mask reduces inhalation of dusts, pollens and smoke. Aspirin can trigger asthma

---

Warning
Pirbuterol can cause or worsen high blood pressure. It is especially dangerous for people who have high blood pressure, heart disease, diabetes, or thyroid disease. People over 60 are more likely than younger people to experience effects on the heart and blood pressure, restlessness, nervousness, and confusion.

in people who are aspirin-allergic, as can beta-blockers. Infections aggravate lung problems.

During epidemics of respiratory illnesses, avoid crowded places, and wash your hands to help prevent getting infected. If you have asthma, get a flu vaccination.

Note: The information on this page addresses the care of asthma that is not serious enough to need emergency treatment.

Before You Use This Drug

Tell your doctor if you have or have had
❑ allergies to drugs
❑ convulsions
❑ diabetes
❑ heart problems including angina, and coronary artery disease
❑ stroke
❑ high blood pressure
❑ smoked
❑ thyroid problems

Tell your doctor about any other drugs you take, including aspirin, herbs, vitamins, and other non-prescription products.

When You Use This Drug

◆ **Do not use more often or in a higher dose than that prescribed by your doctor.** If your condition does not improve, or worsens, call your doctor.
◆ Avoid exercises that trigger asthma attacks. Ask your doctor to recommend appropriate exercises.

How To Use This Drug

For the aerosol for oral inhalation:
◆ Invert the can, then shake well.
◆ Exhale as completely as possible.
◆ Place mouthpiece into the mouth. Close lips loosely around it. Tilt inhaler upward and head backward, then inhale slowly and deeply while actuating the inhaler. (Some physicians recommend placing inhaler about 2 inches from the front of the open mouth.) Remove inhaler from mouth. Hold breath a few seconds, then exhale slowly.
◆ Avoid contact with the eyes.

◆ Clean the inhaler and plastic mouthpiece with warm water.
◆ Do not puncture, burn, or incinerate the container. It contains fluorocarbons.
◆ If your dose is more than one inhalation, wait a full minute between inhalations.
◆ Use your pirbuterol inhaler 5 minutes before using any corticosteroid or ipratropium inhaler.
◆ If you miss a dose, take it as soon you remember, but skip it if it is almost time for the next dose.
◆ Do not expose to heat, moisture, or strong light. Do not store in the bathroom. The cannister can burst at 120°F.
◆ When discarded, do not burn in fire or incinerator.

Interactions With Other Drugs

The following drugs are listed in *Evaluations of Drug Interactions,* 1991 as causing "highly clinically significant" or "clinically significant" interactions when used together with this drug. There may be other drugs, especially those in the families of drugs listed below, that also will react with this drug to cause severe adverse effects. Make sure to ask your doctor for a complete listing of them and let her or him know if you are taking any of these interacting drugs:

FLUOTHANE; guanethidine; halothane; imipramine; INDERAL; ISMELIN; propranolol; timolol; TIMOPTIC; TOFRANIL.

Adverse Effects

Call your doctor immediately:
❑ bruising
❑ chest pain
❑ dizziness
❑ rapid heartbeat
❑ numbness in hands or feet
❑ tremors

Call your doctor if these symptoms continue:
❑ abdominal cramps or pain
❑ cough
❑ diarrhea

❑ dry mouth
❑ headache
❑ loss of appetite
❑ mood changes

❑ nausea
❑ nervousness
❑ sense of smell or taste changes

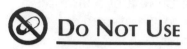 **DO NOT USE**

Alternative treatment: See Cold, Cough, Allergy, and Hay Fever, p. 382.

Chlorpheniramine, Phenyltoloxamine, Phenylpropanolamine, and Phenylephrine (combined)
NALDECON (Bristol)

Family: Cold and Allergy Drugs (see p. 382)

This combination of chlorpheniramine (see p. 391), phenyltoloxamine (fen ill tole *ox* a meen), phenylpropanolamine (fen ill proe pa *nole* a meen), and phenylephrine (fen ill *ef* rin) is marketed as a drug that relieves congestion and other problems caused by allergies and the common cold. Naldecon, a brand-name product, is advertised as a remedy for sneezing, runny nose, and other symptoms of nasal congestion. You should not use it, for two reasons.

First, fixed-combination products containing antihistamines (chlorpheniramine and phenyltoloxamine) and decongestants (phenylpropanolamine and phenylephrine) exemplify the "shotgun" approach to treating cold and allergy symptoms, which are better treated with individual drugs for individual symptoms. **The combination lacks clinical evidence of effectiveness.** Second, this product contains duplicates from each class of drugs. There is no reason to believe that two nasal decongestants or two antihistamines in a product make it any more effective than an adequate amount of one. Increasing the number of drugs increases the chance of unwanted side effects, without increasing the effectiveness.

If you want to treat congestion caused by an allergy, the best treatment is an antihis-

---

Warning

Phenylpropanolamine (PPA) can cause or worsen high blood pressure. It is especially dangerous for people who have high blood pressure, heart disease, diabetes, or thyroid disease. People over 60 are more likely than younger people to experience effects on the heart and blood pressure, restlessness, nervousness, and confusion.

Warning: Special Mental and Physical Adverse Effects

Older adults are especially sensitive to the harmful anticholinergic effects of antihistamines such as chlorpheniramine and phenyltoloxamine. Drugs in this family should not be used unless absolutely necessary.

Mental Effects: confusion, delirium, short-term memory problems, disorientation, and impaired attention.

Physical Effects: dry mouth, constipation, difficulty urinating (especially for a man with an enlarged prostate), blurred vision, decreased sweating with increased body temperature, sexual dysfunction, and worsening of glaucoma.

tamine such as chlorpheniramine or phenyltoloxamine. If you want to treat congestion caused by a cold, the best treatment is a decongestant nose spray or nose drops. There is no reason to combine an antihistamine and a decongestant in one product.

Either chlorpheniramine or phenyltoloxamine is an effective antihistamine for treating hay fever and other allergies, although only chlorpheniramine is available as a single-drug product. If you have congestion caused by an allergy, taking chlorpheniramine or another antihistamine alone will help. There is no satisfactory evidence that allergy patients benefit from adding a decongestant such as phenyl-

propanolamine or phenylephrine to an antihistamine. Chlorpheniramine and phenyltoloxamine can cause drowsiness, loss of coordination, mental inattention, and dizziness.

If your congestion is caused by a cold rather than an allergy, you can use decongestant nasal sprays or drops such as phenylephrine, oxymetazoline, or xylometazoline, all available without a prescription. Any of these is a better choice than a drug like phenylpropanolamine, which can have dangerous side effects because you take it by mouth and it affects your whole body. Do not use decongestant nasal sprays or drops longer than 3 days (see p. 382).

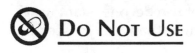 **Do Not Use**

Alternative treatment: See Cold, Cough, Allergy, and Hay Fever, p. 382.

Chlorpheniramine and Pseudoephedrine (combined)
NOVAFED A (Merrell Dow)
DECONAMINE (Berlex)

Family: Cold and Allergy Drugs (see p. 382)

This combination of chlorpheniramine (see p. 391) and pseudoephedrine (soo doe e *fed* rin) is marketed as a drug that relieves

congestion and other problems caused by allergies and the common cold. Novafed A

> ### Warning
> Pseudoephedrine can cause or worsen high blood pressure. It is especially dangerous for people who have high blood pressure, heart disease, diabetes, or thyroid disease. People over 60 are more likely than younger people to experience effects on the heart and blood pressure, restlessness, nervousness, and confusion. Do not use pseudoephedrine during or within 14 days following adminstration of monoamine oxidase (MAO) inhibitors.

> ### Warning: Special Mental and Physical Adverse Effects
> Older adults are especially sensitive to the harmful anticholinergic effects of antihistamines such as chlorpheniramine. Drugs in this family should not be used unless absolutely necessary.
> *Mental Effects*: confusion, delirium, short-term memory problems, disorientation, and impaired attention.
> *Physical Effects*: dry mouth, constipation, difficulty urinating (especially for a man with an enlarged prostate), blurred vision, decreased sweating with increased body temperature, sexual dysfunction, and worsening of glaucoma.

and Deconamine, two brand name products, are advertised as remedies for sneezing, runny nose, and other symptoms of nasal congestion. **You should not use them.** Fixed-combination products containing an antihistamine (chlorpheniramine) and a decongestant (pseudoephedrine) exemplify the "shotgun" approach to treating cold and allergy symptoms, which are better treated with individual drugs for individual symptoms. **The combination of drugs lacks clinical evidence of effectiveness.**

If you want to treat congestion caused by an allergy, the best treatment is an antihistamine such as chlorpheniramine. If you want to treat congestion caused by a cold, the best treatment is a decongestant nose spray or nose drops. There is no reason to combine an antihistamine and a decongestant in one product.

Chlorpheniramine is an effective antihistamine for treating hay fever and other allergies. If you have congestion caused by an allergy, taking chlorpheniramine or another antihistamine alone will help. There is no satisfactory evidence that allergy patients benefit from adding a decongestant such as pseudoephedrine to an antihistamine. Chlorpheniramine can cause drowsiness, loss of coordination, mental inattention, and dizziness.

If your congestion is caused by a cold rather than an allergy, you can use decongestant nasal sprays or drops such as phenylephrine, oxymetazoline, or xylometazoline, all available without a prescription. Any of these is a better choice than a drug like pseudoephedrine, which can have dangerous side effects because you take it by mouth and it affects your whole body. Do not use decongestant nasal sprays or drops longer than 3 days (see p. 382).

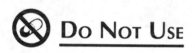 DO NOT USE

Alternative treatment: See Cold, Cough, Allergy, and Hay Fever, p. 382.

Codeine and Pseudoephedrine (combined)
NUCOFED Capsules and Syrup (Beecham)

Codeine, Pseudoephedrine, Guaifenesin, and Alcohol (combined)
NUCOFED Expectorant Syrup (Beecham)

Family: Cold and Allergy
Cough Suppressants

These combination products with codeine (*koe* deen), pseudoephedrine (soo doe eh *fed* rin), guaifenesin (gwye *fen* e sin), and alcohol are promoted to relieve cough and congestion due to respiratory illnesses. Taking the capsule or syrup form is taking two drugs, each with its own cautions, adverse effects, and drug interactions. Taking the expectorant syrup is taking four drugs, each with its own cautions, adverse effects, and drug interactions. Fixed-combination products curtail the ability to vary doses of each drug.

Codeine effectively suppresses a cough, allowing for more rest. Codeine is best reserved for dry coughs. Productive cough clears mucous plugs and thick secretions from your airways and opens collapsed segments of your lungs. Drinking lots of liquids, especially soup and other hot drinks, and inhaling steam from hot showers and warms baths helps loosen secretions and cleans and soothes mucous membranes.

Ordinarily, it is inadvisable for people with asthma or emphysema to take codeine. Do not use codeine if you have a history of serious constipation.

Guaifenesin is the most widely used expectorant. An expectorant thins mucus in the airways so it can be coughed up more easily. No well-designed study has shown that guaifenesin works, despite the efforts of drug manufacturers to convince people that it does.

Products combining both a cough suppressant and an expectorant offer no advantage over a product containing only one of these ingredients.

If you have a dry, irritating cough that is not producing mucus and that interferes

One hazard of taking codeine continuously for longer than several weeks is addiction. **Do not stop taking your drug suddenly.** With the help of your doctor, work out a schedule for slowly lowering the amount of the drug you take by about 5 to 10% each day. Keep a written record of the dosage reduction schedule with you. These steps will make it much easier to become drug free without developing distressing symptoms of drug withdrawal.

A Food and Drug Administration advisory panel review of expectorants found that all nonprescription expectorants on the market lack evidence of effectiveness.

with your sleep, you may benefit from a cough suppressant. The best non-narcotic treatment is dextromethorphan, which you can get without a prescription. **If your cough persists, see your doctor or other health professional, especially if you are a smoker.**

If your congestion is caused by a cold, rather than an allergy, you can use decongestant nasal sprays or drops such as phenylephrine, oxymetazoline, or xylometazoline, all available without prescription. Any of these is a better choice than a drug like pseudoephedrine, which can have dangerous side effects because you take it by mouth and it affects your whole body. Do not use decongestant nasal sprays or drops longer than 3 days (see p. 382).

Warning
Pseudoephedrine can cause or worsen high blood pressure. It is especially dangerous for people who have high blood pressure, heart disease, diabetes, or thyroid disease. People over 60 are more likely than younger people to experience effects on the heart and blood pressure, restlessness, nervousness, and confusion. Do not use pseudoephedrine during or within 14 days following administration of monoamine oxidase (MAO) inhibitors.

Alcohol is present in Nucofed Expectorant Syrup at 12.5%, about the same as fortified wines. A limited amount of alcohol may help you rest. However, if you are taking other medications, alcohol might interact with these. In this formulation alcohol is one of three ingredients that depresses the central nervous system. Older people, especially, should avoid these "shotgun" preparations.

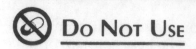 **DO NOT USE**

Alternative treatment: See Cold, Cough, Allergy, and Hay Fever, p. 382.

Iodinated Glycerol
ORGANIDIN (Wallace)

Family: Expectorants (see p. 382)

Iodinated glycerol (*eye* oh di nay ted *gli* ser ole) is promoted as an expectorant that will thin the mucus in the airways so that it can be coughed up more easily. No well-designed study has shown that this drug works, despite the efforts of drug manufacturers to convince people that it does. In addition, iodine can cause thyroid problems, and you may get a skin rash and sores if you take iodinated glycerol for a long time. This reaction may be severe or cause death in rare instances. **Do not waste your money on this drug or on any product containing iodinated glycerol.**

If you have a cough, it is not necessarily a good idea to take a cough suppressant. Coughing clears mucous plugs and thick secretions from your airways and opens collapsed segments of your lungs. Drinking lots of liquids, especially soup and other hot drinks, and inhaling steam from hot showers and warm baths will help to loosen secretions and clean and soothe mucous membranes.

If you have a dry, irritating cough that is not producing mucus and that interferes with your sleep, you may benefit from a cough suppressant. The best non-narcotic treatment is generic dextromethorphan, which you can get without a prescription. **If your cough persists, you should see a doctor or other health professional, especially if you are a smoker.**

A Food and Drug Administration advisory panel review of expectorants found that all nonprescription expectorants on the market lack evidence of effectiveness.

Warning

An unpublished study, done under the direction of the National Toxicology Program (Department of Health and Human Services) shows that iodinated glycerol, the ingredient in Organidin, causes cancer in animals. Male rats fed this compound had an increased incidence of leukemia and thyroid cancer while female mice had increased occurrence of pituitary tumors. Organidin is a classic example of risks without benefits.

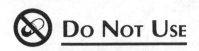 **DO NOT USE**

Alternative treatment: See Cold, Cough, Allergy, and Hay Fever, p. 382.

Chlorpheniramine and Phenylpropanolamine (combined)
ORNADE (Smith Kline & French)

Family: Cold and Allergy Drugs (see p. 382)

This combination of chlorpheniramine (see p. 391) and phenylpropanolamine (fen ill proe pa *nole* a meen) is marketed as a drug that relieves congestion and other problems caused by allergies and the common cold. Ornade, a brand-name product, is advertised as a remedy for sneezing, runny nose, and other symptoms of nasal congestion. You should not use it, for two reasons.

First, the long-lasting capsule form of this drug is unacceptable because your body does not absorb it gradually at an even rate. This means that levels of the drug in your body may vary significantly over time rather than staying constant. Second, fixed-combination products containing an antihistamine (chlorpheniramine) and a decongestant (phenylpropanolamine) exemplify the "shotgun" approach to treating cold and allergy symptoms, which are better treated with individual drugs for individual symptoms. **The combination lacks clinical evidence of effectiveness.**

If you want to treat congestion caused by an allergy, the best treatment is an antihistamine such as chlorpheniramine. If you want to treat congestion caused by a cold, the best treatment is a decongestant nose spray or nose drops. There is no reason to combine an antihistamine and a decongestant in one product.

Chlorpheniramine is an effective antihistamine for treating hay fever and other allergies. If you have congestion caused by an allergy, taking chlorpheniramine or another antihistamine alone will help. There is no satisfactory evidence that allergy patients benefit from adding a decongestant such as phenylpropanolamine to an antihistamine. Chlorpheniramine can cause drowsiness, loss of coordination, mental inattention, and dizziness.

If your congestion is caused by a cold rather than an allergy, you can use decongestant nasal sprays or drops such as phenylephrine, oxymetazoline, or xylometazoline, all available without a prescription. Any of these is a better choice

---

Warning
Phenylpropanolamine (PPA) can cause or worsen high blood pressure. It is especially dangerous for people who have high blood pressure, heart disease, diabetes, or thyroid disease. People over 60 are more likely than younger people to experience effects on the heart and blood pressure, restlessness, nervousness, and confusion.

Warning: Special Mental and Physical Adverse Effects
Older adults are especially sensitive to the harmful anticholinergic effects of antihistamines such as chlorpheniramine. Drugs in this family should not be used unless absolutely necessary.

Mental Effects: confusion, delirium, short-term memory problems, disorientation, and impaired attention.

Physical Effects: dry mouth, constipation, difficulty urinating (especially for a man with an enlarged prostate), blurred vision, decreased sweating with increased body temperature, sexual dysfunction, and worsening of glaucoma.

than a drug like phenylpropanolamine, which can have dangerous side effects because you take it by mouth and it affects your whole body. Do not use decongestant nasal sprays or drops longer than 3 days (see p. 382).

Cyproheptadine
PERIACTIN (Merck Sharp & Dohme)

Generic: available

Family: Antihistamines (see p. 382)

Cyproheptadine (si proe *hep* ta deen) relieves the symptoms of hay fever and other allergies. **Do not use it to stimulate appetite, and do not use it to treat a cold.** Colds and allergies have different causes, and cyproheptadine is not effective against either the cause of a cold or its symptoms. In fact, the drug can make a cold or cough worse by thickening nasal secretions and drying mucous membranes. It also causes drowsiness, which is a problem for anyone who must remain alert.

Cyproheptadine can cause harmful side effects, and these are more common in people over 60 than in younger people. They include confusion; dizziness; fainting;

Warning: Special Mental and Physical Adverse Effects

Older adults are especially sensitive to the harmful anticholinergic effects of antihistamines such as cyproheptadine. Drugs in this family should not be used unless absolutely necessary.

Mental Effects: confusion, delirium, short-term memory problems, disorientation, and impaired attention.

Physical Effects: dry mouth, constipation, difficulty urinating (especially for a man with an enlarged prostate), blurred vision, decreased sweating with increased body temperature, sexual dysfunction, and worsening of glaucoma.

---

difficult or painful urination; dry mouth, nose, or throat; nightmares; unusual excitement, nervousness, restlessness, or irritability. If you have any of these while taking cyproheptadine, ask your doctor about changing or discontinuing this drug.

Before You Use This Drug
Tell your doctor if you have or have had
❑ allergies to drugs
❑ asthma
❑ problems with urination
❑ glaucoma
❑ enlarged prostate
Tell your doctor about any other drugs you take, including aspirin, herbs, vitamins, and other non-prescription products.

When You Use This Drug
◆ **Do not use more often or in a higher dose than prescribed. Overuse increases your risk of side effects.**
◆ Do not drink alcohol or use other drugs that can cause drowsiness.
◆ Until you know how you react to this drug, do not drive or perform other activities requiring alertness.
◆ If you plan to have any surgery, including dental, tell your doctor that you take this drug.

How To Use This Drug
◆ Do not expose to heat, moisture, or strong light. Do not store in the bathroom. Do not allow liquid form to freeze.
◆ Take with food, water, or milk to avoid stomach upset.
◆ Swallow extended-release forms whole.

◆ If you miss a dose, take it as soon as you remember, but skip it if it is almost time for the next dose. **Do not take double doses.**

Interactions With Other Drugs

The following drugs are listed in *Evaluations of Drug Interactions*, 1991 as causing "highly clinically significant" or "clinically significant" interactions when used together with this drug. There may be other drugs, especially those in the families of drugs listed below, that also will react with this drug to cause severe adverse effects. Make sure to ask your doctor for a complete listing of them and let her or him know if you are taking this interacting drug:

DILANTIN; phenytoin.

Adverse Effects

Call your doctor immediately:

❑ **if you experience signs of overdose:** clumsiness or unsteadiness; dry mouth, nose, or throat; flushed or red face; shortness of breath; trouble breathing; seizures; hallucinations; trouble sleeping; severe drowsiness; faintness or lightheadedness

❑ sore throat and fever
❑ unusual bleeding or bruising
❑ unusual tiredness or weakness

Call your doctor if these symptoms continue:

❑ thickening bronchial secretions
❑ change in vision
❑ confusion
❑ difficult or painful urination
❑ nightmares
❑ loss of appetite
❑ unusual excitement, nervousness, restlessness, or irritability
❑ ringing or buzzing in ears
❑ skin rash
❑ stomach upset or pain
❑ increased sweating
❑ unusually fast heartbeat
❑ increased sensitivity to sun (rash, hives, skin reactions)

Albuterol
PROVENTIL (Schering) VENTOLIN (Glaxo)
Terbutaline
BRETHAIRE, BRETHINE, (Geigy)
BRICANYL (Lakeside/Merrell Dow)

Generic: available

Family: Asthma Drugs (see p. 388)

Inhaled albuterol (al *byoo* ter ole) and terbutaline (ter *byoo* ta leen) are used to treat asthma, as well as chronic bronchitis and emphysema. Within five minutes it begins to subdue wheezing and improve breathing.

They belong to the same family as pirbuterol (Maxair). According to Goodman and Gilman's *The Pharmacological Basis of Therapeutics*, there is little basis to choose one of this drug family over another.[51]

Albuterol and terbutaline can cause tremors, jitters, and nervousness, especially in older adults.[52] Albuterol has also been found to cause benign tumors in the ligament surrounding the ovaries in rats.[53]

If you are taking one of these drugs and are suffering from side effects, ask your doctor to change your prescription to the other one. **If you are over 60, you will generally need to take less than the usual adult dose of these drugs, especially if you have heart disease.**

Whichever of these drugs you take, use only the inhaled form. Do not take the tablets, capsules, or liquids. Because these forms are swallowed, the drug is distributed throughout your body, increasing the risk of side effects. An inhaler deposits most of the drug in the lungs, where it is needed.

Avoid exposure to things which trigger your allergies or asthma, such as animals, bedding, chemicals, cosmetics, drugs, dust, mold, foods, pollens or smoke.

Wearing a mask reduces inhalation of drugs, pollens and smoke. Aspirin can trigger asthma in people who are aspirin-allergic, as can beta-blockers. Infections aggravate lung problems.

During epidemics of respiratory illnesses, avoid crowded places, and wash your hands to help prevent getting infected. If you have asthma, get a flu vaccination.

Note: The information on this page addresses the care of asthma that is not serious enough to need emergency treatment.

Warning

Albuterol and terbutaline can cause or worsen high blood pressure. It is especially dangerous for people who have high blood pressure, heart disease, diabetes, or thyroid disease. People over 60 are more likely than younger people to experience effects on the heart and blood pressure, restlessness, nervousness, and confusion.

Before You Use This Drug
Do not use if you have or have had
❑ an allergy to other sympathomimetic drugs such as the decongestants pseudoephedrine or phenylpropanolamine (PPA)
Tell your doctor if you have or have had
❑ allergies to drugs
❑ heart or blood vessel disease
❑ high blood pressure
❑ diabetes
❑ enlarged prostate
❑ enlarged thyroid
❑ history of seizures, *for terbutaline*

Tell your doctor about any other drugs you take, including aspirin, herbs, vitamins, and other non-prescription products.

When You Use This Drug
◆ **Do not use more often or in a higher dose than that prescribed by your doctor. Call your doctor if you do not feel better after taking the usual dose, if you still have trouble breathing 1 hour after a dose, if symptoms return within 4 hours, or if your condition worsens.** If you plan to have any surgery, including dental, tell your doctor that you take an asthma drug.
Do not take other drugs without talking to your doctor first — especially non-prescription drugs for appetite control, asthma, colds, coughs, hay fever, or sinus problems.

How To Use This Drug
Do not expose to heat, moisture, or strong light. Do not store in the bathroom. Do not allow inhaled form to freeze.

To prevent dryness of the mouth and throat, gargle and rinse your mouth out with water after each time you use the inhaled form.

If you use more than one inhalant, use them at least 15 minutes apart. Aerosol inhalants contain chemicals called chlorofluorocarbons, which can be harmful to your health.

Be careful not to get medicine in your eyes.
◆ If you miss a dose, take it as soon as you remember, but skip it if it is almost time for the next dose. **Do not take double doses.**

For the aerosol for oral inhalation:
◆ Invert the can, then shake well. Exhale as completely as possible.
◆ Place mouthpiece into the mouth. Close lips loosely around it. Tilt inhaler upward and head backward, then inhale slowly and deeply while actuating the inhaler. (Some physicians recommend placing inhaler about 2 inches from the front of the open mouth.) Remove inhaler from mouth. Hold breath a few seconds, then exhale slowly.
◆ Avoid contact with the eyes.
◆ Clean the inhaler and plastic mouthpiece with warm water.
◆ Do not puncture, burn, or incinerate the container. It contains fluorocarbons.

Interactions With Other Drugs
The following drugs are listed in *Evaluations of Drug Interactions,* 1991 as causing "highly clinically significant" or "clinically significant" interactions when used together with this drug. There may be other drugs, especially those in the families of drugs listed below, that also will react with this drug to cause severe adverse effects. Make sure to ask your doctor for a complete listing of them and let her or him know if you are taking any of these interacting drugs:

flecainide; FLUOTHANE; halothane; imipramine; INDERAL; propranolol; TAMBOCOR; TOFRANIL.

Adverse Effects
Call your doctor immediately:
❑ **if you experience signs of overdose:** chest pain; dizziness; severe or persistent headache; increased blood pressure; persistent nausea or vomiting; fast or pounding heartbeat; nervousness or restlessness; muscle cramps
Call your doctor if these symptoms continue:
❑ nervousness, trembling
❑ difficult urination
❑ dryness or irritation of mouth or throat
❑ heartburn
❑ restlessness, trouble sleeping
❑ heartburn and unusual taste in mouth, *for albuterol*

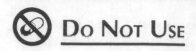 **DO NOT USE**

Alternative treatment: See Theophylline, p. 401.

Guaifenesin and Theophylline (combined)
QUIBRON (Mead Johnson)

Family: Asthma Drugs (see p. 388)

This combination of guaifenesin (gwye *fen* e sin) (see p. 425) and theophylline (see p. 401) is used to treat spasms of the airways (bronchospasm) in people with asthma, bronchitis, and emphysema. Theophylline is effective for this purpose. We do not recommend this combination because it contains an ineffective ingredient, guaifenesin.

Guaifenesin is marketed as an expectorant, a drug which supposedly thins the mucus in the airways so that it can be coughed up more easily. Although guaifenesin is the most widely used expectorant, no well-designed study has shown that it works, despite the efforts of drug manufacturers to convince people that it does. The best expectorant is water. If you have a cough or lung congestion, drinking lots of liquid (especially soup and other hot drinks) and inhaling steam from hot showers and warm baths will help to loosen secretions and clean and soothe mucous membranes.

If you have bronchospasms caused by asthma, bronchitis, or emphysema, theophylline alone is effective and is less expensive than this combination. It opens airways narrowed by bronchospasm, increasing the flow of air through them and making breathing easier. Since there is a narrow range between a helpful and a harmful amount of theophylline in your body, your doctor should monitor your dose and the level of the drug in your bloodstream. Too little theophylline may not work, bringing on an asthma attack. Too much may produce headache, nervousness, nausea, rapid heartbeats, and other side effects.[54]

A Food and Drug Administration advisory panel review of expectorants found that all nonprescription expectorants on the market lack evidence of effectiveness.

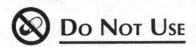 **DO NOT USE**

Alternative treatment: See Cold, Cough, Allergy, and Hay Fever, p. 382.

Guaifenesin
ROBITUSSIN (Robins)

Family: Expectorants (see p. 382)

Guaifenesin (gwye *fen* e sin) is the most widely used expectorant. An expectorant thins mucus in the airways so it can be coughed up more easily. No well-designed study has shown that guaifenesin works, despite the efforts of drug manufacturers to convince people that it does.

If you have a cough, it is not necessarily a good idea to take a cough suppressant. Coughing clears mucous plugs and thick secretions from your airways and opens collapsed segments of your lungs. Drinking lots of liquids, especially soup and other hot drinks, and inhaling steam from hot showers and warm baths will help to loosen secretions and clean and soothe mucous membranes.

If you have a dry, irritating cough that is not producing mucus and that interferes with your sleep, you may benefit from a cough suppressant. The best non-narcotic treatment is generic dextromethorphan, which you can get without a prescription. **If your cough persists, you should see a doctor or other health professional, especially if you are a smoker.**

> A Food and Drug Administration advisory panel review of expectorants found that all nonprescription expectorants on the market lack evidence of effectiveness.

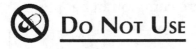 **DO NOT USE**

Alternative treatment: See Cold, Cough, Allergy, and Hay Fever, p. 382.

Guaifenesin and Dextromethorphan (combined)
ROBITUSSIN-DM (Robins)

Family: Expectorants
　　　　　Cough Suppressants (see p. 382)

This combination of guaifenesin (gwye *fen* e sin) (see p. 425) and dextromethorphan (dex troe meth *or* fan) is promoted as a cough suppressant and an expectorant. An expectorant thins mucus in the airways so that it may be coughed up more easily. Dextromethorphan is an effective cough suppressant, but there is no convincing evidence that adding guaifenesin increases

the effectiveness of dextromethorphan in any way. No well-designed study has shown that guaifenesin works as an expectorant, despite the efforts of drug manufacturers to convince people that it does.

> A Food and Drug Administration advisory panel review of expectorants found that all nonprescription expectorants on the market lack evidence of effectiveness.

If you have a cough, it is not necessarily a good idea to take a cough suppressant. Coughing clears mucous plugs and thick secretions from your airways and opens collapsed segments of your lungs. Drinking lots of liquids, especially soup and other hot drinks, and inhaling steam from hot showers and warm baths will help to loosen secretions and clean and soothe mucous membranes.

If you have a dry, irritating cough that is not producing mucus and that interferes with your sleep, you may benefit from a cough suppressant. The best non-narcotic treatment is generic dextromethorphan, which you can get without a prescription. **If your cough persists, you should see a doctor or other health professional, especially if you are a smoker.**

Terfenadine
SELDANE (Merrell Dow)

Generic: not available

Family: Antihistamines (See p. 382)

Terfenadine (ter *fen* a deen) can relieve symptoms of hay fever and other allergies. Although less sedating than older antihistamines, it has not been shown to be more effective than older antihistamines, and is potentially more dangerous, as well as more expensive.

The advent of these less-sedating but, as it turns out, potentially more dangerous antihistamines has lessened the tendency of physicians and patients to use the lowest possible dose of the older, less expensive and safer antihistamines such as chlorpheniramine maleate (see p. 391), the active ingredient in Chlor-Trimeton and dozens of other prescription and over-the-counter allergy medicines. By trying a lower dose, you may find that you significantly reduce the sedating effects and avoid the possible danger and expense of terfenadine.

Do not use terfenadine to treat a cold. Colds and allergies have different causes, and terfenadine is not effective against either the cause of a cold or its symptoms. In fact, the drug can make a cold or cough worse by thickening nasal secretions and drying mucous membranes.

Terfenadine causes less drowsiness than other antihistamines but can cause other unwanted effects, especially if you take a higher dose than necessary. Certain side effects that are more common in people

> *Warning*
> The Food and Drug Administration (FDA) recently required manufacturers to warn doctors and patients about serious heart problems caused by terfenadine. The most serious problems involve abnormal heart rhythms (arrhythmias) increasing significantly with higher blood levels of the drug. Dangerous levels of terfenadine in your blood can occur without your taking more than prescribed if you are also using erythromycin or ketoconazole with terfenadine — which raises the blood levels of terfenadine — or if you have liver disease, which impairs your ability to clear the drugs out of your body. Dizziness or fainting may be an early warning signal of a serious heart arrhythmia. Fainting should lead to immediate discontinuation of products containing terfenadine, and full evaluation of potential arrhythmias. People with liver disease or those who take erythromycin or ketoconazole should not take either Seldane or Seldane-D.

over 60 include headaches; difficult or painful urination; dry mouth, nose, or throat; nightmares; unusual excitement, nervousness, restlessness, and irritability. If you experience any of these symptoms while taking terfenadine, ask your doctor about changing or discontinuing this drug.

Since older people can be more sensitive to the usual adult dose, start with a low dose. This may decrease adverse effects.

Avoid exposure to things which trigger your allergy, such as animals, bedding, chemicals, cosmetics, drugs, dust, foods, molds, pollens or smoke. Many people with mildly red, itching eyes require no treatment. Cold compresses to the eyes may prove helpful. Using eye drops with vasoconstrictors whitens eyes for a while, but rebound redness can occur. Misuse of vasoconstrictors sets up a vicious cycle.

Warning: Special Mental and Physical Adverse Effects

Older adults are especially sensitive to the harmful anticholinergic effects of antihistamines, such as terfenadine. Drugs in this family should not be used unless absolutely necessary.

Mental Effects: confusion, delirium, short-term memory problems, disorientation, and impaired attention.

Physical Effects: dry mouth, constipation, difficulty urinating (especially for a man with an enlarged prostate), blurred vision, decreased sweating with increased body temperature, sexual dysfunction, and worsening of glaucoma.

Before You Use This Drug

Do not use if you have or have had:
❑ liver disease
❑ if you are taking erythromycin or ketoconazole

Tell your doctor if you have or have had
❑ allergies to drugs
❑ asthma
❑ glaucoma
❑ heart problems

❑ enlarged prostate
❑ problems with urination

Tell your doctor about any other drugs you take, including aspirin, herbs, vitamins, and other non-prescription products.

When You Use This Drug

◆ **Do not use more often or in a higher dose than prescribed. Overuse increases your risk of side effects.**
◆ Do not drink alcohol or use other drugs that can cause drowsiness.
◆ Until you know how you react to this drug, do not drive or perform other activities requiring alertness.
◆ If you plan to have any surgery, including dental, tell your doctor that you take this drug.

How To Use This Drug

◆ Do not expose to heat, moisture, or strong light. Do not store in the bathroom.
◆ Take with food, water, or milk to decrease stomach upset.
◆ If you miss a dose, take it as soon as you remember, but skip it if it is almost time for the next dose. **Do not take double doses.**

Interactions With Other Drugs

The following drugs are listed in *Evaluations of Drug Interactions*, 1991 as causing "highly clinically significant" or "clinically significant" interactions when used together with this drug. There may be other drugs, especially those in the families of drugs listed below, that also will react with this drug to cause severe adverse effects. Make sure to ask your doctor for a complete listing of them and let her or him know if you are taking this interacting drug:

ketoconazole; NIZORAL.

Additionally, consultants of *The Medical Letter* recommend caution when using terfenadine with drugs which affect its breakdown in the liver:

ANTABUSE; BIAXIN; cimetidine; CIPRO; ciprofloxacin; clarithromycin; disulfiram; E-MYCIN; EES; erythromycin; PCE DISPERTAB; TAGAMET; TAO; troleandomycin.

Adverse Effects
Call your doctor immediately:
- ❏ **if you experience signs of overdose**: clumsiness or unsteadiness; dry mouth, nose or throat; flushed or red face; shortness of breath; trouble breathing; seizures; hallucinations; trouble sleeping; severe drowsiness; faintness or lightheadedness
- ❏ dizziness, fainting
- ❏ sore throat or fever
- ❏ unusual bleeding or bruising
- ❏ unusual tiredness or weakness

Call your doctor if these symptoms continue:
- ❏ thickening bronchial secretions
- ❏ change in vision
- ❏ confusion
- ❏ difficult or painful urination
- ❏ nightmares
- ❏ appetite changes
- ❏ unusual excitement, nervousness, restlessness or irritability
- ❏ ringing or buzzing in ears
- ❏ skin rash
- ❏ stomach upset or pain
- ❏ increased sweating
- ❏ unusually fast heartbeat
- ❏ increased sensitivity to sun (rash, hives, skin reactions)
- ❏ cough
- ❏ drowsiness
- ❏ headache
- ❏ nausea or vomiting

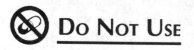 **DO NOT USE**

Alternative Treatments: See Cold, Coughs, Allergy and Hay Fever, p. 382.

Terfenadine and Pseudoephedrine (combined)
SELDANE-D (Marion Merrell Dow)

Generic: not available

Family: Cold and Allergy Drugs

This combination of terfenadine (ter *fen* a deen) and pseudoephedrine (soo doe e *fed* rin) is promoted to relieve symptoms of congestion due to allergies.

Taking this product is the same as taking two drugs, each with its own cautions, side effects, and drug interactions. Fixed combinations of an antihistamine (terfenadine) and a decongestant (pseudoephedrine) exemplify the "shotgun"

> ### Warning
> The Food and Drug Administration (FDA) recently required manufacturers to warn doctors and patients about serious heart problems caused by terfenadine. The most serious problems involve abnormal heart rhythms (arrhythmias) increasing significantly with higher blood levels of the drug. Dangerous levels of terfenadine in your blood can occur without your taking more than prescribed if you are also using erythromycin or ketoconazole with terfenadine — which raises the blood levels of terfenadine — or if you have liver disease, which impairs your ability to clear the drugs out of your body. Dizziness or fainting may be an early warning signal of a serious heart arrhythmia. Fainting should lead to immediate discontinuation of products containing terfenadine, and full evaluation of potential arrhythmias. People with liver disease or those who take erythromycin or ketoconazole should not take either Seldane or Seldane-D.

approach to treating allergy symptoms, better treated with individual drugs for individual symptoms. Fixed-combination products and long-acting forms curtail the ability to vary doses of each drug.

If you want to treat congestion caused by an allergy the best treatment is an antihistamine, whether terfenadine (see p. 426), available by prescription, or chlorpheniramine, available without prescription as a generic.

If your congestion is caused by a cold,

rather than an allergy, you can use decongestant nasal sprays or drops such as phenylephrine, oxymetazoline, or xylometazoline, all available without prescription. Any of these is a better choice than a drug like pseudoephedrine, which can have dangerous side effects because you take it by mouth and it affects your whole body. Do not use decongestant nasal sprays or drops longer than 3 days (see p. 382).

In this fixed-combination product, only the pseudoephedrine is long-acting. So if adverse effects occur, these will be harder to control.

Warning: Special Mental and Physical Adverse Effects

Older adults are especially sensitive to the harmful anticholinergic effects of antihistamines, such as terfenadine. Drugs in this family should not be used unless absolutely necessary.

Mental Effects: confusion, delirium, short-term memory loss, disorientation, and impaired attention.

Physical Effects: dry mouth, constipation, difficulty urinating (especially for a man with an enlarged prostate), blurred vision, decreased sweating with increased body temperature, sexual dysfunction, and worsening of glaucoma.

Warning

Pseudoephedrine can cause or worsen high blood pressure. It is especially dangerous for people who have high blood pressure, heart disease, diabetes, or thyroid disease. People over 60 are more likely than younger people to experience effects on the heart and blood pressure, restlessness, nervousness, and confusion. Do not use pseudoephedrine during or within 14 days following administration of monoamine oxidase (MAO) inhibitors.

LIMITED USE

Clemastine
TAVIST, TAVIST-1 (Sandoz)

Generic: available

Family: Antihistamines

Clemastine (clem *as* tine) is used to treat symptoms of allergies and hay fever, such as itching, nasal congestion, runny nose, sneezing, or watery eyes. It does not cure an allergy. **Do not use it to treat a cold.** In

fact the drug can make a cold worse by thickening nasal secretions and drying mucous membranes. It also causes drowsiness, which is a problem for anyone who must remain alert.

Clemastine can cause other harmful side effects, and these are more common in people over 60 than in younger people. They include confusion; dizziness; fainting;

difficult or painful urination; dry mouth, nose, or throat; nightmares; unusual excitement, nervousness, restlessness, or irritability. If you have any of these symptoms while taking clemastine, ask your doctor about changing or discontinuing this drug.

Since older people can be more sensitive to the usual adult dose, start with a low dose. This may decrease adverse effects. Avoid exposure to things which trigger your allergy, such as animals, bedding, chemicals, cosmetics, drugs, dust, foods, molds, pollens or smoke. Many people with mildly red, itching eyes require no treatment. Cold compresses to the eyes may prove helpful. Using eye drops with vasoconstrictors whitens eyes for a while, but rebound redness can occur. Misuse of vasoconstrictors sets up a vicious cycle.

If you need an antihistamine, chlorpheniramine or diphenhydramine are available without a prescription. The adverse effects are similar to clemastine, but the price is less (see p. 398).

> ### Warning: Special Mental and Physical Adverse Effects
>
> Older adults are especially sensitive to the harmful anticholinergic effects of antihistamines such as clemastine. Drugs in this family should not be used unless absolutely necessary.
>
> *Mental Effects*: confusion, delirium, short-term memory problems, disorientation, and impaired attention.
>
> *Physical Effects*: dry mouth, constipation, difficulty urinating (especially for a man with an enlarged prostate), blurred vision, decreased sweating with increased body temperature, sexual dysfunction, and worsening of glaucoma.

Before You Use This Drug
Tell your doctor if you have or have had
- [ ] allergies to drugs
- [ ] asthma
- [ ] problems with urination
- [ ] glaucoma
- [ ] enlarged prostate
- [ ] heart problems
- [ ] high blood pressure
- [ ] hyperthyroidism
- [ ] nasal polyps
- [ ] ulcers or other stomach problems

Tell your doctor about any other drugs you take, including aspirin, herbs, vitamins, and other non-prescription products.

When You Use This Drug
- ◆ **Do not use more often or in a higher dose than prescribed. Overuse increases your risk of side effects.**
- ◆ Do not drive or perform other activities that require alertness because this drug may make you drowsy, dizzy, or lightheaded.
- ◆ You may feel dizzy when rising from a lying or sitting position. If you are lying down, hang your legs over the side of the bed for a few minutes, then get up slowly. When getting up from a chair, stay by the chair until you are sure that you are not dizzy. (See p. 14.)
- ◆ If you plan to have any surgery, including dental, tell your doctor that you take this drug.

How To Use This Drug
- ◆ Swallow tablet whole, or break tablets in half to ease swallowing. Take with food, water or milk to decrease stomach upset.
- ◆ If clemastine causes you to be drowsy, schedule at least one dose at bedtime.
- ◆ If you miss a dose, take it as soon as you remember, but skip it if it is almost time for the next dose. **Do not take double doses.**

Interactions With Other Drugs
The following drugs are listed in *Evaluations of Drug Interactions*, 1991 as causing "highly clinically significant" or "clinically significant" interactions when used together with this drug. There may be other drugs, especially those in the families of drugs listed below, that also will react with this drug to cause severe adverse effects.

Make sure to ask your doctor for a complete listing of them and let her or him know if you are taking any of these interacting drugs:

alcohol (note: clemastine syrup contains 5% alcohol); DILANTIN; phenytoin; RESTORIL; temazepam. Additionally, the *United States Pharmacopeia Drug Information*, 1992 lists these drugs as having interactions of major significance:

amitriptyline; ELAVIL; EUTONYL; furazolidone; FUROXONE; LUDIOMIL; maprotiline; MATULANE; monoamine oxidase (MAO) inhibitors (wait at least two days after discontinuing a MAO inhibitor before taking clemastine); pargyline; procarbazine.

Adverse Effects

Call your doctor immediately:
- ❑ **if you experience signs of overdose:** clumsiness or unsteadiness; dry mouth, nose, or throat; flushed or red face; shortness of breath; trouble breathing; seizures; hallucinations; trouble sleeping; severe drowsiness; faintness or lightheadedness
- ❑ sore throat or fever
- ❑ bleeding or bruising
- ❑ unusual tiredness, weakness
- ❑ chills

Call your doctor if these symptoms continue:
- ❑ change in vision
- ❑ confusion
- ❑ difficult or painful urination
- ❑ nightmares
- ❑ appetite changes
- ❑ unusual excitement, nervousness, restlessness or irritability
- ❑ ringing or buzzing in ears
- ❑ skin rash
- ❑ stomach upset or pain
- ❑ increased sweating
- ❑ unusually fast heartbeat
- ❑ increased sensitivity to sun (rash, hives, skin reactions)
- ❑ drowsiness
- ❑ headache
- ❑ nausea
- ❑ dizziness

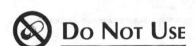 **Do Not Use**

Alternative treatment: See Cold, Cough, Allergy, and Hay Fever, p. 382.

Clemastine and Phenylpropanolamine (combined)
TAVIST-D (Sandoz)

Family: Cold and Allergy Drugs (see p. 382)

This combination of clemastine (klem *as* teen) and phenylpropanolamine (fen ill proe pa *nole* a meen) is marketed as a drug that relieves congestion and other problems caused by allergies and the common cold. Tavist-D, a brand-name product, is advertised as a remedy for sneezing, runny nose, and other symptoms of nasal congestion. **You should not use it.** Fixed-combination products containing an antihistamine (clemastine) and a decongestant (phenylpropanolamine) exemplify the "shotgun" approach to treating cold and allergy symptoms, which are better treated with individual drugs for individual symptoms. **The combination lacks clinical evidence of effectiveness.**

If you want to treat congestion caused by an allergy, the best treatment is an antihistamine such as clemastine. If you want to treat congestion caused by a cold, the best treatment is a decongestant nose spray or nose drops. There is no reason to combine an antihistamine and a decongestant in one product.

Clemastine is an effective antihistamine for treating hay fever and other allergies. If you have congestion caused by an allergy, taking clemastine or another antihistamine alone will help. There is no satisfactory evidence that allergy patients benefit from adding a decongestant such as

---

Warning: Special Mental and Physical Adverse Effects

Older adults are especially sensitive to the harmful anticholinergic effects of antihistamines such as clemastine. Drugs in this family should not be used unless absolutely necessary.

Mental Effects: confusion, delirium, short-term memory problems, disorientation, and impaired attention.

Physical Effects: dry mouth, constipation, difficulty urinating (especially for a man with an enlarged prostate), blurred vision, decreased sweating with increased body temperature, sexual dysfunction, and worsening of glaucoma.

---

phenylpropanolamine to an antihistamine. Clemastine can cause drowsiness, loss of coordination, mental inattention, and dizziness.

If your congestion is caused by a cold rather than an allergy, you can use decongestant nasal sprays or drops such as phenylephrine, oxymetazoline, or xylometazoline, all available without a prescription. Any of these is a better choice than a drug like phenylpropanolamine, which can have dangerous side effects because you take it by mouth and it affects your whole body. Do not use decongestant nasal sprays or drops longer than 3 days (see p. 382).

Warning

Phenylpropanolamine (PPA) can cause or worsen high blood pressure. It is especially dangerous for people who have high blood pressure, heart disease, diabetes, or thyroid disease. People over 60 are more likely than younger people to experience effects on the heart and blood pressure, restlessness, nervousness, and confusion.

LIMITED USE

Benzonatate
TESSALON (Du Pont)

Generic: not available

Family: Cough Suppressants (see p. 382)

Benzonatate (ben *zone* a tate) is a cough suppressant. It may be used for short-term treatment (no more than 1 week) of an unproductive cough, a dry cough bringing up no mucus, or a cough that is preventing you from sleeping. However, dextromethorphan, a less expensive cough

suppressant that is available without a prescription, is a better choice.

You should not use benzonatate or any other drug to treat a cough that is producing mucus, because this is the body's way of ridding itself of secretions and decreasing infection. If you have this kind of cough, drinking lots of liquids, especially soup and other hot drinks, and inhaling steam from hot showers and warm baths will help to loosen secretions and clean and soothe mucous membranes. For more information on treating coughs, see Cold, Cough, Allergy, and Hay Fever, p. 382.

Before You Use This Drug

Tell your doctor if you have or have had
❏ allergies to drugs
❏ asthma
Tell your doctor about any other drugs you take, including aspirin, herbs, vitamins, and other non-prescription products.

When You Use This Drug

◆ Do not use more often or in a higher dose than prescribed. Call your doctor if your cough continues after taking this drug for 1 week, or if you get a high fever, skin rash, or persistent headache.

How To Use This Drug

◆ **Swallow capsules whole. Do not chew or break them.** If this drug is released in your mouth, it can temporarily numb your mouth and throat.

◆ Do not expose to heat, moisture, or strong light. Do not store in the bathroom.

Interactions With Other Drugs

Some other drugs that you may be taking (either over-the-counter or prescription drugs) can interact with this one, causing adverse effects. Find out from your doctor what these drugs are and let him or her know if you are taking any of them.

Adverse Effects

Call your doctor immediately:
❏ skin rash, itching
❏ numbness in the chest
❏ burning sensation in the eyes
Call your doctor if these symptoms continue:
❏ drowsiness
❏ dizziness, lightheadedness
❏ nausea or vomiting
❏ stomach pain
❏ nasal congestion
❏ constipation
❏ headache

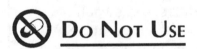 **DO NOT USE**

Alternative Treatment: See Cold, Cough, Allergy, and Hay Fever, p. 382.

Azatadine and Pseudoephedrine (combined)
TRINALIN (Key Pharmaceuticals)

Family: Cold and Allergy Drugs (see p. 382)

This combination of azatadine (a *zat* ah deen) and pseudoephedrine (soo doe e *fed* rin) is marketed as a drug to relieve congestion and other problems caused by allergies and the common cold. When taking this product you are taking two drugs, each with its own cautions, adverse effects, and drug interactions. Fixed-combinations of an antihistamine (azatadine) and a decongestant (pseudoephedrine) exemplify the "shotgun" approach to treating cold

and allergy symptoms, which are better treated with individual drugs for individual symptoms.

If you want to treat congestion caused by an allergy, the best treatment is an antihistamine, whether azatadine (Optimine) available by prescription, or chlorpheniramine, available as a non-prescription generic.

If you want to treat congestion caused by a cold the best treatment is a decongestant nose spray or nose drops. There is no reason to combine an antihistamine and a decongestant in one product. For colds, the effectiveness of anticholinergics, such as azatadine, has not been established when used in combination products. In fact, fixed-combinations and long-acting forms curtail the ability to individualize doses and adjust doses in response to adverse effects.

Used separately, azatadine is an effective antihistamine, for hay fever and other allergies. If you have congestion caused by an allergy, taking azatadine or other antihistamines available without a prescription, will help. There is no satisfactory evidence that allergy patients benefit from adding a decongestant, such as pseudoephedrine to an antihistamine. Antihistamines can cause drowsiness, loss of concentration, mental inattention, and dizziness. If your congestion is caused by a cold, rather than an allergy, you can use decongestant nasal sprays or drops such as phenylephrine, oxymetazoline, or xylometazoline, all available without prescription. Do not use decongestant nasal sprays or drops longer than 3 days. Any of these is a better choice than a drug like pseudoephedrine, which can have dangerous side effects because you take it by mouth and it affects your whole body.

Warning

Pseudoephedrine can cause or worsen high blood pressure. It is especially dangerous for people who have high blood pressure, heart disease, diabetes, or thyroid disease. People over 60 are more likely than younger people to experience effects on the heart and blood pressure, restlessness, nervousness, and confusion. Do not use pseudoephedrine during or within 14 days following administration of monoamine oxidase (MAO) inhibitors.

Warning: Special Mental and Physical Adverse Effects

Older adults are especially sensitive to the harmful anticholinergic effects of antihistamines such as azatadine. Drugs in this family should not be used unless absolutely necessary.

Mental Effects: confusion, delirium, short-term memory problems, disorientation, and impaired attention.

Physical Effects: dry mouth, constipation, difficulty urinating (especially for a man with an enlarged prostate), blurred vision, decreased sweating with increased body temperature, sexual dysfunction, and worsening of glaucoma.

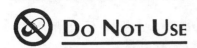 **DO NOT USE**

Alternative treatment: See Cold, Cough, Allergy, and Hay Fever, p. 382.

Iodinated Glycerol and Codeine (combined)
TUSSI-ORGANIDIN (Wallace)

Family: Cough Suppressants (see p. 382)

This combination of iodinated glycerol (see p. 418), and codeine (see p. 276) is promoted as a cough suppressant, but it should not be used.

This combination contains a narcotic cough suppressant (codeine) blended with an expectorant (iodinated glycerol). Codeine is an effective cough suppressant, but there is no evidence that adding iodinated glycerol increases the effectiveness of codeine in any way.

Iodinated glycerol is supposed to thin the mucus in the airways so that it can be coughed up more easily, but no well-designed study has shown that it does this, despite the efforts of drug manufacturers to convince people that it does. **Do not waste your money on this drug or on any product containing iodinated glycerol.** Also, iodine can cause thyroid problems, and you may get a skin rash and sores if you take iodinated glycerol for a long time. This reaction may be severe or cause death in rare instances.

If you have a cough, it is not necessarily a good idea to take a cough suppressant. Coughing clears mucous plugs and thick secretions from your airways and opens collapsed segments of your lungs. Drinking lots of liquids, especially soup and other hot drinks, and inhaling steam from hot showers and warm baths will help to loosen secretions and clean and soothe mucous membranes.

If you have a dry, irritating cough that is not producing mucus and that interferes with your sleep, you may benefit from a cough suppressant. The best non-narcotic treatment is generic dextromethorphan, which you can get without a prescription. **If your cough persists, you should see a doctor or other health professional, especially if you are a smoker.**

A Food and Drug Administration advisory panel review of expectorants found that all nonprescription expectorants on the market lack evidence of effectiveness.

Warning
An unpublished study, done under the direction of the National Toxicology Program (Department of Health and Human Services) shows that iodinated glycerol, an ingredient in Tussi-Organidin, causes cancer in animals. Male rats fed this compound had an increased incidence of leukemia and thyroid cancer while female mice had increased occurrence of pituitary tumors. Tussi-Organidin is a classic example of risks without benefits.

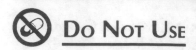 **DO NOT USE**

Alternative treatment: See Cold, Cough, Allergy, and Hay Fever, p. 382.

Iodinated Glycerol and Dextromethorphan (combined)
TUSSI-ORGANIDIN DM (Wallace)

Family: Cough Suppressants (see p. 382)

This combination of iodinated glycerol (see p. 418) and dextromethorphan (dex troe meth *or* fan) is promoted as a cough suppressant but should not be used.

This combination contains a cough suppressant (dextromethorphan) blended with an expectorant (iodinated glycerol). Dextromethorphan is an effective cough suppressant, but there is no evidence that adding iodinated glycerol increases the effectiveness of dextromethorphan in any way.

Iodinated glycerol is supposed to thin the mucus in the airways so that it can be coughed up more easily, but no well-designed study has shown that it does this, despite the efforts of drug manufacturers to convince people that it does. **Do not waste your money on this drug or on any product containing iodinated glycerol.** Also, iodine can cause thyroid problems, and you may get a skin rash and sores if you take iodinated glycerol for a long time. This reaction may be severe or cause death in rare instances.

If you have a cough, it is not necessarily a good idea to take a cough suppressant. Coughing clears mucous plugs and thick secretions from your airways and opens collapsed segments of your lungs. Drinking lots of liquids, especially soup and other hot drinks, and inhaling steam from hot showers and warm baths will help to loosen secretions and clean and soothe mucous membranes.

If you have a dry, irritating cough that is not producing mucus and that interferes with your sleep, you may benefit from a cough suppressant. The best non-narcotic treatment is generic dextromethorphan, which you can get without a prescription. **If your cough persists, you should see a doctor or other health professional, especially if you are a smoker.**

A Food and Drug Administration advisory panel review of expectorants found that all nonprescription expectorants on the market lack evidence of effectiveness.

Warning

An unpublished study, done under the direction of the National Toxicology Program (Department of Health and Human Services) shows that iodinated glycerol, an ingredient in Tussi-Organidin DM, causes cancer in animals. Male rats fed this compound had an increased incidence of leukemia and thyroid cancer while female mice had increased occurrence of pituitary tumors. Tussi-Organidin DM is a classic example of risks without benefits.

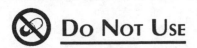 **Do Not Use**

Alternative treatment: See Cold, Cough, Allergy, and Hay Fever, p. 382.

Hydrocodone and Phenyltoloxamine (combined)
TUSSIONEX (Pennwalt)

Family: Cough Suppressants (see p. 382)

This combination of hydrocodone (hye droe *koe* done) and phenyltoloxamine (fen ill tole *ox* a meen) is promoted as a cough suppressant. The narcotic hydrocodone is an effective cough suppressant, but there is no convincing evidence that adding the antihistamine phenyltoloxamine improves the cough-suppressing action of hydrocodone in any way. In fact, antihistamines thicken lung secretions and may actually create problems for people who produce mucus with their coughs or who have difficulty breathing.

Phenyltoloxamine can cause drowsiness, loss of coordination, mental inattention, and dizziness. Hydrocodone, which is similar to codeine, can be addictive. If you have a cough that needs to be treated with drugs (see p. 382), the best non-narcotic treatment is generic dextromethorphan, which you can get without a prescription.

> *Warning: Special Mental and Physical Adverse Effects*
>
> Older adults are especially sensitive to the harmful anticholinergic effects of antihistamines such as phenyltoloxamine. Drugs in this family should not be used unless absolutely necessary.
>
> *Mental Effects:* confusion, delirium, short-term memory problems, disorientation, and impaired attention.
>
> *Physical Effects:* dry mouth, constipation, difficulty urinating (especially for a man with an enlarged prostate), blurred vision, decreased sweating with increased body temperature, sexual dysfunction, and worsening of glaucoma.

> The National Academy of Sciences-National Research Council rated this drug ineffective as a fixed combination.

Notes for Cough, Cold, Allergy, and Asthma Drugs

1. These are 1992 costs to the pharmacists for the highest recommended adult treatment as reported in *The Medical Letter on Drugs and Therapeutics*. New York: The Medical Letter, Inc., 1993; 35:7-10. Older adults will usually take lower doses.

2. *The Medical Letter on Drugs and Therapeutics*. New York, The Medical Letter, Inc., 1987; 29:11-6.

3. Ibid.

4. Newhouse MT, Dolovich MB. Control of asthma by aerosols. *New England Journal of Medicine* 1986; 315:870.

5. AMA Department of Drugs. *AMA Drug Evaluations*. 5th ed. Chicago: American Medical Association, 1983:1478.

6. Dukes MNG, ed. *Side Effects of Drugs Annual* 10. New York: Elsevier 1986:11.

7. *USP DI, Drug Information for the Health Care Provider*. 7th ed. Rockville Md.: The United States Pharmacopeial Convention, Inc., 1987:1552.

8. Grasela TH, Dreis MW. An evaluation of the quinolone-theophylline interaction using the Food and Drug Administration Spontaneous Reporting System. *Archives of Internal Medicine* 1992; 152:617-21.

9. Dukes MNG, Beeley L, eds. *Side Effects of Drugs Annual* 15, Amsterdam: Elsevier, 1991:137.

10. Randall T. International consensus report urges sweeping reform in asthma treatment. *Journal of the American Medical Association* 1992; 267:2153-4.

11. Pras E, Stienlauf S, Pinkhas J, Sidi Y. Urinary retention associated with ipratropium bromide. *DICP, The Annals of Pharmacology* 1991; 25:939-40.

12. AMA Department of Drugs. *AMA Drug Evaluations Annual* 1992. Chicago: American Medical Association, 1992:489.

13. Humphreys DM. Acute angle closure glaucoma associated with nebulised ipratropium bromide and salbutamol (letter). *British Medical Journal* 1992; 304:320.

14. Shah P, Dhurjon L, Metcalfe T, Gibson JM. Acute angle closure glaucoma associated with nebulised ipratropium bromide and salbutamol. *British Medical Journal* 1992; 304:40-1.

15. Weinberg. Asthma in primary care patients. Challenges and controversies. *Postgraduate Medicine* 1990; 88:107-10, 113-4.

16. Kastrup EK, ed. *Facts and Comparisons*. St. Louis: J.B. Lippincott Co., January 1986:173a.

17. AMA, 1983, op. cit., p. 580.

18. *USP DI*, 1987, op. cit.

19. Grasela, op. cit.

20. Kastrup EK, ed. *Facts and Comparisons*. St. Louis: J.B. Lippincott Co., July 1987:178e-179b.

21. *USP DI*, 1987, op. cit.

22. Orgel HA, Meltzer EO, Kemp JP, Ostrom NK, Welch MJ. Comparison of intranasal cromolyn sodium, 4%, and oral terfenadine for allergic rhinitis: symptoms, nasal cytology, nasal ciliary clearance, and rhinomanometry. *Annals of Allergy* 1991; 66:237-44.

23. Randall, op. cit.

24. Friedlaender MH. Current concepts in ocular allergy. *Annals of Allergy* 1991; 67:5-10.

25. Kalpaxis JG, Thayer TO. Double-blind trial of penigetide ophthalmic solution, 0.5%, compared with cromolyn sodium, 4%, ophthalmic solution for allergic conjunctivitis. *Annals of Allergy* 1991; 66:393-8.

26. Weinberg, op. cit.

27. AMA Department of Drugs. *AMA Drug Evaluations Annual* 1991. Chicago: American Medical Association, 1991:455-6.

28. Gilman AG, Rall TW, Nies AS, Taylor P, eds. *The Pharmacological Basis of Therapeutics.* 8th ed. New York: Pergamon Press, 1990:630-2.

29. Hoag JE, McFadden ER. Long-term effect of cromolyn sodium on nonspecific bronchial hyperresponsiveness: a review. *Annals of Allergy* 1991; 66:53-63.

30. Schuller DE, Selcow JE, Joos TH, Hannaway PJ, Hirsch SR, Schwartz HJ, Filley WV, Fink JN. A multicenter trial of nedocromil sodium, 1% nasal solution, compared with cromolyn sodium and placebo in ragweed seasonal allergic rhinitis. *Journal of Allergy and Clinical Immunology* 1990; 85:554-61.

31. Weinberg, op. cit.

32. O'Connell EJ, Rojas AR, Sachs MI. Cough-type asthma: a review. *Annals of Allergy* 1991; 66:278-85.

33. Ibid.

34. Weinberg, op. cit.

35. AMA, 1991, op. cit., p. 455-6.

36. Gilman, op. cit.

37. Emm T, Metcalf JE, Lesko LJ, Chai MF. Update on the physical-chemical compatibility of cromolyn sodium nebulizer solution: bronchodilator inhalant solution admixtures. *Annals of Allergy* 1991; 66:185-9.

38. *The Medical Letter on Drugs and Therapeutics.* New York: The Medical Letter, Inc., 1992; 34:9-10.

39. AMA, 1991, op. cit., p. 1609.

40. *The Medical Letter on Drugs and Therapeutics,* 1992, op. cit.

41. *USP DI, Drug Information for the Health Care Professional.* 12th ed. Rockville MD: The United States Pharmacopeial Convention, Inc., 1992:398.

42. Dukes MNG, ed. *Side Effects of Drugs Annual* 12, New York: Elsevier, 1988:142.

43. *Physicians' Desk Reference.* 46th ed. Mountvale, NJ: Medical Economics Company, 1992:113-9.

44. *USP DI,* 1992, op. cit.

45. Kaufman HS, Chang P, Chang G. Astemizole-induced paresthesia. *The New England Journal of Medicine* 1990; 323:684.

46. Gilman, op. cit.

47. Olin BR, ed. *Facts and Comparisons.* St. Louis: J.B. Lippincott Co., September 1992:173b.

48. Neilly JB, Carter R, Tweddel A, Martin W, Hutton I, Banham SW, Stevenson RD. Long term haemodynamic, pulmonary function and symptomatic effects of pirbuterol in COPD. *Respiratory Medicine* 1989; 83:59-65.

49. Windom H, Grainger J, Burgess C, Crane J, Pearce N, Beasley R. A comparison of the haemodynamic and hypokalaemic effects of inhaled pirbuterol and salbutamol. *New Zealand Medical Journal* 1990; 103:259-61.

50. Randall, op. cit.

51. Gilman, op. cit.

52. *The Medical Letter on Drugs and Therapeutics.* New York: The Medical Letter, Inc.,1982; 24:84.

53. *Physicians' Desk Reference.* 41st ed. Oradell, N.J.: Medical Economics Company, 1987:1948.

54. *USP DI*, 1987, op. cit.

Drugs For Infections

Antibiotics

For eye antibiotics, see p. 580.

Anti-Tuberculosis Drugs

Antifungal Drugs

Antiviral Drugs

Antiparasites

Antibiotics

Antibiotics (drugs used to treat bacterial infections) are overwhelmingly misprescribed in the United States. After congressional hearings and numerous academic studies on this issue, it has become the general consensus that 40 to 60% of all antibiotics in this country are misprescribed.[1] To put it simply, the majority of antibiotics are given in situations in which the infection cannot be treated by any antibiotic or a more effective and appropriate antibiotic should be used instead. This should be a major concern, since the misprescribing of antibiotics poses some real dangers to the population at large, as well as to the individuals taking them, especially older adults.

Problems from Misuse of Antibiotics

The problems resulting from misuse are adverse side effects from the drugs, exposure to additional complications from ineffective treatment of an infection, and bacterial resistance to antibiotics. In addition, misprescribing is a waste of money.

Adverse Side Effects

Although the numbers of side effects and problems with antibiotics are often low compared with other drugs, there are still some serious side effects that can occur. For example, an allergic reaction to penicillin can cause death, although this is uncommon. Use of antibiotics taken by mouth can cause stomach irritation and diarrhea, which can progress to a severe intestinal condition caused by very resistant bacteria that are difficult to kill.

Other antibiotics can cause problems with the liver and kidneys, which is a real concern when prescribing for older adults. The best way to avoid these side effects is not to use antibiotics unless they are indicated and to avoid especially dangerous ones whenever possible. This is not the current practice, however.

Chloramphenicol, for example, is one antibiotic that has a particular danger. In rare instances, this drug can cause irreversible bone marrow depression, which can be fatal. In 1983, **49% of all prescriptions of chloramphenicol were for conditions in which the drug was clearly not indicated, such as tonsillitis and infection-prevention after surgery. This meant that half the prescriptions for chloramphenicol exposed people unnecessarily to a serious danger.**

Exposure to Additional Complications

Antibiotics are often misused to treat the common cold or flu. In 1983, more than 51% of the more than 3 million patients who saw doctors for treatment of the common cold were *unnecessarily* given a prescription for an antibiotic.[2] Since both the cold and the flu are caused by viruses, there is absolutely no possible way antibiotics can help cure these diseases or speed up the natural cure. They can, however, make a person more susceptible to a dangerous bacterial super-infection, such as a pneumonia, which could be resistant to the antibiotic the person is taking.

Germs that are not killed by the antibiotics can cause an infection, such as candidiasis, a fungal infection. Oral candidiasis is fairly common in older adults who wear dentures. A sore mouth or tongue or soreness of the vagina are possible symptoms.

Bacterial Resistance

This is becoming an ever-expanding problem. After antibiotics are used for a period of time, certain bacteria develop methods that enable them to become resistant to some antibiotics. The resistant bacteria are the ones that survive after antibiotic treatment, and after time they become the dominant force via a process of natural selection. For example, the staphylococcus, a common bacterium causing skin infections, used to be exquisitely sensitive to penicillin when the drug was first introduced. Twenty years later, penicillin was no longer anywhere near as effective against the staphylococcus. A new drug, called methicillin, was designed to combat the "staph bug," and it was widely used. Over time, strains of methicillin-resistant "super-staph" have also emerged. This illustrates that newer, improved antibiotics are not the final answer to bacterial resistance. **If new antibiotics are developed but then overused, bacteria will find new ways to develop resistance, making the drugs ineffective.**

Many bacteria in the hospital setting have now become resistant to multiple antibiotics, and, as a result, infections with these bacteria have become a very dangerous occurrence. The only way to help stop the development of bacterial resistance is by discouraging the gross misuse and overuse of antibiotics. It makes sense to use these "magic bullets," especially the newer ones, only when necessary so that their power will still be effective when it is truly needed.

Thus, there are both dangers and benefits to antibiotics. When you have an infection that can be cured with the proper antibiotic, the benefit of taking the drug is much, much greater than its dangers. But since there are dangers, there are compelling reasons to avoid unnecessary use of antibiotics and to select the safest and most effective ones.

Avoiding Unnecessary Use of Antibiotics

There are several basic principles that should be followed in determining the correct antibiotic:

1. *Establish that an antibiotic is necessary.* This means that your infection has to be the type that can be effectively treated by an antibiotic. Antibiotics are used to specifically treat bacterial infections. Antibiotics do *not* treat viral infections, such as the common cold. (Although there has been some heartening progress in the development of specific antiviral agents such as acyclovir, ribavirin, AZT, and amantadine, viral infections, for the most part, cannot be treated with drugs.)

2. *Choose the correct antibiotic.* It must be effective against the most likely organisms that can cause your infection. In our drug pages on individual antibiotics, we state the types of infections for which each antibiotic is best suited.

3. *Take a culture before using an antibiotic.* A culture should be taken from where you have an infection, such as your throat, urine, or blood, and then grown to determine the specific organism that is causing your infection and whether it is susceptible to the preferred antibiotic. For example, if you have a urinary tract infection, the doctor should take a urine specimen and send it for culture before treating your infection. This does not mean that your infection cannot be treated right away, only that a culture is sent before you start antibiotics. In this way, if your infection persists, your doctor can determine which alternative antibiotic can be used against the bacteria. Your doctor may find out that you do not have an infection and do not require antibiotics.

4. *Consider the cost of the antibiotic.* This should be done when everything else is equal. If several antibiotics are equally effective, their cost should be taken into consideration when selecting a drug to use. Newer drugs on patent are much more expensive than older antibiotics that have been on the market for some time. For example, the oral cephalosporin cefuroxime (Ceftin) is often used to treat urinary tract infections. There is no advantage between using this drug and using a generic drug such as trimethoprim and sulfamethoxazole. Cefuroxime, however, costs 12 times as

much for 2 weeks of treatment.[3] Clearly, in the case of a simple infection, the less expensive drug is preferred as an initial choice.

The Importance of Completing a Full Course of Therapy

It is important with any antibiotic to **take the entire amount of the drug that your doctor prescribes.** Oftentimes, after the first few days of taking antibiotics, you will begin to feel better. Perhaps you think that you do not have to finish your course of treatment, since you are, after all, feeling healthy. This is not the case, however. The length of the regimen that your doctor prescribes for you is designed to eliminate *all* of the bacteria that are causing your illness. If you do not take all of your medication, the bacteria will not be completely eliminated and can quickly multiply, causing another infection. This infection may then be resistant to the original antibiotic.

In general, antibiotics taken by mouth are preferred if you do not require hospitalization and can take the pills without any problem. There is no advantage to having an injection of an antibiotic.

Newer Versus Older Antibiotics

There is often a question in people's minds as to whether the newer antibiotics are better than the older ones. Newer antibiotics cannot eradicate any additional types of "bugs" that the older and less expensive antibiotics cannot. The newer ones are primarily designed to fight resistant bacteria. This does not mean that the older antibiotics, such as penicillin, are less effective than the new ones. There are many situations in which bacteria have not yet developed resistance, and in these cases, the older antibiotics are preferred. In most cases, they have fewer adverse side effects. For example, the organism that causes strep throat, the streptococcus, remains exquisitely sensitive to oral penicillin V, which is the drug of choice. In this case, newer is not better.

In summary, antibiotics can make a world of difference when the right antibiotic is chosen for the right situation. Unfortunately, in the United States today, this is only being done a minority of the time. Questioning your doctor about why he or she is prescribing an antibiotic is a step in the right direction toward safer and better antibiotic use.

Penicillins and Cephalosporins

The following chart lists the penicillins and cephalosporins that are discussed in this book. It does not identify the ones that are given mainly as injections or intravenously, most of which are used primarily in the hospital.

Penicillins (oral)
Amoxicillin/TRIMOX; POLYMOX
Amoxicillin and Clavulanate/
    AUGMENTIN
Ampicillin/OMNIPEN; POLYCILLIN
Cloxacillin/CLOXAPEN; TEGOPEN
Dicloxacillin/DYCILL; DYNAPEN
Penicillin G/PENTIDS
Penicillin V/PEN VEE K

Cephalosporins (oral)
Cefaclor/CECLOR
Cefadroxil/DURICEF; ULTRACEF
Cefixime/SUPRAX
Cefuroxime/CEFTIN
Cephalexin/KEFLEX
Cephradine/ANSPOR; VELOSEF

Penicillins are a group of antibiotics used to kill bacteria or prevent infections. They are probably the least toxic of all the antibiotics. The penicillins are some of the most commonly prescribed antibiotics and are often the drugs of choice for people who are not allergic to them.

Cephalosporins are relatives of the penicillins and have a similar, if slightly expanded, range of action. They have a good safety record,[4] but certain problems can occur with their use. Diarrhea is the most common side effect, and it may become so bad that treatment must be stopped.

Types of Allergic Reactions

Allergic reactions are the most common adverse effects observed with penicillins. Between 5 and 10% of the general public are allergic to them. If you are allergic to penicillins you should carry a card or wear an ID bracelet stating that you are allergic. Make sure to tell your doctor if you think you have an allergy to penicillin so that the information will be recorded.

There are three kinds of allergic reactions to penicillin: immediate, accelerated, and delayed.

Immediate reactions, also known as anaphylaxis, usually happen within 20 minutes of receiving the drug. Symptoms range from skin rash and itching to swelling, difficulty breathing, and even death. Immediate anaphylactic reactions are very rare, occurring in less than 1% of the people who are allergic to penicillins.[5]

Accelerated reactions usually happen between 20 minutes and 2 days after taking penicillin. Itching, rash, and fever are some of the symptoms.

Delayed reactions usually happen at least 2 days to 1 month after taking penicillin. Symptoms can include fever, feeling sick or uncomfortable, skin rash, muscle or joint pain, or pain in the abdomen.

Similar allergies can occur in people who take cephalosporins since the drugs are related to penicillins. If you experience any of the above symptoms, call your doctor immediately. Although penicillin and cephalosporin allergies are more common in people who have had such a reaction previously, they also can occur in people who have repeatedly taken penicillin without prior incident.

Some people who are allergic to penicillin may also be allergic to a cephalosporin; this occurs about 5% of the time. Cephalosporins should *not* be used for people who have had immediate reactions to penicillins. People who have had delayed reactions, such as a rash, should discuss with their doctors whether they should take a cephalosporin.

In older adults, caution must be used with high doses of penicillins and cephalosporins to prevent damage to the nervous system resulting in seizures, drowsiness, and confusion.[6] The dose of most penicillins and cephalosporins must be reduced when the kidneys do not function normally in order to prevent other complications. For example, a normal dose of 20 million units of penicillin G potassium injection in someone with kidney problems could lead to a severe or even fatal increase of potassium (hyperkalemia). Older adults and people with decreased kidney function are more likely to have damage to the kidney when a cephalosporin and an aminoglycoside antibiotic (gentamicin, tobramycin, and neomycin, for example) are used at the same time.

Almost any antibiotic can cause antibiotic-associated colitis (inflammation of the colon). Clindamycin, lincomycin and ampicillin are thought to cause this disease most frequently. Other penicillins and cephalosporins are implicated less often but this reaction is still common. Risk of this disease seems to increase with the age of the user.

Dosage Forms, Effects, and Uses

Oral forms of cefaclor, a cephalosporin, and most penicillins should be taken on an empty stomach (1 hour before or 2 hours after meals) with a full glass (8 ounces) of water. Most other cephalosporins and amoxicillin can be taken on a full stomach. Try to take your doses at evenly spaced times during the day and night so that the amount of drug in your body will stay constant. Store liquid forms in the refrigerator, but do not allow them to freeze.

Capsules may be opened to facilitate swallowing. Oral penicillins and cephalosporins may cause nausea, vomiting, or diarrhea.

Injectable forms of penicillins and cephalosporins can cause pain and swelling at the site of injection. Diabetics may not absorb these drugs well when they are given in the muscle. Tell your doctor if you are on a salt restricted (sodium) diet because injected penicillins and cephalosporins contain sodium. People who have congestive heart failure may have a hard time getting rid of extra sodium.[7]

People who are elderly, have poor nutrition, or are alcoholic may have a greater risk of developing bleeding problems (blood takes longer to clot, for example) that are associated with some of the cephalosporins.[8] Vitamin K supplements, as pills or injections, may prevent this complication.

Cephalosporins are often used to prevent infections caused by surgery. In most operations where an artificial part is used, such as open heart surgery, and in gynecologic and gastrointestinal surgery, the use of cephalosporins before surgery is generally justified.[9] For many operations, an older cephalosporin, such as cephalexin (Keflex) is preferred. An exception to this is pelvic and gastrointestinal surgery, for which cefoxitin (Mefoxin) may be a better choice.[10]

Cephalosporins are widely overused in the United States. They are not the first-choice drugs to treat most infections. Usually when a cephalosporin is chosen to treat an infection, an equally effective and less expensive antibiotic is available. The newer cephalosporins are relatively expensive, but some of them have become the drugs of choice for some serious infections.[11]

Fluoroquinolones

The following list of fluoroquinolones are discussed in this book:

Ciprofloxacin/CIPRO
Norfloxacin/NOROXIN, CHIBROXIN
Ofloxacin/FLOXIN

One of the biggest selling and most over-prescribed new classes of drugs in the United States is the family called fluoroquinolones. One clue that a drug your doctor wants to give you is in this class is the fact that the generic names of all such drugs approved in the United States include the sequence *floxacin*. These drugs are alternatives for individuals allergic to or with infections resistant to other antibiotics. Common infections for which many of these drugs, especially ciprofloxacin, are misprescribed are colds, sore throats or community-acquired (as opposed to hospi-

tal-acquired) pneumonia. No antibiotic should be prescribed for the common cold, and penicillin or — if allergic — erythromycin is the drug of choice for a strep throat, and no fluoroquinolone is the drug of choice for treatment of bronchitis or pneumonia that could be caused by pneumococcal bacteria, the commonest cause of community-acquired pneumonia. With rare exceptions, fluoroquinolones are not the drug of choice for other infections. A 7-day course of treatment with one of the fluoroquinolone drugs can cost between 7 and 21 times more than equally effective (for most infections) treatment with other drugs, for example generic ampicillin or trimethoprim/sulfamethoxazole (the generic version of Bactrim/Septra). Both resistance and allergy to one drug in this family usually cross to the rest of the fluoroquinolones and sometimes even occur during therapy.[12,13] Overgrowth of normal bacteria may cause yeast infections, especially when antibiotics are used for long periods. The fluoroquinolones can cause central nervous system problems and psychosis.[14] Severe, even fatal, allergic reactions have happened after just one dose. Collapse of the circulatory system has occurred. As a group, the fluoroquinolones are expensive, resistance is increasing, and many effective alternatives are available.[15]

> ### *Warning*
> In mid-1992, only a few months after it was initially approved for marketing in the U.S., Abbott's OMNIFLOX, generic name temafloxacin, was pulled off the market worldwide because of an unacceptably high number of cases of serious anemia, kidney failure and life-threatening anaphylactic (allergic) shock including a number of deaths.

Tetracyclines

Tetracyclines are rarely the antibiotics of choice to treat bacterial infections that are common in older adults. In general, tetracyclines are used to treat such infections as urethritis (inflammation of the urinary tract), prostate infections, pelvic inflammatory disease, acne, Rocky Mountain spotted fever, acute bronchitis in people with chronic lung disease, "walking" pneumonia and other miscellaneous infections.[16]

Considerations When Prescribing for Older Adults

Since a decrease in kidney function is one of the normal changes associated with the aging process, tetracyclines must be used with this in mind. With the exception of doxycycline, these drugs should *not* be used for someone with impaired kidney function, as they can damage the kidneys further. Tetracyclines also can cause liver damage. This is more likely to happen when they are injected into the blood (intravenously) in people who already have liver or kidney impairment.[17]

Dosage Forms, Uses, and Effects

The oral forms — tablet, capsule, suspension—should be taken with a full glass (8 ounces) of water. The last dose of the day should be taken at least an hour before bedtime.[18] **Esophageal ulcers (irritation of the esophagus, the tube leading from the throat to the stomach) have occurred in people who have taken doxycycline at bedtime with insufficient water to wash it down.** Liquid forms should be shaken well before use. Do not freeze them. Try to take your doses at evenly spaced times during the day and night so that the amount of drug in your body will stay constant. If you miss a dose, take it as soon as possible. If it is almost time for the next dose and you are supposed to take your medicine:

❑ once a day: space missed dose and next dose about 12 hours apart.
❑ twice a day: space missed dose and next dose about 6 hours apart.
❑ 3 or more times a day: space missed dose and next dose about 3 hours apart or double the next dose.

Then go back to your regular schedule.

The injected forms should only be used when the oral forms are not adequate or not tolerated. The intramuscular injection of the tetracyclines should be used rarely, as it is very painful and not well absorbed. The intravenous forms should be used only when the oral forms are not appropriate, as severe vein inflammation or clotting commonly occurs.[19]

Tetracyclines applied externally as ointments or creams are of little value except for treatment of some eye infections and possibly some skin conditions. Two types of eye (ophthalmic) preparations are available — ointment and drops. (See p. 582 for directions on applying eye preparations.)

Sometimes when tetracyclines are used, microbes that are not killed by these drugs cause infection. An example is candidiasis, a fungal infection. (Some of its symptoms are sore mouth and tongue and itching in the genital or rectal area.) Candidiasis in the mouth is fairly common in older adults who wear dentures.

Tell your doctor that you take a tetracycline before you have any tests done. These drugs may interfere with your urine test results. Talk to your doctor before you change your diet or any medication.

LIMITED USE

Tetracycline
ACHROMYCIN (Lederle) PANMYCIN (Upjohn)

Generic: available

Family: Antibiotics (see p. 444)
Tetracyclines (see p. 449)

Tetracycline (te tra *sye* kleen) is used to treat chronic (long-term) infections of the prostate gland, urinary tract infections, pelvic inflammatory disease, and acute bronchitis (in people with chronic lung disease). **Tetracycline will not help a cold or the flu.**

Tetracycline is sometimes used to treat bacterial infections that are common in older adults, but it is rarely the best antibiotic for this purpose.[20] Penicillin would be a better choice. Also, tetracycline can worsen existing kidney damage, so you should not take it if you have significant kidney impairment. If you have kidney damage and you do need to take a drug in this family (tetracyclines), doxycycline (see p. 505) is preferred.[21] **People with liver disease may need to take less than the usual adult dose of tetracycline.**

Before You Use This Drug
Tell your doctor if you have or have had
❏ allergies to drugs
❏ an unusual reaction to tetracycline or another drug in its family, such as doxycycline
❏ kidney or liver disease
Tell your doctor about any other drugs you take, including aspirin, herbs, vitamins, and other non-prescription products.

When You Use This Drug
◆ Stay out of the sun as much as possible, and call your doctor if you get a rash, hives, or any other skin reaction. Tetracycline makes you more sensitive to the sun.
◆ Do not eat or drink milk or other dairy products, and do not take antacids or iron, vitamin, or mineral supplements for a few hours before and after you take each dose of tetracycline. These substances can keep your body from absorbing the drug, which makes it less effective.
◆ Call your doctor if your symptoms do not improve in 2 or 3 days or if you get diarrhea. Do not treat the diarrhea yourself.
◆ **Take all the tetracycline your doctor prescribed, even if you feel better before you run out. If you stop too soon, your symptoms could come back.**

◆ Do not give the drug to anyone else. Throw away outdated drugs.

◆ If you plan to have any surgery, including dental, tell your doctor that you take this drug.

How To Use This Drug

◆ Take on an empty stomach (at least 1 hour before or 2 hours after a meal) with **a full glass (8 ounces) of water**. Take your last dose of the day at least an hour before bedtime.

◆ Keep the container closed tightly and in a dry place. Do not store in the bathroom or expose to heat, strong light, or moisture. **Do not use if the appearance or taste has changed.**

◆ Take tetracycline at least 2 hours apart from any other drug you are taking.

◆ If you miss a dose, take it as soon as you remember, but skip it if it is almost time for your next dose. **Do not take double doses unless you are taking it 3 or more times a day.**

Interactions With Other Drugs

The following drugs are listed in *Evaluations of Drug Interactions*, 1991 as causing "highly clinically significant" or "clinically significant" interactions when used together with this drug. There may be other drugs, especially those in the families of drugs listed below, that also will react with this drug to cause severe adverse effects. Make sure to ask your doctor for a complete listing of them and let her or him know if you are taking any of these interacting drugs:

ALAGEL; ALTERNAGEL; aluminum hydroxide; AMPHOJEL; digoxin; ESKALITH; ether; FEOSOL; ferrous sulfate; insulin; LANOXICAPS; LANOXIN; lithium carbonate; LITHOBID; LITHONATE; methoxyflurane; penicillin G; PENTHRANE; PENTIDS; SLOW FE.

Adverse Effects

Call your doctor if these symptoms continue:

❏ stomach cramps or burning sensation in the stomach

❏ diarrhea

❏ skin rash, increased sensitivity of skin to sun (increased sunburn)

❏ sore or discolored mouth or tongue

❏ itching in the genital or rectal area

❏ nausea or vomiting

❏ dizziness or clumsiness

Cephradine
ANSPOR (Smith Kline & French)
VELOSEF (Squibb)

Generic: not available

Family: Antibiotics (see p. 444)
Cephalosporins (see p. 446)

Cephradine (*sef* ra deen) is used to treat certain infections caused by bacteria, such as infections of the bladder and soft tissues (puncture wounds or deep cuts). For most of these infections, though, you could take an antibiotic from a different family that would be just as effective as cephradine and much less expensive.[22] Oral cephradine (taken by mouth) is also used to help prevent infection after some types of surgery.[23] **Cephradine will not help a cold or the flu.**

Sometimes doctors prescribe cephradine or another drug in its family because the person taking the drug is allergic to penicillin. However, there is a chance that someone allergic to penicillin will also be allergic to drugs in this family (cephalosporins).

If you have kidney disease, you may need to take less than the usual adult dose of cephradine.

Before You Use This Drug

Tell your doctor if you have or have had
❑ allergies to drugs
❑ a reaction to any penicillin or cephalosporin (see p. 447 for examples)
❑ other allergies
❑ stomach or intestinal disease
❑ kidney or liver disease
❑ a salt (sodium)-restricted diet (the injected form of cephradine contains sodium)

Tell your doctor about any other drugs you take, including aspirin, herbs, vitamins, and other non-prescription products.

When You Use This Drug

Call your doctor if your symptoms do not improve in 2 or 3 days or if you get diarrhea. Do not treat the diarrhea yourself. **Take all the cephradine your doctor prescribed, even if you feel better before you run out. If you stop too soon, your symptoms could come back. Caution diabetics:** see p. 516.

Do not give the drug to anyone else. Throw away outdated drugs.

If you plan to have any surgery, including dental, tell your doctor that you take this drug.

How To Use This Drug

Taking cephradine with food may help prevent stomach upset.

Store liquid form in the refrigerator but do not freeze. Shake well before using.
◆ Do not store capsules in the bathroom, and do not expose to heat, moisture, or strong light.

Capsules may be opened and mixed with food or water.

If you miss a dose, take it as soon as you remember, but skip it if it is almost time for the next dose. **Do not take double doses.**

Interactions With Other Drugs

The following drugs are listed in *Evaluations of Drug Interactions*, 1991 as causing "highly clinically significant" or "clinically significant" interactions when used together with this drug. There may be other drugs, especially those in the families of drugs listed below, that also will react with this drug to cause severe adverse effects. Make sure to ask your doctor for a complete listing of them and let her or him know if you are taking any of these interacting drugs:

BENEMID; COUMADIN; GARAMYCIN; gentamicin; probenecid; warfarin.

Adverse Effects

Call your doctor immediately:
❑ **if you have signs of severe allergic reaction (anaphylactic shock):** severe asthma (wheezing); extreme weakness; abdominal pain; nausea or vomiting; diarrhea; rash

Call your doctor immediately, even if it has been a month since you stopped taking cephradine:
❑ pain, cramps, or bloating in the abdomen or stomach
❑ severe, watery diarrhea (may contain blood)
❑ fever
❑ nausea or vomiting
❑ increased thirst
❑ abnormal weakness or tiredness
❑ abnormal weight loss
❑ dizziness or headache
❑ joint pain

Call your doctor if these symptoms continue:
❑ mild diarrhea
❑ sore mouth or tongue
❑ mild stomach pain
❑ itching of the genital or rectal area
❑ skin rash, hives, or itching

Trimethoprim and Sulfamethoxazole (combined)
BACTRIM (Roche)
SEPTRA (Burroughs Wellcome)
COTRIM (Lemmon)

Generic: available

Family: Antibiotics (see p. 444)

Trimethoprim (see p. 492) and sulfamethoxazole (sulfa meth *ox* a zole) are antibiotics that can be used separately to treat various infections. This combination of trimethoprim and sulfamethoxazole is a rational combination that offers more benefit than either drug alone. The combination is used to treat ear, prostate, intestinal, and urinary tract infections, and acute bronchitis in people with chronic lung disease. **Trimethoprim and sulfamethoxazole will not help a cold or the flu.** Rarely, this drug may cause severe blood disorders, especially in older adults.[24]

If you have either liver or kidney impairment, you might need to take less than the usual adult dose of this drug.

Practice measures to prevent urinary tract infections. Drink plenty of fluids, especially water. While cranberry juice is unreliable as a cure for urinary tract infections, the juice may reduce odor from incontinence.[25] Practice meticulous hygiene. After using the toilet, wipe backwards, not forwards, then wash your hands. Prepare and store foods properly, especially when traveling to prevent diarrhea. Restrict caffeine, which widens the urethra. Indwelling catheters invite urinary tract infections. However, unless there are symptoms of urinary infection, it is not always necessary to take medication just because bacteria are found in a urine test.[26] Women are particularly prone to repeated urinary tract infections. If urinary tract symptoms occur often, ask your doctor about keeping a supply of medication on hand. Ideally,

the antibiotic you use should be the most effective, least toxic, and least costly.[27,28]

Before You Use This Drug
Tell your doctor if you have or have had
- allergies to drugs
- an unusual reaction to other sulfonamides (sulfa drugs), furosemide, thiazide diuretics, or diabetes or glaucoma drugs taken by mouth
- glucose-6-phosphate dehydrogenase deficiency
- liver or kidney disease
- porphyria

Tell your doctor about any other drugs you take, including aspirin, herbs, vitamins, and other non-prescription products.

When You Use This Drug
- **Drink a full glass (8 ounces) of water with each dose, and drink several additional glasses of water every day, unless your doctor tells you differently.**
- Call your doctor if your symptoms do not get better in 2 or 3 days.
- **Take all the medication your doctor prescribed, even if you feel better before you run out. If you stop too soon, your symptoms could come back.**
- Do not give the drug to anyone else. Throw away outdated drugs.
- **Caution diabetics:** see p. 516.
- Stay out of the sun as much as possible, and call your doctor if rash, hives, or skin reaction develops. This drug makes you more sensitive to the sun.
- Ask your doctor if you need to get more vitamin K than usual.
- If you plan to have any surgery, including dental, tell your doctor that you take this drug.

How To Use This Drug

◆ Take with **a full glass of water (8 ounces) on an empty stomach** (at least 1 hour before or 2 hours after meals). Tablets may be crushed and mixed with the water. Shake liquid form before using.

◆ Do not store in the bathroom or expose to heat, moisture, or strong light. Do not let the liquid form freeze.

◆ If you miss a dose, take it as soon as you remember. If you are taking two doses a day of this drug, take the dose you missed and then wait at least 5 or 6 hours before taking the next one. If you are taking this drug 3 or more times a day, you can take the missed dose and the next one at the same time.

Interactions With Other Drugs

The following drugs are listed in *Evaluations of Drug Interactions*, 1991 as causing "highly clinically significant" or "clinically significant" interactions when used together with this drug. There may be other drugs, especially those in the families of drugs listed below, that also will react with this drug to cause severe adverse effects. Make sure to ask your doctor for a complete listing of them and let her or him know if you are taking any of these interacting drugs:

COUMADIN; DILANTIN; FOLEX; methotrexate; ORINASE; PENTOTHAL; phenytoin; thiopental; tolbutamide; warfarin.

Adverse Effects

Call your doctor immediately:
❑ increased sensitivity of skin to sun
❑ skin rash or itching
❑ aching joints or muscles
❑ difficulty swallowing
❑ fever, pale skin, sore throat, or abnormal bleeding or bruising
❑ abnormal tiredness or weakness
❑ yellow eyes or skin

Call your doctor if these symptoms continue:
❑ diarrhea
❑ dizziness or headache
❑ loss of appetite
❑ nausea or vomiting

Periodic Tests

Ask your doctor which of these tests should be done periodically while you are taking this drug:
❑ complete blood counts during long-term therapy

LIMITED USE

Mupirocin
BACTROBAN (Beecham)

Generic: not available

Family: Antibiotics (see p. 444)

Mupirocin (mu *pir* o sin) is an ointment used to treat impetigo and other skin infections. A recent review concluded that penicillin or erythromycin should be used to treat non-bullous (simple) impetigo,[29] and some doctors prefer to use oral antibi-otics to treat it. If the impetigo affects only a small skin area and you prefer not to take oral therapy, consider mupirocin.

Resistance and secondary infection with mupirocin can occur with prolonged use.[30,31] Mupirocin is for external use, so do not use if your skin is broken or you have a burn, since you could absorb the drug internally and cause kidney problems.[32]

Before You Use This Drug

Tell your doctor if you have or have had

❑ allergies to drugs or polyethylene glycol (PEG)

When You Use This Drug

◆ Call your doctor if no improvement occurs within 3-5 days.

◆ **Use all the mupirocin your doctor prescribed, even if you feel better before you run out. If you stop too soon, your symptoms could come back.**

How To Use This Drug

◆ Wash the affected area with soap and water, then dry.

◆ Rub a small amount gently onto the skin. To avoid rubbing ointment off the skin and to protect your clothing, you may cover the site with a gauze dressing.

◆ If you miss a dose apply it as soon as you remember but skip it if it is almost time for the next application.

◆ Do not use in the eyes.

◆ Recap the tube. Store at room temperature. Do not store at high temperatures or freezing temperatures.

Interactions With Other Drugs

Some other drugs that you may be taking (either over-the-counter or prescription drugs) can interact with this one, causing adverse effects. Find out from your doctor what these drugs are and let him or her know if you are taking any of them.

When using topical products it is advisable not to apply other topical preparations, including cosmetics, to the same site. This prevents interactions that could irritate your skin.

Adverse Reactions

Call your doctor immediately:

❑ rash, swelling, burning, itching, or pain

Call your doctor if these symptoms continue:

❑ dry skin

❑ nausea

LIMITED USE

Clarithromycin
BIAXIN (Abbott)

Generic: not available

Family: Antibiotics (see p. 444)

Clarithromycin (clare *ith* row mycin) is approved to treat infections, such as Legionnaire's disease, pneumonia, skin and soft tissue infections. **Clarithromycin will not help a cold**, but may be effective in treating bronchitis or sinusitis.[33,34]

If you are allergic to penicillin, your doctor may prescribe clarithromycin for other infections.

Clarithromycin belongs to the same family of antibiotics as erythromycin.

For most infections, clarithromycin is similar in effectiveness to amoxicillin, erythromycin, cloxacillin, or penicillin. Clarithromycin, however, costs much

> *Warning*
> **If you are using clarithromycin do not use SELDANE, SELDANE-D or HISMANAL.** These allergy drugs, when used in combination with clarithromycin can accumulate to dangerous levels in the body and can cause life-threatening, sometimes fatal heart arrhythmias.[35]

more than these alternative antibiotics. Some experts recommend that it be reserved, in most instances, to treat AIDS-related infections.

If you have kidney disease you may require less than the usual adult dose of clarithromycin.

Before You Use This Drug

Tell your doctor if you have or have had
❑ allergies to drugs
❑ liver or kidney problems
Tell your doctor about any other drugs you take, including aspirin, herbs, vitamins, and other non-prescription products.

When You Use This Drug

Call your doctor if your symptoms do not improve in 2 or 3 days or if you get diarrhea. Do not treat the diarrhea yourself.
Take all the clarithromycin your doctor prescribed, even if you feel better before you run out. If you stop too soon, your symptoms could come back.
◆ If you plan to have any surgery, including dental, tell your doctor that you take this drug.

How To Use This Drug

◆ Do not store tablets in the bathroom, and do not expose to heat, moisture, or strong light.
If you miss a dose, take it as soon as you remember, but skip it if it is almost time for the next dose. **Do not take double doses.**
Take tablets with **a full glass (8 ounces) of water.**

Interactions With Other Drugs

The following drugs are listed in *Evaluations of Drug Interactions*, 1991 as causing "highly clinically significant" or "clinically significant" interactions when used together with this drug. There may be other drugs, especially those in the same families of drugs listed below, that also will react with this drug to cause severe adverse effects. Make sure to ask your doctor for a complete listing of them and let her or him know if you are taking any of these drugs:
alfentanil; CAFERGOT; carbamazepine; COUMADIN; cyclosporine; digoxin; disopyramide; ELIXOPHYLLIN; ergot; LANOXIN; MEDROL; methylprednisolone; NORPACE; SANDIMMUNE; TEGRETOL; THEO-DUR; theophylline; warfarin.

Additionally, *The Medical Letter* and the *United States Pharmacopeia Drug Information*, 1992 lists these drugs as having interactions of major significance:
AZT; zidovudine.
The following drugs should not be taken with clarithromycin (see warning box):
astemizole; HISMANAL; SELDANE; SELDANE-D; terfenadine.

Adverse Effects

Call your doctor immediately:
❑ severe, watery diarrhea
❑ skin rash
Call your doctor if these symptoms continue:
❑ abdominal discomfort or pain
❑ dizziness
❑ headache
❑ nausea
❑ taste change

Cefaclor
CECLOR (Lilly)

Generic: not available

Family: Antibiotics (see p. 444)
        Cephalosporins (see p. 446)

Cefaclor (*sef* a clor) is used to treat some infections caused by bacteria, such as infections of the ear or soft tissues (puncture wounds or deep cuts). For most of these infections, though, you could take an antibiotic from a different family that would be just as effective as cefaclor and much less expensive.[36]

For example, if you have an ear infection, taking cefaclor for 10 days will be four times as expensive as taking another antibiotic, amoxicillin (see p. 500), for 10 days.[37] **Cefaclor will not help a cold or the flu.**

Sometimes doctors prescribe cefaclor or another drug in its family because the person taking the drug is allergic to penicillin. However, there is a chance that someone allergic to penicillin will also be allergic to drugs in this family (cephalosporins).

If you have kidney disease, you may need to take less than the usual adult dose of cefaclor.

Before You Use This Drug
Tell your doctor if you have or have had
❑ allergies to drugs
❑ a reaction to any penicillin or cephalosporin (see p. 447 for examples)
❑ allergies
❑ stomach or intestinal disease
❑ kidney or liver disease
❑ a salt (sodium)-restricted diet (the injected form of cefaclor contains sodium)
Tell your doctor about any other drugs you take, including aspirin, herbs, vitamins, and other non-prescription products.

When You Use This Drug
◆ Call your doctor if your symptoms do not improve in 2 or 3 days or if you get diarrhea. Do not treat the diarrhea yourself.
◆ **Take all the cefaclor your doctor prescribed, even if you feel better before you run out. If you stop too soon, your symptoms could come back.**
◆ **Caution diabetics:** see p. 516.
◆ Do not give the drug to anyone else. Throw away outdated drugs.
◆ If you plan to have any surgery, including dental, tell your doctor that you take this drug.

How To Use This Drug
◆ Taking cefaclor with food may help prevent stomach upset.
◆ Store liquid form in the refrigerator but do not freeze. Shake well before using.
◆ Do not store capsules in the bathroom, and do not expose to heat, moisture, or strong light.
◆ Capsules may be opened and mixed with food or water.
◆ If you miss a dose, take it as soon as you remember, but skip it if it is almost time for the next dose. **Do not take double doses.**

Interactions With Other Drugs
The following drugs are listed in *Evaluations of Drug Interactions*, 1991 as causing "highly clinically significant" or "clinically significant" interactions when used together with this drug. There may be other drugs, especially those in the families of drugs listed below, that also will react with this drug to cause severe adverse effects. Make sure to ask your doctor for a complete listing of them and let her or him know if you are taking any of these interacting drugs:
    BENEMID; COUMADIN; GARAMYCIN; gentamicin; probenicid; warfarin.

Adverse Effects
Call your doctor immediately:
❏ if you have any signs of severe allergic reaction (anaphylactic shock): severe asthma (wheezing); extreme weakness; abdominal pain; nausea or vomiting; diarrhea; rash

Call your doctor immediately, even if it has been a month since you stopped taking cefaclor:
❏ pain, cramps, or bloating in the abdomen or stomach
❏ severe, watery diarrhea (may contain blood)

❏ fever
❏ nausea or vomiting
❏ increased thirst
❏ abnormal weakness or tiredness
❏ abnormal weight loss

Call your doctor if these symptoms continue:
❏ mild diarrhea
❏ sore mouth or tongue
❏ mild stomach pain
❏ skin rash, hives, or itching
❏ itching of genital or rectal area

LIMITED USE

Cefuroxime Axetil
CEFTIN (Allen & Hanburys)

Generic: not available

Family: Antibiotics (see p. 444)
         Cephalosporins (see p. 446)

Cefuroxime (seff ur *ox* ime) is an antibiotic, belonging to the family of second generation cephalosporins, used to cure infections caused by susceptible bacteria. The oral form is used to treat bronchitis, and ear, urinary tract and skin infections. Although prior to surgery, cefuroxime is sometimes used to prevent an infection. *The Medical Letter* does not list it as the drug of choice for any infection.[38]

Like all antibiotics, it does not help a cold. A sensitivity test should justify use of cefuroxime. Otherwise, other antibiotics, including less costly cephalosporins, are likely to be as effective.

Sometimes doctors prescribe cefuroxime or another drug in its family because the person taking the drug is allergic to penicillin. However, there is a chance that some-one allergic to penicillin will also be allergic to drugs in this family (cephalosporins).

If you have kidney disease, you may need to take less than the usual adult dose of cefuroxime. Cefuroxime may lower your vitamin K, especially if you are malnour-ished, prolonging bleeding.

Before You Use This Drug
Tell your doctor if you have or have had
❏ allergies to drugs
❏ a reaction to any penicillin or cephalos-porin (see p. 447 for examples)
❏ allergy or rash after taking any paraben-containing products such as sun screens
❏ kidney or liver disease
❏ a salt (sodium)-restricted diet (injected form of cefuroxime contains sodium)
Tell your doctor about any other drugs you take, including aspirin, herbs, vitamins, and other non-prescription products.

When You Use This Drug
◆ Call your doctor if your symptoms do not improve in 2 or 3 days or if you get diarrhea. Do not treat the diarrhea yourself.

◆ **Take all the cefuroxime your doctor prescribed, even if you feel better before you run out. If you stop too soon, your symptoms could come back.**

◆ **Caution diabetics:** see p. 516.

◆ Do not give the drug to anyone else. Throw away outdated drugs.

◆ If you plan to have any surgery, including dental, tell your doctor that you take this drug.

How To Use This Drug

◆ Swallow tablets whole. Take with food or milk. You may crush tablets and mix with food such as applesauce, chocolate milk, ice cream, or milk to mask the bitter taste. Or, pour 2 to 3 ounces of apple juice, or grape juice, and let it warm to room temperature. Then add your dose to the juice. After the tablets disintegrate, stir, then swallow immediately. Follow with more juice without the drug.

◆ If you miss a dose, take it as soon as possible. If it is almost time for the next dose adjust your schedule. If you take one dose a day, take the missed dose, then the next dose 10 to 12 hours later. If you take 2 doses a day, take the missed dose, then the next dose 5 to 6 hours later. If you take 3 or more doses a day, take the missed dose and the next dose 2 to 4 hours later.

◆ Do not store in the bathroom, and do not expose to heat, moisture, or strong light.

Interactions With Other Drugs

The following drugs are listed in *Evaluations of Drug Interactions*, 1991 as causing "highly clinically significant" or "clinically significant" interactions when used together with this drug. There may be other drugs, especially those in the families of drugs listed below, that also will react with this drug to cause severe adverse effects. Make sure to ask your doctor for a complete listing of them and let her or him know if you are taking any of these interacting drugs:

BENEMID; COLBENEMID; COUMADIN; GARAMYCIN; gentamicin; probenecid; warfarin.

Adverse Effects
Call your doctor immediately:
❑ severe abdominal or stomach cramps
❑ breathing difficulty
❑ convulsions
❑ severe diarrhea
❑ fever
❑ joint pain
❑ low blood pressure
❑ skin rash, blistering, hives, peeling, or swelling
❑ unusual bleeding or bruising
❑ decrease in amount of urine
Call your doctor if these symptoms continue:
❑ cramps
❑ diarrhea
❑ nausea or vomiting
❑ sore mouth or tongue
❑ vaginal itching

Periodic Tests
Ask your doctor which of these tests should be done periodically while you are taking this drug:
❑ bleeding or prothrombin time
❑ stool exam

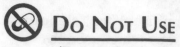

Do Not Use
(Except in the Hospital)

Chloramphenicol
CHLOROMYCETIN (Parke-Davis)

Family: Antibiotics (see p. 444)

Although chloramphenicol (klor am *fen* i kole) **is effective in treating many conditions, it should be used only in a very limited number of situations because it is so dangerous.** It can cause an irreversible depression of the bone marrow (where blood cells and platelets are produced), which usually results in death.

Chloramphenicol should be used to treat serious diseases for which there is no better antibiotic available. Most of these diseases require hospital treatment, so there is rarely any reason to take chloramphenicol at home. The only exception is that you may need to take it at home to finish treatment that was begun in the hospital.

Oral chloramphenicol (taken by mouth) is usually prescribed inappropriately to treat trivial infections.[39] **Chloramphenicol should not be used for minor infections, and it will not help a cold or the flu.**

Limited Use

Ciprofloxacin
CIPRO (Miles)

Generic: not available

Family: Antibiotics (see p. 444)
　　　　Fluoroquinolones (see p. 448)

Ciprofloxacin (sip row *flocks* a sin) is used to treat infections, such as urinary tract infections, osteomyelitis, infectious diarrhea, and gonorrhea. **Since older people tend to have reduced kidney function, they are usually prescribed low doses of ciprofloxacin.**

Ciprofloxacin belongs to a family of drugs called fluoroquinolones. These drugs are alternatives for individuals allergic to or with infections resistant to other antibiotics. A 7-day course of ciprofloxacin costs 5 to 10 times more than drugs such as amoxicillin or trimethoprim-sulfamethoxazole (Septra), which are equally effective for most infec-

---

Warning
Extreme caution should be used when fluoroquinolones such as ciprofloxacin are to be prescribed in conjunction with aminophylline or theophylline, particularly in elderly patients. Prudence would suggest that aminophylline doses be adjusted, perhaps reduced by 30% to 50% at the initiation of fluoroquinolone therapy. The reduction in dose must be guided by the clinical conditions of the patient, the use of other concomitant medication, and the baseline value of the theophylline serum concentration. In addition, serum theophylline levels should be obtained following the initiation of a fluoroquinolone no later than 2 days into therapy.[40]

tions. Both resistance and allergy to one drug in this family usually cross to the rest of the fluoroquinolones and sometimes even occur during therapy.[41,42] Overgrowth of normal bacteria may cause yeast infections, especially when antibiotics are used for long periods. The fluoroquinolones can cause central nervous system problems and psychosis.[43] Severe, even fatal, allergic reactions have happened after just one dose. Collapse of the circulatory system has occurred. As a group fluoroquinolones are expensive, resistance is increasing, and effective alternatives are available.[44]

The Journal of the American Medical Association reports widespread misuse of ciprofloxacin. Ciprofloxacin is inappropriate for common sinus and ear infections and community-acquired pneumonias. For most pneumonias and streptococcal infections penicillin or a cephalosporin remain drugs of choice.[45,46,47] **Ciprofloxacin will not help a cold.**

Practice measures to prevent urinary tract infections. Drink plenty of fluids, especially water. While cranberry juice is unreliable as a cure for urinary tract infections, the juice may reduce odor from incontinence.[48] Practice meticulous hygiene. After using the toilet, wipe backwards, not forwards, then wash your hands. Prepare and store foods properly, especially when traveling, to prevent diarrhea. Restrict caffeine, which widens the urethra. Indwelling catheters invite urinary tract infections. However, unless there are symptoms of urinary infection, it is not always necessary to take medication just because bacteria are found in a urine test.[49] Women are particularly prone to repeated urinary tract infections. If urinary tract symptoms occur often, ask your doctor about keeping a supply of medication on hand. Ideally, the antibiotic you use should be the most effective, least toxic, and least costly.[50,51]

Before You Use This Drug
Tell your doctor if you have or have had
❑ allergies to drugs
❑ colitis

❑ diabetes
❑ epilepsy or seizures
❑ kidney or liver problems
❑ myasthenia gravis[52]
❑ an implanted metal device[53]
Tell your doctor about any other drugs you take, including aspirin, herbs, vitamins, and other non-prescription products. It is especially important you tell your doctor if you take any theophylline drug (See p. 401).

When You Use This Drug
◆ **Take all the ciprofloxacin your doctor prescribed, even if you feel better before you run out. If you stop too soon, your symptoms could come back.**
◆ Do not drive or perform other activities that require alertness because this drug may make you drowsy, dizzy, or lightheaded.
◆ Drink plenty of fluids.
◆ Protect yourself from sunburn. Do not use a sunlamp.
◆ If you plan to have any surgery, including dental, tell your doctor that you take this drug.

How To Use This Drug
◆ Swallow tablet whole with **a full glass (8 ounces) of water**.
◆ If you miss a dose, take it as soon as you remember, but skip it if it is almost time for the next dose. **Do not take double doses.**
◆ Do not store in the bathroom, and do not expose to heat, moisture, or strong light.

Interactions With Other Drugs
The following drugs are listed in *Evaluations of Drug Interactions,* 1991 as causing "highly clinically significant" or "clinically significant" interactions when used together with this drug. There may be other drugs, especially those in the families of drugs listed below, that also will react with this drug to cause severe adverse effects. Make sure to ask your doctor for a complete listing of them and let her or him

know if you are taking any of these interacting drugs:

aluminum; caffeine (beverages or drugs); CARAFATE; COUMADIN; cyclosporine; ELIXOPHYLLIN; SANDIMMUNE; sucralfate; THEO-DUR; theophylline (older people are more likely to experience interactions with theophylline.)[54]

Additionally, the *United States Pharmacopeia Drug Information*, 1992 lists these drugs as having interactions of major significance:

antacids; calcium.

Caution should be taken when the following drugs are used with this one (see warning box):

aminophylline; AMOLINE; BRONKODYL; CONSTANT-T; ELIXOPHYLLIN; QUIBRON-T-SR; SLO-BID; SLO-PHYLLIN;

SOMOPHYLLIN; SUSTAIRE; THEO-24; THEOLAIR; theophylline.

Adverse Effects

Call your doctor immediately:
❑ agitation
❑ breathing difficulty
❑ confusion, hallucinations
❑ fever
❑ rash, itching
❑ seizure
❑ swelling of face, neck
❑ tremors
❑ blurred vision

Call your doctor if these symptoms continue:
❑ dizziness, lightheadedness
❑ drowsiness
❑ headache
❑ insomnia, restlessness
❑ nausea, vomiting, diarrhea
❑ pain in abdomen, stomach, joints

LIMITED USE

Clindamycin
CLEOCIN (Upjohn)

Generic: available

Family: Antibiotics (See p. 444)

Clindamycin (klin da *mye* sin) is used to treat life-threatening infections that do not respond to penicillin or other antibiotics, such as bone or abdominal infections. **Clindamycin will not help a cold or the flu, and it is too dangerous to use for sore throats and other upper respiratory infections.**

Clindamycin can have serious side effects. It can cause serious inflammation of the large intestine, abdominal cramps, and severe diarrhea, sometimes with passage of blood and mucus. These side effects can

happen up to several weeks after you stop using the drug. Because of the possibility of these serious side effects, your doctor should prescribe a drug less toxic than clindamycin if at all possible. If you are taking clindamycin, watch closely for the serious side effects listed. If any occur, call your doctor immediately, stop taking clindamycin, and **do not take any other medication to treat your side effects.** When you take antidiarrheal drugs to treat diarrhea caused by clindamycin, they can prolong or worsen the diarrhea instead of helping.

If you have combined liver and kidney disease, you should take less than the usual adult dose of clindamycin.

Before You Use This Drug

Tell your doctor if you have or have had
❑ allergies to drugs
❑ an unusual reaction to clindamycin or lincomycin (see p. 480)
❑ kidney or liver impairment
❑ stomach or intestinal disease
❑ allergies to tartrazine (a food dye) or aspirin
❑ diarrhea

Tell your doctor about any other drugs you take, including aspirin, herbs, vitamins, and other non-prescription products.

When You Use This Drug

◆ Call your doctor if your symptoms do not improve in 2 or 3 days or if you get diarrhea.
◆ **Take all the medication your doctor prescribed, even if you feel better before you run out. If you stop too soon, your symptoms could come back.**
◆ Do not give this drug to anyone else. Throw away outdated drugs.
◆ If you plan to have any surgery, including dental, tell your doctor that you take this drug.

How To Use This Drug

◆ **Take capsules with a full glass (8 ounces) of water or with food to avoid irritation or ulcers in the esophagus** (the tube that carries food from your mouth to your stomach).
◆ Do not refrigerate the liquid form. Shake well before using.

◆ If you miss a dose, take it as soon as you remember. If it is almost time for your next dose, space missed dose and next dose 2 to 4 hours apart.

Interactions With Other Drugs

The following drugs are listed in *Evaluations of Drug Interactions*, 1991 as causing "highly clinically significant" or "clinically significant" interactions when used together with this drug. There may be other drugs, especially those in the families of drugs listed below, that also will react with this drug to cause severe adverse effects. Make sure to ask your doctor for a complete listing of them and let her or him know if you are taking any of these interacting drugs:

ether; pancurmonium; PAULILON.

Adverse Effects

Call your doctor immediately even if these symptoms occur up to a month after you stop taking clindamycin:
❑ stomach cramps or abdominal pain
❑ severe, watery diarrhea (may contain blood)
❑ fever
❑ nausea or vomiting
❑ increased thirst
❑ abnormal weakness or tiredness
❑ abnormal weight loss

Call your doctor if these symptoms continue:
❑ mild diarrhea
❑ skin rash or itching
❑ itching in the genital or rectal area
❑ sore mouth or tongue

Cloxacillin
CLOXAPEN (Beecham) TEGOPEN (Bristol)
Dicloxacillin
DYNAPEN (Bristol) DYCILL (Beecham)

Generic: available

Family: Antibiotics (see p. 444)
Penicillins (see p. 446)

Cloxacillin (klox a *sill* in) and dicloxacillin (dye *klox* a sill in) are used to treat bacterial infections that are resistant to penicillin, such as certain infections of the skin, soft tissue (such as puncture wounds or deep cuts), and joints and to prevent infection after hip surgery. Your doctor should usually do lab tests before prescribing either of these drugs, and should prescribe one of them only if tests show that the bacteria causing your infection are resistant to penicillin. If the bacteria are not resistant to penicillin, your doctor should prescribe penicillin instead. **These drugs will not help a cold or the flu.**

It should be used with caution in people who are over age 70, or people with impaired kidney function.[55]

Before You Use This Drug
Tell your doctor if you have or have had
❑ allergies to drugs
❑ a reaction to any penicillin or cephalosporin (see p. 446 for examples)
❑ allergies
❑ stomach or intestinal disease
❑ kidney disease
Tell your doctor about any other drugs you take, including aspirin, herbs, vitamins, and other non-prescription products.

When You Use This Drug
◆ Call your doctor if your symptoms do not improve in 2 or 3 days or if you get diarrhea. Do not treat the diarrhea yourself.

◆ Take all the cloxacillin or dicloxacillin your doctor prescribed, even if you feel better before you run out. If you stop too soon, your symptoms could come back.
◆ **Caution diabetics:** see p. 516.
◆ If you plan to have any surgery, including dental, tell your doctor that you take this drug.

How To Use This Drug
◆ Take on an empty stomach (at least 1 hour before or 2 hours after meals) with **a full glass (8 ounces) of water.** Capsules may be opened and mixed with water.
◆ Store liquid form in the refrigerator but do not freeze. Shake well before using.
◆ Do not store capsules in the bathroom, and do not expose to heat, moisture, or strong light.
◆ If you miss a dose, take it as soon as you remember, but skip it if it is almost time for the next dose. **Do not take double doses.**

Interactions With Other Drugs
The following drugs are listed in *Evaluations of Drug Interactions*, 1991 as causing "highly clinically significant" or "clinically significant" interactions when used together with this drug. There may be other drugs, especially those in the families of drugs listed below, that also will react with this drug to cause severe adverse effects. Make sure to ask your doctor for a complete listing of them and let her or him know if you are taking any of these interacting drugs:
AUREOMYCIN; chlortetracycline; COUMADIN; GARAMYCIN; gentamicin; heparin; warfarin.

Adverse Effects
Call your doctor immediately:
- ❏ **if you have signs of severe allergic reaction (anaphylactic shock):** severe asthma (wheezing); extreme weakness; abdominal pain; nausea or vomiting; diarrhea; rash

Call your doctor immediately, even if it has been a month since you stopped taking this drug:
- ❏ pain, cramps, or bloating in the abdomen or stomach

- ❏ severe, watery diarrhea (may contain blood)
- ❏ fever
- ❏ nausea or vomiting
- ❏ increased thirst
- ❏ abnormal weakness or tiredness
- ❏ abnormal weight loss
- ❏ skin rash, hives, or itching

Call your doctor if these symptoms continue:
- ❏ mild diarrhea
- ❏ sore mouth or tongue
- ❏ darkened or discolored tongue

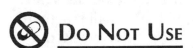 **DO NOT USE**

Alternative treatment: An antibiotic alone, if necessary.

Neomycin, Polymyxin B, and Hydrocortisone (combined)
CORTISPORIN EAR DROPS (OTIC) (Burroughs Wellcome)

Family: Antibiotics (see p. 444)
Corticosteroids (see p. 609)

This combination of the drugs neomycin (nee oh *mye* sin), polymyxin (pol i *mix* in) B, and hydrocortisone (see p. 616) is used to treat ear infections caused by bacteria and allergies. **There is no persuasive proof that it is beneficial for this purpose.**

One of the drugs in this product, hydrocortisone, generally should not be used for treating infections at all, because it can hide the signs of an infection or make it spread. The other two drugs in this product,

neomycin and polymyxin B, are antibiotics and are unnecessary unless your ear problem is caused by a bacterial infection. If it is caused by a bacterial infection, you should be taking an antibiotic alone rather than this combination with hydrocortisone.

Neomycin commonly causes skin rashes in 8% of the people who use it. Using neomycin can also make it hard for you to use other drugs in its family (amino-glycoside antibiotics, such as gentamicin and tobramycin, see p. 594) that may be needed later in life for serious infections.

Fluconazole
DIFLUCAN (Roerig)

Generic: not available

Family: Antifungals

Fluconazole (flu *con* as ol) is used to treat severe fungal infections, such as meningitis and infections of the mouth or esophagus.[56,57] Often these infections occur when another condition, such as cancer, organ transplant, or HIV infection, reduces your immunity to infections. You may also be more prone to these fungal infections if you have been exposed to contaminated air conditioners, or certain animals or geographic areas. Outbreaks have occurred during remodeling of hospitals.[58] The drug should not be used to treat trivial fungal skin infections.

Before You Use This Drug
Tell your doctor if you have or have had
❏ allergies to drugs
❏ cancer
❏ diabetes
❏ kidney or liver problems
❏ seizures
❏ tuberculosis
Tell your doctor about any other drugs you take, including aspirin, herbs, vitamins, and other non-prescription products.

When You Use This Drug
◆ Take all the fluconazole your doctor prescribed, even if you feel better before you run out. If you stop too soon, your symptoms could come back.

How To Use This Drug
◆ If you miss a dose, take it as soon as you remember, but skip it if it is almost time for the next dose. **Do not take double doses.**
◆ Do not store capsules in the bathroom, and do not expose to heat, moisture, or strong light.

Interactions With Other Drugs
The following drugs are listed in *Evaluations of Drug Interactions*, 1991 as causing "highly clinically significant" or "clinically significant" interactions when used together with this drug. There may be other drugs, especially those in the families of drugs listed below, that also will react with this drug to cause severe adverse effects. Make sure to ask your doctor for a complete listing of them and let her or him know if you are taking any of these interacting drugs:
COUMADIN; cyclosporine; DECADRON; dexamethasone; DILANTIN; phenytoin; QUINAGLUTE; QUINIDEX; quinidine; RIFADIN; rifampin; SANDIMMUNE; SELDANE; terfenadine; warfarin.
Additionally, the *United States Pharmacopeia Drug Information,* 1992 lists this drug as having interactions of major significance:
glipizide; GLUCOTROL.

Adverse Effects
Call your doctor immediately:
❏ unusual bleeding or bruising
❏ abdominal pain, especially on right side under ribs
❏ dizziness
❏ fever
❏ seizures
❏ yellowing of eyes or skin
❏ reddened, blistering, itching or peeling skin
❏ dark, amber urine
Call your doctor if these symptoms continue:
❏ abdominal discomfort
❏ fatigue

❑ headache
❑ nausea, vomiting, diarrhea

Periodic Tests
Ask your doctor which of these tests should

be done periodically while you are taking this drug:
❑ blood creatinine
❑ blood urea nitrogen (BUN)
❑ liver function tests

Cefadroxil
DURICEF (Mead Johnson)
ULTRACEF (Bristol)

Generic: available

Family: Antibiotics (see p. 444)
Cephalosporins (see p. 446)

Cefadroxil (sef a *drox* ill) is used to treat some infections caused by bacteria, such as infections of the bladder or soft tissues (puncture wounds or deep cuts). For most of these infections, though, you could take an antibiotic from a different family that would be just as effective as cefadroxil and much less expensive.[59] For example, if you have an ordinary urinary tract infection and take cefadroxil, your treatment could cost 25 times as much as if you took another drug, generic sulfisoxazole (see p. 474), which works just as well.[60] **Cefadroxil will not help a cold or the flu.**

Sometimes doctors prescribe cefadroxil or another drug in its family because the person taking the drug is allergic to penicillin. However, there is a chance that someone allergic to penicillin will also be allergic to drugs in this family (cephalosporins).

If you have kidney disease, you may need to take less than the usual adult dose of cefadroxil.

Before You Use This Drug
Tell your doctor if you have or have had
❑ allergies to drugs
❑ a reaction to any penicillin or cephalosporin (see p. 447 for examples)

❑ stomach or intestinal disease
❑ kidney or liver disease
❑ a salt (sodium)-restricted diet (injected form of cefadroxil contains sodium)
Tell your doctor about any other drugs you take, including aspirin, herbs, vitamins, and other non-prescription products.

When You Use This Drug
◆ Call your doctor if your symptoms do not improve in 2 or 3 days or if you get diarrhea. Do not treat the diarrhea yourself.
◆ **Take all the cefadroxil your doctor prescribed, even if you feel better before you run out. If you stop too soon, your symptoms could come back.**
◆ **Caution diabetics:** see p. 516.
◆ Do not give this drug to anyone else. Throw away outdated drugs.
◆ If you plan to have any surgery, including dental, tell your doctor that you take this drug.

How To Use This Drug
◆ Taking cefadroxil with food may help prevent stomach upset. Capsules may be opened and mixed with food or water.
◆ Store liquid form in the refrigerator but do not freeze. Shake well before using.
◆ Do not store capsules in the bathroom, and do not expose to heat, moisture, or strong light.
◆ If you miss a dose, take it as soon as

you remember, but skip it if it is almost time for the next dose. **Do not take double doses.**

Interactions With Other Drugs

The following drugs are listed in *Evaluations of Drug Interactions*, 1991 as causing "highly clinically significant" or "clinically significant" interactions when used together with this drug. There may be other drugs, especially those in the families of drugs listed below, that also will react with this drug to cause severe adverse effects. Make sure to ask your doctor for a complete listing of them and let her or him know if you are taking any of these interacting drugs:

BENEMID; COUMADIN; GARAMYCIN; gentamicin; probenecid; warfarin.

Adverse Effects

Call your doctor immediately:
❑ if you have signs of severe allergic

reaction (anaphylactic shock): severe asthma (wheezing); extreme weakness; abdominal pain; nausea or vomiting; diarrhea; rash

Call your doctor immediately, even if it has been a month since you stopped taking cefadroxil:
❑ pain, cramps, or bloating in abdomen or stomach
❑ severe, watery diarrhea (may contain blood)
❑ fever
❑ nausea or vomiting
❑ increased thirst
❑ abnormal weakness or tiredness
❑ abnormal weight loss

Call your doctor if these symptoms continue:
❑ mild diarrhea
❑ sore mouth or tongue
❑ mild stomach pain
❑ muscle or joint pain
❑ skin rash, hives, or itching
❑ itching in the genital or rectal area

Erythromycin
ERYTHROCIN (Abbott) ETHRIL (Squibb)
E-MYCIN (Upjohn) EES (Abbott)

Generic: available

Family: Antibiotics (see p. 444)

Erythromycin (eh rith roe *mye* sin) is used to treat infections such as diphtheria and some kinds of pneumonia. Your doctor may also prescribe erythromycin for other infections if you are allergic to penicillin. **Erythromycin will not help a cold or the flu.**

Erythromycin is one of the safest antibiotics available. However, people who use a particular type of erythromycin called erythromycin estolate (Ilosone) are about 20 times more likely to suffer liver damage (toxicity) from the drug than people who use other forms.[61]

Therefore, you should not take erythromycin estolate (Ilosone, see p. 476).[62] **If you have liver disease, you should be taking less than the usual adult dose of erythromycin.**

> *Warning*
> **If you are using erythromycin do not use SELDANE, SELDANE-D or HISMANAL.** These allergy drugs, when used in combination with erythromycin can accumulate to dangerous levels in the body and can cause life-threatening, sometimes fatal heart arrhythmias.[63]

Before You Use This Drug

Tell your doctor if you have or have had
- allergies to drugs
- an unusual reaction to erythromycin
- liver disease

Tell your doctor about any other drugs you take, including aspirin, herbs, vitamins, and other non-prescription products.

When You Use This Drug

- Call your doctor if your symptoms do not improve in 2 or 3 days or if you get diarrhea. Do not treat the diarrhea yourself.
- **Take all the erythromycin your doctor prescribed, even if you feel better before you run out. If you stop too soon, your symptoms could come back.**
- Do not give this drug to anyone else. Throw away outdated drugs.
- If you plan to have any surgery, including dental, tell your doctor that you take this drug.

How To Use This Drug

Erythromycin taken by mouth:
- Most types must be taken on an empty stomach (at least 1 hour before or 2 hours after meals) with **a full glass (8 ounces) of water**.
- Some brands of enteric-coated erythromycin and erythromycin ethyl succinate can be taken on either a full or an empty stomach. Ask your doctor if you are taking one of these types.
- Chewable tablets should be chewed or crushed, not swallowed whole. Enteric-coated tablets (coated so they won't dissolve in your stomach) or capsules should be swallowed whole.
- Do not store in the bathroom, and do not expose to heat, moisture, or strong light. Store liquid erythromycin in the refrigerator (do not freeze) and shake well before using.
- If you miss a dose, take it as soon as you remember. If you are on a twice-a-day schedule, take the dose you missed and then wait 6 hours before taking the next

one. If you are on a schedule of 3 doses or more a day, you can take the dose you missed and the next one at the same time.

Erythromycin eye ointment:
- If you are using eye ointment, see instructions on p. 582.
- If you miss an application, do it as soon as you remember, but skip it if it is almost time for the next application.

Interactions With Other Drugs

The following drugs are listed in *Evaluations of Drug Interactions*, 1991 as causing "highly clinically significant" or "clinically significant" interactions when used together with this drug. There may be other drugs, especially those in the families of drugs listed below, that also will react with this drug to cause severe adverse effects. Make sure to ask your doctor for a complete listing of them and let her or him know if you are taking any of these interacting drugs:

ALFENTA; alfentanil; BRONKODYL; CAFERGOT; carbamazepine; CONSTANT-T; COUMADIN; cyclosporine; digoxin; disopyramide; ELIXOPHYLLIN; ergotamine; LANOXIN; MEDROL; methylprednisolone; NORPACE; QUIBRON-T-SR; SANDIMMUNE; SLO-BID; SLOPHYLLIN; SOMOPHYLLIN; SUSTAIRE; TEGRETOL; THEO-24; THEOLAIR; theophylline; tubocurarine; warfarin.

The following drugs should not be taken with erythromycin (see warning box):
astemizole; HISMANAL; SELDANE; SELDANE-D; terfenadine.

Adverse Effects

Call your doctor immediately:
- severe, watery diarrhea (may contain blood)
- dark or colored urine
- light-colored stools
- severe stomach pain
- abnormal tiredness or weakness
- yellow eyes or skin

❑ temporary hearing loss (rare)
Call your doctor if these symptoms continue:
❑ nausea or vomiting

❑ sore mouth or tongue
❑ mild stomach pain

LIMITED USE

Metronidazole
FLAGYL (Searle)

Generic: available

Family: Antibiotics (see p. 444)

Metronidazole (me troe *ni* da zole) is used to treat some serious infections caused by bacteria or protozoa, including trichomonas, amoebiasis, and giardiasis. **This drug will not help a cold or the flu.**

Metronidazole has been shown to cause cancer in mice and rats. Because of this connection, you should only be using metronidazole if you have a serious infection. Doctors sometimes prescribe metronidazole for a vaginal infection called trichomonas ("trich"), but you should not be using this drug for this kind of infection until you have tried other treatments such as taking a tub bath twice a day, wearing cotton underwear, and not wearing panty hose. If you have tried these treatments and you still have symptoms of a trichomonas infection, then metronidazole may be prescribed.[64]

If you are taking metronidazole for a vaginal trichomonas infection, it is best to use the form that must be taken for one day only. **If you are taking metronidazole for any reason and you have kidney or severe liver impairment, you may need to take less than the usual adult dose.[65]**

The information on this page deals mostly with the forms of metronidazole taken by mouth — tablets and capsules.

Before You Use This Drug
Tell your doctor if you have or have had
❑ allergies to drugs
❑ an unusual reaction to metronidazole
❑ disease of the central nervous system
❑ epilepsy
❑ severe liver disease
Tell your doctor about any other drugs you take, especially an anticoagulant such as warfarin or heparin, and including aspirin, herbs, vitamins, and other non-prescription products.

When You Use This Drug
◆ Do not drink alcohol. If you do, you may get abdominal cramps, nausea, vomiting, headaches, flushing, or low blood sugar.
◆ Call your doctor if your symptoms do not get better in 2 or 3 days.
◆ **Take all the metronidazole your doctor prescribed, even if you feel better before you finish. If you stop too soon, your symptoms could come back.**
◆ Do not give this drug to anyone else. Throw away outdated drugs.
◆ If you are going to have any medical tests done, first tell your doctor that you are taking metronidazole.
◆ Metronidazole may cause your urine to get darker. This is normal and not dangerous.

How To Use This Drug

◆ If you are taking metronidazole by mouth, eat something at the same time to prevent stomach irritation.

◆ Always take your doses of metronidazole the same number of hours apart, even at night, to keep the amount of the drug in your body constant.

◆ Do not store in the bathroom, and do not expose to strong light, heat, or moisture.

◆ If you miss a dose, take it as soon as you remember, but skip it if it is almost time for the next dose. **Do not take double doses.**

Interactions With Other Drugs

The following drugs are listed in *Evaluations of Drug Interactions*, 1991 as causing "highly clinically significant" or "clinically significant" interactions when used together with this drug. There may be other drugs, especially those in the families of drugs listed below, that also will react with this drug to cause severe adverse effects. Make sure to ask your doctor for a complete listing of them and let her or him know if you are taking any of these interacting drugs:

alcohol, ethyl; ANTABUSE; ARALEN; choloroquine; COUMADIN; disulfiram; ESKALITH; lithium; LUMINAL; phenobarbital; warfarin.

Adverse Effects

Call your doctor immediately:

❑ numbness, tingling, pain, or weakness in hands or feet

❑ clumsiness or unsteadiness

❑ seizures

❑ confusion, irritability, depression, weakness, or trouble sleeping

❑ mood or mental changes

❑ skin rash, redness, hives, or itching

❑ sore throat or fever

❑ vaginal dryness, discharge, or irritation

Call your doctor if these symptoms continue:

❑ nausea or vomiting

❑ diarrhea (even if you stopped taking the drug a month ago)

❑ dizziness or lightheadedness

❑ headache

❑ loss of appetite

❑ stomach cramps or pain

❑ sore mouth or tongue

❑ problems urinating

❑ constipation, dark urine, dry mouth, bad taste in mouth, or abnormal tiredness or weakness

❑ joint pain

Periodic Tests

Ask your doctor which of these tests should be done periodically while you are taking this drug:

❑ total and differential white blood cell counts (before and after long-term treatment)

LIMITED USE

Ofloxacin
FLOXIN (Ortho/McNeil)

Generic: not available

Family: Antibiotics (see p. 444)
Fluoroquinolones (see p. 448)

Ofloxacin (oh *flocks* a sin) kills a broad spectrum of bacteria and can cure infections caused by susceptible bacteria. Ofloxacin is primarily used to treat complicated infections of the urinary tract and prostate. It is also used for chronic bronchitis, pneumonia, soft skin infections, and uncomplicated gonorrhea. Ofloxacin is not a drug of choice for community-acquired pneumonias. Length of therapy varies from a few days to several weeks or months. Treatment of other conditions, or to prevent urinary tract infections is still under study.

Ofloxacin belongs to a family of drugs called fluoroquinolones. These drugs are alternatives for individuals allergic to or with infections resistant to other antibiotics. A 7-day course of ofloxacin costs 5 to 10 times more than drugs such as amoxicillin (see p. 500) or trimethoprim and sulfamethoxazole (see p. 453), which are equally effective for most infections. Both resistance and allergy to one drug in this family usually cross to the rest of the fluoroquinolones and sometimes even occur during therapy.[67,68] Overgrowth of normal bacteria may cause yeast infections, especially when antibiotics are used for long periods. The fluoroquinolones can cause central nervous system problems and psychosis.[69] Severe, even fatal, allergic reactions have happened after just one dose. Collapse of the circulatory system has occurred. As a group fluoroquinolones are expensive, resistance is increasing, and effective alternatives are available.[70]

In people over age 65 ofloxacin is excreted more slowly, so a lower dose is usually used.[71] One-dose therapies with ofloxacin are often followed by a recurrence of the infection.[72] Ofloxacin should not be used for minor infections. *The Medical Letter* also finds ofloxacin to be interchangeable with ciprofloxacin for most uses.

Practice measures to prevent urinary tract infections. Drink plenty of fluids, especially water. While cranberry juice is unreliable as a cure for urinary tract infections, the juice may reduce odor from incontinence.[73] Practice meticulous hygiene. After using the toilet, wipe backwards, not forwards, then wash your hands. Prepare and store foods properly, especially when traveling to prevent diarrhea. Restrict caffeine, which widens the urethra. Indwelling catheters invite urinary tract infections. However, unless there are symp-

---

Warning
Extreme caution should be used when fluoroquinolones such as ofloxacin are to be prescribed in conjunction with aminophylline or theophylline, particularly in elderly patients. Prudence would suggest that aminophylline doses be adjusted, perhaps reduced by 30% to 50% at the initiation of fluoroquinolone therapy. The reduction in dose must be guided by the clinical conditions of the patient, the use of other concomitant medication, and the baseline value of the theophylline serum concentration. In addition, serum theophylline levels should be obtained following the initiation of a fluoroquinolone no later than 2 days into therapy.[66]

toms of urinary infection, it is not always necessary to take medication just because bacteria are found in a urine test.[74] Women are particularly prone to repeated urinary tract infections. If urinary tract symptoms occur often, ask your doctor about keeping a supply of medication on hand. Ideally, the antibiotic you use should be the most effective, least toxic, and least costly.[75,76]

Before You Use This Drug

Tell your doctor if you have or have had
- ❑ allergies to any drugs
- ❑ cataracts
- ❑ colitis[77]
- ❑ diabetes
- ❑ heart problems
- ❑ involuntary movement of the eye
- ❑ kidney or liver problems
- ❑ low blood pressure
- ❑ myasthenia gravis
- ❑ seizures
- ❑ difficulty swallowing
- ❑ white blood cell counts that were very low

Tell your doctor about any other drugs you take, including aspirin, herbs, vitamins, and other non-prescription products.

When You Use This Drug

- ◆ Do not drive or perform other activities that require alertness because this drug may make you drowsy, dizzy, or lightheaded.
- ◆ Drink plenty of fluids (water, fruit and vegetable juices) to prevent crystals of ofloxacin forming in your urine.
- ◆ **Take all the ofloxacin your doctor prescribed, even if you feel better before you run out. If you stop too soon, your symptoms could come back.**
- ◆ Protect yourself from sunburn. Wear protective clothing, headgear, sunglasses, and use a sunscreen.

How To Use This Drug

- ◆ Swallow whole tablet. Take with **a full (8 ounce) glass of water**. Do not take with food.

- ◆ If you miss a dose, take it as soon as you remember, but skip it if it is almost time for the next dose. **Do not take double doses.**
- ◆ Do not store tablets in the bathroom, and do not expose to heat, moisture, or strong light.

Interactions With Other Drugs

The following drugs are listed in *Evaluations of Drug Interactions*, 1991 as causing "highly clinically significant" or "clinically significant" interactions when used together with this drug. There may be other drugs, especially those in the families of drugs listed below, that also will react with this drug to cause severe adverse effects. Make sure to ask your doctor for a complete listing of them and let her or him know if you are taking any of these interacting drugs:

aluminum; antacids; caffeine (beverages, drugs); CARAFATE; COUMADIN; cyclosporine; ELIXOPHYLLIN; magnesium; QUINAGLUTE; QUINIDEX; quinidine; SANDIMMUNE; sucralfate; THEO-DUR; theophylline; warfarin.

Caution should be taken when the following drugs are used with this one (see warning box):

aminophylline; AMOLINE; BRONKODYL; CONSTANT-T; ELIXOPHYLLIN; QUIBRON-T-SR; SLO-BID; SLO-PHYLLIN; SOMOPHYLLIN; SUSTAIRE; THEO-24; THEOLAIR; theophylline.

Adverse Effects

Call your doctor immediately:
- ❑ difficulty breathing or swallowing
- ❑ chest pain
- ❑ confusion, disorientation
- ❑ convulsions
- ❑ diarrhea, severe
- ❑ dizziness, fainting
- ❑ fever
- ❑ hallucinations
- ❑ rapid heartbeat[78]

- ❑ itching
- ❑ muscle pain
- ❑ numbness or tingling sensation
- ❑ skin rash, hives
- ❑ swelling of face or throat
- ❑ tremors[79]

Call your doctor if these symptoms continue:
- ❑ abdominal pain
- ❑ diarrhea
- ❑ dry mouth

- ❑ fatigue
- ❑ gas
- ❑ headache
- ❑ hearing lessens, or ringing in ears
- ❑ insomnia
- ❑ loss of appetite
- ❑ nausea and vomiting
- ❑ nervousness
- ❑ taste changes
- ❑ vaginal discharge or itching
- ❑ vision change, inability to see red, blue[80]

Sulfisoxazole
GANTRISIN (Roche)

Generic: available

Family: Antibiotics (see p. 444)
Sulfonamides

Sulfisoxazole (sul fi *sox* a zole) is used to treat urinary tract infections and some other infections. **If you have kidney or liver damage, you should take less than the usual adult dose. Sulfisoxazole will not help a cold or the flu.**

Sulfisoxazole is available in several forms. It is often taken by mouth. Another form is a vaginal cream that is used to treat vaginitis, but there is no evidence that this is an effective treatment. For eye infections, there is an eye ointment and eye solution, which are similar to sulfacetamide (see p. 582).

Practice measures to prevent urinary tract infections. Drink plenty of fluids, especially water. While cranberry juice is unreliable as a cure for urinary tract infections, the juice may reduce odor from incontinence.[81] Practice meticulous hygiene. After using the toilet, wipe backwards, not forwards, then wash your hands. Prepare and store foods properly, especially when traveling to prevent diarrhea. Restrict caffeine, which widens the urethra.

Indwelling catheters invite urinary tract infections. However, unless there are symptoms of urinary infection, it is not always necessary to take medication just because bacteria are found in a urine test.[82] Women are particularly prone to repeated urinary tract infections. If urinary tract symptoms occur often, ask your doctor about keeping a supply of medication on hand. Ideally, the antibiotic you use should be the most effective, least toxic, and least costly.[83,84]

Before You Use This Drug
Tell your doctor if you have or have had
- ❑ allergies to drugs
- ❑ an unusual reaction to other sulfonamides (sulfa drugs), furosemide, thiazide diuretics, or diabetes or glaucoma drugs taken by mouth
- ❑ glucose-6-phosphate dehydrogenase deficiency
- ❑ liver or kidney disease
- ❑ porphyria

Tell your doctor about any other drugs you take, including aspirin, herbs, vitamins, and other non-prescription products.

When You Use This Drug
- ◆ **Take each dose with a full glass (8 ounces) of water, and drink a few more**

glasses of water every day, unless your doctor tells you differently.

◆ Call your doctor if your symptoms do not improve in 2 or 3 days.
Take all the sulfisoxazole your doctor prescribed, even if you feel better before you finish. If you stop too soon, your symptoms could come back.
Do not give the drug to anyone else.
Throw away outdated drugs.
Caution diabetics: see p. 516.
Stay out of the sun as much as possible, and call your doctor if you get a rash, hives, or any other skin reaction. Sulfisoxazole makes you more sensitive to the sun.
While taking this drug, you may need more vitamin K than usual. Ask your doctor.
If you plan to have any surgery, including dental, tell your doctor that you take this drug.

How To Use This Drug

◆ Take with **a full glass of water (8 ounces) on an empty stomach** (at least 1 hour before or 2 hours after meals). Tablets can be crushed and mixed with the water. Shake liquid form before using.
If you are using sulfisoxazole eye drops or ointment, see instructions on p. 582.
Do not store in the bathroom or expose to heat, moisture, or strong light. Do not allow liquid form to freeze.
If you miss an oral dose, take it as soon as you remember. If you are on a twice-a-day schedule for taking sulfisoxazole, take the dose you missed and then wait at least 5 or 6 hours before taking the next one. If you are taking sulfisoxazole 3 times a day or more, you can take the missed dose and the next one at the same time.

◆ If you miss an application of eye ointment or eye drops, do it as soon as you remember, but skip it if it is almost time for the next application.

Interactions With Other Drugs

The following drugs are listed in *Evaluations of Drug Interactions*, 1991 as causing "highly clinically significant" or "clinically significant" interactions when used together with this drug. There may be other drugs, especially those in the families of drugs listed below, that also will react with this drug to cause severe adverse effects. Make sure to ask your doctor for a complete listing of them and let her or him know if you are taking any of these interacting drugs:

COUMADIN; DILANTIN; FOLEX; methotrexate; ORINASE; phenytoin; tolbutamide; warfarin.

Adverse Effects

Call your doctor immediately:
❑ increased sensitivity of skin to sun (increased sunburn)
❑ skin rash or itching
❑ aching joints or muscles
❑ difficulty swallowing
❑ fever, pale skin, or sore throat
❑ abnormal bleeding or bruising
❑ abnormal tiredness or weakness
❑ yellow eyes or skin
Call your doctor if these symptoms continue:
❑ diarrhea
❑ dizziness or headache
❑ loss of appetite
❑ nausea or vomiting

Periodic Tests

Ask your doctor which of these tests should be done periodically while you are taking this drug:
❑ complete blood counts, if you take the drug for a long time

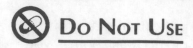 **Do Not Use**

Alternative treatment: See erythromycin, p. 468.

Erythromycin Estolate
ILOSONE (Dista)

Family: Antibiotics (see p. 444)

Erythromycin is one of the safest antibiotics available. However, people who use a particular type of erythromycin called erythromycin estolate (Ilosone) are about 20 times more likely to suffer liver damage (toxicity) from the drug than people who use other forms.[85] Therefore, you should not take erythromycin estolate (Ilosone).[86] **If you have liver disease, you should be taking less than the usual adult dose of erythromycin.**

> *Warning*
> **If you are using erythromycin do not use SELDANE, SELDANE-D or HISMANAL.** These allergy drugs, when used in combination with erythromycin can accumulate to dangerous levels in the body and can cause life-threatening, sometimes fatal heart arrhythmias.[87]

Isoniazid
INH (CIBA)

Generic: available

Family: Antibiotics (see p. 444)
(for tuberculosis)

Isoniazid (eye soe *nye* a zid) is used to treat and prevent tuberculosis (TB). If you are an older adult who has had a positive TB skin test, you do not necessarily need preventive treatment for TB. You should be treated *only* if you are at special risk, for example if you have cancer, if you are taking high doses of corticosteroid drugs on a long-term basis, or if you had a negative TB skin test until recently. If you have sudden, serious liver disease, you should not get preventive TB treatment. If you have confirmed tuberculosis, you should always get a second drug, rifampin (see p. 494), along with isoniazid, rather than taking only one. If you take only one, you may develop bacteria that are resistant to one of these drugs.[88]

Isoniazid can cause serious damage to your liver. Some people who have taken this drug, especially people over age 50, have developed severe and even fatal hepatitis (a liver disease). You are more likely to get hepatitis if you drink alcohol daily, so do not drink while taking this drug. Call your doctor immediately if you have any of the symptoms of hepatitis: fatigue, weakness, malaise (vague feeling of being unwell), loss of appetite, nausea, vomiting, or yellow eyes or skin. **Schedule monthly visits with your doctor while taking this drug. If you have impaired liver function or severe kidney failure, you should probably be taking less than the usual adult dose of isoniazid.**

A small number of people using isoniazid develop nerve pain and tenderness in their hands and feet. Taking 15 to 50 milligrams of vitamin B$_6$ every day can prevent this problem. If necessary, your doctor can give you a prescription for vitamin B$_6$ along with the isoniazid prescription.

Warning

If you have nausea, vomiting, yellow eyes, dark urine, unexplained fatigue, or abdominal pain, don't take this medication — call your doctor.[89]

Warning

There have been a number of case reports of liver damage involving a possible drug interaction between isoniazid, a medication used to prevent and treat tuberculosis, and acetaminophen, an over-the-counter painkiller and the active ingredient in Tylenol. Each drug alone is known to cause liver damage. Isoniazid alone, especially as people get older, has been documented to cause liver damage. Acetaminophen, alone in large doses or probably in combination with alcohol, also increases the risk of liver damage. The combination of acetaminophen with isoniazid, according to the authors of these case reports, may also be dangerous.

If you are taking isoniazid for tuberculosis or have a positive TB skin test and are using the drug, consult your physician before using acetaminophen or any combination product containing acetaminophen. Discuss alternatives to acetaminophen with your physician.[90,91]

Before You Use This Drug

Tell your doctor if you have or have had
- allergies to drugs
- an unusual reaction to isoniazid, ethionamide, pyrazinamide, or niacin
- liver disease
- alcohol dependence
- epilepsy or seizures
- severe kidney disease

Tell your doctor about any other drugs you take, including aspirin, herbs, vitamins, and other non-prescription products.

When You Use This Drug

- ◆ Do not drink alcohol.
- ◆ Call your doctor if your symptoms do not get better in 2 or 3 weeks or if they get worse.
- ◆ You may need more vitamin B$_6$ and niacin than usual. Ask your doctor.
- ◆ Call your doctor if you get symptoms of a food reaction (see Adverse Effects).
- ◆ **Caution diabetics:** see p. 516.
- ◆ **Take all the isoniazid your doctor prescribes, even if you feel better in a few weeks. You might have to take it every day for a year or more. Do not miss doses. If you stop too soon, your symptoms could come back.**
- ◆ Do not give this drug to anyone else. Throw away outdated drugs.
- ◆ If you plan to have any surgery, including dental, tell your doctor that you take this drug.

How To Use This Drug

- ◆ Take with **a full glass (8 ounces) of water** on an empty stomach (at least 1 hour before or 2 hours after meals). If isoniazid upsets your stomach, try taking it with food. Tablets may be crushed and mixed with water.
- ◆ If you take antacids, take them at least 1 hour before or after you take your isoniazid.
- ◆ Do not store in the bathroom or expose to heat, moisture, or direct light. Do not let the liquid form freeze.
- ◆ If you miss a dose, take it as soon as you remember, but skip it if it is almost time for the next dose. **Do not take double doses.**

Interactions With Other Drugs

The following drugs are listed in *Evaluations of Drug Interactions*, 1991 as causing "highly clinically significant" or "clinically significant" interactions when used to-

gether with this drug. There may be other drugs, especially those in the families of drugs listed below, that also will react with this drug to cause severe adverse effects. Make sure to ask your doctor for a complete listing of them and let her or him know if you are taking any of these interacting drugs:

carbamazepine; DILANTIN; phenytoin; RIFADIN; rifampin; RIMACTANE; TEGRETOL.

The following acetaminophen-containing drugs should not be taken with isoniazid (see warning box):

acetaminophen; BANCAP-HC; ESGIC; FIORICET; PERCOCET; TYLENOL; TYLENOL 3; TYLOX; VICODIN.

Adverse Effects

Call your doctor immediately:

❑ **if you experience signs of overdose:** *early signs* are nausea; vomiting; dizziness; slurred speech; blurred vision; and hallucinations, including bright colors and strange designs; *late signs* are seizures; trouble breathing; stupor and coma

❑ numbness, tingling, pain, or weakness of hands or feet

❑ clumsiness or unsteadiness

❑ dark urine

❑ yellow eyes or skin

❑ loss of appetite

❑ light colored stools

❑ headache

❑ pain in stomach or abdomen

❑ unexplained fatigue

❑ nausea or vomiting

❑ abnormal tiredness or weakness

❑ blurring or changes in vision

❑ **if you have signs of food reaction:** red or itching skin, fast or pounding heartbeat, sweating, chills, or headache after eating certain foods such as cheese, fermented sausages, fish, herring, or sauerkraut. If you have such a reaction, you may have to avoid these foods while you are using isoniazid.

Call your doctor if these symptoms continue:

❑ dizziness or upset stomach

❑ breast enlargement in men

❑ fever or joint pain

❑ skin rash

Periodic Tests

Ask your doctor which of these tests should be done periodically while you are taking this drug:

❑ liver function tests, before treatment and regularly thereafter. (During 9 months of treatment, you should have them at the end of months 1, 3, 6, and 9.)

Cephalexin
KEFLEX (Lilly)

Generic: available

Family: Antibiotics (see p. 444)
                Cephalosporins (see p. 446)

Cephalexin (sef a *lex* in) is used to treat some infections caused by bacteria, such as infections of the bladder or soft tissues (puncture wounds or deep cuts). For most of these infections, though, you could take an antibiotic from a different family that would be just as effective as cephalexin and much less expensive.[92] **Cephalexin will not help a cold or the flu.**

Sometimes doctors prescribe cephalexin or another drug in its family because the person taking the drug is allergic to penicillin. However, there is a chance that someone allergic to penicillin will also be allergic to drugs in this family (cephalosporins).

If you have kidney disease, you may need to take less than the usual adult dose of cephalexin.

Before You Use This Drug
Tell your doctor if you have or have had
❑ allergies to drugs
❑ a reaction to any penicillin or cephalosporin (see p. 447 for examples)
❑ stomach or intestinal disease
❑ kidney or liver disease
❑ a salt (sodium)-restricted diet (the injected form of cephalexin contains sodium)
Tell your doctor about any other drugs you take, including aspirin, herbs, vitamins, and other non-prescription products.

When You Use This Drug
◆ Call your doctor if your symptoms do not improve in 2 or 3 days or if you get diarrhea. Do not treat the diarrhea yourself.
◆ Take all the cephalexin your doctor prescribed, even if you feel better before you run out. If you stop too soon, your symptoms could come back.
◆ **Caution diabetics:** see p. 516.
◆ Do not give this drug to anyone else. Throw away all outdated drugs.
◆ If you plan to have any surgery, including dental, tell your doctor that you take this drug.

How To Use This Drug
◆ Taking cephalexin with food may help prevent stomach upset.
◆ Store liquid form in the refrigerator but do not freeze. Shake well before using.
◆ Do not store capsules in the bathroom, and do not expose to heat, moisture, or strong light. Capsules may be opened and mixed with food or water.
◆ If you miss a dose, take it as soon as you remember, but skip it if it is almost time for the next dose. **Do not take double doses.**

Interactions With Other Drugs
The following drugs are listed in *Evaluations of Drug Interactions*, 1991 as causing "highly clinically significant" or "clinically significant" interactions when used together with this drug. There may be other drugs, especially those in the families of drugs listed below, that also will react with this drug to cause severe adverse effects. Make sure to ask your doctor for a complete listing of them and let her or him know if you are taking any of these interacting drugs:

BENEMID; colistimethate; COLY-MYCIN; COUMADIN; GARAMYCIN; gentamicin; probenecid; warfarin.

Adverse Effects
Call your doctor immediately:
❑ if you have signs of severe allergic

reaction (anaphylactic shock): severe asthma (wheezing); extreme weakness; abdominal pain; nausea or vomiting; diarrhea; rash

Call your doctor immediately, even if it has been a month since you stopped taking cephalexin:
- ❑ pain, cramps, or bloating in the abdomen or stomach
- ❑ severe, watery diarrhea (may contain blood)

- ❑ fever
- ❑ nausea or vomiting
- ❑ increased thirst
- ❑ abnormal weakness or tiredness
- ❑ abnormal weight loss

Call your doctor if these symptoms continue:
- ❑ mild diarrhea
- ❑ sore mouth or tongue
- ❑ mild stomach pain
- ❑ itching in the genital or rectal area

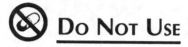 **DO NOT USE**

Alternative treatment: See Clindamycin, p. 462.

Lincomycin
LINCOCIN (Upjohn)

Family: Antibiotics (see p. 444)

Lincomycin (lin koe *mye* sin) is similar to another antibiotic called clindamycin (see p. 462) and is also used to treat infections.

Lincomycin does *not* have any advantage over clindamycin.[93] It is hard for your body to absorb, and it has more unwanted side effects than clindamycin. It should not be used.

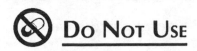 **DO NOT USE**

Alternative treatment: See Ampicillin, p. 489, Trimethoprim, p. 492, and Trimethoprim and Sulfamethoxazole, p. 453.

Nitrofurantoin
MACRODANTIN, FURADANTIN (Norwich Eaton)

Family: Antibiotics (see p. 444)

Nitrofurantoin (nye troe fyoor *an* toyn) is used to treat certain urinary tract infections. **It is a dangerous drug and should not be used.** People over 60 who take this drug have such a high risk of harmful side effects that the World Health Organization has said older adults should not use it.

Because your kidneys normally work less effectively as you grow older, they do not eliminate this drug from your body fast enough. Because of this, nitrofurantoin accumulates to dangerously high levels in your bloodstream, causing side effects. Two of the possible side effects, a nerve disease called peripheral neuropathy and scarring of the lungs, may be irreversible, and deaths from these side effects have been reported.[94] Almost always, you can take another drug that will be just as effective as nitrofurantoin and much safer. **If you are taking this drug, ask your doctor to change your prescription.**

Miconazole
MONISTAT-DERM (Ortho)
MONISTAT 7 (Ortho)

Generic: available

Family: Antifungals

Miconazole (mi *kon* a zole) is used to treat fungal infections and is available in several forms, including a cream, a lotion, and tablets. Since older adults most often use miconazole for skin and vaginal infections, the information here deals mostly with these forms of the drug.

Mild vaginal infections are often self-limiting.[95] For some women a bland cream (without drugs) relieves symptoms until infection spontaneously goes away.[96] Preventive measures include less sugar in the diet, and avoiding tightfitting pants and panty hose. Cotton is preferable to synthetics.[97] Dry the vaginal area thoroughly after bathing or swimming.

Before You Use This Drug
Tell your doctor if you have or have had
❏ allergies to drugs
❏ an unusual reaction to miconazole
❏ other allergies
Tell your doctor about any other drugs you take, including aspirin, herbs, vitamins, and other non-prescription products.

When You Use This Drug
◆ **Take all the miconazole your doctor prescribed, even if you feel better before you finish. If you stop too soon, your symptoms could come back.**
◆ Do not give this drug to anyone else. Throw away outdated drugs.
◆ Do not store in the bathroom, and do not expose to strong light, heat, or moisture.

Using miconazole lotion, skin cream, liquid, or aerosol powder:

◆ Call your doctor if your skin problem does not improve within 4 to 6 weeks. (It will usually improve in the first week.)

◆ Call your doctor immediately if new symptoms appear—skin rash, itching, swelling, or other signs of skin irritation. This is rare.

Using miconazole vaginal cream or tablets:

◆ Call your doctor immediately if you develop new symptoms of vaginal burning, a skin rash, or abdominal cramps, or if your sex partner feels burning or irritation of his penis after you start this treatment.

◆ Wear freshly washed cotton underwear. Wearing a sanitary napkin will protect your clothes from fluids draining from your vagina.

◆ Ask your doctor if you have questions about douching or having sex during treatment.

How To Use This Drug

Using miconazole lotion, skin cream, liquid, or aerosol powder:

◆ Apply enough to cover the affected area of skin and the surrounding area, and rub in gently.

◆ Do not apply an airtight dressing unless your doctor recommends it.

◆ Shake lotion and aerosol powder well before using.

◆ If you miss a dose, apply it as soon as you remember, but skip it if it is almost time for the next dose.

◆ Avoid getting this drug in your eyes.

Using miconazole vaginal cream or tablets:

◆ If you miss a dose, insert it as soon as you remember, but skip it if you don't remember until the next day.

Interactions With Other Drugs

The following drugs are listed in *Evaluations of Drug Interactions*, 1991, as causing "highly clinically significant" or "clinically significant" interactions when used together with this drug. There may be other drugs that also will react with this drug to cause less severe adverse effects. Make sure to ask your doctor for a complete listing of them and let her or him know if you are taking any of these interacting drugs:

COUMADIN; cyclosporine; DILANTIN; phenytoin; SANDIMMUNE; warfarin.

When using topical products it is advisable not to apply other topical preparations, including cosmetics, to the same site. This prevents interactions that could irritate your skin.

Clotrimazole
MYCELEX (Miles)
LOTRIMIN (Schering)
GYNE-LOTRIMIN (Schering)

Generic: available

Family: Antifungals

Clotrimazole (kloe *trim* a zole) is used to treat fungal infections in different parts of the body. For skin infections, you may be given clotrimazole cream, lotion, or liquid to apply externally; for vaginal infections, vaginal cream or tablets placed in the vagina; and for mouth and throat infections, lozenges placed in the mouth. Since older adults most often use clotrimazole for skin and vaginal infections, the information here deals mostly with these forms of the drug.

Mild vaginal infections are often self-limiting.[98] For some women a bland cream (without drugs) relieves symptoms until infection spontaneously goes away.[99] Preventive measures include less sugar in the diet, and avoiding tightfitting pants and panty hose. Cotton is preferable to synthetics.[100] Dry the vaginal area thoroughly after bathing or swimming.

Before You Use This Drug
Tell your doctor if you have or have had
❏ allergies to drugs
❏ an unusual reaction to clotrimazole
❏ other allergies
Tell your doctor about any other drugs you take, including aspirin, herbs, vitamins, and other non-prescription products.

When You Use This Drug
◆ **Take all the clotrimazole your doctor prescribed, even if you feel better before you finish. If you stop too soon, your symptoms could come back.**
◆ Do not give this drug to anyone else. Throw away outdated drugs.

How To Use This Drug
◆ Do not store in the bathroom, and do not expose to strong light, heat, or moisture.
Using clotrimazole skin cream, lotion, and liquid:
◆ Apply enough to cover the affected skin and the surrounding area, and rub in gently.
◆ Do not use an airtight bandage unless your doctor recommends it.
◆ If you miss a dose, apply it as soon as you remember, but skip it if it is almost time for the next dose.
◆ Avoid getting this drug in your eyes.
◆ Call your doctor if your skin problem does not improve within 4 weeks. (Usually it will improve in the first week.)
◆ Call your doctor immediately if new symptoms appear—skin rash, itching, swelling, or other signs of skin irritation. This is rare.
Using clotrimazole vaginal cream or tablets:
◆ If you miss a dose, insert it as soon as you remember, but skip it if you don't remember until the next day.
◆ Call your doctor immediately if you get new symptoms of vaginal burning, a skin rash, or abdominal cramps, or if your sex partner feels burning or irritation of his penis after you start this treatment.
◆ Wear freshly washed cotton underwear. Wearing a sanitary napkin will protect your clothes from fluid draining from your vagina.
◆ Ask your doctor if you have questions about douching or having sex during treatment.

Interactions With Other Drugs
The following drugs are listed in *Evaluations of Drug Interactions,* 1991 as causing

"highly clinically significant" or "clinically significant" interactions when used together with this drug. There may be other drugs, especially those in the families of drugs listed below, that also will react with this drug to cause severe adverse effects. Make sure to ask your doctor for a complete listing of them and let her or him know if you are taking any of these interacting drugs:

cyclosporine; DILANTIN; phenytoin; SANDIMMUNE.

When using topical products it is advisable not to apply other topical preparations, including cosmetics, to the same site. This prevents interactions that could irritate your skin.

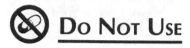 **DO NOT USE**

Alternative treatment: Separate antifungal and corticosteroid ointments or creams.

Nystatin and Triamcinolone (combined)
MYCOLOG II (Squibb)

Family: Antifungals
Corticosteroids (see p. 609)

This combination of nystatin (see p. 485) and triamcinolone (see p. 614) is commonly prescribed by dermatologists (skin doctors) to treat fungal skin infections, such as the yeast infection called candidiasis. However, *one* of its ingredients, triamcinolone, may actually be dangerous to an infection because drugs in its family can hide the signs of an infection or make it spread. Therefore, this drug product is an irrational combination for treating an infection. Instead, your doctor should prescribe nystatin alone.

If you have a fungal skin infection that is inflamed, itching, or scaly, it may be appropriate to use hydrocortisone (see p. 616) in addition to an antifungal ointment such as nystatin for a few days. Each drug should be applied *separately* in a ratio determined by your doctor.

This drug, sold under the brand name Mycolog II, also has an older form which is called Mycolog cream. Mycolog cream is a combination of neomycin and gramacidin, and it should not be used either. Neomycin commonly causes skin rashes in 8% of the people who use it.[101] Using neomycin can also make it hard for you to use other drugs in its family (aminoglycoside antibiotics, such as gentamicin and tobramycin, see p. 594) that may be needed later in life for serious infections.[102]

Nystatin
MYCOSTATIN (Squibb)
NILSTAT (Lederle)

Generic: available

Family: Antifungals

Nystatin (nye *stat* in) is used to treat fungal infections in different parts of the body. For infections in your mouth, you may be given a liquid or powder form of nystatin; for intestinal infections, tablets that are swallowed; for a vaginal infection, tablets that are inserted in the vagina; and for skin infections, a powder that you apply to your skin.

Before You Use This Drug
Tell your doctor if you have or have had
❑ allergies to drugs
❑ an unusual reaction to nystatin
Tell your doctor about any other drugs you take, including aspirin, herbs, vitamins, and other non-prescription products.

When You Use This Drug
◆ **Take all the nystatin your doctor prescribed, even if you feel better before you finish. If you stop too soon, your symptoms could come back.**
◆ Do not give this drug to anyone else. Throw away outdated drugs.

How To Use This Drug
◆ Do not store in the bathroom, and do not expose to moisture, strong light, or heat. Do not let the liquid form freeze.
◆ If you miss a dose, take it as soon as you remember, but skip it if it is almost time for the next dose. **Do not take double doses.**
Taking nystatin by mouth:
◆ *Dry powder*: When it is time to take a dose, add about 1/8 teaspoon of dry powder to a glass of water and stir well.

Take one mouthful of this mixture and hold it in your mouth, swishing it around for as long as you can before swallowing. Continue, one mouthful at a time, until the whole glass is gone.
◆ *Liquid (suspension):* Shake well. Measure out the dose and put half of it in each side of your mouth. Hold it in your mouth or swish it around as long as you can before swallowing.
Using nystatin skin cream, ointment, or powder:
◆ Apply enough to cover the affected area.
◆ Do not use an airtight bandage unless your doctor recommends it.
◆ For fungal infection of the feet, dust powder onto feet, socks, and shoes.
◆ Call your doctor immediately if new symptoms appear—skin rash, itching, swelling, or other signs of skin irritation. This is rare.
◆ Do not let cream or ointment freeze.
Using nystatin vaginal tablets:
◆ If you miss a dose, insert it as soon as you remember, but skip it if you don't remember until the next day.
◆ Call your doctor immediately if you get new vaginal burning, a skin rash, or abdominal cramps.
◆ Wear freshly washed cotton underwear. Wearing a sanitary napkin will protect your clothes from fluid draining from your vagina.
◆ Ask your doctor if you have questions about douching or having sex during treatment.

Interactions With Other Drugs
Some other drugs that you may be taking (either over-the-counter or prescription drugs) can interact with this one, causing adverse effects. Find out from your doctor

what these drugs are and let him or her know if you are taking any of them. When using topical products it is advisable not to apply other topical preparations, including cosmetics, to the same site. This prevents interactions that could irritate your skin.

Adverse Reactions
Call your doctor immediately:
For forms of nystatin taken by mouth:
❑ diarrhea
❑ nausea or vomiting
❑ stomach pain

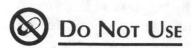 **Do Not Use**

Alternative treatment: Cleaning the infected area well and taking antibiotics by mouth or as injections, if necessary.

Neomycin, Polymyxin B, and Bacitracin (combined)
NEOSPORIN (Burroughs Wellcome)
MYCITRACIN (Upjohn)

Family: Antibiotics (see p. 444)

This combination of three antibiotics — neomycin (nee oh *mye* sin), polymyxin (pol i *mix* in) B, and bacitracin (bass i *tray* sin) — is used to treat a wide variety of skin infections. It is also used to prevent infection in burns or broken skin. It is available as an aerosol spray, powder, and ointment.

There is no satisfactory evidence that antibiotics applied directly to the skin (as opposed to injected or swallowed) help healing or prevent infection. Uninfected, well-cleaned wounds usually heal by themselves. If a wound is infected and antibiotics are needed, they should be given by mouth or by injection.

Despite the controversy over external use of antibiotics, dermatologists (skin doctors) often prescribe this combination drug to treat some superficial skin infections, such as inflammation of hair follicles (folliculitis) and impetigo.

Neomycin commonly causes skin rashes in 8% of the people who use it.[103] Using neomycin can also make it hard for you to use other drugs in its family (aminoglycoside antibiotics, such as gentamicin and tobramycin, see p. 594) that may be needed later in life for serious infections.

LIMITED USE

Norfloxacin
*NOROXIN tablets (Merck)
CHIBROXIN eye drops (Merck)

Generic: not available

Family: Antibiotics (see p. 444)
Fluoroquinolones (see p. 448)
** Do not confuse this drug with
Noroxine, a thyroid hormone de-
scribed on p. 660.*

Norfloxacin (nor *flocks* a sin) kills a broad
spectrum of bacteria and can cure infections
caused by susceptible bacteria. Oral
norfloxacin is primarily used to treat infections in the urinary tract. Drops of
norfloxacin are used to treat eye infections.
Treatment of other conditions, or to prevent
urinary tract infections is still under study,
and not yet approved in the U.S.

Elderly people have suffered more
severe adverse effects, fatalities, and harmful interactions from norfloxacin.[104,105] **Since
in people over age 65 norfloxacin is
excreted more slowly, a lower dose
is usually used.**

Norfloxacin belongs to a family of drugs
called fluoroquinolones. These drugs are
alternatives for individuals allergic to or
with infections resistant to other antibiotics.
A 7-day course of norfloxacin costs 5 to 10
times more than drugs such as amoxicillin
or trimethoprim sulfamethoxazole (see
p. 453), which are equally effective for most
infections. Both resistance and allergy to
one drug in this family usually cross to the
rest of the fluoroquinolones and sometimes
even occur during therapy.[106,107] Overgrowth of normal bacteria may cause yeast
infections, especially when antibiotics are
used for long periods. The fluoroquinolones
can cause central nervous system reactions
and psychosis.[108] Severe, even fatal, allergic

reactions have happened after just one
dose. Collapse of the circulatory system has
occurred. As a group fluoroquinolones are
expensive, resistance is increasing, and
effective alternatives are available.[109]

The same adverse effects of norfloxacin
can result from either oral tablets or
eye drops.

Practice measures to prevent urinary
tract infections. Drink plenty of fluids,
especially water. While cranberry juice is
unreliable as a cure for urinary tract infections, the juice may reduce odor from
incontinence.[110] Practice meticulous hygiene. After using the toilet, wipe backwards, not forwards, then wash your
hands. Prepare and store foods properly,
especially when traveling to prevent diarrhea. Restrict caffeine, which widens the

---

Warning
Extreme caution should be used
when fluoroquinolones such as
norfloxacin are to be prescribed in
conjunction with aminophylline or
theophylline, particularly in elderly
patients. Prudence would suggest that
aminophylline doses be adjusted,
perhaps reduced by 30% to 50% at the
initiation of fluoroquinolone therapy.
The reduction in dose must be guided
by the clinical conditions of the patient,
the use of other concomitant medication, and the baseline value of the
theophylline serum concentration. In
addition, serum theophylline levels
should be obtained following the
initiation of a fluoroquinolone no later
than 2 days into therapy.[111]

urethra. Indwelling catheters invite urinary tract infections. However, unless there are symptoms of urinary infection, it is not always necessary to take medication just because bacteria are found in a urine test.[112] Women are particularly prone to repeated urinary tract infections. If urinary tract symptoms occur often, ask your doctor about keeping a supply of medication on hand. Ideally, the antibiotic you use should be the most effective, least toxic, and least costly.[113,114]

Before You Use This Drug

Tell your doctor if you have or have had
❑ allergies to drugs
❑ epilepsy
❑ kidney or liver problems
❑ seizures
Tell your doctor about any other drugs you take, including aspirin, herbs, vitamins, and other non-prescription products.

When You Use This Drug

Do not drive or perform other activities that require alertness because this drug may make you drowsy, dizzy, or lightheaded.

Take all the norfloxacin your doctor prescribed, even if you feel better before you run out. If you stop too soon, your symptoms could come back.
Drink several glasses of fluids (water, fruit, and vegetable juices) each day. This flushes bacteria out of your bladder and prevents crystals of norfloxacin from forming.
Restrict your use of caffeine.
Limit exposure to bright light. Protect yourself from sunburn by wearing protective clothing, headgear, and sunglasses, and using a sunblock.
If you plan to have any surgery, including dental, tell your doctor that you take this drug.

How To Use This Drug

Swallow tablet whole. Take with **a full glass (8 ounces) of water,** one hour before or two hours after meals. Space doses evenly apart.
◆ Instill eyedrops according to instructions on p. 582.
◆ Avoid touching the tip of the container in or around your eye.
◆ Do not take antacids, sucralfate (Carafate), or products containing iron or zinc within 2 hours of taking norfloxacin.
◆ Do not store in the bathroom, and do not expose to heat, moisture, or strong light.

Interactions With Other Drugs

The following drugs are listed in *Evaluations of Drug Interactions,* 1991 as causing "highly clinically significant" or "clinically significant" interactions when used together with this drug. There may be other drugs, especially those in the families of drugs listed below, that also will react with this drug to cause severe adverse effects. Make sure to ask your doctor for a complete listing of them and let her or him know if you are taking any of these interacting drugs:

aluminum; antacids; caffeine (beverages, drugs); CARAFATE; cyclosporine; ELIXOPHYLLIN; magnesium; SANDIMMUNE; sucralfate; THEO-DUR; theophylline.

Additionally, the *United States Pharmacopeia Drug Information,* 1992 lists this drug as having an interaction of major significance:

calcium.

A report in the *Archives of Internal Medicine* adds this interaction as one most frequently reported in older people:[115]

COUMADIN; warfarin.

Caution should be taken when the following drugs are used with this one (see warning box):

aminophylline; AMOLINE; BRONKODYL; CONSTANT-T; ELIXOPHYLLIN; QUIBRON-T-SR; SLO-BID; SLO-PHYLLIN; SOMOPHYLLIN; SUSTAIRE; THEO-24; THEOLAIR; theophylline.

Adverse Effects

Call your doctor immediately:
- ❏ difficulty breathing or swallowing
- ❏ confusion, disorientation
- ❏ depression
- ❏ fainting
- ❏ fever
- ❏ hallucinations
- ❏ numbness
- ❏ seizures
- ❏ skin rash, itching or redness
- ❏ swelling of face, neck, tongue, fingers, or joints
- ❏ tremors

Call your doctor if these symptoms continue:
- ❏ abdominal pain
- ❏ anxiety, irritability, restlessness
- ❏ constipation, diarrhea
- ❏ dizziness, lightheadedness
- ❏ drowsiness, fatigue
- ❏ dry mouth
- ❏ headache
- ❏ indigestion
- ❏ insomnia, unusual dreams
- ❏ loss of appetite
- ❏ nausea or vomiting
- ❏ sensitivity to light, sunburn
- ❏ stomach pain
- ❏ bitter taste

Ampicillin
OMNIPEN (Wyeth) POLYCILLIN (Bristol)

Generic: available

Family: Antibiotics (see p. 444)
    Penicillins (see p. 446)

Ampicillin (am pi *sill* in) is used to treat some bacterial infections such as ear, sinus, bladder, and intestinal infections, and to treat people with chronic lung disease who have acute bronchitis. **Ampicillin will not help if you have a cold or the flu. If you have kidney disease, you may need to take less than the usual adult dose of ampicillin.**

Many people who take ampicillin develop a slight skin rash. This may or may not be a sign that you are allergic to the drug. If you get a skin rash, call your doctor. Some of ampicillin's side effects can appear as much as a month after you stop taking it (see Adverse Effects).

Before You Use This Drug

Tell your doctor if you have or have had
- ❏ allergies to drugs
- ❏ a reaction to any penicillin or cephalosporin (see p. 447 for examples)
- ❏ other allergies
- ❏ stomach or intestinal disease
- ❏ kidney disease
- ❏ infectious mononucleosis
- ❏ a salt (sodium)-restricted diet (the injected form of ampicillin contains sodium)

Tell your doctor about any other drugs you take, including aspirin, herbs, vitamins, and other non-prescription products.

When You Use This Drug

- ◆ Call your doctor if your symptoms do not improve in 2 or 3 days or if you get diarrhea. Do not treat the diarrhea yourself.
- ◆ **Take all the ampicillin your doctor prescribed, even if you feel better before you run out. If you stop too soon, your symptoms could come back.**
- ◆ Do not give the drug to anyone else. Throw away outdated drugs.
- ◆ **Caution diabetics:** see p. 516.
- ◆ If you plan to have any surgery, including dental, tell your doctor that you take this drug.

How To Use This Drug

◆ Take ampicillin on an empty stomach (at least 1 hour before or 2 hours after meals) with **a full glass (8 ounces) of water.** Capsules may be opened and mixed with water.

◆ Store liquid form in the refrigerator but do not freeze. Shake well before using.

◆ Do not store capsules in the bathroom, and do not expose to heat, moisture, or strong light.

◆ If you miss a dose, take it as soon as you remember, but skip it if it is almost time for the next dose. **Do not take double doses.**

Interactions With Other Drugs

The following drugs are listed in *Evaluations of Drug Interactions*, 1991 as causing "highly clinically significant" or "clinically significant" interactions when used together with this drug. There may be other drugs, especially those in the families of drugs listed below, that also will react with this drug to cause severe adverse effects. Make sure to ask your doctor for a complete listing of them and let her or him know if you are taking any of these interacting drugs:

AUREOMYCIN; chlortetracycline; COUMADIN; GARAMYCIN; gentamicin; heparin; warfarin.

Adverse Effects

Call your doctor immediately:

❏ **if you have signs of severe allergic reaction (anaphylactic shock):** severe asthma (wheezing); extreme weakness; abdominal pain; nausea or vomiting; diarrhea; rash

Call your doctor immediately, even if it has been a month since you stopped taking ampicillin:

❏ pain, cramps, or bloating in the abdomen or stomach

❏ severe, watery diarrhea (may contain blood)

❏ fever

❏ nausea or vomiting

❏ increased thirst

❏ abnormal weakness or tiredness

❏ abnormal weight loss

❏ skin rash, hives, or itching

Call your doctor if these symptoms continue:

❏ mild diarrhea

❏ sore mouth or tongue

❏ darkened or discolored tongue

Penicillin G
PENTIDS (Squibb)
Penicillin V
PEN VEE K (Wyeth)

Generic: available

Family: Antibiotics (see p. 444)
Penicillins (see p. 446)

These two forms of penicillin (pen i *sill* in) are taken by mouth (orally). They are used to treat some infections caused by bacteria, including strep throat, some other oral (mouth) infections, and skin infections. Your doctor may also prescribe oral penicillin for you to take at home if you are just getting out of the hospital and were getting antibiotic shots while you were in the hospital. **Penicillin will not help if you have a cold or the flu.**

If you are taking penicillin by mouth, penicillin V is the better form to take because your body absorbs it better. **If you have kidney damage, you may need to take less than the usual adult dose.**

Before You Use This Drug
Tell your doctor if you have or have had
❑ allergies to drugs
❑ a reaction to any penicillin or cephalosporin (see p. 447 for examples)
❑ other allergies
❑ stomach or intestinal disease
❑ kidney disease
Tell your doctor about any other drugs you take, including aspirin, herbs, vitamins, and other non-prescription products.

When You Use This Drug
◆ Call your doctor if your symptoms do not improve in 2 or 3 days or if you get diarrhea. Do not treat the diarrhea yourself.
◆ **Take all the penicillin your doctor** prescribed, even if you feel better before you run out. **If you stop too soon, your symptoms could come back.**
◆ Do not give the drug to anyone else. Throw away outdated drugs.
◆ If you plan to have any surgery, including dental, tell your doctor that you take penicillin.

How To Use This Drug
◆ Taking penicillin with food may help prevent stomach upset.
◆ Store liquid form of penicillin in the refrigerator but do not freeze. Shake well before using.
◆ Do not store capsules in the bathroom, and do not expose to heat, moisture, or strong light. Capsules may be opened and mixed with water or food.
◆ If you miss a dose, take it as soon as you remember, but skip it if it is almost time for the next dose. **Do not take double doses.**

Interactions With Other Drugs
The following drugs are listed in *Evaluations of Drug Interactions*, 1991 as causing "highly clinically significant" or "clinically significant" interactions when used together with this drug. There may be other drugs, especially those in the families of drugs listed below, that also will react with this drug to cause severe adverse effects. Make sure to ask your doctor for a complete listing of them and let her or him know if you are taking any of these interacting drugs:

AUREOMYCIN; chlortetracycline; COUMADIN; GARAMYCIN; gentamicin; heparin; warfarin.

Adverse Effects
Call your doctor immediately:
❑ **if you have signs of severe allergic reaction (anaphylactic shock):** severe asthma (wheezing); extreme weakness; abdominal pain; nausea or vomiting; diarrhea; rash

Call your doctor immediately, even if it has been a month since you stopped taking penicillin:
❑ pain, cramps, or bloating in the abdomen or stomach

❑ severe, watery diarrhea (may contain blood)
❑ fever
❑ nausea or vomiting
❑ increased thirst
❑ abnormal weakness or tiredness
❑ abnormal weight loss
❑ skin rash, hives, or itching
❑ seizures

Call your doctor if these symptoms continue:
❑ mild diarrhea
❑ darkened or discolored tongue

Trimethoprim
PROLOPRIM (Burroughs Wellcome)
TRIMPEX (Roche)

Generic: available

Family: Antibiotics (see p. 444)
Urinary anti-infectives

Trimethoprim (trye *meth* oh prim) is used mainly to treat some urinary tract infections. **It will not help a cold or the flu.**

If you have severe kidney impairment, you should use caution in taking trimethoprim.[116] **If you have impaired kidney function, you may need to take less than the usual adult dose.** While taking trimethoprim, you may suffer a rash or itching.

Practice measures to prevent urinary tract infections. Drink plenty of fluids, especially water. While cranberry juice is unreliable as a cure for urinary tract infections, the juice may reduce odor from incontinence.[117] Practice meticulous hygiene. After using the toilet, wipe backwards, not forwards, then wash your hands. Prepare and store foods properly, especially when traveling to prevent diarrhea. Restrict caffeine, which widens the urethra. Indwelling catheters invite urinary tract infections. However, unless there are symptoms of urinary infection, it is not always necessary to take medication just because bacteria are found in a urine test.[118] Women are particularly prone to repeated urinary tract infections. If urinary tract symptoms occur often, ask your doctor about keeping a supply of medication on hand. Ideally, the antibiotic you use should be the most effective, least toxic, and least costly.[119,120]

Before You Use This Drug
Tell your doctor if you have or have had
❑ allergies to drugs
❑ an unusual reaction to trimethoprim
❑ folic acid (folate) deficiency
❑ kidney or liver disease
Tell your doctor about any other drugs you take, including aspirin, herbs, vitamins, and other non-prescription products.

When You Use This Drug
◆ Call your doctor if your symptoms do not get better in 2 or 3 days.
◆ **Take all the trimethoprim your doctor**

prescribed, even if you feel better before you run out. If you stop too soon, your symptoms could come back.
- Do not give this drug to anyone else. Throw away outdated drugs.
- Schedule regular doctor's visits to check your progress.
- If you take trimethoprim for a long time, ask your doctor if you need a folic acid supplement.
- If you plan to have any surgery, including dental, tell your doctor that you take this drug.

How To Use This Drug
- Always take doses the same number of hours apart.
- If the drug irritates your stomach, try taking it with food.
- Tablets may be crushed and mixed with food or water.
- Do not store in the bathroom or expose to heat, moisture, or strong light.
- If you miss a dose, take it as soon as you remember. If you are taking trimethoprim only once a day, take the dose you missed and wait about 12 hours before taking the next one. If you are taking trimethoprim twice a day, take the dose you missed and wait about 6 hours before taking the next one.

Interactions With Other Drugs
The following drugs are listed in *Evaluations of Drug Interactions*, 1991 as causing "highly clinically significant" or "clinically significant" interactions when used together with this drug. There may be other drugs, especially those in the families of drugs listed below, that also will react with this drug to cause severe adverse effects. Make sure to ask your doctor for a complete listing of them and let her or him know if you are taking any of these interacting drugs:

COUMADIN; DILANTIN; FOLEX; methotrexate; phenytoin; warfarin.

Adverse Effects
Call your doctor immediately:
- fever or sore throat
- abnormal bleeding or bruising
- abnormal paleness, tiredness, or weakness
- bluish fingernails, lips, or skin
- trouble breathing

Call your doctor if these symptoms continue:
- skin rash or itching
- headache
- unusual taste in mouth
- diarrhea
- loss of appetite
- nausea or vomiting
- sore mouth or tongue
- stomach cramps or pain

Periodic Tests
Ask your doctor which of these tests should be done periodically while you are taking this drug:
- complete blood counts (monthly, if you are on long-term therapy)

Rifampin
RIMACTANE (CIBA)
RIFADIN (Merrell Dow)

Generic: not available

Family: Antibiotics (see p. 444)
        (for tuberculosis)

Rifampin (rif *am* pin) is often used together with other drugs, such as isoniazid (see p. 476), to treat tuberculosis (TB). Rifampin and isoniazid are the most effective drugs to fight TB. If you test positive for TB in a skin test but do not have a confirmed case of the disease, and your doctor decides you need preventive treatment, your treatment will probably be isoniazid alone. If you are carrying a type of bacteria called meningitis but you have no symptoms, you may be prescribed a short course of rifampin alone. However, if you have confirmed tuberculosis, you should always take both of these drugs together. If you take only one, you may develop bacteria that are resistant to one of these drugs.[121]

Some people have developed severe and even fatal liver disease while taking rifampin. You increase your risk of liver disease if you drink alcohol daily, so do not drink while taking this drug. Call your doctor immediately if you have any symptoms of liver disease: fatigue, weakness, malaise (vague feeling of being unwell), loss of appetite, nausea, vomiting, or yellow eyes or skin. If you have impaired liver function, you will probably need to take less than the usual adult dose of rifampin.

Before You Use This Drug
Tell your doctor if you have or have had
❑ allergies to drugs
❑ an unusual reaction to rifampin
❑ alcohol dependence
❑ liver disease
Tell your doctor about any other drugs you take, including aspirin, herbs, vitamins, and other non-prescription products.

When You Use This Drug
◆ Do not drink alcohol.
◆ Call your doctor if your symptoms don't get better in 2 or 3 weeks or if they get worse.
◆ **Take all the rifampin your doctor prescribed, even if you feel better in a few weeks. You may have to take rifampin every day for a year or more. If you stop too soon, your symptoms might come back.**
◆ **Do not miss doses. If you do not keep to your schedule for taking rifampin, you are more likely to have serious side effects. Stopping and starting the drug can cause kidney failure, although this is rare.**
◆ Do not give this drug to anyone else. Throw away outdated drugs.
◆ Your urine, stools, saliva, sweat, and tears might turn red or orange. This is no cause for alarm, but let your doctor know that it has happened and watch for signs of overdose (see Adverse Effects). If you wear soft contact lenses, they may be permanently discolored.
◆ If you plan to have any surgery, including dental, tell your doctor that you take this drug.

How To Use This Drug
◆ Take with **a full glass (8 ounces) of water** on an empty stomach (at least 1 hour before or 2 hours after meals). If it upsets your stomach, try taking it with food.
◆ Capsules may be opened and mixed with food such as applesauce or jelly.
◆ Do not store in the bathroom or expose to heat or direct light.

◆ If you miss a dose, take it as soon as you remember, but skip it if it is almost time for the next dose. **Do not take double doses.**

Interactions With Other Drugs

The following drugs are listed in *Evaluations of Drug Interactions*, 1991 as causing "highly clinically significant" or "clinically significant" interactions when used together with this drug. There may be other drugs, especially those in the families of drugs listed below, that also will react with this drug to cause severe adverse effects. Make sure to ask your doctor for a complete listing of them and let her or him know if you are taking any of these interacting drugs:

CALAN; CATAPRES; chloramphenicol; CHLOROMYCETIN; clonidine; COUMADIN; CRYSTODIGIN; cyclosporine; digitoxin; digoxin; DILANTIN; DOLOPHINE; DURAQUIN; ELIXOPHYLLIN; FLUOTHANE; halothane; HYDELTRA-TBA; INH; isoniazid; ketoconazole; LANOXICAPS; LANOXIN; LOPRESSOR; methadone; metoprolol; METRETON; NIZORAL; phenytoin; PRED FORTE; prednisolone; QUINAGLUTE DURA-TABS; quinidine; SANDIMMUNE; theophylline; verapamil; warfarin.

Adverse Effects

Call your doctor immediately:
❏ **if you experience signs of overdose:** nausea; vomiting; extreme tiredness; malaise; abdominal pain
❏ **if you experience flu-like symptoms:** fever; chills; trouble breathing; dizziness; headache; muscle or joint aches; shivering
❏ confusion or inability to concentrate
❏ loss of appetite
❏ nausea or vomiting
❏ abnormal tiredness or weakness
❏ bloody or cloudy urine
❏ noticeable decrease in frequency of urinating or amount of urine
❏ sore throat
❏ abnormal bruising or bleeding
❏ yellow eyes or skin

Call your doctor if these symptoms continue:
❏ diarrhea
❏ stomach cramps or heartburn
❏ itching, redness, or skin rash
❏ sore mouth or tongue
❏ blurring or any change in vision

Periodic Tests

Ask your doctor which of these tests should be done periodically while you are taking this drug:
❏ liver function tests

Silver Sulfadiazine
SILVADENE (Marion)

Generic: available

Family: Antibiotics (see p. 444)
Sulfonamides

Silver sulfadiazine (sul fa *dye* a zeen) is a cream that is used on burns, to prevent and treat infection. **If you have decreased kidney and liver function, you may need to use less than the usual adult dose to prevent dangerous levels of this drug from accumulating in your body.** When you use this cream on burns over large areas of your body, your doctor should be carefully watching your kidney function and the levels of the drug in your body, and your urine should be tested for sulfa crystals.

Before You Use This Drug
Tell your doctor if you have or have had
❑ allergies to drugs
❑ an unusual reaction to silver sulfadiazine
❑ glucose-6-phosphate dehydrogenase deficiency
❑ liver or kidney disease
Tell your doctor about any other drugs you take, including aspirin, herbs, vitamins, and other non-prescription products.

Interactions With Other Drugs
The following drugs are listed in *Evaluations of Drug Interactions,* 1991 as causing "highly clinically significant" or "clinically significant" interactions when used together with this drug. There may be other drugs, especially those in the families of drugs listed below, that also will react with this drug to cause severe adverse effects. Make sure to ask your doctor for a complete listing of them and let her or him know if you are taking any of these interacting drugs:
COUMADIN; DILANTIN; FOLEX; methotrexate; ORINASE; phenytoin; tolbutamide; warfarin.

Adverse Effects
Call your doctor immediately:
❑ burning, itching, or rash (rare)
❑ worsening of condition, or no improvement
Because silver sulfadiazine is absorbed into the body, you may have other side effects like those that occur with the sulfonamides (sulfa drugs). See sulfisoxasole, p. 474, for examples.

LIMITED USE

Cefixime
SUPRAX (Lederle)

Generic: not available

Family: Antibiotics (see p. 444)
Cephalosporins (see p. 446)

Cefixime (sef *ix* ime) is an antibiotic used for certain infections, such as uncomplicated urinary tract infections, gonorrhea, respiratory, sinus, or ear infections. Cefixime has no demonstrated clinical advantage over other antibiotics, some of which cost much less **and does not help a cold, or staph infections.** Gastrointestinal toxicity, mainly diarrhea, appears to be more frequent with cefixime than with some other drugs, such as amoxicillin (see p. 500) or cefaclor (see p. 457).[122]

Before You Use This Drug
Tell your doctor if you have or have had
❑ allergies to drugs
❑ colitis
❑ diabetes
❑ kidney or liver problems
❑ stomach disorders
❑ a salt (sodium)-restricted diet (injected form of cefixime contains sodium)
Tell your doctor about any other drugs you take, including aspirin, herbs, vitamins, and other non-prescription products.

When You Use This Drug
◆ Call your doctor if your symptoms do not improve in 2 or 3 days or if you get diarrhea. Do not treat the diarrhea yourself.
◆ **Take all the cefixime your doctor prescribed, even if you feel better before you run out. If you stop too soon, your symptoms could come back.**
◆ **Caution diabetics: see p. 516.**
◆ Do not give the drug to anyone else. Throw away outdated drugs.

◆ If you plan to have any surgery, including dental, tell your doctor that you take this drug.

How To Use This Drug
◆ Swallow tablet whole. If you take the liquid form, shake it well before measuring. Since the liquid contains sugar, rinse your mouth after swallowing a dose.
◆ If you miss a dose, take it as soon as you remember, but skip it if it is almost time for the next dose. **Do not take double doses.**
◆ Do not store tablets in the bathroom, and do not expose to heat, moisture, or strong light. The oral liquid may be refrigerated, but avoid freezing. Discard liquid after two weeks.

Interactions With Other Drugs
The following drugs are listed in *Evaluations of Drug Interactions,* 1991 as causing "highly clinically significant" or "clinically significant" interactions when used together with this drug. There may be other drugs, especially those in the families of drugs listed below, that also will react with this drug to cause severe adverse effects. Make sure to ask your doctor for a complete listing of them and let her or him know if you are taking this interacting drug:
BENEMID; COLBENEMID; probenecid.
Additionally, the *United States Pharmacopeia Drug Information,* 1992 lists these drugs as having interactions of major significance:
COUMADIN; heparin; warfarin.

Adverse Effects
Call your doctor immediately, even if it has been a month since you stopped taking cefixime:
❑ abdominal cramps

- ❏ bleeding, bruising
- ❏ breathing difficulty
- ❏ severe diarrhea
- ❏ dizziness
- ❏ fever
- ❏ headache
- ❏ seizures
- ❏ skin rash, blistering, itching
- ❏ decrease in amount of urine

Call you doctor if these symptoms continue:
- ❏ loss of appetite
- ❏ changes in stool or diarrhea
- ❏ dry mouth

- ❏ fatigue
- ❏ gas, heartburn
- ❏ insomnia
- ❏ pain in joints
- ❏ nausea, vomiting, mild diarrhea
- ❏ sore mouth or tongue

Periodic Tests
Ask your doctor which of these tests should be done periodically while you are taking this drug:
- ❏ bleeding time or prothrombin time
- ❏ stool exam

Amantadine
SYMMETREL (Du Pont)

Generic: available

Family: Antivirals
Antiparkinsonians

Amantadine (a *man* ta deen) is used to treat two different problems: diseases caused by a virus, such as flu, and Parkinson's disease. **If you are over 60, you will probably need to take less than the usual adult dose.** For use against flu, **a lower dose of no more than 100 mg is recommended for older people,** even less if your kidney is impaired, or you are underweight.[123,124]

For the flu (influenza), it is best to get a flu shot early in the season. However, if you cannot get a flu shot because it is unavailable or you have a medical condition that prevents it, you can use amantadine. During outbreaks of the flu, amantadine may be prescribed in addition to earlier flu shots. For amantadine to be effective against the flu, you must take it within 48 hours of your first flu symptoms.[125]

Your doctor may also prescribe amantadine if you have Parkinson's disease, usually as a supplement to another drug. A combination drug of two drugs called levodopa and carbidopa (see p. 537) is the best treatment for Parkinson's disease. Amantadine is often effective only for a limited time (less than 6 months), and it often produces side effects such as confusion, lightheadedness, hallucinations, and anxiety, which reduce its usefulness.[126] When you are taking amantadine, especially if you are a woman, the skin of your legs may become mottled (this is known as livedo reticularis). This will go away when you stop taking the drug.

If you have symptoms of parkinsonism, you should know that they might be caused by a drug that you are taking for another problem. As many as half of older adults with these symptoms may have developed them as a side effect of one of their drugs. A list of drugs that can cause symptoms of parkinsonism appears on p. 30. If you are taking any of the drugs on this list, discuss the possibility of drug-induced parkinsonism with your doctor, and ask to have your prescription changed or stopped.

Before You Use This Drug
Tell your doctor if you have or have had
- ❏ allergies to drugs

❏ blood vessel disease of the brain
❏ congestive heart failure
❏ eczema (recurring)
❏ heart disease, swelling of feet
  and ankles
❏ kidney disease
❏ mental illness
❏ seizures, epilepsy
❏ stomach ulcers

Tell your doctor about any other drugs you take, including aspirin, herbs, vitamins, and other non-prescription products.

When You Use This Drug

◆ **Keep to the schedule and dose your doctor prescribed for you. Do not use more or less often, or in a higher or lower dose, than was prescribed.**

◆ Avoid driving and other activities requiring alertness until you know how you react to this drug. Amantadine can cause fainting and confusion.

◆ You may feel dizzy when rising from a lying or sitting position. If you are lying down, hang your legs over the side of the bed for a few minutes, then get up slowly. When getting up from a chair, stay by the chair until you are sure that you are not dizzy. (See p. 14.)

◆ Do not drink alcohol.

◆ Take measures to prevent falls. Hold on to handrails or steps, avoid using throw rugs.

How To Use This Drug

◆ Do not store in the bathroom or expose to heat, strong light, or moisture. Do not let the liquid form freeze.

◆ If you miss a dose, take it as soon as you remember, but skip it if it is less than 4 hours until the next dose. **Do not take double doses.**

Interactions With Other Drugs

Some other drugs that you may be taking (either over-the-counter or prescription drugs) can interact with this one, causing adverse effects. Find out from your doctor what these drugs are and let him or her know if you are taking any of them.

Adverse Effects

Call your doctor immediately:
❏ **if you experience signs of overdose:** severe confusion or other mental changes; seizures; severe nightmares; trouble sleeping
❏ confusion or hallucinations
❏ mood or mental changes
❏ problems urinating
❏ fainting
❏ slurred speech
❏ uncontrolled rolling of eyes
❏ sore throat and fever
❏ swelling of feet or lower legs
❏ shortness of breath
❏ rapid weight gain
Call your doctor if these symptoms continue:
❏ difficulty concentrating
❏ dizziness, lightheadedness
❏ irritability
❏ loss of appetite
❏ nausea, vomiting
❏ nervousness
❏ red, blotchy spots on skin
❏ nightmares, trouble sleeping
❏ blurred vision
❏ constipation
❏ dry mouth, nose, and throat
❏ headache
❏ rash

Periodic Tests

Ask your doctor which of these tests should be done periodically while you are taking this drug:
❏ blood pressure

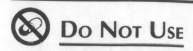 **DO NOT USE**

Alternative treatment: See Clotrimazole (p. 483) and Miconazole (p. 481).

Terconazole
TERAZOL 3 Vaginal Cream or Suppositories (Ortho)
TERAZOL 7 Vaginal Cream (Ortho)

Family: Antifungals

Terconazole (ter *kone* a zole) is used to treat vaginal fungal infections. It is equally as effective as some other antifungal creams (for example clotrimazole and miconazole), but it is absorbed into the body much more than miconazole or clotrimazole, and can cause flu-like symptoms of headache, chills, fever, and a drop in blood pressure.[127,128] If you are using this drug, or if your doctor recommends it, ask your doctor to change your prescription.

Mild vaginal infections are often self-limiting.[129] For some women a bland cream (without drugs) relieves symptoms until infection spontaneously goes away.[130] Preventive measures include less sugar in the diet, and avoiding tightfitting pants and panty hose. Cotton is preferable to synthetics.[131] Dry the vaginal area thoroughly after bathing or swimming.

Amoxicillin
TRIMOX (Squibb) POLYMOX (Bristol)
Amoxicillin and Clavulanate (combined)
AUGMENTIN (Beecham)

Generic: available for Amoxicillin
          not available for Augmentin

Family: Antibiotics (see p. 444)
         Penicillins (see p. 446)

Amoxicillin (a mox i *sill* in) is used to treat certain infections caused by bacteria, such as ear, sinus, and bladder infections. It is also prescribed for bronchitis in people with chronic lung disease and for gonorrhea. A second drug, clavulanate, is sometimes combined with amoxicillin. It helps amoxicillin work better by preventing bacteria from resisting the drug. **Amoxicillin will not help a cold or the flu.**

If you have kidney disease, you may need to take less than the usual adult dose of amoxicillin. In rare instances older people may develop hepatitis if taking the combination of amoxicillin and clavulanate. This is reversible but the hepatitis often does not occur until after the drug is stopped.[132,133]

Before You Use This Drug
Tell your doctor if you have or have had
❑ allergies to drugs
❑ a reaction to any penicillin or cephalosporin (see p. 446 for examples)
❑ allergies
❑ stomach or intestinal disease
❑ kidney disease
❑ liver disease (*for amoxicillin and clavulanate*)
❑ infectious mononucleosis

❑ a salt (sodium)-restricted diet (the injected form of amoxicillin contains sodium)

Tell your doctor about any other drugs you take, including aspirin, herbs, vitamins, and other non-prescription products.

When You Use This Drug

◆ Call your doctor if your symptoms do not improve in 2 or 3 days or if you get diarrhea. Do not treat the diarrhea yourself.

◆ **Take all the amoxicillin your doctor prescribed, even if you feel better before you run out. If you stop too soon, your symptoms could come back.**

◆ Do not give this drug to anyone else. Throw away outdated drugs.

◆ If you plan to have any surgery, including dental, tell your doctor that you take amoxicillin.

How To Use This Drug

◆ Taking amoxicillin with food may help prevent stomach upset. Capsules may be opened and mixed with water or food.

◆ Store liquid form in the refrigerator but do not freeze. Shake well before using.

◆ Do not store capsules in the bathroom, and do not expose to heat, moisture, or strong light.

◆ If you miss a dose, take it as soon as you remember, but skip it if it is almost time for the next dose. **Do not take double doses.**

Interactions With Other Drugs

The following drugs are listed in *Evaluations of Drug Interactions,* 1991 as causing "highly clinically significant" or "clinically significant" interactions when used to-

gether with this drug. There may be other drugs, especially those in the families of drugs listed below, that also will react with this drug to cause severe adverse effects. Make sure to ask your doctor for a complete listing of them and let her or him know if you are taking any of these interacting drugs:

COUMADIN; GARAMYCIN; gentamicin; heparin; warfarin.

Adverse Effects

Call your doctor immediately:

❑ **if you have signs of severe allergic reaction (anaphylactic shock):** severe asthma (wheezing); extreme weakness; abdominal pain; nausea or vomiting; diarrhea; rash

Call your doctor immediately, even if it has been a month since you stopped taking amoxicillin:

❑ pain, cramps, or bloating in abdomen or stomach

❑ severe, watery diarrhea (may contain blood)

❑ fever

❑ nausea or vomiting

❑ increased thirst

❑ abnormal weakness or tiredness

❑ abnormal weight loss

❑ skin rash, hives, or itching

❑ dark urine

❑ yellow eyes or skin

❑ light-colored stools

❑ loss of appetite

❑ itching

Call your doctor if these symptoms continue:

❑ mild diarrhea

❑ sore mouth or tongue

❑ darkened or discolored tongue

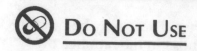 **DO NOT USE**

Alternative treatment: See Ampicillin, p. 489, Trimethoprim, p. 492, and Trimethoprim and Sulfamethoxazole, p. 453.

Atropine, Hyoscyamine, Methenamine, Methylene Blue, Phenyl Salicylate, and Benzoic Acid (combined)
URISED (Webdon)

Family: Antibiotics (see p. 444)
Antispasmodics
Painkillers

This combination of six drugs — atropine (see p. 336), hyoscyamine (hye oh *sye* a meen), methenamine (meth *en* a meen), methylene (*meth* i leen) blue, phenyl salicylate (*fen* ill sa *li* si late), and benzoic (ben *zoe* ik) acid — is used to treat symptoms of urinary tract infections. **This combination of drugs is irrational and too complex, and it should not be used.** Part of the problem is that because the dosage of each individual drug is fixed, your doctor cannot adjust dosages to ensure that the product will be safe and effective. And one drug in this combination, **atropine, causes side effects so severe that people over 60 should not take it at all.**

Some of the ingredients in this product may cause excitement, agitation, drowsiness, or confusion in older adults, even at the usual dose. Call your doctor if you have any of these symptoms. Also, in people over 40, this drug may cause glaucoma, an eye disease that often remains hidden.

Warning: Special Mental and Physical Adverse Effects

Older adults are especially sensitive to the harmful anticholinergic effects of a family of drugs known as belladonna alkaloids. Atropine and hyoscyamine are both in this family. Drugs in this family should not be used unless absolutely necessary.

Mental Effects: confusion, delirium, short-term memory problems, disorientation, and impaired attention.

Physical Effects: dry mouth, constipation, difficulty urinating (especially for a man with an enlarged prostate), blurred vision, decreased sweating with increased body temperature, sexual dysfunction, and worsening of glaucoma.

Mebendazole
VERMOX (Janssen)

Generic: not available

Family: Antiparasites

Mebendazole (meb *n* dah zoll) is a drug of choice for hookworms, lungworm, pinworms, porkworms, roundworms, threadworms, and whipworms, as well as filiarsis caused by Mansonella perstans, and gnathomiasis. It is an alternative drug to treat creeping eruption. Mebendazole is also preferred for mixed infestations of two or more parasites. It deprives the invaders of sugar needed for energy, thereby killing or immobilizing the eggs, larvae, or adult form, depending on the parasite.

It is very important that these conditions be treated since if worms escape from the intestines, they can be unsettling under the skin, and dangerous in the heart, mouth, liver, or joints.[134,135] Masses of roundworms have blocked the intestines or bile duct during therapy.[136] In high doses mebendazole has suppressed the bone marrow. Mebendazole is not approved in the U.S. for tapeworm or hydatid diseases.

Effectiveness of mebendazole depends on whether the infestation is minor or severe, how long it takes worms to pass through your digestive tract, whether or not you have diarrhea, and the susceptibility of the worms. It may take a few days for the body to expel dead forms in the stool. Length of therapy varies from three days to several months, according to the type and number of parasites. At times treatment needs to be repeated at least once. In severe infections, use of mebendazole may prevent the need for a blood transfusion or surgery. Compared to some other pinworm medicine, mebendazole has an advantage of not staining clothing or bedding.

At times individuals recover spontaneously from lungworm.[137] However, it can persist in the body for decades.[138] You may be more susceptible to parasites if you take immunosuppressant drugs or corticosteroids.[139]

Several measures can prevent infestation. Wear shoes. Do not go barefoot where human or animal feces may be on the ground, including beaches, children's sandboxes, and fertilized gardens. Wash fruits and vegetables thoroughly. Eat meat that is completely cooked. Wash your hands before preparing food, eating, and after going to the toilet. Use sanitary conditions to dispose of human feces. Be cautious when traveling to areas with dense shade, high humidity, and sandy soil, coupled with poor sanitation.

Before You Use This Drug
Tell your doctor if you have or have had
❏ allergies to drugs
❏ AIDS[140]
❏ anemia
❏ Crohn's ileitis or colitis
❏ persistent or bloody diarrhea
❏ "ground itch" of feet or hands
❏ inflammatory bowel disease
❏ itching of anal area
❏ liver disease
❏ organ transplant[141]
❏ peptic ulcer
❏ stomach surgery[142]
❏ ulcerative colitis

Inform your doctor of activities, places, or work that may have exposed you to parasites:
❏ lived or traveled in tropical or subtropical areas, especially the Southeastern United States, the Caribbean, Central and South America, the Phillipines, Africa, Thailand, Vietnam, Burma, Turkey, and Eastern Europe.
❏ worked in agriculture, mining, plumbing, tunneling, or with foreign missions, immigrants, refugees, foreign visitors, or been duck hunting.

Tell your doctor about any other drugs you take, including aspirin, herbs, vitamins, and other non-prescription products.

When You Use This Drug

◆ **Take all the mebendazole your doctor prescribed, even if you feel better before you run out. If you stop too soon, your symptoms could come back.**

Prevent reinfection and transmission
Disinfect toilets
Wash your hands often, especially before eating and after using the toilet. Use soap and water and clean under your fingernails.
Change undergarments, bedding, towels, and nightclothes daily.
Launder bedding, towels, and nightclothes to prevent reinfection of pinworms. Merely shaking bedding and clothes is not sufficient.
Observe stools for signs of parasites. If you think there is reinfection, take a stool sample to your doctor.

Also,
Ask your doctor about any diet changes, especially if you are on a low-fat diet.
Ask your doctor if you need to take iron or folic acid supplements.
Do not fast or use enemas or laxatives unless your doctor advises you to do so.
Check with your doctor if there is no improvement within a few days.

How To Use This Drug

Chew tablets, or swallow whole. If desired you may crush the tablets and mix with food. For severe whipworm infections, doctors sometimes order an enema of mebendazole for the pharmacist to compound.[143] If your doctor orders this follow the instructions on your prescription label.
If your dose is high or your course of therapy long, then mebendazole should be taken with a fatty meal which allows your system to absorb the drug more efficiently.

◆ If you miss a dose, take it as soon as you remember. If it is almost time for the next dose, space according to the number of doses you take each day. For 2 doses a day, space the missed dose and the next dose at least 4 hours apart. If you take 8 doses a day, space the missed dose and the next dose at least one and one-half hours apart.
◆ Do not store in the bathroom, and do not expose to heat, moisture, or strong light.

Interactions With Other Drugs

Some other drugs that you may be taking (either over-the-counter or prescription drugs) can interact with this one, causing adverse effects. Find out from your doctor what these drugs are and let him or her know if you are taking any of them.

Adverse Effects

Call your doctor immediately:
❏ fever
❏ itching
❏ skin rash
❏ sore throat
❏ unusual tiredness or weakness

Call your doctor if these symptoms continue:
❏ abdominal pain
❏ diarrhea
❏ dizziness
❏ hair loss
❏ headache
❏ nausea and vomiting
❏ numbness
❏ ringing in the ears

Periodic Tests

Ask your doctor which of these tests should be done periodically while you are taking this drug:
❏ blood levels of mebendazole
❏ complete blood count (CBC)
❏ perianal exam
❏ stool exam

Doxycycline
VIBRAMYCIN (Pfizer) DOXYCHEL (Rachelle)

Generic: available

Family: Antibiotics (see p. 444)
        Tetracyclines (see p. 449)

Doxycycline (dox i *sye* kleen) is used to treat chronic infections of the prostate gland, urinary tract infections, pelvic inflammatory disease, and acute bronchitis (in people with chronic lung disease). **Doxycycline will not help a cold or the flu.**

Doxycycline is sometimes used to treat bacterial infections that are common in older adults, but it is rarely the best antibiotic for this purpose.[144] Penicillin would be a better choice. People with kidney damage who need to take a tetracycline drug are better off taking doxycycline than any other, but they should have their kidney function monitored carefully by their doctor while they are taking this drug. **People with liver failure might need to take less than the usual adult dose of doxycycline.**

When you take doxycycline, make sure that you either drink at least one full glass of water or take it with food. **Some people who have taken doxycycline at bedtime, without sufficient water to wash it down, have gotten esophageal ulcers (irritation of the esophagus, the tube leading from the throat to the stomach).**[145] Doxycycline is more likely than any other pill to lead to this problem.

Before You Use This Drug
Tell your doctor if you have or have had
❑ allergies to drugs
❑ an unusual reaction to doxycycline, tetracycline or other drugs in this family
❑ liver disease
Tell your doctor about any other drugs you take, including aspirin, herbs, vitamins, and other non-prescription products.

When You Use This Drug
◆ Stay out of the sun as much as possible, and call your doctor if you get a rash, hives, or any other skin reaction. Doxycycline makes you more sensitive to the sun.
◆ Do not eat or drink milk or other dairy products, and do not take antacids or iron, vitamin, or mineral supplements for a few hours before and after you take each dose of doxycycline. These substances can stop your body from absorbing the drug, which makes it less effective.
◆ Call your doctor if your symptoms do not improve in 2 or 3 days or if you get diarrhea. Do not treat the diarrhea yourself.
◆ **Take all the doxycycline your doctor prescribed, even if you feel better before you run out. If you stop too soon, your symptoms could come back.**
◆ Do not give this drug to anyone else. Throw away outdated drugs.
◆ If you plan to have any surgery, including dental, tell your doctor that you take this drug.

How To Use This Drug
◆ Take on an empty stomach (at least 1 hour before or 2 hours after meals) with **a full glass (8 ounces) of water.** Take your last dose of the day with **a full glass of water** at least an hour before bedtime. If your stomach gets irritated when you take this drug, you can take it with food to help prevent that.
◆ Keep the container closed tightly and in a dry place. Do not store in the bathroom or expose to heat, strong light, or moisture. **Do not use if the appearance or taste has changed.**
◆ Take doxycycline at least 2 hours apart from any other drug you are taking.

◆ If you miss a dose, take it as soon as you remember, but skip it if it is almost time for your next dose. **Do not take double doses unless you are taking it 3 or more times a day (see p. 449).**

Interactions With Other Drugs

The following drugs are listed in *Evaluations of Drug Interactions*, 1991 as causing "highly clinically significant" or "clinically significant" interactions when used together with this drug. There may be other drugs, especially those in the families of drugs listed below, that also will react with this drug to cause severe adverse effects. Make sure to ask your doctor for a complete listing of them and let her or him know if you are taking any of these interacting drugs:

aluminum hydroxide; carbamazepine; DILANTIN; HISMANAL; LUMINAL; PBR/12; phenobarbital; phenytoin; SOLFOTON; TEGRETOL.

Adverse Effects
Call your doctor if these symptoms continue:
❑ stomach irritation or cramps
❑ diarrhea
❑ skin rash or increased sensitivity of skin to sun
❑ sore or discolored mouth or tongue
❑ itching in the genital or rectal area
❑ nausea or vomiting
❑ dizziness or clumsiness

LIMITED USE

Azithromycin
ZITHROMAX (Pfizer)

Generic: not available

Family: Antibiotics (see p. 444)

Azithromycin (a *zyth* row my sin) is approved to treat infections, such as chlamydia, urethritis, and pneumonia. Your doctor may prescribe azithromycin for other infections if you are allergic to penicillin. **Azithromycin will not help a cold,** but may be effective in the treatment of bronchitis and sinusitis.[146]

Azithromycin belongs to the same family of antibiotics as erythromycin (see p. 468). For many infections azithromycin is similar in effectiveness to amoxicillin (see p. 500) and erythromycin. However, azithromycin costs much more than these alternative antibiotics. Some experts recommend that it be reserved, in most instances, to treat AIDS-related infections.

Before You Use This Drug
Tell your doctor if you have or have had
❑ allergies to drugs
❑ chronic bronchitis
❑ liver or kidney problems
Tell your doctor about any other drugs you take, including aspirin, herbs, vitamins, and other non-prescription products.

Warning
If you are using azithromycin do not use SELDANE, SELDANE-D or HISMANAL. These allergy drugs, when used in combination with azithromycin can accumulate to dangerous levels in the body and can cause life-threatening, sometimes fatal heart arrhythmias.[147]

When You Use This Drug

◆ Call your doctor if your symptoms do not improve in 2 or 3 days or if you get diarrhea. Do not treat the diarrhea yourself.

◆ **Take all the azithromycin your doctor prescribed, even if you feel better before you run out. If you stop too soon, your symptoms could come back.**

◆ Do not give this drug to anyone else. Throw away outdated drugs.

◆ If you plan to have any surgery, including dental, tell your doctor that you take this drug.

How To Use This Drug

◆ Take with **a full glass (8 ounces) of water** on an empty stomach, (at least 1 hour before or 2 hours after meals. Do not take with food, or at the same time as antacids containing aluminum or magnesium.[148,149,150]

◆ If you miss a dose, take it as soon as you remember, but skip it if it is almost time for the next dose. **Do not take double doses.**

◆ Do not store in the bathroom, and do not expose to heat, moisture, or strong light.

Interactions With Other Drugs

The following drugs are listed in *Evaluations of Drug Interactions*, 1991 as causing "highly clinically significant" or "clinically significant" interactions when used together with this drug. There may be other drugs, especially those in the families of those listed below, that also will react with this drug to cause severe adverse effects. Make sure to ask your doctor for a complete listing of them and let her or him know if you are taking any of these interacting drugs:

alfentanil; CAFERGOT; carbamazepine; COUMADIN; cyclosporine; digoxin; disopyramide; ELIXOPHYLLIN; ergot; LANOXIN; MEDROL; methylprednisolone; NORPACE; SANDIMMUNE; TEGRETOL; THEO-DUR; theophylline; warfarin.

The following drugs should not be taken with azithromycin (see warning box):

astemizole; HISMANAL; SELDANE; SELDANE-D; terfenadine.

Adverse Effects

Call your doctor immediately:

❑ severe, watery diarrhea
❑ skin rash

Call your doctor if these symptoms continue:

❑ abdominal discomfort or pain
❑ dizziness
❑ headache
❑ nausea or vomiting
❑ taste change
❑ vaginal itching

Acyclovir
ZOVIRAX (Burroughs Wellcome)

Generic: not available

Family: Antivirals

Acyclovir (ay *sye* kloe veer) is used mostly to treat genital herpes infections the first time they appear, and to prevent them from coming back. The benefits and risks of using acyclovir to prevent recurrence have not been precisely determined. If you have genital herpes, you should discuss this issue with your doctor. Side effects from this drug are rare, but are more common in people with kidney disease.

You should use acyclovir as soon as herpes symptoms appear. The earlier you use it, the better it works. When you have a herpes outbreak, avoid irritating the sores, wear loose clothing, and keep the infected area dry and clean. To protect your sex partner from infection, do not have sex during an outbreak, and use condoms at all other times. Using condoms for sex during an outbreak can lower the risk that you will infect your partner, but it is not foolproof. Women with genital herpes may be more likely to get cancer of the cervix (the opening of the uterus) and should have an annual Pap smear to check for this.

Before You Use This Drug
Tell your doctor if you have or have had
❑ allergies to drugs
❑ kidney or liver disease
❑ nerve disease
Tell your doctor about any other drugs you take, including aspirin, herbs, vitamins, and other non-prescription products.

When You Use This Drug
◆ **Keep to the schedule and dose your doctor prescribed for you. Do not use more or less often, or in a higher or lower dose, than was prescribed.**

◆ Avoid driving and other activities requiring alertness until you know how you react to this drug. Acyclovir can cause confusion and dizziness.

How To Use This Drug
◆ Capsules may be taken with food.
◆ Do not store in the bathroom or expose to heat, strong light, or moisture.
◆ If you miss a dose, take it as soon as you remember, but skip it if it is almost time for the next dose. **Do not take double doses.**

Interactions With Other Drugs
The following drugs are listed in *Evaluations of Drug Interactions*, 1991 as causing "highly clinically significant" or "clinically significant" interactions when used together with this drug. There may be other drugs, especially those in the families of drugs listed below, that also will react with this drug to cause severe adverse effects. Make sure to ask your doctor for a complete listing of them and let her or him know if you are taking any of these interacting drugs:

aluminum hydroxide; ALTERNAGEL; AMPHOJEL; CARAFATE; carbamazepine; digoxin; DILANTIN; ESKALITH; FEOSOL; ferrous sulfate; insulin; LANOXIN; lithium; LUMINAL; methoxyflurane; penicillin; PENTHRANE; PENTIDS; phenobarbital; phenytoin; sucralfate; TEGRETOL.

Adverse Effects
Call your doctor immediately:
If you take acyclovir by mouth
❑ skin rash
If you get acyclovir injections
❑ rash or hives
❑ blood in urine

❑ confusion or hallucinations
❑ trembling
❑ abdominal pain
❑ trouble breathing
❑ decreased urination
❑ nausea, vomiting, loss of appetite
❑ unusual thirst
❑ seizures
❑ unusual tiredness or weakness

Call your doctor if these symptoms continue:
If you take acyclovir by mouth
❑ diarrhea
❑ dizziness
❑ headache
❑ joint pain

❑ nausea, vomiting
❑ acne
❑ trouble sleeping
If you get acyclovir injections
❑ lightheadedness
❑ headache
❑ unusual sweating

Periodic Tests

Ask your doctor which of these tests should be done periodically while you are taking this drug:
❑ Pap smears
❑ kidney function tests (during long-term, continuous treatment)

Notes for Drugs for Infections

1. Kunin CM. Problems in Antibiotic Usage. In *Principles and Practice of Infectious Diseases*. New York: Wiley, 1985:301-7.

2. *National Disease and Therapeutic Index*, I.M.S., Ambler, Pennsylvania, 1983.

3. *The Medical Letter on Drugs and Therapeutics*. New York: The Medical Letter Inc., 1992; 34:64.

4. Gleckman R, Esposito A. Antibiotics in the elderly: skating on therapeutic thin ice. *Geriatrics* 1980; 35:26-8,33-7.

5. James PR. Untoward effects of antimicrobial drugs. *Post-Graduate Medicine* 1971; 50:193-200.

6. Moellering RC. Factors influencing the clinical use of antimicrobial agents in elderly patients. *Geriatrics* 1978; 33:83-91.

7. Ibid.

8. Beam TR. The third generation of cephalosporins, Part II. *Rational Drug Therapy* 1982; 16:1-5.

9. DiPiro JT, Bowden TA, Hooks VH. Prophylactic parenteral cephalosporins in surgery: Are the newer agents better? *Journal of the American Medical Association* 1984; 252:3277.

10. *The Medical Letter on Drugs and Therapeutics*. New York: The Medical Letter Inc., 1985; 27:107.

11. *The Medical Letter on Drugs and Therapeutics*. New York: The Medical Letter Inc., 1986; 28:33-40.

12. American Society of Hospital Pharmacists. *American Hospital Formulary Service Drug Information*, Bethesda, MD, 1992: 2352-63.

13. Todd A, Faulds D. Ofloxacin a reappraisal of its antimicrobial activity, pharmacology and therapeutic use. *Drugs* 1991; 42:825-76.

14. *The Medical Letter on Drugs and Therapeutics*. New York: The Medical Letter Inc., 1991; 33:71-3.

15. *The Medical Letter on Drugs and Therapeutics.* New York: The Medical Letter Inc., 1992; 34: 58-60.

16. Orland MJ, Saltman RJ, eds. *Manual of Medical Therapeutics.* 25th ed. Boston: Little, Brown and Company, 1986:205.

17. AMA Department of Drugs. *AMA Drug Evaluations.* 5th ed. Chicago: American Medical Association, 1983:1674.

18. Kastrup EK, ed. *Facts and Comparisons.* St. Louis: J.B. Lippincott Co., July 1987:341.

19. Patrick J, Panzer JD. Neomycin sensitivity in the normal (nonatopic) individual. *Archives of Dermatology* 1970; 102:532.

20. Gleckman, op. cit.

21. Moellering, op. cit.

22. AMA, 1983, op. cit., p. 1620.

23. *The Medical Letter on Drugs and Therapeutics,* 1985, op. cit.

24. Keisu M, Wiholm BE, Palmblad J. Trimethoprim-sulphamethoxazole-associated blood dyscrasias. Ten years' experience of the Swedish spontaneous reporting system. *Journal of Internal Medicine* 1990; 228:353-60.

25. Marderosian AD, Liberti L. *Natural Product Medicine,* George F. Stickley Co., Philadelphia, PA, 1988:282.

26. AMA Department of Drugs. *AMA Drug Evaluations.* Chicago: American Medical Association, 1992:1182.

27. Sarma PSA, Durairaj P. Randomized treatment of patients with typhoid and paratyphoid fevers using norfloxacin or chloramphenicol. *Transactions of the Royal Society of Tropical Medicine and Hygiene* 1991; 85:670-1.

28. Schubert ML, Sanyal AJ, Wong ES. Antibiotic prophylaxis for prevention of spontaneous bacterial peritonitis? *Gastroenterology* 1991; 101:550-1.

29. Feder HM, Abrahamian LM, Grant-Kels JM. Is penicillin still the drug of choice for non-bullous impetigo? *The Lancet* 1991; 338:803-5.

30. AMA Department of Drugs. *AMA Drug Evaluations.* Chicago: American Medical Association, 1991:1409-10.

31. Slocombe B, Perry C. The antimicrobial activity of mupirocin — an update on resistance. *Journal of Hospital Infection* 1991; 19 (Supplement B):19-25.

32. *USP DI, Drug Information for the Health Care Professional.* 12th ed. Rockville MD: The United States Pharmacopeial Convention, Inc., 1992:1963-4.

33. Anderson G. Clarithromycin in the treatment of community-acquired lower respiratory tract infections. *Journal of Hospital Infection* 1991; 19(Supplement A):21-27.

34. Gu JW, Scully BE, Neu HC. Bactericidal activity of clarithromycin and its 14-hydroxy metabolite against Haemophilus influenzae and streptococcal pathogens. *Journal of Clinical Pharmacology* 1991; 31:1146-50.

35. Warning Letters from Manufacturers.

36. AMA, 1983, op. cit., p. 1620.

37. *The Medical Letter on Drugs and Therapeutics,* 1979, op. cit.

38. *The Medical Letter on Drugs and Therapeutics.,* 1992, op. cit., p. 49-56.

39. Ray W, Federspiel C, Schaffner W. Prescribing of chloramphenicol in ambulatory practice. *Annals of Internal Medicine* 1976; 84:266.

40. Grasela TH, Dreis MW. An evaluation of quinolone-theophylline using the Food and Drug Administration spontaneous reporting system. *Archives of Internal Medicine* 1992; 152:617-21.

41. American Society of Hospital Pharmacists, op. cit.

42. Todd, op. cit.

43. *The Medical Letter on Drugs and Therapeutics* 1991, op. cit., p. 71-3

44. *The Medical Letter on Drugs and Therapeutics* 1992, op. cit., p. 58-60.

45. Frieden T, Mangi R. Inappropriate use of oral ciprofloxacin. *Journal of the American Medical Association* 1990; 264:1438-40.

46. *The Medical Letter on Drugs and Therapeutics* 1991, op. cit., p. 53.

47. *The Medical Letter on Drugs and Therapeutics* 1991, op. cit., p. 75-6.

48. Marderosian, op. cit.

49. AMA Department of Drugs, 1992, op. cit.

50. Sarma, op. cit.

51. Schubert, op. cit.

52. Mumford CJ, Ginsberg L. Ciprofloxacin and myasthenia gravis. *British Medical Journal* 1990; 301:818.

53. American Society of Hospital Pharmacists, 1992, op. cit., p. 417-26.

54. Hansten and Horn. *Drug Interactions & Updates*. Malvern, PA: Lea Febiger, 1990, Updates of July, 1991:291-92.

55. Hedstrom SA, Hybbinette CH. Nephrotoxicity in isoxazolypenicillin prophylaxis in hip surgery. *Acta Orthopedic Scandinavia* 1988; 59:44-7.

56. Brown AE. Overview of fungal infections in cancer patients. *Seminars in Oncology* 1990; 17(Suppl. 6):2-5.

57. Evans TG, Mayer J, Cohen S, Classen D, Carroll K. Fluconazole failure in the treatment of invasive mycoses. *The Journal of Infectious Diseases* 1991; 164:1232-5.

58. Brown, op. cit.

59. AMA, 1983, op. cit., p. 1620.

60. *The Medical Letter on Drugs and Therapeutics*, 1979, op. cit.

61. 46 *Federal Register* 14355, February 27, 1981.

62. Orland, op. cit.

63. Warning Letters from Manufacturers.

64. *The Medical Letter on Drugs and Therapeutics*. New York: The Medical Letter Inc., 1975;17:53.

65. AMA, 1983, op. cit., p. 1717.

66. Grasela, op. cit.

67. American Society of Hospital Pharmacists, op. cit., p. 2352-63.

68. Todd, op. cit.

69. *The Medical Letter on Drugs and Therapeutics*, 1991, op. cit., p. 71-3.

70. *The Medical Letter on Drugs and Therapeutics*, 1992, op. cit., p. 58-60.

71. Todd, op. cit.

72. Hooton TM, Johnson C, Winter C, Kuwamura L, Rogers ME, Roberts PL, Stamm WE. Single-dose and three-day regimens of ofloxacin versus trimethoprim-sulfamethoxazole for acute cystitis in women. *Antimicrobial Agents and Chemotherapy* 1991; 35:1479-83.

73. Marderosian, op. cit.

74. AMA, 1992, op. cit.

75. Sarma, op. cit.

76. Schubert, op. cit.

77. Dukes MNG, Beeley L. *Side Effects of Drugs Annual* 15, Amsterdam: Elsevier, 1991:313-4.

78. American Society of Hospital Pharmacists, op. cit., p. 2352-63.

79. Sanders WE, Morris JF, Alessi L, Makris AT, McClosky RV, Trenholme GM, Iannini P, Bittner MJ. Oral ofloxacin for the treatment of acute bacterial pneumonia: use of a nontraditional protocol to compare experimental therapy with 'Usual Care' in a multicenter clinical trial. *The American Journal of Medicine* 1991; 91:261-6.

80. Dukes, op. cit.

81. Marderosian, op. cit.

82. AMA, 1992, op. cit.

83. Sarma, op. cit.

84. Schubert, op. cit.

85. 46 *Federal Register* 14355, February 27, 1981.

86. Orland, op. cit.

87. Warning Letters from Manufacturers.

88. Gilman AG, Goodman LS, Rall TW, Murad F, eds. *The Pharmacological Basis of Therapeutics.* 7th ed. New York: Macmillan, 1985:1203-5.

89. Moulding TS, Redeker AG, Kanel GC. Twenty isoniazid-associated deaths in one state. *American Review of Respiratory Disease* 1989; 140:700-5.

90. Murphy R, Swartz R, Watkins PB. Severe acetaminophen toxicity in a patient receiving isoniazid. *Annals of Internal Medicine* 1990; 113:799-800.

91. Moulding TS, Redeker AG, Kanel GC. Acetaminophen, isoniazid, and hepatic toxicity. *Annals of Internal Medicine* 1991; 114:431.

92. AMA, 1983, op. cit., p. 1620.

93. Ibid, p. 1663.

94. *Physicians' Desk Reference.* 40th ed. Oradell, N.J.: Medical Economics Company, 1986: 1278.

95. Thomason JL. Clinical evaluation of terconazole United States experience. *Journal of Reproductive Medicine* 1989; 34:597-601.

96. Doering PL, Santiago TM. Drugs for treatment of vulvovaginal candidiasis: comparative efficacy of agents and regimens. *DICP, The Annals of Pharmacotherapy* 1990; 24:1078-83.

97. *USP DI*, op. cit., p. 1558-62.

98. Thomason, op. cit.

99. Doering, op. cit.

100. *USP DI*, op. cit., p. 1558-62.

101. Patrick, op. cit.

102. Ibid

103. Ibid.

104. Jolson M, Tanner LA, Green L, Grasela TH. Adverse reaction reporting of interaction between warfarin and fluoroquinolones. *Archives of Internal Medicine* 1991; 151:1003-4.

105. Dukes, op. cit., p. 312-3.

106. American Society of Hospital Pharmacists, op. cit., 2352-63.

107. Todd, op. cit.

108. *The Medical Letter on Drugs and Therapeutics*, 1991, op. cit., p. 71-3

109. *The Medical Letter on Drugs and Therapeutics*, 1992, op. cit., p. 58-60.

110. Marderosian, op. cit.

111. Grasela, op. cit.

112. AMA, 1992, op. cit.

113. Sarma, op. cit.

114. Schubert, op. cit.

115. Jolson, op. cit.

116. *Physicians' Desk Reference*, op. cit., p. 759.

117. Marderosian, op. cit.

118. AMA, 1992, op. cit.

119. Sarma, op. cit.

120. Schubert, op. cit.

121. Gilman, 1985, op. cit.

122. *The Medical Letter on Drugs and Therapeutics*. New York: The Medical Letter Inc., 1989; 31:73-5.

123. Degelau J, Somani S, Cooper SL, Irvine PW. Occurrence of adverse effects and high amantadine concentrations with influenza prophylaxis in the nursing home. *Journal of American Geriatric Society* 1990; 38:428-32.

124. Stange KC, Little DW, Blatnik B. Adverse reactions to amantadine prophylaxis of influenza in a retirement home. *Journal of American Geriatric Society* 1991; 33:700-5

125. AMA, 1983, op. cit., p. 1457.

126. Vestal, RE, ed. *Drug Treatment in the Elderly*. Sydney, Australia: ADIS Health Science Press, 1984:311.

127. Hirsch HA. Clinical evaluation of terconazole: European experience. *Journal of Reproductive Medicine* 1989; 34:594-6.

128. Moebius UM. Influenza-like syndrome after terconazole. *The Lancet* 1988; ii:966-7.

129. Thomason, op. cit.

130. Doering, op. cit.

131. *USP DI*, op. cit., p. 1558-62.

132. Larrey D, Vial T, Micaleff A, Babany B et al. Hepatitis associated with amoxycillin - clavulanic acid combination report of 15 cases. *Gut* 1992; 33:368-71.

133. Reddy KR, Brilliant P, Schiff ER. Amoxicillin-clavulanate potassium-associated cholestasis. *Gastroenterology* 1989; 96:1135-41.

134. Chippaux J. Mebendazole treatment of dracunculiasis. *Transactions of the Royal Society of Tropical Medicine* 1991; 85:280.

135. Walden J. Other roundworms trichuris, hookworm, and strongyloides. *Primary Care* 1991; 18:53-74.

136. Gilman AG, Rall TW, Nies AS, Taylor P, eds. *The Pharmacological Basis of Therapeutics.* 8th ed. New York: Pergamon Press, 1990:971.

137. *The Medical Letter on Drugs and Therapeutics,* 1992, op. cit., p. 17-26.

138. Walden, op. cit.

139. Ibid.

140. Ibid.

141. Ibid.

142. Ibid.

143. Ibid.

144. Gleckman, op. cit.

145. Amendola M, Spera TD. Doxycycline-induced esophagitis. *Journal of the American Medical Association* 1985; 253: 1009-11.

146. Bahal N, Nahata MC. The new macrolide antibiotics: azithromycin, clarithromycin, dirithromycin, and roxithromycin. *The Annals of Pharmacology* 1992; 26:46-55.

147. Warning Letters from Manufacturers.

148. Drew RH, Gallis HA. Azithromycin — spectrum of activity, pharmacokinetics, and clinical applications. *Pharmacotherapy* 1992; 12:161-73.

149. Foulds G, Hilligoss DM, Henry EB, Gerber N. The effects of an antacid or cimetidine on the serum concentrations of azithromycin. *Journal of Clinical Pharmacology* 1991; 31:164-7.

150. Whitman MS, Tunkel AR. Azithromycin and clarithromycin: overview and comparison with erythromycin. *Infection Control and Hospital Epidemiology* 1992; 13:357-68.

Drugs For Diabetes

Diabetes and Its Treatment

What is Diabetes?

Diabetes (diabetes mellitus) is a malfunction of the control system that the body uses to supply the cells with energy. In a normal body, sweets and starches (carbohydrates) are broken down in the intestines to simple sugars, mostly glucose. Glucose circulates in the blood and enters cells all over the body to be stored or burned to produce energy. But diabetics respond inappropriately to sweet and starchy foods. Glucose cannot enter the cells normally and accumulates in the blood in high concentrations.

High blood sugar stems from a defect in insulin production and/or a defect in insulin action. Insulin is a hormone made in the pancreas, released into the bloodstream, and carried throughout the body. It enables the body's organs to take sugar from the bloodstream and use it for energy. When there isn't enough insulin or when cells have too few receptors that recognize insulin, sugar is not removed from the bloodstream. High blood sugar levels accumulate.

Diabetes can lead to kidney disease, damage to the retina leading to blindness, nerve damage, foot ulcers, hardening of the arteries, heart disease, and bacterial or fungal infections. Three out of four diabetics die of cardiovascular (heart and blood vessel) disease related to their diabetes, and two of those three deaths are from heart disease.

Juvenile-onset (Type-1) Diabetes

Diabetes can be divided into two categories which differ in both cause and treatment, juvenile-onset and adult-onset. Juvenile-onset diabetics, a small fraction of all diabetics, require insulin to live. With insulin, many live to an old age. Although this type of diabetes most commonly appears in childhood or adolescence, the term "juvenile-onset" is misleading. Juvenile-onset diabetes can first occur in much older patients as well. Therefore, physicians often use the non-age-restricted term *type-1 diabetes* to refer to this type.

In type-1 diabetes, the pancreas cannot produce insulin. When a diabetic eats carbohydrates, the blood sugar rises sharply. This is because glucose, without insulin, can only move into the cells very slowly. While a diabetic's blood contains high concentrations of sugar, the cells starve because there is no insulin to help the sugar get into the cells. Unable to obtain glucose, the cells may be forced to burn fat at an abnormally fast rate, a process that in turn floods the body with substances called ketones. Symptoms of ketoacidosis include vomiting, weakness, stomach pain, dehydration, and very low blood pressure. Untreated, it may even lead to coma and death.

Treatment

To prevent toxic levels of ketones from accumulating in the blood, a type-1 diabetic needs insulin injections daily. By adhering strictly to the American Diabetes Association's diet, a type-1 diabetic can regulate the amount and type of sugar taken into the body at various times throughout the day. The type-1 diabetic needs both insulin injections and a regimented diet to live.

Adult-onset (Type-2) Diabetes

Of the millions of older Americans who have diabetes, 85 to 90% have adult-onset type. The vast majority of these people are obese, averaging about one and one-half times ideal body weight. It is thought that type-2 diabetics have a hereditary tendency toward diabetes which usually reveals itself only when they become overweight. The symptoms of adult-onset diabetes involve, at the worst, increased urination, excessive eating and drinking, and perhaps occasional dizziness. Often this condition can be spotted only with blood tests. Adult-onset diabetes injures its victims in the long run, however, even if it does not endanger them day to day. The many long-term complications of diabetes make it the third leading cause of death in this country behind heart and blood vessel disease and cancer.

Like their type-1 counterparts, type-2 diabetics cannot absorb sugar into their cells at a normal rate, but for a different reason. Unlike type-1 diabetics, these people *do* produce enough insulin — but because they overeat (most adult-onset diabetics are overweight),* their cells lose the ability to respond to insulin. How does this happen? When people consistently overeat, two problems occur. First, the number of insulin receptors (places on the cell where the insulin must bind to take effect) decreases. The insulin receptors return to a normal number when a diabetic stops overeating. Second, in response to this insulin resistance by the cells, obesity forces the overweight person's pancreas to put out as much as three times more insulin than a thin person's. In nondiabetic overweight people, the pancreas merely shifts into high gear and keeps pace with the increased demand for insulin. But in the potential diabetic, the pancreas cannot keep up with demand.

Treatment

Treatment of type-2 diabetes can be one of three kinds: diet, oral hypoglycemic pills (antidiabetes drugs taken by mouth), or insulin injections, as well as diet plus a

---

* Obesity has a damaging effect on glucose metabolism and on insulin receptors not due to the excess fat, but rather due to the overeating that maintains the obese state. Thus — of practical importance physically and psychologically — the benefits of a low calorie diet are achieved early in the diet (often within days) when patients are still overweight.[3]

diabetes pill or diet plus insulin. Are all three treatments equally safe and effective? No. Below is a ranking of treatments from most hazardous to safe.

Diabetes pills, although the easiest therapy to follow, actually undermine the purpose of treating diabetes because they may *increase* your chances of dying from cardiovascular disease. The University Group Diabetes Program (UGDP) study, a study done on insulin and antidiabetes drugs, failed to prove that diabetes pills prevent the long-term complications of diabetes, such as heart disease, kidney disease, and blindness.[1] Moreover, it is probable that these drugs cause premature deaths from cardiovascular disease.[2]

Unlike insulin, oral hypoglycemics are only somewhat effective in lowering blood sugar. They fail to adequately control blood sugar in 20 to 40% of patients. But even if they work at first, they may fail later in as many as 30% of patients per year.[4]

After the UGDP report was released, two clinics that stopped using oral hypoglycemics found no change in blood sugar in about one-third to one-half of patients after stopping the drug, indicating that these people did not need to be on the drug in the first place.[5] The remaining patients were able to lower their blood sugar with diet alone or diet plus insulin. These results suggest that a majority of the people who take oral hypoglycemics could get along with mild dietary changes and not risk premature cardiovascular death.

Two oral hypoglycemics pose additional problems for older people. Chlorpropamide (Diabinese) may cause dangerous, long-lasting periods of low blood sugar. It may also produce trouble breathing; drowsiness; muscle cramps; seizures; swelling of face, hands, or ankles; and unconsciousness, water retention, or weakness that could be life-threatening in people who tend to retain water (people who have congestive heart failure or cirrhosis of the liver).[6] For these reasons, the World Health Organization recommends that it not be used by people 60 years and older. Acetohexamide (Dymelor) is eliminated from the body predominantly by the kidneys. Since kidney function decreases steadily with age, there is a possiblity that toxic amounts of this drug may accumulate in older people.

Chlorpropamide and acetohexamide should not be used in older people. Other diabetes pills should *only* be used by people whose diabetes is not controlled by diet and who cannot inject insulin. Below is an informed consent statement containing information that Public Citizen's Health Research Group believes all patients should receive and sign before they are prescribed diabetes pills.

Insulin, like the diabetes pills, only alters the symptoms of the disease without treating the cause. In too large a dose, it may cause trembling, hunger, weakness, and irritability — symptoms of low blood sugar that can progress to insulin shock. Unlike the diabetes pills, however, insulin has not been shown to increase your chance of cardiovascular disease.

It is very important that you understand the use of the correct needle and syringe and instructions that come in the insulin package. **Ask for help if you are not sure about any part of your treatment.** Your doctor can help you or guide you to help. Improper cleansing or injection technique may cause skin problems. Tell your doctor if you are having skin problems or difficulty injecting insulin. Disposable syringes and needles are meant to be used only once. United States Pharmacopeia medical panels do not recommend reusing them. However, if you do reuse them, the syringe and needle must be used for only one person. After each use, wipe the needle with alcohol and replace the cap. These needles should definitely not be used more than a few times. Glass syringes need to be sterilized each time they are used.

Insulin should be refrigerated but *not frozen*. It can be kept at room temperature for a month, but it is better to keep it in the refrigerator. Do not expose it to hot temperatures or sunlight.

Insulin is available in a wide variety of preparations. Some last longer than others. Local allergy is more common with the less pure, older insulins and may be recognized by a hard, red, itching area at the injection site. If you have a problem with allergy, ask your doctor if you should change to a more highly purified kind of insulin. Some people experience more serious allergic reactions (skin rash, swelling, stomach upset, trouble breathing, and very rarely, low blood pressure or even death).[7] Call your doctor immediately if you think you may be experiencing an allergic reaction.

Diet is the safest, most effective treatment available

Informed Consent For Use of Oral Diabetes Drugs

1. I have participated in a program of dietary control and physical exercise including at least 25 hours of instruction.
2. This program did not succeed in weight reduction or control of blood sugar. Dr. _____ told me that insulin was the preferred drug if one had to be used.
3. I refuse (or am physically unable) to take insulin.
4. I am aware of the increased risk of cardiovascular death from taking oral diabetes drugs and of the animal study showing that one of them (tolbutamide) causes a significant increase in coronary artery disease and that therapeutic efficacy has not been proven.

In light of the above, I agree to take _____ (oral diabetes drug).

_____   _____
date   patient's signature

for the vast majority of adult-onset diabetics. More than 90% of type-2 diabetics are overweight. In most cases, blood sugar levels return to normal and symptoms go away when the diabetic loses weight.

Since a large proportion of diabetics can be treated by diet alone, why are so many people taking pills? There are three reasons: drug companies, doctors, and patients. When the oral hypoglycemic agents became available, they were intended to serve as substitutes for insulin in the few adult-onset diabetics who need diet plus insulin to control their diabetes. Instead, the pills became substitutes for the diet. With the availability of oral drugs, experts stopped stressing the role of diet in controlling the disease, mostly in those very people whose diabetes could have been controlled by an appropriate diet. Doctors found it easier to prescribe a pill than to prod and nag patients into losing weight. Some assume that older people won't change their diet or lose weight. They may not even suggest a trial weight loss period, but rather begin treatment by prescribing an oral hypoglycemic pill. Patients, handed a complex diet by their physician and referred to a dietitian for instructions on weighing food portions and memorizing food choices, often find it easier to take a pill than to change eating habits.

However, it is foolhardy to increase the already present risk of heart and blood vessel disease for the convenience of popping a pill when proper instruction, limited dietary changes, and a little encouragement can help you to reach optimal weight, better health, and normal blood sugar. Below are some suggestions for successful weight loss, guidelines for developing a more healthy diet, and details of some of the common pitfalls that cause people to become discouraged and discontinue dietary therapy for diabetes.

Diets that are very complicated or very different from what you are used to are hard to follow. The American Diabetes Association (ADA) diet is a highly structured plan based on exchange lists. Although it serves its purpose of regulating calorie and sugar intake quite well, the ADA diet may be difficult for older people to use. Successful use of this diet requires considerable time spent teaching meal patterns and food portions. Older people often have trouble with this diet because the food lists are long and complicated and require considerable memorization. The amount of patience and manual dexterity necessary to properly weigh and measure foods prove difficult, especially in older people. Rigid control, such as that provided by the ADA diet, is not always necessary in type-2 diabetics. Often more gradual dietary change will reduce weight and lower blood sugar. See if your doctor or a dietitian can help you plan an easy to follow diet that will help to control your diabetes. The diet for a type-2 diabetic is based on the same nutritional principles as for a nondiabetic. Special foods ("dietetic") and imbalanced fad diets are unnecessary and sometimes dangerous. The basic plan should be to avoid sugar and instead eat starch and fiber.

Many people are already eating a diet that is partly appropriate for diabetics. Only small changes may be needed. For example, if you normally have a glass of orange juice, a scrambled egg, and toast with butter for breakfast, you do not need to redefine this in terms of one fruit, one meat, one bread, and one fat exchange because you would still be eating the same thing.

You do need to eat fewer simple sugars. Instead of soft drinks, snack foods, and cookies, substitute sugar-free drinks, graham crackers, or bread sticks. To reduce your risk of atherosclerosis (hardening of the blood vessels) ask your doctor for a list of foods to avoid to reduce your intake of cholesterol and saturated fat. Start by cutting back meals that contain red meat (beef, pork, lamb) to three or fewer per week. These can be replaced with fish, chicken, turkey, or vegetable dishes.

A regular exercise program is recommended for people who have diabetes. Exercise helps both to lower blood sugar and to reduce weight. It does not have to be strenuous; walking is often the best form of exercise.

Health Care for Diabetics

Because diabetes is such a complex disease, your overall health and your response to treatment need to be checked periodically. Schedule regular appointments with your doctor.

Diabetics often measure the amount of sugar in the urine. This is used as an indication of the amount of sugar in their blood. If blood sugar goes high enough, the kidneys cannot hold the sugar any longer, and some sugar spills out into the urine. A doctor should periodically check that the urine measurements accurately reflect sugar levels in the blood.

Foot care is a particular problem for diabetics. Between appointments be sure to check your feet regularly for sores, infections, and ulcers. These need prompt medical attention. Use cotton socks and wear well-fitted shoes.

Diabetic eye disease is one of the major causes of blindness in our country. Schedule an appointment with an eye doctor (ophthalmologist) at least every 6 months.

A number of drugs may raise blood sugar as a side effect. The most common are clonidine, corticosteroids, diuretics, gemfibrozil, narcotics, progesterone, and theophylline. If you are taking one of these drugs, ask your doctor whether you still need the medicine or if there is an alternative.

Most American diabetics have type-2, or adult-onset, diabetes. Weight reduction and mild dietary change is the safest treatment for this type of diabetes and is sufficient to reduce blood sugar in 85 to 90% of type-2 diabetics. Unlike insulin and pills, a diet carries no risk of low blood sugar. Unfortunately, many doctors are prescribing diabetes pills which may increase the already-present risk of heart and blood vessel disease. Pills should *only* be used by diabetics whose blood sugar is not controlled with diet alone *and* who cannot inject insulin. Older people should not use chlorpropamide or acetohexamide.

LIMITED USE

INSULINS
Beef Insulin, Pork Insulin, Human Insulin
HUMULIN, ILETIN (Lilly)
INSULATARD, MIXTARD, NOVOLIN, VELOSULIN (Novo Nordisk)

Generic: available

Family: Antidiabetic Drugs (see p. 516)

Insulin (*in* sull in), a drug that is injected under the skin, controls diabetes that cannnot be controlled by diet alone. **The dose of insulin may have to be adjusted as a person ages.**

Early insulin came from the pancreas of cows or pigs. Human insulin does not come from the human pancreas, but is prepared from bacteria with DNA technology. Human insulin is not necessarily an advantage over animal insulins. Most doctors do not recommend automatically switching from animal to human insulin. When people do switch insulin types, the dose may change. Human insulin is preferred for people who use insulin intermittently.

There are two types of diabetes, type-1 (also called juvenile-onset) and type-2 (adult-onset). People with type-1 diabetes need to take insulin. People with type-2 diabetes need to take insulin only if their disease cannot be controlled by diet alone. Most diabetics with adult-onset disease can control their diabetes without drugs if they follow their prescribed diet (see p. 516). Only about 10-15% cannot control the disease by diet and must use a blood sugar-lowering medicine. There is a decline in tolerance of glucose in normal aging. No absolute criteria exist for diagnosing diabetes in the elderly, and many studies on diabetes have not involved the elderly.[8,9] In a study of doctors, increased physical exercise showed promise as an approach to preventing non-insulin-dependent diabetes mellitus.[10] For a discussion of the two types of diabetes and their treatment see p. 516.

Insulin works by regulating the amount of sugar (glucose) in the blood and the speed at which sugar moves into cells. In diabetics, instead of moving into the cells, the sugar accumulates in the blood so that blood sugar levels become very high.

Your diet affects your cells' need for insulin and the insulin's ability to lower blood sugar when necessary. Therefore, for insulin to do its work, you must also follow a prescribed diet: **Insulin is not a replacement for such a diet.**

Too much insulin may cause low blood sugar (hypoglycemia). This happens most often in people who are over 60, especially if they have reduced kidney function. You may be more likely to suffer hypoglycemia if you skip or delay eating meals, exercise more than usual, or drink a significant amount of alcohol.

To prevent or delay severe consequences of diabetes, such as blindness, cataracts, gangrene, heart, circulatory, and kidney problems, lowering high blood sugar (hyperglycemia) is standard medical practice. Although there is a new emphasis on stricter glucose control than before, there are still concerns about the hazards of low blood sugar (hypoglycemia) if control is *too* strict.[11,12,13,14,15,16,17] Overly strict glucose control also involved diabetics in more auto accidents due to sudden episodes of hypoglycemia.[18,19] Studies conflict on whether severe and frequent episodes of low blood sugar hasten decline in intellectual ability.[20,21,22] Prior objections to frequent testing centered on making people too preoccupied with being ill.

Diabetic therapy must be individualized.

Before You Use This Drug

Tell your doctor if you have or have had
❑ allergies to drugs, beef, or pork
❑ adrenal or pituitary gland problems[23]
❑ eating disorders
❑ kidney or liver problems
❑ loss of consciousness
❑ nausea, vomiting, or diarrhea
❑ severe infections
❑ severe injuries
❑ thyroid problems

Tell your doctor about any other drugs you take, including aspirin, herbs, vitamins, and other non-prescription products.

When You Use This Drug

◆ Know the warning signs of low blood sugar, high blood sugar and ketoacidosis (see Adverse Effects).
◆ Keep sugar on hand. Tubes of glucose, a piece of fruit, pure orange juice, cheese, soda crackers, or one or two cups of milk will suffice. Honey, sugar candy, or syrup can also be used. Carry some with you at all times.
◆ Monitor your blood glucose. Some glucose strips can be divided to prolong the supply. If you use a machine to monitor blood glucose, be sure you receive adequate instruction. Do not hesitate to ask or repeat questions until you feel comfortable using the device.
◆ Eat a diet high in complex carbohydrates and fiber, but low in saturated fats. Avoid sugar, alcohol, and smoking. Distribute your calories over several small meals, or meals and snacks to prevent low blood sugar. Actually, little

information is available on the effect of diets in the elderly.[24]

◆ Whenever you cannot eat properly due to illness (fever, nausea, vomiting), continue your insulin, but realize your insulin requirements may change.
◆ If you plan to have any surgery, including dental, tell your doctor that you are diabetic, and take insulin.
◆ Carry identification stating your condition and the type of insulin(s) you use.
◆ When you travel, pack an extra supply of insulin, syringes, glucose and ketone testing materials, snacks, and a prescription. Carry your supplies instead of checking them.
◆ Exercise regularly. Inconsistent exercise risks low blood sugar on days you exert more.
◆ Keep your feet clean, warm, and dry. If you cannot cut your toenails, find a community group that provides the service. Call your doctor if signs of infection appear.
◆ Wear well-fitting shoes, and break in new shoes gradually. Avoid thongs, chemical corn and callous removers, and hot soaks or pads.
◆ Be cautious driving. Do not drive when your glucose levels are unstable.
◆ Choose non-prescription drugs and vitamins without sugar and alcohol. Lists of acceptable products are generally available from diabetes associations, your doctor and pharmacy. Check with your doctor if you have any doubts.

How To Use This Drug

◆ Obtain insulin syringes corresponding to your concentration and dose of insulin. Always use the same brand of syringes. Switching brands may result in using a different amount of insulin, due to differences in the unmeasured volume between the needle point and bottom calibration. Although it is not recommended, if you do reuse disposable syringes wipe the needle with alcohol, then recap. Reuse only for a limited number of injections.[25] Reusable glass syringes and metal needles can still be ordered. Before each use the syringe, plunger, and needle must be boiled in water for 5 minutes, or immersed in 91% isopropyl alcohol for at least 5 minutes, then air dried. Insulin pen cartridges with replaceable needles are another alternative. Do not use conventional insulin syringes in those devices. Needleless jet injectors are available, but are limited by lack of predictability.[26] If you use an insulin pump, obtain instructions on how to fill the pump, check the tubing, and maintain the infusion site. Pumps have no well-documented advantage over other diabetic therapy.[27,28] If you cannot see well enough to measure insulin, contact community agencies to find someone to predraw your insulin. In plastic syringes, insulin is stable for 2 weeks; in glass, it is stable for 1 week when refrigerated.[29]

Verify the label on your insulin and examine appearance of the insulin. Do not use regular insulin if it is cloudy or thick. Other insulins should appear uniformly milky, but not lumpy, grainy, stuck on the bottle, or unable to shake into suspension. Return questionable, unopened vials to your pharmacy. Wash your hands. Swab the top of the vial with alcohol.

Except for regular (short-acting) insulin, roll the vial slowly between the palms of the hands until the insulin is uniformly mixed.

◆ Do not shake vigorously, or bubbles may interfere with a correct measurement of insulin.

Draw air into the syringe equal to your insulin dose. Insert needle into the vial, then expel the air. Draw insulin into the syringe, check for air bubbles. Double check your dose.

If you use more than 1 type of insulin, always draw in the same order. Draw regular (short-acting) insulin first. Before injecting, roll the syringe to remix. Several premixed insulins are now available. Do not mix buffered insulins with lente (longer-acting) insulins. Store prefilled syringes of mixtures vertically with the needle upwards to avoid plugging the needle.

◆ Select a site to inject insulin in the abdomen, buttocks, front thigh, or back of the arm. Stick to one area, then rotate sites within that area to prevent breakdown of fat tissue.[30] Maintain the same posture each time you inject. Avoid inflamed or infected sites.

◆ Clean the site before injecting. Inject needle at a 90 degree angle just under the skin (subcutaneously). Pull back on the plunger. If blood appears, try again. Inject in less than 5 seconds. Massaging the site after injection may speed absorption of the insulin.[31]

◆ Insulin comes in a variety of forms with different lengths of action. Do not change brands, strength, or type of insulin without checking with your doctor. Switches may call for a change in your insulin dose. If you use a less common form of insulin, deal with a pharmacy that promises to keep some in stock.

◆ Refrigeration prolongs stability, and prevents contamination of insulin. According to the International Diabetes Institute, unopened insulin, properly stored, loses 5% potency in 10 years.[32] Insulin (even old style) may be stored at room temperature. Once assembled, NovolinPen or PenFill must be stored at room temperature and must not be refrigerated. Today, at home, most people with diabetes refrigerate insulin vials until opened, then store the vial being used at room temperature. Do not expose to high temperatures, or sunlight. Never freeze insulin or warm it in a microwave. Once opened, vials should be discarded after several weeks.[33] Policies for storing insulin in congregate living and institutions may differ from home practices.

◆ Dispose of your syringes according to local waste disposal regulations.

Interactions With Other Drugs

The following drugs are listed in *Evaluations of Drug Interactions*, 1991 as causing "highly clinically significant" or "clinically significant" interactions when used together with this drug. There may be other drugs, especially those in the families of drugs listed below, that also will react with this drug to cause severe adverse effects. Many other drugs can contribute to or prolong low or high blood sugar, or mask signs of low blood sugar. Make sure to ask your doctor for a complete listing of them and let her or him know if you are taking any of these interacting drugs:

alcohol; ATROMID; clofibrate; fenfluramine; guanethidine; INDERAL; ISMELIN; l-thyroxine; NARDIL; oxytetracycline; phenelzine; PONDIMIN; propranolol; SYNTHROID; TERRAMYCIN; thyroid; timolol; TIMOPTIC.

Additionally, the *United States Pharmacopeia Drug Information*, 1992 lists this drug as having interactions of major significance:

DELTASONE; prednisone.

Adverse Effects

All insulins may cause allergies in a few individuals.[34,35] Skin cleansers and preservatives in the insulin also can cause local allergic reactions.[36]

Call your doctor:
- ❏ **if you experience allergic reactions:** itching; rapid heartbeat; shortness of breath; swelling at injection site

Call your doctor immediately and get assistance:
- ❏ blood sugar is out of control
- ❏ severe vomiting
- ❏ symptoms of low or high blood sugar are severe

Low Blood Sugar
- ❏ **symptoms of low blood sugar:** anxiety; blurred vision; cold sweats; confusion; difficulty concentrating; drowsiness; fainting; excessive hunger; headache; irritability; nausea; nervousness; numbness;[37] cool, pale skin; rapid pulse; seizures; shakiness; abnormal tiredness or weakness; unsteady gait

- ◆ Low blood sugar can be caused by:
    Missed meals, increased exercise, consuming alcohol, changes in insulin dose, use of long-acting insulins, use of continuous infusion pumps[38,39] and certain illnesses.[40] An increase of even one unit of insulin can cause low blood sugar.[41] If you have low blood sugar often call your doctor. Hunger, sweating, and trembling are signs most diabetics rely on as a warning.[42,43] However, warnings vary with the individual, and whether or not an insulin pump is used. Warning signs may change if low blood sugar occurs often.[44] There is debate as to whether animal and human insulins differ in warnings each provide.[45,46,47,48,49,50,51,52,53,54] Every instance of these symptoms does not mean you have low blood sugar. So do not rely only on warning signs, but also test your blood sugar to see if it actually is low, if time permits.[55]

- ◆ Over half of episodes of low blood sugar happen during the night.[56] Testing blood glucose at bedtime is advisable.[57] So is keeping a source of sugar by your bed. However, you may not always be aware of low blood sugar that happened during the night. Clues on waking up are:[58]
- ❏ morning headaches
- ❏ night sweats
- ❏ symptoms of hypothermia (see glossary, p. 689)

High blood sugar or ketoacidosis
- ❏ **symptoms of high blood sugar in the elderly may vary[59] but they can include:** deep, rapid breathing; breath smells of fruit; dizziness; drowsiness; dry mouth; dry, flushed skin; unusual thirst; increased urinating; headaches; loss of appetite; stomach ache, nausea, vomiting; tiredness; swelling of feet, legs[60]

- ◆ High blood sugar is often due to severe lack of insulin or infection.

Periodic Tests

Ask your doctor which of these tests should be done periodically while you are taking this drug and how often they should be done:

❑ blood levels of glucose, ketones and potassium

❑ blood pH
❑ blood pressure
❑ glycosylated hemoglobin test
❑ urine ketone

ORAL HYPOGLYCEMICS

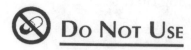 ## DO NOT USE

Chlorpropamide (klor *proe* pa mide)
DIABINESE (Pfizer)
Acetohexamide (a set oh *hex* a mide)
DYMELOR (Lilly)

LIMITED USE

Tolbutamide (tole *byoo* ta mide)
ORINASE (Upjohn)
Glyburide (*glye* byoo ride)
DIABETA (Hoechst-Roussel)
MICRONASE (Upjohn)
Glipizide (*glip* i zide)
GLUCOTROL (Roerig)
Tolazamide (tole *az* a mide)
TOLINASE (Upjohn)

Generic: available except for glyburide and glipizide

Family: Antidiabetic Drugs (see p. 516)

These drugs are taken by mouth (orally) to lower high blood sugar levels caused by adult-onset (type-2) diabetes (see p. 516). **Very few people should use these drugs.** Most type-2 diabetics can control their disease by following a prescribed diet, or, if diet alone does not work, by following a diet and injecting insulin (see p. 516). **The main reason to use these drugs is if diet alone fails to control your diabetes *and* you cannot inject insulin.** If you do use these drugs, it is best to use them *temporarily*, while losing weight, *not permanently*.

If you have type-2 diabetes, before taking any of these pills, you should try following a prescribed diet to reduce your blood sugar levels and, if you are overweight, to lose weight. If this does not work and you need to take a drug, insulin is a better choice than any of these pills. Although taking these pills is easier and more convenient than injecting insulin, they have significant risks, including an increased risk of death from heart attacks and blood vessel disease.

If you do take a diabetes pill, you should make sure that you are taking the safest possible one. **Tolbutamide** is less likely than the other diabetes pills to cause low blood sugar (see Adverse Effects) and takes less time to be eliminated from your body. It is also available in an inexpensive generic form.

Acetohexamide should *not* be used by people who have impaired kidney function.[61] Since many older adults do have impaired kidney function, we do not recommend this drug for people over 60. We also recommend that you do not use **chlorpropamide** because it takes a long time to be eliminated from the body and is more likely than other diabetes pills to cause serious side effects associated with low blood sugar (see Adverse Effects). Chlorpropamide appears on a World Health Organization list of drugs that older adults should not use.[62]

If you are over 60 and you use a diabetes pill, your doctor should start you off at no more than half the usual adult dose.

Before You Use This Drug

Do not use if you have or have had recent
- ❑ severe burns or injuries
- ❑ severe infection
- ❑ major surgery
- ❑ high ketone levels

Tell your doctor if you have or have had
- ❑ allergies to drugs
- ❑ adrenal gland disease
- ❑ kidney or liver disease
- ❑ thyroid disease
- ❑ pituitary gland disease
- ❑ recent nausea, vomiting, or high fever
- ❑ an unusual reaction to another diabetes drug, a sulfonamide (sulfa) antibiotic, or a thiazide diuretic (water pill)
- ❑ heart disease and water retention, *for chlorpropamide*

Tell your doctor about any other drugs you take, including aspirin, herbs, vitamins, and other non-prescription products.

When You Use This Drug

◆ **Call your doctor immediately and eat or drink something with sugar in it if you experience symptoms of low blood sugar (see Adverse Effects, below).**

   For chlorpropamide only: Someone should check on you regularly for at least 3 to 5 days after this happens.

◆ **Do not stop taking your drug without** talking to your doctor.

◆ **If you have a high fever, nausea and vomiting, severe infection, or any severe injury, tell your doctor. Your treatment may have to be changed.**

◆ Do not drink alcohol. The combination of alcohol and diabetes pills may cause abdominal cramps, nausea, vomiting, headaches, flushing, and low blood sugar.

◆ If you plan to have any surgery, including dental, tell your doctor that you take an oral hypoglycemic.

Heat Stress Alert

These drugs can affect your body's ability to adjust to heat, putting you at risk of "heat stress." If you live alone, ask a friend to check on you several times during the day. Early signs of heat stress are dizziness, light-headedness, faintness, and slightly high temperature. Call your doctor if you have any of these signs.

Drink more fluids (water, fruit and vegetable juices) than usual, even if you're not thirsty, unless your doctor has told you otherwise. Do not drink alcohol.

How To Use This Drug

◆ If you miss a dose, take it as soon as you remember, but skip it if it is almost time for the next dose. **Do not take double doses.**

Interactions With Other Drugs

The following drugs are listed in *Evaluations of Drug Interactions,* 1991 as causing "highly clinically significant" or "clinically significant" interactions when used together with one of the oral hypoglycemics. They may interact with any oral hypoglycemic. There may be other drugs, especially those in the families of drugs listed below, that also will react with oral hypoglycemics to cause severe adverse effects. Make sure to ask your doctor for a complete listing of them and let her or him know if you are taking any of these interacting drugs:

ADAPIN; alcohol, ethyl; aspirin; ATROMID-S; BUTAZOLIDIN; charcoal; chloramphenicol; CHLOROMYCETIN; cholestyramine; cimetidine; clofibrate; cortisone; CORTONE; dicumarol; doxepin; EASPRIN; ECOTRIN; EMPIRIN; ESIDRIX; fenfluramine; gemfibrozil; hydrochlorothiazide; HYDRODIURIL; INDERAL; LOPID; NARDIL; oxytetracycline; phenelzine; phenylbutazone; PONDERAL; propanolol; QUESTRAN; SINEQUAN; sulfamethizole; SYNTHROID; TAGAMET; TERRAMYCIN; THIOSULFIL; thyroid; URIBIOTIC-250.

Adverse Effects
Call your doctor immediately:
- **if you experience signs of low blood sugar:** anxiety; chills; cold sweats or cool, pale skin; blurred vision; confusion; seizures; difficulty concentrating; drowsiness; increased hunger; headache; nausea; nervousness; rapid heartbeat; shakiness; unsteady walk; abnormal tiredness or weakness
- **if you experience signs of high blood sugar:** drowsiness; dry, flushed skin;
- chronic high blood sugar levels;

breath smells of fruit; increased urination; loss of appetite; tiredness; abnormal thirst; deep rapid breathing; dizziness; dry mouth; headache; stomach ache; nausea; vomiting; swelling of feet, legs
- dark urine or pale stools
- itching skin
- yellow eyes and skin
- sore throat and fever
- unusual bleeding or bruising
- weakness, fever, fatigue

For chlorpropamide only: difficulty breathing; shortness of breath; muscle cramps; swollen or puffy face, hands, or ankles; water retention
Call your doctor if these symptoms continue:
- diarrhea
- dizziness
- headache
- heartburn
- nausea, vomiting, loss of appetite
- stomach pain
- skin rash

Periodic Tests
Ask your doctor which of these tests should be done periodically done while you are taking this drug:
- blood cell counts
- blood sugar levels
- urine levels of sugar and ketones

Notes for Drugs for Diabetes

1. *Diabetes* 1970; 19 (Suppl 2):813.

2. Chalmers T. Settling the UGDP controversy. *Journal of the American Medical Association* 1975; 231:624.

3. *Diabetes*, op. cit.

4. Vestal RE, ed. *Drug Treatment in the Elderly*. Sydney, Australia: ADIS Health Science Press, 1984:231.

5. Chalmers, op. cit.

6. AMA Department of Drugs. *AMA Drug Evaluations*. 5th ed. Chicago: American Medical Association, 1983:1045.

7. Ibid, p. 1036.

8. Lorenz RA, Santiago JV, Siebert C, Cleary PA, Heyse S, DCCT Research Group. Epidemiology of severe hypoglycemia in the Diabetes Control and Complications Trial. *The American Journal of Medicine* 1991; 90:450-9.

9. Porte D, Kahn SE. What geriatricians should know about diabetes mellitus. *Diabetes Care* 1990; 13 (suppl. 2):47-54.

10. Manson JE, Nathan DM, Krolewski AS, Stampfer MJ, Willett WC, Hennekens CH. A prospective study of exercise and incidence of diabetes among U.S. male physicians. *Journal of the American Medical Association* 1992; 268:63-7.

11. Feingold KR. Hypoglycemia — a major risk of insulin therapy. *The Western Journal of Medicine* 1991; 154:469-71.

12. Lorenz, op. cit.

13. Porte, op. cit.

14. Ratner RE, Whitehouse FW. Motor vehicles, hypoglycemia, and diabetic drivers. *Diabetes Care* 1989; 12:217-22.

15. Reichard P, Berglund A, Britz A, Levander S, Rosenqvist U. Hypoglycaemic episodes during intensified insulin treatment: increased frequency but no effect on cognitive function. *Journal of Internal Medicine* 1991; 229:9-16.

16. Dukes MNG, Beeley L. *Side Effects of Drugs Annual* 15, Amsterdam: Elsevier, 1991:451.

17. Wolff SP. Is hyperglycemia risky enough to justify the increased risk of hypoglycemia linked with tight diabetes control? *Biochemical Medicine and Metabolic Biology* 1991; 46:129-39.

18. Lorenz, op. cit.

19. Ratner, op. cit.

20. Kerr D, Reza M, Smith N, Leatherdale BA. Importance of insulin in subjective, cognitive, and hormonal responses to hypoglycemia in patients with IDDM. *Diabetes* 1991; 40:1057-62.

21. Langan SJ, Deary IJ, Hepburn DA, Frier BM. Cumulative cognitive impairment following recurrent severe hypoglycemia in adult patients with insulin-treated diabetes mellitus. *Diabetologia* 1991; 34:337-44.

22. Reichard, op. cit.

23. Feingold, op. cit.

24. Porte, op. cit.

25. *USP DI, Drug Information for the Health Care Professional.* 12th ed. Rockville MD: The United States Pharmacopeial Convention, Inc., 1992:1580-6.

26. *Manual of Medical Therapeutics,* 26th Edition, Washington University, St. Louis, MO, 1989:381.

27. AMA Department of Drugs. *AMA Drug Evaluations.* Chicago: American Medical Association, 1991:874-87.

28. Gilman AG, Rall TW, Nies AS, Taylor P, eds. *The Pharmacological Basis of Therapeutics.* 8th ed. New York: Pergamon Press, 1990:1463-95.

29. Olin BR, ed. *Facts and Comparisons.* St. Louis: J.B. Lippincott Co., September 1992:129f-130d.

30. Gilman, op. cit.

31. *Manual of Medical Therapeutics,* op. cit.

32. Raab RS. Letter from the International Diabetes Institute, May 4, 1990.

33. American Society of Hospital Pharmacists. *American Hospital Formulary Service Drug Information.* Bethesda, MD, 1992:1883-8.

34. Balsells MC, Corcoy RM, Lleonart RB, Pujol RV, Mauricio DP, Garcia AP, Pou JM, Cistero AB. Primary allergy to human insulin in patients with gestational diabetes. *Diabetes Care* 1991; 14:423-4.

35. Dukes MNG, Beeley L. *Side Effects of Drugs Annual* 14, Amsterdam: Elsevier, 1990:372-3.

36. Olin, op. cit.

37. Kern W, Lieb K, Kerner W, Born J, Fehm HL. Differential effects of human and pork insulin-induced hypoglycemia on neuronal functions in humans. *Diabetes* 1990; 39:1091-8.

38. Dukes, 1990, op. cit.

39. Lorenz, op. cit.

40. Feingold, op. cit.

41. Gin H, Aparicio M, Potaux L, Merville P, Combe CH, de Precigout V, Bouchet JL, Aubertin J. Low-protein, low-phosphorus diet and tissue insulin sensitivity in insulin-dependent diabetic patients with chronic renal failure. *Nephron* 1991; 57:411-5.

42. Egger M, Smith GD, Teuscher AU, Teuscher A. Influence of human insulin on symptoms and awareness of hypoglycaemia: a randomised double blind crossover trial. *British Medical Journal* 1991; 303:622-6.

43. Muhlhauser I, Heinemann L, Fritsche E, von Lennep K, Berger M. Hypoglycemic symptoms and frequency of severe hypoglycemia in patients treated with human and animal insulin preparations. *Diabetes Care* 1991; 14:745-9.

44 Reichard, op. cit.

45. Bendtson I, Binder C. Counterregulatory hormonal response to insulin-induced hypoglycaemia in insulin-dependent diabetic patients: a comparison of equimolar amounts of porcine and semisynthetic human insulin. *Journal of Internal Medicine* 1991; 229:293-6.

46. Cherfas J. UK diabetics plan insulin suit. *Science* 1991; 253:1090.

47. Egger M, Smith GD, Imhoof H, Teuscher A. Risk of severe hypoglycaemia in insulin treated diabetic patients transferred to human insulin: a case control study. *British Medical Journal* 1991; 303:617-21.

48. Egger, Influence of Human Insulin, op. cit.

49. Human insulin (letters). *British Medical Journal* 1991; 303:1265-8.

50. Jick SS, Derby LE, Gross KM, Jick H. Hospitalizations because of hypoglycemia in users of animal and human insulins. 2. Experience in the United States. *Pharmacotherapy* 1990; 1:398-9.

51. Lorenz, op. cit.

52. Muhlhauser, op. cit.

53. Dukes, 1990, op. cit.

54. Confusion over human insulin (letters). *The Lancet* 1991; 338:1213-4.

55. Feingold, op. cit.

56. Lorenz, op. cit.

57. Reichard, op. cit.

58. Gilman, op. cit.

59. Porte, op. cit.

60. Gilman, op. cit.

61. Peden N, Newton RW, Feely J. Oral hypoglycaemic agents. *British Medical Journal* 1983; 286:1566.

62. *Drugs for the Elderly.* Denmark: World Health Organization, 1985:41.

Drugs For Neurological Disorders

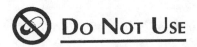 **DO NOT USE**

Alternative treatment: An antihistamine, see below.

Trihexyphenidyl
ARTANE (Lederle) TRIHEXANE (Rugby)

Family: Antiparkinsonians

Trihexyphenidyl (try hex ee *fen* i dill) **should not be used to treat Parkinson's disease** because it can cause several serious side effects more frequently in older adults. These effects include memory impairment, confusion, hallucinations, and retention of urine. If you use trihexyphenidyl, ask your doctor to change your prescription to an antihistamine such as diphenhydramine (Benadryl, see p. 398). Antihistamines work in the same way as trihexyphenidyl, yet have milder side effects in older adults.[1,2] They are usually either used alone, to treat people with mild symptoms of Parkinson's disease, or combined with another antiparkinsonian drug such as levodopa with carbidopa (see p. 537).

If you have symptoms of parkinsonism (tremor, rigid muscles, and disturbances in posture, walking, balance, speech, swallowing and muscle strength), there is a good chance that they are caused by a drug you are taking. As many as half of older adults with symptoms of parkinsonism may have developed them as side effects of a drug. A list of drugs that can cause symptoms of parkinsonism appears on p. 30. If you take any of the drugs on this list, discuss the possibility of drug-induced parkinsonism with your doctor, and ask to have your prescription changed or stopped.

Warning: Special Mental and Physical Adverse Effects

Older adults are especially sensitive to the harmful anticholinergic effects of antiparkinsonian drugs such as trihexyphenidyl. Drugs in this family should not be used unless absolutely necessary.

Mental Effects: confusion, delirium, short-term memory problems, disorientation, and impaired attention.

Physical Effects: dry mouth, constipation, difficulty urinating (especially for a man with an enlarged prostate), blurred vision, decreased sweating with increased body temperature, sexual dysfunction, and worsening of glaucoma.

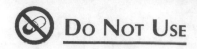 **DO NOT USE**

Alternative treatment: An antihistamine, see below.

Benztropine
COGENTIN (Merck)

Family: Antiparkinsonians

Benztropine (*benz* troe peen) **should not be used to treat Parkinson's disease** because it can cause several serious side effects more frequently in older adults. These effects include memory impairment, confusion, hallucinations, and retention of urine. If you use benztropine, ask your doctor to change your prescription to an antihistamine such as diphenhydramine (Benadryl, see p. 398). Antihistamines work in the same way as benztropine, yet have milder side effects in older adults.[3,4] They are usually either used alone, to treat people with mild symptoms of Parkinson's disease, or combined with another antiparkinsonian drug such as levodopa with carbidopa (see p. 537).

If you have symptoms of parkinsonism (tremor, rigid muscles, and disturbances in posture, walking, balance, speech, swallowing, and muscle strength), there is a good chance that they are caused by a drug you are taking. As many as half of older adults with symptoms of parkinsonism may have developed them as side effects of a drug. A list of drugs that can cause symptoms of parkinsonism appears on p. 30. If you take any of the drugs on this list, discuss the possibility of drug-induced parkinsonism with your doctor, and ask to have your prescription changed or stopped.

Warning: Special Mental and Physical Adverse Effects

Older adults are especially sensitive to the harmful anticholinergic effects of antiparkinsonian drugs such as benztropine. Drugs in this family should not be used unless absolutely necessary.

Mental Effects: confusion, delirium, short-term memory problems, disorientation, and impaired attention.

Physical Effects: dry mouth, constipation, difficulty urinating (especially for a man with an enlarged prostate), blurred vision, decreased sweating with increased body temperature, sexual dysfunction, and worsening of glaucoma.

Phenytoin (Diphenylhydantoin)
DILANTIN (Parke-Davis)

Generic: available

Family: Anticonvulsants

Phenytoin (*fen* i toyn) is used to treat most forms of epilepsy, except a form called absence (petit mal) seizures. It is also used to treat a form of excruciating facial pain, called trigeminal neuralgia or tic douloureux, if the preferred drug, carbamazepine (see p. 547), does not work or causes an adverse reaction. **If you are over 60, you generally need to take less than the usual adult dose of phenytoin.** Many adverse effects can be controlled with a lower dose.

Phenytoin has caused serious, often permanent, and sometimes fatal blood cell abnormalities in a few people. If these occur, it is important that they be detected early because occasionally they can be treated. If you are taking phenytoin and have any of the following possible symptoms of a blood disorder, call your doctor immediately: fever and sore throat, ulcers in the mouth, easy bruising, or skin rashes. It is very important that your doctor check the level of phenytoin in your bloodstream frequently and adjust your dosage as needed.

Before You Use This Drug
Do not use if you have or have had
❑ heart disease
Tell your doctor if you have or have had
❑ allergies to drugs
❑ alcohol dependence
❑ blood cell abnormalities
❑ kidney or liver disease
❑ diabetes
❑ thyroid problems
Tell your doctor about any other drugs you take, including aspirin, herbs, vitamins, and other non-prescription products.

When You Use This Drug
◆ Until you know how you react to this drug, do not drive or perform other activities requiring alertness. Phenytoin can cause dizziness, blurred vision, drowsiness, and lack of muscle coordination.
◆ Schedule regular visits with your doctor to check your progress and test for side effects.
◆ Do not drink alcohol.
◆ Schedule frequent visits with your dentist to have your teeth cleaned, to prevent enlarged, tender, and bleeding gums.
◆ Wear a medical identification bracelet or carry a card stating that you take phenytoin.
◆ **Do not stop taking this drug suddenly. This may cause severe convulsions. Check with your doctor before stopping this drug, changing brands or dosage forms, or taking any other drugs (prescription or non-prescription).**
◆ If you plan to have any surgery, including dental, tell your doctor that you take this drug.

How To Use This Drug
◆ Take with food to decrease stomach upset.
◆ For epilepsy, you can take the total daily dose at one time, preferably at the same time each day (in the morning or at bedtime).
◆ Before using the liquid form, shake vigorously.
◆ Do not expose to heat, moisture, or strong light. Do not store in the bathroom.
◆ *If you miss a dose, use the following guidelines:*
  - If you take phenytoin only once a day, take the missed dose as soon as you remember, but skip it if you don't

remember until the next day. **Do not take double doses.**
- If you take phenytoin more than once a day, take the missed dose as soon as possible, but skip it if it is less than 4 hours until your next scheduled dose. **Do not take double doses.**
- Call your doctor immediately if you miss doses for 2 days in a row.

Interactions With Other Drugs

The following drugs are listed in *Evaluations of Drug Interactions*, 1991 as causing "highly clinically significant" or "clinically significant" interactions when used together with this drug. There may be other drugs, especially those in the families of drugs listed below, that also will react with this drug to cause severe adverse effects. Make sure to ask your doctor for a complete listing of them and let her or him know if you are taking any of these interacting drugs:

alcohol, ethyl; ALERMINE; allopurinol; amiodarone; ANTABUSE; AZOLID; BACTRIM; BiCNU; BRONKODYL; BUTAZOLIDIN; CALCIFEROL; CARAFATE; carmustine; charcoal; chloramphenicol; CHLOROMYCETIN; chlorpheniramine; CHLOR-TRIMETON; cimetidine; CONSTANT-T; CORDARONE; COTRIM; cyclosporine; DECADRON; DECONAMINE; DEPAKENE; dexamethasone; diazoxide; dicumarol; DIFLUCAN; digitalis; disulfiram; dopamine; DOXYCHEL; doxycycline; DURAQUIN; EFOL; ELIXOPHYLLIN; ergocalciferol; FEDAHIST; FEOSOL PLUS; fluconazole; FOLEX; folic acid; FOLVITE; GANTANOL; HEXADROL; ibuprofen; INH; isoniazid; LIPO B-C; LOPURIN; methotrexate; methoxsalen; metocurine; METUBINE; methotrexate; miconazole; MONISTAT; MOTRIN; MYSOLINE; nifedipine; omeprazole; OS-CAL-GESIC; OXSORALEN; phenylbutazone; PRILOSEC; primidone; PROCARDIA; PROLOPRIM; QUIBRON-T-SR; QUINAGLUTE DURA-TABS; quinidine; RIFADIN; rifampin; SANDIMMUNE; SEPTRA; SLO-BID; SLO-PHYLLIN; SOMOPHYLLIN; sucralfate; sulfamethizole; sulfamethoxazole; SUSTAIRE; TAGAMET; THEO-24; THEOLAIR; theophylline; THIOSULFIL; trimethoprim; TRIMPEX; valproic acid; VELBAN; VIBRAMYCIN; vinblastine; vitamin D_2; ZYLOPRIM.

Adverse Effects
Call your doctor immediately:
- ❑ **if you experience signs of overdose:** blurred vision; clumsiness or unsteadiness; confusion; severe dizziness or drowsiness; hallucinations; nausea; slurred speech; staggering walk; uncontrolled eye movements
- ❑ behavior, mood, or mental changes
- ❑ clumsiness or unsteadiness
- ❑ confusion
- ❑ uncontrolled eye movements
- ❑ failure to control seizures
- ❑ weakness or numbness of feet or legs
- ❑ slurring of speech
- ❑ enlarged, bleeding, or tender gums
- ❑ fever, sore throat, or enlarged lymph nodes in neck or underarms
- ❑ skin rash
- ❑ unusual bleeding or bruising
- ❑ dark urine, pale stools, yellow skin or eyes, loss of appetite, or stomach pain
- ❑ swelling around eyes and face[5]

Call your doctor if these symptoms continue:
- ❑ constipation
- ❑ dizziness, lightheadedness
- ❑ drowsiness
- ❑ nausea or vomiting
- ❑ excess hair growth on body and face
- ❑ headache
- ❑ muscle twitching

Periodic Tests

Ask your doctor which of these tests should be done periodically while you are taking this drug:
- ❏ blood levels of phenytoin
- ❏ electroencephalogram (EEG)
- ❏ complete blood counts
- ❏ thyroid function tests
- ❏ dental exam, every 3 months
- ❏ liver function tests
- ❏ blood levels of calcium

Levodopa
DOPAR (Norwich Eaton) LARODOPA (Roche)
Levodopa and Carbidopa (combined)
SINEMET (Merck)

Generic: available only for levodopa in capsule form

Family: Antiparkinsonians

Levodopa (*lee* voe doe pa) and the combination of levodopa and carbidopa (*kar* bi doe pa) are both used to treat Parkinson's disease, a condition that produces tremor (shaking), rigid muscles, and disturbances in posture, walking, balance, speech, swallowing, and muscle strength. The combination drug is often a better choice for treating Parkinson's disease than levodopa alone, because carbidopa enhances the desired effects of levodopa and reduces its side effects. If you are taking levodopa alone, ask your doctor to switch you to a levodopa-carbidopa combination.

If you take levodopa alone, you should avoid foods and vitamins that contain vitamin B_6 (pyridoxine), since this vitamin can destroy the drug's effectiveness. To keep your intake of vitamin B_6 down, you should avoid multiple vitamins, avocados, beans, peas, sweet potatoes, dry skim milk, oatmeal, pork, bacon, beef liver, tuna, and cereals fortified with vitamin B_6. If you take carbidopa with levodopa you do not need to worry about this.

If you have symptoms of parkinsonism, there is a good chance that they are caused by a drug you are taking. As many as half of the older adults with symptoms of parkinsonism may have developed them as side effects of a drug. A list of drugs that can cause symptoms of parkinsonism appears on p. 30. If you take any of the drugs on this list, discuss the possibility of drug-induced parkinsonism with your doctor, and ask to have your prescription changed or stopped.

Before You Use This Drug

Tell your doctor if you have or have had
- ❏ allergies to drugs
- ❏ lung disease, bronchial asthma
- ❏ heart or blood vessel disease
- ❏ diabetes
- ❏ hormone problems
- ❏ skin cancer
- ❏ glaucoma
- ❏ stomach ulcer
- ❏ seizure disorder, epilepsy
- ❏ kidney or liver disease
- ❏ mental illness

Tell your doctor about any other drugs you take, including aspirin, herbs, vitamins, and other non-prescription products.

When You Use This Drug

- ◆ **Use only as prescribed.**
- ◆ Until you know how you react to this drug, do not drive or perform other activities requiring alertness. This drug can cause faintness and lightheadedness.

◆ You may feel dizzy when rising from a lying or sitting position. When getting out of bed, hang your legs over the side of the bed for a few minutes, then get up slowly. When getting up from a chair, stay by the chair until you are sure that you are not dizzy. (See p. 14.)

◆ **Caution diabetics:** Levodopa may interfere with urine tests for sugar and ketones.

◆ Urine or sweat may get darker. This is no cause for alarm.

◆ If you plan to have any surgery, including dental, tell your doctor that you take this drug.

Heat Stress Alert

These drugs can affect your body's ability to adjust to heat, putting you at risk of "heat stress." If you live alone, ask a friend to check on you several times during the day. Early signs of heat stress are dizziness, lightheadedness, faintness, and slightly high temperature. Call your doctor if you have any of these signs.

Drink more fluids (water, fruit and vegetable juices) than usual, even if you're not thirsty, unless your doctor has told you otherwise. Do not drink alcohol.

How To Use This Drug

◆ Take on an empty stomach, at least 1 hour before or 2 hours after meals. This drug will not work as well if you take it with or immediately after food. If the drug causes an upset stomach, eat something about 15 minutes after taking it.

◆ Do not store in the bathroom. Do not expose to heat, strong light, or moisture.

◆ If you miss a dose, take it as soon as you remember, but skip it if it is less than 2 hours until your next scheduled dose. **Do not take double doses.**

Interactions With Other Drugs

The following drugs are listed in *Evaluations of Drug Interactions*, 1991 as causing "highly clinically significant" or "clinically significant" interactions when used together with this drug. There may be other drugs, especially those in the families of drugs listed below, that also will react with this drug to cause severe adverse effects. Make sure to ask your doctor for a complete listing of them and let her or him know if you are taking any of these interacting drugs:

FEOSOL; ferrous sulfate; HERPECIN-L; NARDIL; phenelzine; pyridoxine; RODEX; vitamin B_6.

Adverse Effects

Call your doctor immediately:
❑ mental depression
❑ mood changes, aggressive behavior
❑ problems with urination
❑ dizziness or lightheadedness
❑ irregular heartbeat
❑ severe nausea or vomiting
❑ unusual or uncontrolled movements of the body
❑ spasm or closing of eyelids
❑ high blood pressure
❑ stomach pain
❑ unusual tiredness or weakness

Call your doctor if these symptoms continue:
❑ anxiety, confusion, nervousness
❑ constipation or diarrhea
❑ nightmares or trouble sleeping
❑ dry mouth
❑ flushed skin
❑ headache
❑ loss of appetite
❑ muscle twitching

Periodic Tests

Ask your doctor which of these tests should be done periodically while you are taking this drug:
❑ complete blood counts
❑ liver function tests
❑ kidney function tests
❑ eye pressure tests

Selegiline (Deprenyl)
ELDEPRYL (Somerset)

Generic: not available

Family: Antiparkinsonians

Selegiline (sell *edge* ell lean) has been used in the treatment of Parkinson's disease along with levodopa or carbidopa. While taking selegiline, less levodopa/carbidopa is required. The main usefulness of selegiline is thought to be in the early stages of the disease, when it can be used alone to slow the advance of the disease and to delay the need to institute levodopa. Much controversy surrounds this claim.[6,7,8,9,10,11] Selegiline is not recommended for those in the advanced stages of parkinsonism or with dementia.[12,13] Mental side effects are especially a concern in the elderly.[14] Also of concern is the high price of selegiline in the United States.[15,16] (Selegiline has a second generic name, deprenyl (*dep* ren ill).)

If you have symptoms of parkinsonism, there is a good chance that they are caused by a drug you are taking. As many as half of the older adults with symptoms of parkinsonism may have developed them as side effects of a drug. A list of drugs that can cause symptoms of parkinsonism appears on p. 30. If you take any of the drugs on this list, discuss the possibility of drug-induced parkinsonism with your doctor, and ask to have your prescription changed or stopped.

Selegiline belongs to a group of drugs called monoamine oxidase (MAO) inhibitors. Serious side effects and severe dietary restrictions required when taking other types of MAO inhibitors, *type A*, curtailed use of these drugs for depression. Selegiline is a MAO inhibitor, *type B*, purported to have fewer side effects. However, the same side effects can occur, especially at high doses.[17] In order to reduce adverse effects, it is a good practice to start with a low dose of selegiline, then increase the dose gradually.[18,19]

Before You Use This Drug
Tell your doctor if you have or have had
❑ allergies to drugs
❑ ulcers
Tell your doctor about any other drugs you take, including aspirin, herbs, vitamins, and other non-prescription products.

When You Use This Drug
◆ Do not eat highly fermented foods, which contain tyramine: aged cheese, beer and wines (including "alcohol-free" ones), sherry, liqueurs, fava and broad beans, smoked and pickled meats/fish, sausages, caviar, chicken livers, over-ripe fruit, yeast extracts (Marmite, packet soups) .
◆ Avoid or eat moderately: sour cream, yogurt, soy sauce, chocolate, and caffeine. These dietary restrictions extend up to two weeks after you stop taking any MAO inhibitor, such as selegiline.
◆ You may feel dizzy when rising from a lying or sitting position. If you are lying down, hang your legs over the side of the bed for a few minutes, then get up slowly. When getting up from a chair, stay by the chair until you are sure that you are not dizzy. (See p. 14.)
◆ Protect yourself from sunburn.
◆ If you take levodopa, your dose will be reduced gradually.
◆ Take only cold, cough and diet pills recommended by your doctor.
◆ If you plan to have any surgery, including dental, tell your doctor that you take this drug.

How To Use This Drug
◆ Swallow tablet whole or break up. Time doses for morning or noontime. Do not

take in late afternoon or bedtime. Take with meals.

◆ Do not store in the bathroom. Do not expose to heat, strong light, or moisture.

◆ If you miss a dose, take it as soon as you remember but skip it if it is almost time for the next dose. **Do not take double doses.**

Interactions With Other Drugs

The following drugs are listed in *Evaluations of Drug Interactions*, 1991 as causing "highly clinically significant" or "clinically significant" interactions when used together with this drug. There may be other drugs, especially those in the families of drugs listed below, that also will react with this drug to cause severe adverse effects. Make sure to ask your doctor for a complete listing of them and let her or him know if you are taking any of these interacting drugs.

If you stop taking these drugs wait 5 to 6 weeks before starting selegiline. If you go off selegiline, wait 2 weeks before taking these drugs:

DEMEROL; dextromethorphan; fluoxetine; meperidine; PROZAC; ROBITUSSIN-DM.

If a tricyclic antidepressant is used with selegiline, dosage must be carefully monitored.

Additionally, the *United States Pharmacopeia Drug Information*, 1992 lists this drug as having interactions of major significance:

LARODOPA; levodopa (if you already take levodopa your dose should be lowered 2 to 3 days before starting selegiline).

Adverse Effects

Call your doctor immediately:
❑ mood changes
❑ problems with urination
❑ dizziness
❑ chest pain or irregular heartbeat
❑ severe nausea or vomiting
❑ unusual or uncontrolled movements of the body
❑ enlarged pupils, sensitivity to light
❑ stomach pain
❑ difficulty breathing or speaking
❑ convulsions
❑ fever or chills
❑ hallucinations
❑ severe headache
❑ black, tarry stools
❑ increased sweating
❑ swelling of feet or legs

Call your doctor if these symptoms continue:
❑ dry mouth, burning of lips or throat, grinding teeth
❑ insomnia
❑ numbness in feet or toes
❑ ringing in ears
❑ unusual tiredness or weakness
❑ blurred vision
❑ weight change

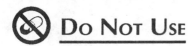 **DO NOT USE**

Alternative treatment: See below.

Ergoloid Mesylates
HYDERGINE, HYDERGINE LC (Sandoz)
DEAPRIL-ST (Mead Johnson)

Family: Drugs used in Alzheimer's Disease

Hydergine has been misleadingly promoted and advertised as effective therapy for "those who would be considered to suffer from some ill-defined process related to aging" and as "the only product for Alzheimer's dementia."[20] The truth is quite the opposite.

According to a recent review on geriatric medicine in the *Journal of the American Medical Association*, "One widely used treatment [for Alzheimer's] (ergoloid mesylates) has been convincingly demonstrated to be of no value. This trial [referring to the study discussed below], along with the absence of a convincing pathophysiologic basis for its use, indicates that this treatment should be abandoned."[21]

Hydergine (ergoloid mesylates), is the only drug approved by the Food and Drug Administration (FDA) for the treatment of mental deterioration in the elderly, and has been on the market for more than 30 years. A study, published in *The New England Journal of Medicine*,[22] shows ergoloid mesylates to be totally ineffective for mild to moderate Alzheimer's, and to actually accelerate patients' mental deterioration. Previous research showing ergoloid mesylates to be effective was flawed. This study was more carefully designed in several ways. Potential participants underwent a rigorous evaluation at the start of the study to screen out patients whose dementia was due to a medical or psychiatric problem other than Alzheimer's. More patients were studied (39 took ergoloid mesylates, and 41 took placebo), and the trial was continued for longer (24 weeks) than most previous studies.

Subjects taking Hydergine-LC, at the recommended dose of 1 mg 3 times daily, did worse than the control group on one measure of appropriate behavior and one measure of IQ. The authors said that the drug may either be directly toxic to the brain, or may somehow accelerate the progression of Alzheimer's.

The term "dementia" describes a collection of symptoms including confusion, disorientation, apathy, and memory loss. More than 60 disorders can cause dementia.[23] Alzheimer's dementia, which is not reversible, accounts for about 50 to 60% of the cases of dementia.[24] A smaller percentage of dementias are reversible.

A person showing signs of dementia should be completely tested to see whether he or she is suffering from one of the dementias that can be cured. These tests include complete physical, neurological, and psychiatric examinations as well as a chest X-ray, CT scan, and blood tests.[25] In addition, many cases of dementia are caused or worsened by prescription drugs such as tranquilizers and sleeping pills (see p. 27). If you are taking one of these drugs, ask your doctor about stopping or changing your prescription.

If, after testing, a physician determines that a person has Alzheimer's dementia, a health-care team — including a doctor, a nurse, and a social worker experienced in working with dementia — can offer practical suggestions to increase the person's safety and comfort at home and can discuss alternative care options. Efforts to improve the mental and physical state of older or senile adults are most beneficial if they address social, physical, nutritional, psychological, occupational, and recreational needs.[26]

Clonazepam
KLONOPIN (Roche)

Generic: not available

Family: Anticonvulsants
         Benzodiazepines

Clonazepam (clawn *az* ah pam) is approved for the control of several types of seizures in which myoclonus is a major element. Myoclonus refers to brusque, lightning-like movements of a muscle or part of a muscle, sometimes sufficiently strong enough to move an entire limb, and characterizes benign absence attacks, atypical petit mal, and the prodromal period of grand mal. Usually, other anticonvulsants are needed as well, to control the non-myoclonic elements of the seizure. Clonazepam is also useful in the control of myoclonus that sometimes follows recovery from anoxic brain damage and in the control of restless movements of the legs during sleep. Though unapproved for the purpose, clonazepam is also used to treat insomnia and a variety of psychiatric problems, such as anxiety and panic attacks. These latter disorders are treated far more effectively by drugs other than clonazepam.

Clonazepam is one of the benzodiazepine drugs (see p. 198), the best known of which are Valium, Xanax, Librium and Halcion. Elderly people are usually more sensitive to the central nervous system effects of these drugs.

Because clonazepam has been prescribed to treat panic attacks, anxiety and sleeplessness, it is important to rule out preventable causes of these problems. The cause of panic attacks may be thyroid disease, low blood sugar, overuse of caffeine and aspirin, or withdrawal from addictive drugs.[27] Before using drugs for panic disorders try controlled breathing, distraction, and relaxation.[28] Anxiety and sleeplessness may be aggravated by alcohol, caffeine, and a number of drugs.

Before You Use This Drug
Do not use if you have or have had
❑ alcohol dependence or drug addiction
❑ cirrhosis or other liver disease
❑ glaucoma (narrow angle)
Tell your doctor if you have or have had
❑ allergies to drugs
❑ asthma
❑ depression
❑ epilepsy
❑ glaucoma, any type
❑ hepatitis
❑ hyperactivity
❑ kidney problems
❑ low albumin
❑ low blood pressure
❑ lung problems
❑ myasthenia gravis
❑ porphyria
❑ smoked
❑ snore
❑ swallowing difficulties
Tell your doctor about any other drugs you take, including aspirin, herbs, vitamins, and other non-prescription products.

One hazard of taking clonazepam continuously for longer than several weeks is addiction. **Do not stop taking your drug suddenly**. With the help of your doctor, work out a schedule for slowly lowering the amount of the drug you take by about 5 to 10% each day. Keep a written record of the dosage reduction schedule with you. These steps will make it much easier to become drug free without developing distressing symptoms of drug withdrawal.

When You Use This Drug
◆ Do not drink alcohol.
◆ Until you know how you react to this drug, do not drive or perform other activities requiring alertness.
◆ You may feel dizzy when rising from a lying or sitting position. If you are lying down, hang your legs over the side of the bed for a few minutes, then get up slowly. When getting up from a chair, stay by the chair until you are sure that you are not dizzy. (See p. 14.)
◆ Carry medical identification stating your condition and that you are taking clonazepam.
◆ If you plan to have any surgery, including dental, tell your doctor that you take this drug.

How To Use This Drug
◆ Swallow tablets whole or break apart. Some experts find taking clonazepam with food lessens adverse effects.[29]
◆ If you take different doses at different times of the day, take the largest dose at night.[30]
◆ If you miss a dose, take it within an hour. Otherwise, wait until time for the next dose. **Do not increase your dose or take double doses.**
◆ Do not store in the bathroom. Do not expose to heat, strong light, or moisture.
◆ Check with your doctor before you stop taking this drug. A gradual lowering of the dose is required to prevent seizures and other signs of withdrawal.
◆ If you need a refill, contact your pharmacy well ahead of time, to allow time for the pharmacist to contact your doctor before refilling.

Interactions With Other Drugs
The following drugs are listed in *Evaluations of Drug Interactions*, 1991 as causing "highly clinically significant" or "clinically significant" interactions when used together with this drug. There may be other drugs, especially those in the families of drugs listed below, that also will react with this drug to cause severe adverse effects. Make sure to ask your doctor for a complete listing of them and let her or him know if you are taking any of these interacting drugs:

alcohol; BENADRYL; cimetidine; digoxin; diphenhydramine; KETALAR; ketamine; LANOXIN; TAGAMET.

Additionally, the *United States Pharmacopeia Drug Information*, 1992 lists these drugs, as well as any drug which depresses the central nervous system (drugs which can make you dizzy or drowsy), as having interactions of major significance:

M S CONTIN; morphine; RETROVIR; zidovudine.

Adverse Effects
Call your doctor immediately:
❑ **if you experience signs of overdose:** confusion; unusual weakness; severe drowsiness; difficulty breathing; slurred speech; staggering; slow heartbeat; slowed reflexes
Call your doctor if these symptoms continue:
❑ confusion, forgetfulness
❑ constipation or diarrhea
❑ dry mouth, increased saliva
❑ headache
❑ rapid heartbeat
❑ increased sensitivity to light, noise
❑ insomnia
❑ irritability
❑ increased sweating
❑ loss of bladder control
❑ nausea or vomiting
❑ runny nose
❑ skin rash
❑ swelling of ankles, face, lymph glands
❑ twitching
❑ unusual eye movements

When you stop taking clonazepam, symptoms of withdrawal may occur, even several days after cessation of the medication. In older people this time may be longer.[31] Tapering off the drug helps prevent these signs:
❑ deep depression

❑ hallucinations
❑ seizures
❑ stomach cramps
❑ excessive sweating
❑ tremors
❑ vomiting

Periodic Tests
Ask your doctor which of these tests should be done periodically while you are taking this drug:
❑ reassessment of efficacy of clonazepam (estimation of serum concentrations)

LIMITED USE

Phenobarbital
LUMINAL (Winthrop-Breon)
SOLFOTON (Poythress) PBR/12 (Scott-Allison)

Generic: available

Family: Barbiturates
Anticonvulsants

Phenobarbital (fee noe *bar* bi tal) is of limited benefit to older adults because it is addictive and has potentially serious side effects. You should not be taking it to promote sleep, relieve nervousness or anxiety, lower blood pressure, or reduce pain. Like other drugs in its family, it is commonly misused as a painkiller, although it can actually increase your sensation of and reaction to pain. **You should only be taking phenobarbital to control convulsions**

One hazard of taking phenobarbital continuously for longer than several weeks is addiction. **Do not stop taking your drug suddenly**. With the help of your doctor, work out a schedule for slowly lowering the amount of the drug you take by about 5 to 10% each day. Keep a written record of the dosage reduction schedule with you. These steps will make it much easier to become drug free without developing distressing symptoms of drug withdrawal.

(seizures). For this purpose, you can take it at doses well below those that cause you to go to sleep.

If your kidney or liver function is impaired, you need to take less than the usual adult dose of phenobarbital.
Phenobarbital causes liver cancer in mice and rats.

Before You Use This Drug
Do not use if you have or have had
❑ porphyria
Tell your doctor if you have or have had
❑ allergies to drugs
❑ mental depression
❑ liver disease
❑ asthma or other breathing difficulties
❑ diabetes
❑ kidney impairment
❑ anemia
❑ long-term pain
❑ adrenal gland problems
❑ overactive thyroid
Tell your doctor about any other drugs you take, including aspirin, herbs, vitamins, and other non-prescription products.

When You Use This Drug
◆ Until you know how you react to this drug, do not drive or perform other activities requiring alertness.

Phenobarbital may cause drowsiness, dizziness, and lightheadedness.
- ◆ Do not drink alcohol or use other drugs that can cause drowsiness.
- ◆ Phenobarbital can worsen symptoms of Parkinson's disease.
- ◆ **Do not stop taking this drug suddenly. Your doctor must lower your dose gradually to prevent withdrawal symptoms.**
- ◆ If you plan to have any surgery, including dental, tell your doctor that you take this drug.

Interactions With Other Drugs

The following drugs are listed in *Evaluations of Drug Interactions*, 1991 as causing "highly clinically significant" or "clinically significant" interactions when used together with this drug. There may be other drugs, especially those in the families of drugs listed below, that also will react with this drug to cause severe adverse effects. Make sure to ask your doctor for a complete listing of them and let her or him know if you are taking any of these interacting drugs:

alcohol, ethyl; BRONKODYL; chlorpromazine; CONSTANT-T; COUMADIN; CRYSTODIGIN; cyclosporine; DECADRON; DEPAKENE; dexamethasone; digitoxin; DOXYCHEL; doxycycline; DURAQUIN; ELIXOPHYLLIN; FLAGYL; HEXADROL; LOPRESSOR; methoxyflurane; metoprolol; metronidazole; MYPROIC ACID; PENTHRANE; QUIBRON-T-SR; QUINAGLUTE DURA-TABS; quinidine; SANDIMMUNE; SLO-BID; SLO-PHYLLIN; SOMOPHYLLIN; SUSTAIRE; THEO-24; THEOLAIR; theophylline; THORAZINE; valproic acid; VIBRAMYCIN; warfarin.

Adverse Effects
Call your doctor immediately:
- ❑ **if you experience signs of overdose:** confusion; severe drowsiness, weakness; difficulty breathing; slurred speech; staggering; slow heartbeat; unusual eye movements; trouble sleeping; unusual irritation
- ❑ confusion
- ❑ hallucinations
- ❑ mental depression
- ❑ skin rash, hives, wheezing
- ❑ swelling of eyelids, face, lips
- ❑ sore throat, fever
- ❑ unusual bleeding or bruising
- ❑ unusual excitement
- ❑ unusual tiredness or weakness
- ❑ yellow eyes or skin

Call your doctor if these symptoms continue:
- ❑ clumsiness, unsteadiness
- ❑ dizziness, lightheadedness
- ❑ drowsiness
- ❑ anxiety, nervousness
- ❑ constipation
- ❑ faintness
- ❑ headache
- ❑ nausea or vomiting
- ❑ nightmares, difficulty sleeping
- ❑ unusual irritability

Periodic Tests
Ask your doctor which of these tests should be done periodically while you are taking this drug:
- ❑ complete blood counts
- ❑ liver function tests
- ❑ kidney function tests
- ❑ blood levels of phenobarbital (when used as an anticonvulsant)

Bromocriptine
PARLODEL (Sandoz)

Generic: not available

Family: Antiparkinsonians

Bromocriptine (broe moe *krip* teen) has several uses. This page discusses its use for Parkinson's disease, for which it is the second-choice drug, after a combination of levodopa and carbidopa (see p. 537). If you have Parkinson's disease, your doctor should first try levodopa with carbidopa, and should prescribe bromocriptine only if the combination drug does not decrease your symptoms or if it causes you too many side effects. Bromocriptine often works best when given with levodopa. **If you are over 60, you should generally be taking less than the usual adult dose.**

In older adults, bromocriptine often causes dizziness, nausea, constipation, and tingling in fingers or toes when exposed to the cold. It can also cause more serious side effects called choreiform movements — unusual and uncontrolled movements in the body, face, tongue, arms, hands, and upper body. About 25% of bromocriptine users in all age groups experience this side effect. If you have any of these symptoms, especially if they are severe or persistent, call your doctor and ask if your dose of bromocriptine should be reduced. Do not take less bromocriptine than your doctor prescribed unless he or she instructs you to do so.

If you have symptoms of parkinsonism (tremor, rigid muscles, and disturbances in posture, walking, balance, speech, swallowing, and muscle strength), there is a good chance that they are caused by a drug you are taking. As many as half of older adults with symptoms of parkinsonism may have developed them as side effects of a drug. A list of drugs that can cause symptoms of parkinsonism appears on p. 30. If you take any of the drugs on this list, discuss the possibility of drug-induced parkinsonism with your doctor, and ask to have your prescription changed or stopped.

Before You Use This Drug
Tell your doctor if you have or have had
❑ allergies to drugs
❑ liver disease
❑ mental illness
Tell your doctor about any other drugs you take, including aspirin, herbs, vitamins, and other non-prescription products.

When You Use This Drug
◆ **Do not use more or less often or in a higher or lower dose than prescribed.** Higher doses increase the risk of side effects, while lower doses may worsen symptoms of parkinsonism.
◆ Until you know how you react to this drug, do not drive or perform other activities requiring alertness. Bromocriptine can cause drowsiness and lightheadedness.
◆ You may feel dizzy when rising from a lying or sitting position. When getting

---

Heat Stress Alert
This drug can affect your body's ability to adjust to heat, putting you at risk of "heat stress." If you live alone, ask a friend to check on you several times during the day. Early signs of heat stress are dizziness, lightheadedness, faintness, and slightly high temperature. Call your doctor if you have any of these signs.

Drink more fluids (water, fruit and vegetable juices) than usual, even if you're not thirsty, unless your doctor has told you otherwise. Do not drink alcohol.

out of bed, hang your legs over the side of the bed for a few minutes, then get up slowly. When getting up from a chair, stay by the chair until you are sure that you are not dizzy. (See p. 14.)

◆ Try to stop smoking to lessen the chance of adverse effects from this drug.[32]

How To Use This Drug

◆ Take with food to decrease stomach upset.

◆ Do not store in the bathroom. Do not expose to heat, strong light, or moisture.

◆ If you miss a dose, take it as soon as you remember, but skip it if it is less than 4 hours until your next scheduled dose. **Do not take double doses.**

Interactions With Other Drugs

The following drugs are listed in *Evaluations of Drug Interactions*, 1991 as causing "highly clinically significant" or "clinically significant" interactions when used together with this drug. There may be other drugs, especially those in the families of drugs listed below, that also will react with this drug to cause severe adverse effects. Make sure to ask your doctor for a complete listing of them and let her or him know if you are taking this interacting drug:

MELLARIL; thioridazine.

Adverse Effects

Call your doctor immediately:

❑ dizziness or lightheadedness
❑ confusion or hallucinations
❑ unusual and uncontrolled movements of the body
❑ tarry stools or bloody vomit
❑ seizures
❑ sudden weakness

Call your doctor if these symptoms continue:

❑ drowsiness
❑ mental depression
❑ headache
❑ nausea or stomach pain
❑ constipation or diarrhea
❑ dry mouth
❑ leg cramps at night
❑ loss of appetite
❑ stuffy nose
❑ tingling in fingers or toes when exposed to cold

Periodic Tests

Ask your doctor which of these tests should be done periodically while you are taking this drug:

❑ blood pressure

Carbamazepine
TEGRETOL (Geigy)

Generic: available

Family: Anticonvulsants

Carbamazepine (kar ba *maz* e peen) is used to treat some forms of epilepsy that have not responded to other drugs and to treat a form of excruciating facial pain called trigeminal neuralgia or tic douloureux. This drug is *not* a simple painkiller and should *not* be used to treat general aches or pains.

If you are over 60, you will generally need to take less than the usual adult dose. Ask your doctor about starting with a daily dose of 50 milligrams to prevent harmful side effects, especially mental confusion and slowed pulse. Call your doctor if either of these side effects occurs. If you are taking carbamazepine for neuralgia, your doctor should try reducing your dose every few months to see if a smaller dose will relieve your symptoms.

Carbamazepine can cause serious and sometimes fatal abnormalities of blood cells. If these occur, it is important that they be detected early because usually they can be treated. If you have any of the following possible symptoms of a blood disorder, call your doctor immediately: fever and sore throat, ulcers in the mouth, easy bruising, or skin rashes.[33] Before you start using carbamazepine, you should have a complete blood count, to be certain that you don't have any potential blood abnormalities that could be worsened by the drug.

Carbamazepine causes malignant liver tumors in female rats and benign tumors of the testicles in male rats.[34]

Before You Use This Drug

Do not use if you have or have had
❑ heart block
❑ blood disorders
❑ bone marrow depression
Tell your doctor if you have or have had
❑ allergies to drugs
❑ kidney, heart, or liver disease
❑ diabetes
❑ glaucoma
❑ alcohol dependence
❑ retention of urine
❑ a reaction to tricyclic antidepressant drugs (see p. 196)
Tell your doctor about any other drugs you take, including aspirin, herbs, vitamins, and other non-prescription products.

When You Use This Drug

◆ Until you know how you react to this drug, do not drive or perform other activities requiring alertness. Carbamazepine can cause dizziness, drowsiness, and lack of muscle coordination.
◆ **Schedule regular visits with your doctor to check your progress and test for side effects.**
◆ Wear a medical identification bracelet or carry a card stating that you take carbamazepine.
◆ **Do not stop taking this drug suddenly. This may cause convulsions.**

◆ If you plan to have any surgery, including dental, tell your doctor that you take this drug.

How To Use This Drug

◆ Take with food to decrease stomach upset.
◆ Do not expose to heat, moisture, or strong light. Do not store in the bathroom.
◆ If you miss a dose, take it as soon as you remember, but skip it if it is almost time for the next dose. **Do not take double doses.** Call your doctor immediately if you miss more than 1 dose in a day.

Interactions With Other Drugs

The following drugs are listed in *Evaluations of Drug Interactions*, 1991 as causing "highly clinically significant" or "clinically significant" interactions when used together with this drug. There may be other drugs, especially those in the families of drugs listed below, that also will react with this drug to cause severe adverse effects. Make sure to ask your doctor for a complete listing of them and let her or him know if you are taking any of these interacting drugs:

ARM A CHAR; CALAN; charcoal; cimetidine; cyclosporine; danazol; DANOCRINE; DARVON; DARVON-N; DECADRON; DEPAKENE; dexamethasone; dicumarol; DOXYCHEL; doxycycline; EES; ELIXOPHYLLIN; E-MYCIN; erythromycin; ESKALITH; HALDOL; haloperidol; ILOSONE; INH; isoniazid; lithium carbonate; LITHOBID; LITHONATE; MYPROIC ACID; propoxyphene; SANDIMMUNE; TAGAMET; THEO-DUR; theophylline; valproic acid; verapamil; VIBRAMYCIN.

Adverse Effects

Call your doctor immediately:
❑ if you experience signs of overdose: seizures; severe dizziness or drowsiness;

irregular, slow, or shallow breathing; trembling; fast heartbeat
- ❏ blurred vision
- ❏ confusion, slurred speech, or hallucinations
- ❏ mental depression
- ❏ ringing or buzzing in the ears
- ❏ unusual or uncontrolled movements
- ❏ dark urine, yellow skin and eyes, or pale stools
- ❏ fainting
- ❏ irregular or slow pulse
- ❏ sudden increase or decrease in urine production
- ❏ numbness, tingling, pain, or weakness in hands or feet
- ❏ chest pain
- ❏ pain, tenderness, bluish color, or swelling of legs or feet
- ❏ unusual tiredness or weakness

Call your doctor if these symptoms continue:
- ❏ clumsiness or unsteadiness
- ❏ dizziness, lightheadedness
- ❏ drowsiness
- ❏ nausea or vomiting
- ❏ aching joints or muscles

- ❏ constipation or diarrhea
- ❏ dry mouth
- ❏ headache
- ❏ increased sensitivity to sunlight
- ❏ irritation or inflammation of tongue
- ❏ appetite loss
- ❏ hair loss
- ❏ sexual problems
- ❏ skin rash
- ❏ stomach pain or discomfort
- ❏ increased sweating

Periodic Tests

Ask your doctor which of these tests should be done periodically while you are taking this drug:
- ❏ blood levels of carbamazepine
- ❏ complete blood counts: before using the drug, weekly during the first 3 months of treatment, and monthly thereafter for at least 2 to 3 years
- ❏ kidney function tests
- ❏ liver function tests
- ❏ eye pressure tests
- ❏ complete urinalysis

Notes for Drugs for Neurological Disorders

1. AMA Department of Drugs. *AMA Drug Evaluations.* 5th ed. Chicago: American Medical Association, 1983:333.

2. Vestal RE, ed. *Drug Treatment in the Elderly.* Sydney, Australia: ADIS Health Science Press, 1984:310.

3. AMA, op. cit.

4. Vestal, op. cit.

5. Grillone G, Myssiorek D. Otolaryngologic manifestations of phenytoin toxicity. *Clinical Otolaryngology* 1992; 17:185-91.

6. Clough CG. Parkinson's disease: management. *The Lancet* 1991; 337: 1324-7.

7. Cotton P. Many researchers, few clinicians, using drug that may slow, even prevent, Parkinson's. *Journal of the American Medical Association* 1990; 264:1083-4.

8. DATATOP Investigators et al. DATATOP and clinical neuromythology IX special correspondence. *Neurology* 1991; 41:771-7.

9. Deprenyl and the progression of Parkinson's disease (letters). *Science* 1990; 249:303-4.

10. Grimes JD. Deprenyl: the exciting possibility of protective effect. *Canadian Journal of Neurological Sciences* 1991; 18:85-6.

11. Pearce JMS. Progression of Parkinson's disease. *British Medical Journal* 1990; 301:396.

12. Boyson SJ. Psychiatric effects of selegiline. *Archives of Neurology* 1991; 48:902.

13. Gilman AG, Rall TW, Nies AS, Taylor P, eds. *The Pharmacological Basis of Therapeutics.* 8th ed. New York: Pergamon Press, 1990:475.

14. Marsden CD. Parkinson's disease. *The Lancet* 1990; 335:948-52.

15. Cotton, op. cit.

16. Riley D, Devereaux M, Grossman G, Chandar K, Bahntge M. Deprenyl for the treatment of early Parkinson's disease (letter). *The New England Journal of Medicine* 1990; 322:1526-8.

17. Dukes MNG, Beeley L. *Side Effects of Drugs Annual* 14, Amsterdam: Elsevier, 1990:11-2.

18. Boyson, op. cit.

19. Saint-Hilaire M, Feldman RG, Durso R. and Goldstein M, Lew JH. Deprenyl for the treatment of Parkinson's disease (letters). *The New England Journal of Medicine* 1990; 322:1526-8.

20. Advertisement for Hydergine. *Journal of the American Medical Association* 1985; 254:2233.

21. Larson EB. Geriatric medicine. *Journal of the American Medical Association* 1991; 265:1325-6.

22. Thompson TL, Filley CR, Mitchell WD, Culig KM, LoVerde M, Byyny RL. Lack of efficacy of Hydergine in patients with Alzheimer's disease. *The New England Journal of Medicine* 1990; 323:445-8.

23. Haase GR. Disease presenting as dementia. In *Dementia* 2nd ed., edited by CE Wells. Philadelphia: FA Davis, 1977:27-67.

24. Smith JS, Kiloh LF. The investigation of dementia: results in 200 consecutive admissions. *The Lancet* 1981; 1:824-7.

25. Weatherall DJ, Ledingham JGG, Warrel DA, eds. In *Oxford Textbook of Medicine*, 1st ed. New York: Oxford University Press, Inc., 1983; 24:14.

26. *The Medical Letter on Drugs and Therapeutics.* New York: The Medical Letter Inc., 1974; 16:21.

27. Raj A, Sheehan DV. Medical evaluation of panic attacks. *Journal of Clinical Psychiatry* 1987; 48:309-13.

28. DeRubeis R, Beck A. Cognitive Therapy. In *Handbook of Cognitive-Behavioral Therapies.* New York: The Guilford Press, 1988.

29. Davidson JRT. Continuation treatment of panic disorder with high-potency benzodiazepines. *Journal of Clinical Psychiatry* 1990; 51 (12 Supplement A):31-7.

30. American Society of Hospital Pharmacists. *American Hospital Formulary Service Drug Information;* Bethesda, MD, 1992:1196-8.

31. *USP DI, Drug Information for the Health Care Professional.* 12th ed. Rockville MD: The United States Pharmacopeial Convention, Inc., 1992:601-10.

32. Melmed S, Braunstein GD. Bromocriptine and pleuropulmonary disease. *Archives of Internal Medicine* 1989; 149:258-9.

33. *Physicians' Desk Reference.* 40th ed. Oradell, N.J.: Medical Economics Company, 1986:900.

34. *USP DI, Drug Information for the Health Care Provider.* 6th ed. Rockville MD.: The United States Pharmacopeial Convention, Inc., 1986:441.

Nutritional Supplements

Nutritional Supplements

Nutritional supplements are one of ten groups of drugs most commonly used by older adults. The Food and Drug Administration estimates that 40% of adults in this country take a nutritional supplement.[1] This category includes vitamins, minerals, and combinations of the two, as well as supplements for which there are no known daily requirements for the human body, such as carnitine, lecithin, and inositol.

An enormous industry has grown around sales of nutritional supplements. To promote these supplements, companies advertise to make many people worry about whether they are getting enough nutrients. But do most people really need to take vitamins and minerals to supplement their diets? Or are they a waste of money? What better alternatives are there to taking supplements to ensure adequate nutrition? This section will attempt to answer these questions and help you sort through the tangled web of fact and fantasy that invariably surrounds nutritional supplements.

Causes of Nutritional Deficiencies in Older Adults

It is a fact that there are older adults who have nutritional deficiencies, and they fall into three categories:
1. People who do not eat enough food — fewer than 1,500 calories a day.
2. People who eat enough food but have an unbalanced, low-quality diet.
3. People who have medical problems or take drugs that contribute to nutritional deficiencies.

Too Few Calories

The most common cause of inadequate nutrition in older adults is eating too few calories. A diet that provides fewer than 1,500 calories a day does not ensure an adequate intake of all necessary nutrients. There are special reasons why this can happen.

Physical changes occur with aging. A decrease in the sensitivity of smell and taste results in food not tasting as good and a subsequent loss of appetite. Dental problems make eating more difficult, especially raw vegetables and meat. Physical handicaps hinder food preparation and eating.

Economic factors also play a role in preventing people from eating enough. **One out of every six older adults lives in poverty, which makes buying sufficient, wholesome food a difficult task.**

An Unbalanced, Low-quality Diet

Another group of older adults at risk for nutritional deficiencies are those who eat enough food to feel full but eat an inadequate supply of necessary nutrients (vitamins and minerals which ensure your body's good health). Certain changes make a deficiency more likely to happen.

As a person ages, his or her daily requirement for calories decreases because of a reduction in basal metabolic rate and physical activity. In order to maintain a weight of 140 pounds, a 70-year-old must eat fewer calories than he or she did as a 40-year-old. The basal metabolic rate, which determines how many calories your body burns off while resting, can decrease from as much as 15 to 20% between the ages of 30 and 75. As a result, older adults require fewer calories. Less exercise results in a loss of lean body weight with a decrease in muscle and an increase in fat.

Regular exercise is the only way to slow this process down or reverse it. Exercise can increase both your basal metabolic rate and the amount of muscle in your body. It can also quicken the rate at which your food is digested and used. These effects from exercise allow you to eat more food without gaining weight.

Although the number of needed calories decreases with age, nutrient needs remain about the same (unless there is a special situation, such as a physical condition or a drug, that creates a need for more). As a result, a high-quality diet becomes more essential. More attention must be paid to eating quality food rather than eating inadequate food that contains "empty calories," calories with little nutritive value.

A barrier to this goal of adequate nutrition is that older adults often do not shop for or prepare their own food. Eating out often makes it harder to choose a healthy diet. Being immobile or in long-term institutional care reduces control over eating a high-quality diet. Living alone is also a barrier because preparing meals for one and eating alone is not always that appealing.

Medical Problems and Drugs

Nutritional deficiencies can also be caused by medical problems, including alcohol dependence and drugs. For example, diseases of the intestine, pancreas, and liver cause decreased absorption of certain nutrients, and some chronic diseases reduce the appetite.

Certain prescription and nonprescription drugs and alcohol also cause increased requirements of certain nutrients. These are the most common drugs (see the individual drug listings for more details):

❑ Drugs that affect the stomach or intestines such as mineral oil and laxatives
❑ Cholesterol-reducing drugs such as clofibrate and cholestyramine
❑ Antibiotics such as the cephalosporins and isoniazid
❑ Cytotoxic drugs (drugs that cause damage to cells) such as methotrexate, colchicine and many anticancer drugs
❑ Anticonvulsants such as phenytoin and phenobarbital
❑ Blood pressure drugs such as hydrochlorothiazide and hydralazine
❑ Alcohol

If you have any medical problems or use any drugs that increase the demand for certain vitamins and minerals, talk to your doctor about the best ways to increase your nutrient intake.

How to Prevent and Treat a Nutritional Deficiency

Should these three groups of people who have nutritional deficiencies take vitamins or minerals? There is no simple answer to this question because of the various causes of nutritional deficiencies. Sometimes, taking a supplement will help. But supplements are never the complete answer to anyone's nutritional problems. It is far better to address the situation that could cause nutritional deficiency than to take a supplement and do nothing more.

Steps Toward a Better Diet

Eating a well-balanced diet with plenty of variety and high-quality food is the most important way to ensure good nutrition. Here are some healthy suggestions for doing that. If you decide to make changes in your diet, try one at a time; you will have a better chance of succeeding.

1. *Decrease the amount of fat in your diet, particularly saturated fats.* Most Americans eat too much fat, which contributes to heart disease, the nation's number one killer. Fat should contribute only 30% of your total daily caloric intake. You can decrease the amount of fat by
   - trimming fat off meat
   - eating more fish and chicken (without the skin) instead of red meat
   - drinking skim milk instead of whole milk and cutting down on your consumption of whole-milk dairy products
   - eating fewer fried foods
   - steaming or baking food instead of cooking with oils and butter
2. *Decrease the amount of salt in your diet.* Eating a high-salt diet contributes to high blood pressure, thereby increasing your risk of heart disease and stroke. Foods that are high in salt include processed food, condiments, and salted meats. It is possible to buy low-salt crackers, no-salt pretzels, unsalted nuts, and low-sodium canned goods and breakfast cereals.
3. *Eat more fruits, vegetables, and whole grains.* These are the best sources of

complex carbohydrates (starches that provide fiber and essential nutrients) and are also good sources of vitamins and minerals. Carbohydrates should contribute 55% of your total daily caloric intake, with the majority of them being fruits, vegetables, and whole grains. They also provide the best source of natural fiber, which comes from nonprocessed foods that are often more difficult to chew — raw cauliflower, broccoli, carrots, and whole-grain breads, for example. Fiber also promotes regularity (see Psyllium, p. 356), and may help to significantly reduce your cholesterol level and/or blood pressure.[2]

4. *Decrease the amount of simple sugars in your diet.* Replace foods sweetened with refined sugar (sucrose), such as candy, ice cream, pastry, jam, with naturally sweet foods, such as oranges and apples.

5. *Decrease your alcohol intake.* Drink no more than three to five drinks a week, if not fewer.

6. *Increase your fluid intake to 6 to 8 glasses of fluids a day, especially water.* Kidney function is often reduced in older adults. Drinking more fluids helps the kidneys function better and also promotes regularity. However, first ask your doctor if you need to restrict your fluid intake.

7. *Eat a wide variety of foods.* A wide variety of wholesome foods will provide all the nutrients you need. It's not too late to try new foods and get into new habits if your diet has been limited. Change your eating habits a little bit at a time and soon you will notice a difference. If you want to change your diet to get more of a specific nutrient, there is a list of good dietary sources of the individual vitamins and minerals at the end of this section.

Who Needs Vitamin and Mineral Supplements?

Having said that eating good food is the best and only sure way to improve your nutritional health, it should be added that for particular groups of older adults, taking nutritional supplements is entirely reasonable and, at times, necessary:

1. People who eat fewer than 1,500 calories a day.
2. People who are institutionalized.
3. People with certain chronic diseases, including alcoholism, as well as liver, kidney, and intestinal diseases.
4. People who take drugs that interfere with absorption of nutrients.
5. People with a specific diagnosed nutritional deficiency or who are in a high-risk group for developing a deficiency. Examples are postmenopausal women taking calcium to prevent osteoporosis and strict vegetarians who do not eat eggs or milk products taking vitamin B_{12}.

People who fit into these categories may require either a supplement of a specific nutrient or a multivitamin supplement with or without minerals. Either way, supplementation should be started after discussion with and approval by a doctor.

Taking Vitamin and Mineral Supplements as "Insurance"

What about people who do not fall into these categories? For example, what if you eat an inadequate diet and find it hard to make changes toward a healthy diet? Many people in this situation take a vitamin and mineral supplement to provide adequate "insurance" for their diets. Is this a good idea? One needs to look at both sides of the issue. Supplements cannot provide "insurance" from a poor diet because vitamin and mineral deficiencies are not the only problems from eating an unbalanced diet, and may not even be the most important one.

A diet high in fat, cholesterol, and salt, for example, contributes to heart disease. A diet low in fiber causes constipation and irregularity of bowel movements, and contributes to development of diverticulitis, a disease of the intestine that can result in bleeding of the intestine. A vitamin and mineral supplement will not insure against any of these problems. Only changes in your diet can help you to prevent such diseases. Relying on supplements for insurance can give you a false sense of security about your diet. We all have met people who eat a poor diet and justify it by saying, "Well, at least I'm taking vitamins." This sense of security can be harmful in that it may remove any incentive to improve your diet.

What if you realize this, but want to take a supplement anyway? There is no strong medical evidence of benefit from supplements when a specific deficiency does not exist, although it is a fact that people take them for peace of mind.

There is, however, one recent, very well-controlled study done in people 65 and older in which a multiple-vitamin pill with minerals was given to half of the people, and a placebo to the other half. At the end of one year, those who took the balanced supplement had significantly fewer days of illness due to infections than those who took the placebo. Other markers for immune response were also better in the vitamin group. The results were due to the fact that some of those studied actually had previously had deficiencies of one or more vitamins or minerals which were remedied by the supplement. The authors stressed that no large doses of any vitamin or mineral were used since they might actually impair immunity.[3]

On the other hand, there is no evidence that a regular multivitamin supplement with or without minerals taken in a dose less than or equal to the recommended dietary allowance (RDA) is detrimental to your health. This does not hold true, however, for doses that far exceed the RDA (megadoses) of vitamins and minerals. If you decide to use a supplement, there are a few things that you should know.

Guidelines for Selecting Supplements

Be rational about selecting a supplement. If you are not at risk for a specific vitamin or mineral deficiency, choose a basic multi-vitamin plus a mineral supplement. Taking specific pills for specific vitamins is a marketing tactic designed to make supplements more expensive. The average multivitamin pill with close to 100% of the RDA of each of the vitamins is less expensive.

Read the mineral contents on the label if you are concerned about increasing your intake of minerals. Most multivitamin supplements with minerals contain close to 100% of the RDA for vitamins but not for minerals. Mineral deficiency is actually more common than vitamin deficiency, despite what advertising might say. In older postmenopausal women, for example, calcium deficiency is a major health problem. We concur with the National Institutes of Health's recommendation of 1,000 to 1,500 milligrams of calcium a day. If you cannot get this amount through your diet, take a calcium supplement (see p. 561), either singly or in combination with a vitamin supplement.

Do not buy a supplement that contains nutrients for which there are no known requirements or "new" vitamins, such as lecithin, carnitine, and inositol. Supporters of these supplements argue that we do not know all of what the human body really needs. Within the last 10 years, however, people with intestinal problems have been living successfully on injected solutions of protein, carbohydrates, fats, and established vitamins. If there were any unknown nutrients needed, this information would be known by now.

Buy the least expensive supplements. Many products are horrendously overpriced, being marked up to 1,000% over cost! Money that you overspend on supplements is money taken away from buying wholesome food. There is no benefit to be gained from a "natural" supplement versus a synthetic supplement. Brand name vitamins are no better than generic versions. Buy the generics, which will work exactly the same as the more expensive name brands.

Recommended Dietary Allowances (RDA) — What They Really Mean

There is no need to take vitamin or mineral doses above the recommended dietary allowances. There is much confusion about the various recommended allowances.

The National Academy of Sciences is the organization that sets the recommended dietary allowance (RDA) for each vitamin and mineral, and this allowance varies for males, females, and different age groups. Because they are designed to account for differences between older and younger adults, the RDAs are the most appropriate ones for an older adult to use.

There is a prevailing myth that the RDA is no more than the amount of a vitamin or mineral that is needed to prevent deficiencies. This is not the case. When an RDA is set, the committee first decides how much of a vitamin or mineral the average person needs, and then raises this number to cover the needs of 98% of the healthy population. **This number is set at a level that is often two to three times higher than people's needs, resulting in a significant safety margin — the government's own "insurance" for your health.**

The vast majority of people do not need to get 100% of the RDA daily, according to the RDA committee. Thus, there is no need to take supplements that go beyond the RDA.

You may be familiar with two other guidelines, the USRDA and the MDR. Neither of these guidelines is as appropriate as the RDA for older adults. The Food and Drug Administration sets a single U.S. Recommended Daily Allowance (USRDA), which is largely based on the RDA for teenage boys. This allowance is not appropriate for older adults, since it does not account for age differences. Most vitamin supplements will state on the label what percent of the USRDA they provide. The Minimum Daily Requirement (MDR) was a forerunner of the USRDA and is now out of date.

The Myth of Megadose

There is a great deal of advertising that promotes the unproven benefits of taking supplements well beyond the RDA, the so-called megadoses of vitamins and minerals. Sensational claims of health and well-being are made for megadoses — claims that they will "add vitality to your health," "restore the luster to your skin," and "perk up your sex life." When looked at critically, these claims just don't stand up.

To understand what vitamins or minerals can or cannot do, one must first understand their function in the human body. For the most part, a vitamin is a part of an enzyme (protein) which helps the enzyme perform certain chemical functions in the body. For example, many B vitamins help enzymes convert food into energy. Minerals act similarly. Calcium builds bones and also helps enzymes perform their functions. Iron is an essential element of red blood cells and helps them carry oxygen from the lungs to the tissues.

Vitamin functions were originally determined through vitamin deficiency diseases in people who were deprived of certain kinds of food for long periods of time. Sailors who were deprived of citrus fruits developed scurvy, a deficiency of vitamin C. They had such symptoms as bleeding into joints, poor healing of wounds, and emotional changes. Scurvy became known as a disease resulting from vitamin C deficiency when it was found out that the sailors' symptoms dramatically disappeared once they ate citrus fruits.

The vitamin manufacturers take the process of deficiency diseases and vitamins one step further. For example, claims are made that vitamin C will help cure any skin or emotional problems, colds, or cancer. The overwhelming majority of these problems are not caused by vitamin C deficiency, so nothing will improve in to the average person taking vitamin C.

The flaw in this logic can be demonstrated by using food as an example of a deficiency. If you fast for a long time you will begin to develop certain symptoms, such as muscle aches, headaches, nausea, and dizziness, which will disappear dramatically once you begin to eat again. It does not follow from this that if you have symptoms of nausea, headaches, and dizziness while eating normally, that more food will cause them to go away. You know that from experience. But this is the kind of logic most manufacturers use to make claims for the benefits of megadoses of supplements.

The only way to determine a beneficial effect of a supplement is through controlled scientific experiments, in which a supplement's effects are compared with those of a placebo (dummy medication). No extravagant claims made by manufacturers for megadoses of any vitamins have stood up to these tests.

There are a few instances where vitamins have been determined to have specific additional benefits that have been demonstrated by rigorous scientific studies. Most of these therapeutic uses occur at doses not much greater than the RDA. They are discussed on the individual drug pages which follow this section.

There is serious danger from taking megadoses of many vitamins. People who take a multivitamin supplement in low doses have few risks; however, people who take high doses of certain vitamins have a risk of developing serious medical problems. Dangerous, toxic, and occasionally fatal effects have been associated with high doses of the fat-soluble vitamins A, D, E, and K. Even the water-soluble vitamin C and the B vitamins, which normally pass out of the body in your urine, can have side effects at high doses. Vitamin B_6 has been associated with nerve damage,[4] for example. Too much vitamin C can cause stomach cramps or diarrhea.

Some vitamins should not be taken, even in normal doses, if you use certain drugs or have certain medical problems. If you use warfarin (Coumadin) to prevent blood clots, you should not take vitamin K; it will inhibit warfarin's ability to work. If you are B_{12} deficient and take folic acid (folate) without taking B_{12} as well, neurological symptoms can be worsened. So if you are going to take any type of supplement, it is a good idea to discuss it with your doctor before you start.

Nutritional supplements are a booming business in this country. Many people are misled by advertising into thinking that taking a supplement will help get rid of many of their health problems. But this is not the case. The most important step that you can take to maintain your nutritional well-being is to eat a healthy and well-balanced diet.

Certain older adults may need specific vitamin and mineral supplementation and should talk to their doctors about this. If you do not fall into one of these categories and still wish to take a supplement, you should follow a few rules of thumb.

First, realize that supplements are by no means the complete answer to good nutrition. Taking a supplement is not an adequate replacement for eating healthy food. If you do buy supplements there is no need to buy anything more than a regular multivitamin or a mineral supplement. Take supplements less than or equal to the recommended dietary allowance for older adults. Try to buy the generic brands, not the expensive name brands and "natural" supplements. Finally, avoid megadoses of any supplement. They will give you no additional benefits from the supplement, but will greatly increase your chances of toxic side effects.

Dietary Sources of Vitamins and Minerals

Vitamins

A   Beef liver*, carrots, sweet potatoes, tomatoes, green leafy vegetables, broccoli, watermelon, cantaloupe, apricots, peaches, butter*, margarine*, whole milk*, fortified skim milk

D   Some fatty fishes* and fish-liver oils*, vitamin D-fortified milk* and bread, eggs*, chicken livers*

E   Vegetable oils* (corn, cottonseed, soybean, safflower), wheat germ, whole-grain cereals, egg yolk*

K   Green leafy vegetables, beef*, pork*

C   Citrus fruits (oranges, grapefruit, lemons, limes), tomatoes, strawberries, cantaloupe, cabbage, broccoli, cauliflower, potatoes, raw peppers

B_1 (thiamine)   Dried beans, peas, whole-grain or enriched breads and cereals, enriched or brown rice, enriched pasta, noodles, and other flour products, potatoes, pork*, beef liver*, nuts*

B_2 (riboflavin)   Milk*, enriched and whole-grain products, green leafy vegetables, meat*, fish, poultry*, eggs*, liver*, cheese*

B_3 (niacin)   Beans, peas, potatoes, enriched grain products, beef*, poultry*, pork*, liver*, nuts*

B_6 (pyridoxine)   Wheat and corn products, soybeans, lima beans, yeast, beef*, poultry*, pork*, organ meats*

B_{12} (cyanocobalamin)   Shellfish*, tongue*, fish, milk*, eggs*, cheese*, peas, beans, lentils, tofu, nuts*, beef*, poultry*, pork*, organ meats*

Folic Acid (folate)   Dried beans and nuts*, fruits, green leafy vegetables, organ meats*, whole grains, yeast

Minerals

Calcium   Milk*, cheese*, yogurt*, ice cream* — low-fat and nonfat dairy products can be used, canned salmon and sardines, shellfish*, broccoli, green leafy vegetables, including collards, bok choy, mustard and turnip greens

Iron   Organ meats*, red meat*, fish, green leafy vegetables, peas, wheat germ, brewer's yeast, oysters*, dried beans and fruits

* High in fat and/or cholesterol. Keep servings of these foods to a minimum. Ideally, the calories in all of these foods together should be less than 30% of your diet.

Recommended Dietary Allowances For Older Adults
(National Academy of Sciences Recommendations for Adults over 50 Years)
(1989)[5]

	Amount	
Vitamins	**Males**	**Females**
A		
Retinol	1,000 mcg	800 mcg
Beta-carotene	6,000 mcg	4,800 mcg
International Units	3,300 i.u.	2,640 i.u.
D	400 i.u.	200 i.u.
E	10 mg	8 mg
C	60 mg	60 mg
Thiamine (B$_1$)	1.2 mg	1.0 mg
Riboflavin (B$_2$)	1.4 mg	1.2 mg
Niacin (B$_3$)	15 mg	13 mg
B$_6$	2.0 mg	1.6 mg
Folic Acid (folate)	200 mcg	180 mcg
B$_{12}$	2.0 mcg	2.0 mcg
Minerals		
Calcium	800 mg	1,000-1,500 mg*
Phosphorus	800 mg	800 mg
Magnesium	350 mg	280 mg
Iron	10 mg	10 mg
Zinc	15 mg	12 mg
Iodine	150 mcg	150 mcg

i.u.= International Units
mcg = micrograms
mg = milligrams

* This is not the official calcium RDA for women, which is 800 mg. Many experts consider this too low, including the National Institutes of Health which recommends an intake of 1,000-1,500 mg a day for women after menopause (we agree). See Calcium Supplements for further details.

CALCIUM SUPPLEMENTS
Calcium Carbonate
OS-CAL 500 (Marion) SUPLICAL (Warner-Lambert)
CALTRATE (Lederle)
Calcium Gluconate
Calcium Citrate
CITRACAL (Mission)
Calcium Lactate

Generic: available

Family: Nutritional Supplements (see p. 553)

Calcium (*kal* see um) is a mineral that is stored in the bones and is necessary for bone growth and strength. It also benefits the nervous system, muscles, and heart. As your body ages, its ability to absorb calcium decreases and it has less to use, even though its need for calcium does not diminish. If you are older and also have a diet that lacks adequate calcium, both factors limit the amount of the mineral available for your body to use.

Calcium deficiency in older adults causes changes in the bones and diseases that increase the risk of falls, fractures, and deformity. These bone diseases are osteomalacia and osteoporosis. Osteomalacia is an overall decrease in bone density. Osteoporosis, which occurs most frequently in thin, small-boned, and white women, is a condition in which the bones become weak, so that they are more likely to break or become deformed.

How much calcium do you need? The recommended dietary allowance (RDA) for calcium is 800 milligrams per day, but many experts consider that too low for the population as a whole. In 1984, the National Institutes of Health recommended a calcium intake of 1,000 to 1,500 milligrams per day for women after menopause.[6] We think that this is a safe and desirable intake for all older adults. It will not necessarily protect you against the fractures and deformity of osteoporosis, but it may help and it is unlikely to do you any harm. We do not recommend taking more than 1,500 milligrams per day, since the greater amount has no advantages and can cause some dangerous side effects (see Adverse Effects).

The best way to get calcium is to eat foods that are rich in it (see food sources, below). In particular, you can increase your calcium intake by drinking milk and adding liquid or powdered milk to almost any cooked food (you can use low-fat or nonfat milk if you want to keep your fat intake down). If you cannot get enough calcium from your diet, take a calcium supplement. However, if you have a history of kidney stones, do not increase your calcium intake without talking to your doctor first.

Many people, particularly women, take calcium supplements in the hope that it will decrease their risk of getting osteoporosis. While it has been shown that a diet containing adequate calcium can prevent high blood pressure, taking supplements to prevent osteoporosis is controversial. If you want to reduce your risk of osteoporosis, try quitting smoking; drinking alcohol in moderation if at all; and doing weight-bearing exercise such as walking, aerobics, jogging, dancing, tennis, and biking (although biking is less beneficial than the others).

If you decide to take a calcium supplement, some cautions are in order. You should not take calcium supplements that contain bone-meal and dolomite. The Food and Drug Administration reported that they might contain lead in amounts that could present a risk to older adults.[7] Another caution is that your body does not absorb all calcium supplements with equal ease. It is important to know if the tablets you buy will dissolve properly so that your body can use them effectively. Unfortunately, it has not been determined which supplement is absorbed the best. One study showed that calcium citrate was best absorbed, but another showed that there was no significant difference in absorption among various types of supplements.[8,9] Ask your pharmacist or other health professional for suggestions.

When comparing calcium supplements, you should always check how much elemental (pure) calcium they contain. Because calcium supplements contain other ingredients in addition to calcium, a 100-milligram calcium supplement tablet does not contain 100 milligrams of calcium, and a 100-milligram tablet of one supplement does not necessarily have the same amount of calcium as a 100-milligram tablet of another. Calcium carbonate is 40% calcium, calcium gluconate is 9%, and calcium citrate is 24%. Read the label on the container to find out the amount of elemental calcium. This is the only measurement that counts as far as your body is concerned.

Foods high in calcium: milk, liquid or powdered, including low-fat and nonfat milk; low-fat yogurt; ice cream; cheese (some are high in fat and/or cholesterol); canned salmon and sardines; shellfish; broccoli; green leafy vegetables.

1 cup plain low-fat yogurt	415 milligrams
1 cup milk	300 milligrams
3-1/2 ounces canned salmon with bones	198 milligrams

Before You Use This Drug

Do not use if you have or have had
- ❑ high level of calcium in your blood
- ❑ increased parathyroid gland function
- ❑ reduced parathyroid gland function (*only for calcium phosphate*)
- ❑ kidney stones
- ❑ irregular heartbeat

Tell your doctor if you have or have had
- ❑ allergies to drugs
- ❑ symptoms of appendicitis (severe abdominal pain)
- ❑ blood in stool (bowel movement)
- ❑ heart disease
- ❑ hemorrhoids
- ❑ high blood pressure
- ❑ peptic ulcer
- ❑ intestinal blockage
- ❑ kidney disease
- ❑ sarcoidosis

Tell your doctor about any other drugs you take, including aspirin, herbs, vitamins, and other non-prescription products.

When You Use This Drug

- ◆ **Call your doctor immediately if you have black, tarry stools or vomit material that looks like coffee grounds.**
- ◆ After taking a calcium supplement, wait 1 to 2 hours before taking any other drug by mouth.
- ◆ Do not drink milk or eat milk products, spinach, rhubarb, bran, or whole-grain cereals at the same time that you take calcium. They decrease its absorption.

How To Use This Drug

- ◆ Do not expose to heat, moisture, or strong light. Do not store in the bathroom. Do not let liquid form freeze.
- ◆ If you are taking calcium supplements on a fixed schedule and you miss a dose, take it as soon as you remember, but skip it if it is almost time for the next dose. **Do not take double doses.**

Interactions With Other Drugs

The following drugs are listed in *Evaluations of Drug Interactions*, 1991 as causing "highly clinically significant" or "clinically significant" interactions when used together with this drug. There may be other drugs, especially those in the families of drugs listed below, that also will react with this drug to cause severe adverse effects. Make sure to ask your doctor for a complete listing of them and let her or him know if you are taking any of these interacting drugs:

ACHROMYCIN; aspirin; CALAN; chlorothiazide; DIURIL; ECOTRIN; ISOPTIN; tetracycline; verapamil.

Adverse Effects
Call your doctor immediately:
❏ severe constipation

❏ severe abdominal pain or cramping
❏ difficult or painful urination
❏ irregular heartbeat
❏ mood or mental changes
❏ muscle pain or twitching
❏ nervousness or restlessness
❏ unpleasant taste in mouth
❏ unusual tiredness or weakness
❏ slowed breathing

Call your doctor if these symptoms continue:
❏ belching, bloated stomach
❏ chalky taste in mouth

Folic Acid (Folate)
FOLVITE (Lederle)

Generic: available

Family: Nutritional Supplements (see p. 553)

Folic (*foe* lik) acid, also called folate or vitamin B_9, is essential for cell formation and growth, particularly of blood cells. It is found in several foods (see food sources, below). A well-balanced diet with a variety of healthful foods should supply all the folic acid your body needs. The recommended dietary allowance (RDA) of folic acid for older adults is 200 micrograms per day for men, 180 for women.

It is unlikely that you would have a folic acid deficiency just from a diet low in this vitamin. Rather, certain medical conditions or the long-term use of several drugs can lead to a folic acid deficiency. Alcoholism is perhaps the most common cause because alcoholics often eat an inadequate diet. Some diseases of the small intestine can also interfere with your body's absorption of folic acid, so there is less available for the body to use. Long-term treatment with

drugs such as methotrexate, trimethoprim, triamterene, corticosteroids, certain painkillers, sulfasalazine, and some anticonvulsants (phenobarbital, phenytoin, and primidone) can also cause a folic acid deficiency.

If you have to increase your intake of folic acid in order to prevent or treat a deficiency, eat folate-rich foods rather than taking a vitamin supplement. You should only take a supplement when you have a clear need for more folic acid and when you cannot get enough from your diet. You should not take a supplement until your doctor has made sure that you do not have pernicious anemia, a disease resulting in vitamin B_{12} deficiency. Folic acid supplements can hide the easily detected symptoms of pernicious anemia while allowing irreversible nervous system damage to occur undetected.

If you take folic acid without a doctor's supervision, do not exceed the RDA.
Foods high in folic acid (folate): organ meats and nuts (both are high in cholesterol and/or fat); green vegetables; dried beans;

fruits; yeast; whole grains. Cooking may destroy some folic acid.

1/2 cup spinach	110 micrograms
1 ounce chicken liver	108 micrograms
1/2 cup peanuts	60 micrograms
1 ounce shredded wheat	30 micrograms

Before You Use This Drug

Tell your doctor if you have or have had
❑ allergies to drugs
❑ pernicious anemia
Tell your doctor about any other drugs you take, including aspirin, herbs, vitamins, and other non-prescription products.

How To Use This Drug

◆ Do not expose to heat, moisture, or strong light. Do not store in the bathroom. Do not let liquid form freeze.
◆ As with all drugs, it is important to take this one regularly. However, because of the length of time required for a folic acid deficiency to occur, there is no cause for concern if a dose is missed. If you miss a dose, take it when you remember.

Interactions With Other Drugs

The following drugs are listed in *Evaluations of Drug Interactions*, 1991 as causing "highly clinically significant" or "clinically significant" interactions when used together with this drug. There may be other drugs, especially those in the families of drugs listed below, that also will react with this drug to cause severe adverse effects. Make sure to ask your doctor for a complete listing of them and let her or him know if you are taking this interacting drug:

DILANTIN; phenytoin.

Adverse Effects

Folic acid and other water-soluble vitamins seldom cause adverse effects in people whose kidneys function normally. If you have decreased kidney function or are taking large doses of this vitamin, you should *call your doctor immediately* if you have these side effects:
❑ skin rash or itching
❑ fever

IRON SUPPLEMENTS
Ferrous Sulfate
FEOSOL (Menley & James) SLOW FE (CIBA Consumer)
Ferrous Gluconate
FERGON (Winthrop) SIMRON (Merrell Dow)
Ferrous Fumarate
FEOSTAT (Forest) HEMOCYTE (U.S. Pharmaceutical)

Generic: available

Family: Nutritional Supplements (see p. 553)

Iron is a mineral that your body needs to manufacture hemoglobin, a substance found in red blood cells which carries oxygen to cells throughout the body. A lack of iron produces anemia, which means that the body has too few red blood cells, too little hemoglobin, or too little blood. Iron is found in many foods (see food sources below), and a well-balanced diet with a variety of foods should supply all the iron that your body needs. There is no reason to take an iron supplement unless you have a low iron count or iron deficiency anemia. The recommended dietary allowance (RDA) for older adults is 10 milligrams per day.

Adults generally become iron-deficient from blood loss rather than from a lack of iron in their diet. If your doctor says that you have iron deficiency anemia, she or he must determine the site of the blood loss.

If you have iron deficiency anemia due to blood loss, you should add iron-rich foods to your diet as well as take an iron supplement. You should start out with a supplement containing ferrous sulfate, rather than one made of ferrous gluconate or ferrous fumarate.[10] Only if ferrous sulfate upsets your stomach (a side effect that happens about 10 percent of the time) should you switch to ferrous gluconate or ferrous fumarate.

Do not use iron supplements that also contain other minerals such as calcium and magnesium, which can interfere with your body's absorption of iron. Also, do not use enteric-coated tablets (tablets coated so they do not dissolve in your stomach) and timed-release products because your body does not absorb them evenly. Do not take an iron supplement at the same time as eating foods high in fiber or calcium.

Within 2 weeks from when you begin to take an iron supplement, your red blood cell count should improve. If there is no improvement after 3 to 4 weeks, ask your doctor to reevaluate your situation. If you are anemic, you might need to take iron supplements for 6 months or longer to replenish the body's supply. If the cause of your iron deficiency is poor absorption of iron, a rare problem, you may have to take an iron supplement for longer than this.

If you do not have a low iron count or iron deficiency anemia, there is no reason for you to take an iron supplement. Your body saves iron and cannot get rid of extra iron except by bleeding. Taking too much iron can cause an iron overload in the body and damage to your liver, heart, or kidneys.[11]

Foods high in iron: organ meats, red meat, oysters (all are also high in cholesterol and/ or fat); fish; green leafy vegetables; peas; brewer's yeast; wheat germ; certain dried beans and fruits. Iron from meats is absorbed an average of five times better than iron from vegetables.

3 1/2 ounces calves' liver	14 milligrams
1 lean hamburger	3.9 milligrams
3 1/2 ounces chickpeas	3 milligrams
1/2 cup cooked lima beans	3 milligrams

Before You Use This Drug

Do not use if you have or have had
- ❏ diseases of iron overload (hemochromatosis, hemosiderosis)
- ❏ thalassemia (a hereditary anemia)

Tell your doctor if you have or have had
- ❏ allergies to drugs
- ❏ alcohol dependence
- ❏ liver disease (hepatitis)
- ❏ active infections
- ❏ inflammation of the pancreas
- ❏ peptic ulcer
- ❏ disease of the intestines
- ❏ recent blood transfusion

Tell your doctor about any other drugs you take, including aspirin, herbs, vitamins, and other non-prescription products.

When You Use This Drug

- ◆ Do not use calcium carbonate antacids or calcium supplements; drink coffee, tea, or milk; or eat whole-grain breads or cereals, eggs or milk products within 2 hours of taking an iron supplement. They can decrease iron absorption.
- ◆ Your stools will probably turn black. This is a normal side effect and no cause for concern.

How To Use This Drug

- ◆ Take on an empty stomach, at least 1 hour before or 2 hours after meals. If the iron upsets your stomach, try taking it with food instead. If you can, drink a glass of fruit juice with your iron as this will improve its absorption.
- ◆ Liquid form or contents of capsules can be taken alone or can be mixed with juice, cereal, or other food.
- ◆ Do not expose to heat, moisture, or strong light. Do not store in the bathroom. Do not let the liquid form freeze.
- ◆ If you miss a dose, take it as soon as you remember, but skip it if it is almost time for the next dose. **Do not take double doses.**

Interactions With Other Drugs

The following drugs are listed in *Evaluations of Drug Interactions*, 1991 as causing "highly clinically significant" or "clinically significant" interactions when used together with this drug. There may be other drugs, especially those in the families of drugs listed below, that also will react with this drug to cause severe adverse effects. Make sure to ask your doctor for a complete listing of them and let her or him know if you are taking any of these interacting drugs:

ACHROMYCIN; ALDOMET; CUPRIMINE; LARODOPA; levodopa; methyldopa; PANMYCIN; penicillamine; tetracycline.

Adverse Effects

Call your doctor immediately:
- ❏ stomach pain, cramping, soreness
- ❏ fresh red blood in stools

If you know that you or someone else has taken an overdose of an iron supplement, particularly if that person is a child, seek emergency room treatment immediately. Do not wait for symptoms, which may not appear for 1 hour.
- ❏ **early signs of overdose:** diarrhea; nausea or vomiting; sharp stomach pain or cramping
- ❏ **late signs of overdose:** bluish lips, fingernails, and palms; drowsiness; pale, clammy skin; unusual tiredness; weak, fast heartbeat

Call your doctor if these symptoms continue:
- ❏ constipation or diarrhea
- ❏ dark urine
- ❏ heartburn
- ❏ nausea or vomiting

Periodic Tests

Ask your doctor which of these tests should be done periodically while you are taking this drug:
- ❏ hemoglobin tests
- ❏ reticulocyte (young red blood cell) counts

Multivitamin Supplements
(with and without minerals)
THERAGRAN-M (Squibb) UNICAP (Upjohn)

Generic: available

Family: Nutritional Supplements (see p. 553)

The U.S. Food and Drug Administration estimates that 40% of adults in the United States take vitamin supplements daily.[12] Is this necessary?

Vitamin deficiencies are rare in this country. Mineral deficiencies are more common, but taking a multivitamin supplement with minerals is often not the best way to get minerals. These products either do not supply enough of the mineral you lack, or they contain other minerals which reduce your body's ability to absorb the mineral you need. Instead of taking such supplements, try changing your diet so that you get more of the mineral you need, or take a specific mineral supplement. For example, if you have iron deficiency anemia, you should be taking an iron supplement. Calcium deficiency is another example. Most multivitamin supplements with minerals do not supply enough calcium to meet the recommended dietary allowance (RDA), so taking these supplements may give you a false sense of security about your calcium intake. Changes in your diet, combined with a calcium supplement, may be the best way to increase your calcium intake. See the listings for individual minerals and vitamins for more details.

Who needs a multivitamin and mineral supplement? The following groups of older adults are at risk of vitamin deficiency and may need a supplement:

❑ those who eat fewer than 1,500 calories a day and may have a barely adequate vitamin intake

❑ those who live alone, are institutionalized, have recently been discharged from the hospital, or cannot shop for their food

❑ those who have certain medical problems (such as some intestinal disorders) or take certain drugs that interfere with their body's ability to absorb nutrients

❑ those who drink too much alcohol, which can reduce the body's supply of certain vitamins (thiamine, riboflavin, folic acid, vitamins C and B_6)

The more of these groups you belong to, the greater your risk of having a low-calorie, unbalanced, and nutritionally deficient diet. If you have one or more of these factors, you may need a multivitamin supplement, and you and your doctor should discuss the need for one. But a supplement will not completely make up for deficiencies in your diet, since vitamins are only a very small part of proper nutrition. Getting a good balance of protein, fat, carbohydrates, and fiber is also important, and you can only do this through a well-balanced diet.

If you don't fit into the risk categories above, should you take a supplement for "insurance"? If you are eating a well-balanced diet, there is no reason why you need one.

There is, however, one recent very well-controlled study done in people 65 and older in which a multiple-vitamin pill with minerals was given to half of the people, and a placebo to the other half. At the end of one year, those who took the balanced supplement had significantly fewer days of illness due to infections than those who took the placebo. Other markers for immune response were also better in the vitamin group. The results were due to the fact that some of those studied actually had previously had deficiencies of one or more vitamins or minerals which were remedied by the supplement. The authors stressed that no large doses of any vitamin or mineral were used since they might actually impair immunity.[13]

If you take a multivitamin supplement, don't take doses significantly higher than the recommended dietary allowance (RDA). Doses higher than the RDA will either be eliminated from your body in your urine (in the case of water-soluble vitamins such as the B vitamins and vitamin C) or will accumulate in the body tissues and cause harmful side effects (in the case of the fat-soluble vitamins A, D, E, and K). For the vitamins that accumulate, taking more than the RDA may unnecessarily expose you to the risk of a dangerous overdose.

When choosing a multivitamin, keep in mind that many manufacturers use the same general trademark for several products that have different formulas. Some make drastic changes in the formula of a product and keep the same name. Read the labels and compare the contents of several products. Compare the label with the Recommended Dietary Allowances for Older Adults (p. 560). There is not much logic in a formula that contains less than 50% of the RDA for some vitamins and more than 500% for others. Choose a supplement that comes as close as possible to 100% of the RDA for each ingredient.

Buy the least expensive supplement that meets your needs, and buy a generic version if you can. Generic products are cheaper and are just as effective as the brand-name products.

Niacin (Vitamin B₃)
NICOLAR (Rhone-Poulenc)

Generic: available

Family: Nutritional Supplements (see p. 553)
Cholesterol-lowering drugs (see p. 70)

Niacin (*nye* a sin), also called nicotinic acid or vitamin B₃, and its derivative niacinamide (nye a *sin* a mide), also called nicotinamide, are used by the body to help convert food to energy. Niacin is available in many types of foods (see food sources, below), and a well-balanced diet with a variety of healthful foods should supply all the niacin that your body needs. The recommended dietary allowance (RDA) is 15 milligrams for older men and 13 milligrams for older women.

Dietary deficiency of niacin, called pellagra, is rare. If you need to get more niacin, it is better to eat niacin-rich foods than to take a vitamin supplement. You should take niacin supplements to prevent and treat niacin deficiency only when your diet does not provide an adequate amount.

Niacin (nicotinic acid), but not niacinamide, has another use. It can be prescribed as part of a program to lower blood cholesterol or fat, which also includes a modified diet and exercise. The dose for this purpose, 300 milligrams or more, is much higher than the dose as a dietary supplement (10 to 20 milligrams). Taking niacin for this purpose is only an adjunct to weight reduction and exercise, not a substitute. The side effects of niacin, such as blood vessel dilation which produces intense flushing and itching of the face and upper part of the body, may limit the usefulness of this treatment. **One aspirin taken 30 minutes before a dose of niacin may reduce this side effect.**[14]

Niacin is *not* useful in treating schizophrenia and other mental disorders unrelated to niacin deficiency. It has not been proven effective in treating any blood vessel diseases nor in treating acne, leprosy, or motion sickness.

If you use niacin without a doctor's supervision, do not exceed the RDA. Excess niacin, beyond what is needed each day, simply passes through you and is eliminated in the urine without being used by your body. **Avoid taking extended-release forms of niacin, since these may damage your liver (see p. 570).**

Foods high in niacin (vitamin B₃): beef, pork, liver, eggs, nuts, poultry, milk and dairy products (all are high in cholesterol and/or fat); fish; whole-grain and enriched breads and cereals; beans; peas; potatoes. Cooking destroys some niacin.

3 1/2 ounces calves' liver	16.5 milligrams
1 cup wheat flakes	14.7 milligrams
4 ounces halibut	10.4 milligrams
1/4 cup peanuts	10.0 milligrams
3 1/2 ounces roast turkey	7.7 milligrams
1 slice whole wheat bread	0.6 milligrams

Before You Use This Drug

Tell your doctor if you have or have had
❑ allergies to drugs
❑ arterial bleeding or hemorrhage
❑ liver disease
❑ diabetes
❑ gout
❑ glaucoma
❑ ulcer

Tell your doctor about any other drugs you take, including aspirin, herbs, vitamins, and other non-prescription products.

When You Use This Drug

◆ Until you know how you react to this drug, do not drive or perform other activities requiring alertness. Niacin may cause dizziness or fainting.

How To Use This Drug

◆ Take with food to reduce stomach upset.
◆ Do not expose to heat, moisture, or strong light. Do not store in the bathroom. Do not let liquid form freeze.
◆ If you take a high dose of niacin and want to stop using the drug, reduce the dose gradually. If you plan to take a high dose, work up to it gradually.
◆ As with all drugs, it is important to take this one regularly. However, because of the length of time required for niacin deficiency to occur, there is no cause for concern if you are taking niacin to supplement your diet and you miss a dose. Take it when you remember.
◆ If you are taking niacin as a cholesterol-lowering agent and you miss a dose, take it as soon as you remember, but skip it if it is almost time for your next scheduled dose. **Do not take double doses.**

Interactions With Other Drugs

The following drugs are listed in *Evaluations of Drug Interactions*, 1991, as causing "highly clinically significant" or "clinically significant" interactions when used together with this drug. There may be other drugs, especially those in the families of drugs listed below, that also will react with this drug to cause severe adverse effects. Make sure to ask your doctor for a complete listing of them and let her or him know if you are taking this interacting drug:

lovastatin; MEVACOR.

Adverse Effects

Niacin and other water-soluble vitamins seldom cause adverse effects in people whose kidneys function normally. If you have decreased kidney function or are taking large doses of niacin, you should *call your doctor immediately* if you have these side effects:
❑ skin rash or itching
❑ wheezing, an allergic reaction
Call your doctor if these symptoms continue:
❑ flushing of skin, warmth

- ❏ headache
- ❏ diarrhea
- ❏ lighheadedness or dizziness
- ❏ dry skin
- ❏ nausea or vomiting
- ❏ stomach pain
- ❏ joint pain

Periodic Tests

Ask your doctor which of these tests should be done periodically while you are taking this drug:

For high-dose therapy:
- ❏ blood sugar levels
- ❏ liver function tests
- ❏ blood levels of uric acid

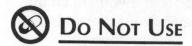 **DO NOT USE**

Alternative treatment: See Non-sustained-release Niacin (p. 568).

Niacin (Vitamin B₃) (All Sustained-release dosage forms of niacin)
NIA-BID (Geriatric Pharmacy)
NICOBID (Rhone-Poulenc)
NIACELS (Hauck)
SLO-NIACIN (Upsher-Smith)

Family: Nutritional Supplements (see p. 553)
Cholesterol-lowering Agents (see p. 70)

Although niacin is useful and effective as a cholesterol-lowering drug (see p. 70), it should only be used in a non-extended dose/sustained-release form because of liver damage caused by the sustained-release dosage forms. In the past several years, a number of studies have documented that liver toxicity, sometimes quite serious, is much more commonly associated with the sustained-release form than with the crystalline or regular form.[15,16]

If you are taking niacin for its lipid-lowering effects, ask your doctor if it is the crystalline (regular) type (see p. 568). Be sure that the prescription is not changed to a slow-release preparation by a pharmacist and do not purchase slow-release pills over the counter. The doses used to lower blood lipids are much higher than the amount needed for normal metabolism, and the slow-release formulas probably promote excessive accumulation of the drug in the liver.

Thiamine (Vitamin B₁)
BETALIN S (Lilly) BIAMINE (Forest)

Generic: available

Family: Nutritional Supplements (see p. 553)

Thiamine (*thye* a min), or vitamin B₁, helps the body use sugars and starches (carbohydrates) effectively. It is available in several kinds of foods (see food sources, below), and a well-balanced diet with a variety of healthful foods should supply all the thiamine that your body needs. The recommended dietary allowance (RDA) of thiamine is 1.2 milligrams per day for older men and 1.0 milligrams per day for older women.

The signs of thiamine deficiency include loss of feeling on areas of the hands and feet, decreased muscle strength, personality disturbances, depression, lack of initiative, and poor memory. Thiamine deficiency is most commonly seen in alcoholics (the condition caused by a severe deficiency is called beriberi). Alcoholics can become thiamine deficient because their diets often do not provide enough thiamine and because alcohol hinders the absorption of what thiamine they have. Chronic diarrhea can also lead to a need for more thiamine.

Thiamine is effective for treating conditions resulting from a thiamine deficiency, as in alcoholism. It has not been proven effective for treating skin problems, persistent diarrhea, fatigue, mental disorders, multiple sclerosis, or ulcerative colitis, or for use as an insect repellant or appetite stimulant.[17]

If you have to increase your intake of thiamine, eat more thiamine-rich foods rather than taking a vitamin supplement. You should take a supplement only when dietary changes are inadequate to treat a deficiency.

If you take thiamine supplements without a doctor's supervision, do not take more than the RDA. Excess thiamine, beyond what is needed each day, simply passes through you and is eliminated in the urine without being used by your body. *Foods high in thiamine (vitamin B₁):* meats (especially pork), organ meats, and nuts (all of which are high in cholesterol and/or fat); dried beans; peas; whole-grain or enriched breads and cereals; enriched or brown rice; enriched pasta, noodles, and other flour products; potatoes. Cooking destroys some thiamine.

1 loin chop	1.18 milligrams
1 ounce wheat germ	0.56 milligrams
3 1/2 ounces roast pork	0.39 milligrams

Before You Use This Drug
Tell your doctor if you have or have had
❑ allergies to drugs
Tell your doctor about any other drugs you take, including aspirin, herbs, vitamins, and other non-prescription products.

When You Use This Drug
◆ Do not drink alcohol. It interferes with your body's absorption of thiamine.

How To Use This Drug
◆ Do not expose to heat, moisture, or strong light. Do not store in the bathroom. Do not let liquid form freeze.
◆ As with all drugs, it is important to take this one regularly. However, because of the length of time required for thiamine deficiency to occur, there is no cause for concern if you miss a dose. Take it when you remember.

Interactions With Other Drugs
Some other drugs that you may be taking (either over-the-counter or prescription drugs) can interact with this one, causing adverse effects. Find out from your doctor

what these drugs are and let him or her know if you are taking any of them.

Adverse Effects

Thiamine and other water-soluble vitamins seldom cause adverse effects in people whose kidneys function normally. If you have decreased kidney function or are taking large doses of thiamine, you should *call your doctor immediately* if you have these side effects:

❑ skin rash or itching
❑ wheezing, an allergic reaction

Limited Use

Vitamin A
ALPHALIN (Lilly) AQUASOL A (Armour)

Generic: available

Family: Nutritional Supplements (see p. 553)

Vitamin A is necessary for growth and bone development, vision, and healthy skin. It is found in many foods (see food sources, below), and a well-balanced diet with a variety of healthful foods should supply all the vitamin A that your body needs. The recommended dietary allowance (RDA) of vitamin A is 1,000 micrograms per day for men and 800 micrograms per day for women.

Vitamin A deficiency is rare, but older adults may develop this deficiency if they have certain intestinal and liver diseases, an overactive thyroid (hyperthyroidism), or diabetes. You may also develop vitamin A deficiency from an inadequate diet or if you take certain drugs such as cholestyramine, colestipol, mineral oil, neomycin, or sucralfate. The liver stores enough vitamin A to last several months, so symptoms of a deficiency may take a few months to develop. The symptoms include night blindness and dry, cracked skin.

If you have to increase your intake of vitamin A to prevent or treat a deficiency, eat more foods that are rich in the vitamin rather than taking a vitamin supplement. You should take a supplement only if your diet does not supply enough vitamin A.

You can get vitamin A from foods in two main forms. Animal sources such as liver, egg yolks, and butter provide a form of vitamin A called retinol. Plant sources such as carrots, squash, and some fruits provide a substance called beta-carotene, which your body converts into vitamin A in the body. Plant sources have several advantages over animal sources, the main one being that they are low in calories, fat, and cholesterol and high in fiber and other nutrients.

Some claim that people who eat large amounts of foods containing beta-carotene have a lower risk of some types of cancer than those who eat less of these foods.[18] Studies are in progress to determine if a beta-carotene supplement will prevent cancer in humans, but current evidence does not support this idea. The evidence does support the recommendation that you should eat foods high in beta-carotene.

If you use vitamin A supplements without a doctor's supervision, do not exceed the RDA. Taking doses only a few times higher than the RDA can be risky. Unlike with some other vitamins, your body cannot eliminate excess vitamin A, so the vitamin can accumulate to dangerous, toxic levels in your body. The toxic effects of too much retinol include liver damage; weakness; increased pressure in the brain; bone and joint pain and damage; and dry, rough skin. The effects from beta-carotene are not as serious.

Foods high in beta-carotene (plant sources): carrots, sweet potatoes, squash, broccoli, tomatoes, green leafy vegetables, cantaloupe, apricots, peaches, margarine.

Foods high in retinol (animal sources): beef liver, butter, egg yolks, fish-liver oils (all four are high in cholesterol and/or fat). Freezing may destroy some vitamin A in both types of food sources.

1 large carrot	11,000 International Units
1 ounce calves' liver	9,340 International Units
1/2 cup cooked spinach	7,300 International Units
2/3 cup cooked broccoli	2,500 International Units
1/4 cup cantaloupe	2,000 International Units
1 cup milk	300–500 International Units

Before You Use This Drug

Tell your doctor if you have or have had
❑ allergies to drugs
❑ diseases of the intestines
❑ diseases of the liver
❑ overactive thyroid
❑ kidney problems

Tell your doctor about any other drugs you take, including aspirin, herbs, vitamins, and other non-prescription products.

How To Use This Drug

◆ Take with food to reduce stomach upset.
◆ Do not crush, break, or chew extended-release capsules or tablets. Swallow whole, or mix capsule contents with jam, applesauce or other foods.
◆ Liquid form can be taken alone or mixed with juice, cereal, or any other food.
◆ Do not expose to heat, moisture, or strong light. Do not store in the bathroom. Do not let liquid form freeze.
◆ As with all drugs, it is important to take this one regularly. However, because of the length of time required for a vitamin A deficiency to occur, there is no cause for concern if you miss a dose. Take it when you remember.

Interactions With Other Drugs

Some other drugs that you may be taking (either over-the-counter or prescription drugs) can interact with this one, causing adverse effects. Find out from your doctor what these drugs are and let him or her know if you are taking any of them.

Adverse Effects

Call your doctor immediately:
❑ pain in your bones or joints
❑ dizziness, weakness
❑ headaches, irritability
❑ dry, rough skin
❑ orange skin, *for beta-carotene*
❑ vomiting, diarrhea
❑ tiredness
❑ loss of appetite
❑ increased sensitivity of skin to sunlight

LIMITED USE

Vitamin B$_{12}$
BETALIN 12 (Lilly) RUBRAMIN PC (Squibb)

Generic: available

Family: Nutritional Supplements (see p. 553)

Vitamin B$_{12}$, also called cyanocobalamin (sye an oh koe *bal* a min), is essential for cell growth and normal formation of blood cells. It is found in several kinds of foods (see food sources, below), and a well-balanced diet with a variety of healthful foods should supply all the vitamin B$_{12}$ that your body needs. The recommended dietary allowance (RDA) of vitamin B$_{12}$ for older adults is 2.0 micrograms per day.

Even if you do not get enough vitamin B$_{12}$ in your diet, a vitamin B$_{12}$ deficiency may take years to develop because the liver stores a vast supply of this vitamin. You may develop a deficiency from certain physical conditions or from an inadequate diet. In adults, a vitamin B$_{12}$ deficiency usually comes from a defect in the digestive tract's absorption of the vitamin, a condition called pernicious anemia. You may also develop a deficiency if you have had parts of your stomach or small intestine removed, which prevents the digestive tract from adequately absorbing the vitamin. In both of these cases, you need vitamin B$_{12}$ injections. Since plants do not contain vitamin B$_{12}$, strict vegetarians who do not eat eggs or milk products also need a vitamin B$_{12}$ supplement, and can take one by mouth.

Vitamin B$_{12}$ deficiency can lead to anemia and to slow, progressive, irreversible damage to the nervous system. This damage will cause loss of feeling in the hands and feet, unsteadiness, loss of memory, confusion, and moodiness. To prevent these changes, people who require life-long treatment with monthly B$_{12}$ injections should be reevaluated at 6 to 12 month intervals by their doctor if they are otherwise well.[19]

If you have to increase your intake of vitamin B$_{12}$ to prevent and treat a deficiency, unless you have one of the conditions that requires B$_{12}$ injections, you should eat more food that is rich in this vitamin rather than taking a vitamin supplement. You should take a supplement only if your diet does not provide an adequate amount.

The claims made for vitamin B$_{12}$ as a remedy for numerous conditions are unfounded. There is no evidence that supplements can provide more pep or counter depression or fatigue in people who do not have a deficiency.

Foods high in vitamin B$_{12}$: tongue, beef, pork, organ meats, eggs, nuts, milk, shellfish, poultry (all may be high in cholesterol and/or fat); fish; cheese; peas; beans; lentils; tofu. Cooking is not likely to destroy vitamin B$_{12}$.

1 ounce beef liver	9–34 micrograms
3 1/2 ounces round roast	4 micrograms
3 1/2 ounces fillet of sole	1.3 micrograms
1 ounce Swiss cheese	0.9 micrograms
1 cup whole milk	0.5 micrograms

Before You Use This Drug
Tell your doctor if you have or have had
❏ allergies to drugs
❏ gout
Tell your doctor about any other drugs you take, including aspirin, herbs, vitamins, and other non-prescription products.

How To Use This Drug

◆ Do not expose to heat, moisture, or strong light. Do not store in the bathroom. Do not let liquid form freeze.

◆ As with all drugs, it is important to take this one regularly. However, because of the length of time required for a vitamin B$_{12}$ deficiency to occur, there is no cause for concern if you miss a dose. Take it when you remember.

Interactions With Other Drugs

Some other drugs that you may be taking (either over-the-counter or prescription drugs) can interact with this one, causing adverse effects. Find out from your doctor what these drugs are and let him or her know if you are taking any of them.

Adverse Effects

Vitamin B$_{12}$ and other water-soluble vitamins seldom cause adverse effects in people whose kidneys function normally. If you have decreased kidney function or are taking large doses of this vitamin, you should *call your doctor immediately* if you have any of these side effects:

❑ skin rash or itching
❑ wheezing
❑ persistent diarrhea

Periodic Tests

Ask your doctor which of these tests should be done periodically while you are taking this drug:

❑ blood levels of folic acid, potassium, and vitamin B$_{12}$
❑ reticulocyte (young red blood cell) count

LIMITED USE

Vitamin C (Ascorbic Acid)
ARCO-CEE (Arco) CEVI-BID (Geriatric)

Generic: available

Family: Nutritional Supplements (see p. 553)

Ascorbic (a *skor* bic) acid, also called vitamin C, helps bind cells together and promotes healing. It is found in certain fruits and vegetables (see food sources, below), and a well-balanced diet with a variety of healthful foods should supply all the vitamin C that you need. The recommended dietary allowance (RDA) for older adults is 60 milligrams per day.

Vitamin C deficiency, known as scurvy, is rare. It is seen occasionally in people whose diet does not supply enough vitamin C — some older adults who live alone, alcoholics, and drug abusers, for example.

Symptoms of scurvy include anemia, loose teeth, red and swollen gums, wounds that do not heal, and small broken blood vessels that cause tiny purplish-red spots in the skin. Scurvy is easily prevented and is treated by increasing the intake of vitamin C through diet and a supplement.

You should take a vitamin C supplement only if your diet does not supply enough to prevent and treat a vitamin C deficiency, or if your body has a special demand for more vitamin C due to surgery, smoking, or an infectious disease, for example. Although doses that far exceed the RDA are touted as remedies for many conditions from the common cold to cancer, research does not support such claims.

If you use a vitamin C supplement without a doctor's supervision, do not take more than the RDA. Higher doses have few beneficial effects except in people with scurvy, and high-dose products are more expensive. Also, taking high doses of vitamin C is risky for people with a history of kidney stones and for people who use anticoagulants (drugs that prevent blood clots from forming in the blood vessels) such as warfarin (Coumadin).[20] If you are taking high doses of vitamin C and want to stop, do not stop suddenly. Reduce your dose gradually because your body needs time to adjust to the reduction.

Foods high in ascorbic acid (vitamin C): citrus fruits and juices (oranges, lemons, limes, grapefruit), tomatoes, strawberries, cantaloupe, cabbage, broccoli, cauliflower, potatoes, and raw peppers. Vitamin C in foods is reduced by drying, salting, and ordinary cooking. Mincing fresh vegetables and mashing potatoes also reduces the vitamin C content.

6 or 7 brussel sprouts	87 milligrams
1 cup cauliflower	62 milligrams
1 medium orange or 1/2 cup orange juice	60 milligrams
1 cup shredded cabbage	47 milligrams
1 slice watermelon	42 milligrams
1/2 grapefruit or 2/3 cup grapefruit juice	40 milligrams
1 medium potato	30 milligrams

Before You Use This Drug

Tell your doctor if you have or had
❑ allergies to drugs
❑ gout
❑ kidney stones
❑ diabetes
❑ sickle cell anemia
❑ glucose-6-phosphate dehydrogenase deficiency

Tell your doctor about any other drugs you take, including aspirin, herbs, vitamins, and other non-prescription products.

How To Use This Drug

◆ Take with food to reduce stomach upset. Swallow with water.
◆ Do not crush, break, or chew extended-release capsules or tablets. Swallow them whole, or mix capsule contents with jam, applesauce or other food.
◆ Liquid form can be taken alone or can be mixed with juice, cereal, or any other food.
◆ Do not expose to heat, moisture, or strong light. Do not store in the bathroom. Do not let liquid form freeze.
◆ As with all drugs, it is important to take this one regularly. However, because of the length of time required for a vitamin C deficiency to occur, there is no cause for concern if you miss a dose. Take it when you remember.

Interactions With Other Drugs

The following drugs are listed in *Evaluations of Drug Interactions,* 1991 as causing "highly clinically significant" or "clinically significant" interactions when used together with this drug. There may be other drugs, especially those in the families of drugs listed below, that also will react with this drug to cause severe adverse effects. Make sure to ask your doctor for a complete listing of them and let her or him know if you are taking this interacting drug:
flecainide; TAMBOCOR.

Adverse Effects

Call your doctor if these symptoms continue: These can occur if you take more than 1 gram (1,000 milligrams) per day.
❑ diarrhea
❑ flushing of skin, warmth
❑ headache
❑ increase in urination
❑ nausea, vomiting
❑ stomach cramps

LIMITED USE

Vitamin D
CALCIFEROL (Kremers-Urban) DELTALIN (Lilly)

Generic: available

Family: Nutritional Supplements (see p. 553)

Vitamin D maintains normal blood levels of calcium and phosphate, both of which are necessary for bone growth and strength. It is available in several foods (see food sources, below), and your body can also manufacture it (in the skin) if you are out in the sun. If you eat a well-balanced diet with a variety of healthful foods and spend some time in the sun, you should have all the vitamin D that your body needs. The recommended dietary allowance (RDA) for men is 400 International Units per day and is 200 for women.

Vitamin D deficiency in older adults prevents your body from absorbing calcium and phosphate normally. This leads to an overall decrease in bone density and weakening of the bones, called osteomalacia. If you have to increase your intake of vitamin D, eat more foods rich in the vitamin rather than taking a vitamin pill. You should take a supplement only if your diet does not supply enough vitamin D to prevent and treat a deficiency or to treat a low blood level of calcium.

If you use vitamin D without a doctor's supervision, do not take more than the RDA. Unlike with some other vitamins, your body cannot eliminate excess vitamin D, so the vitamin can accumulate to dangerous, toxic levels. This is especially risky for people who take the heart medication digoxin (see p. 134), because vitamin D increases the side effects of digoxin. The signs of vitamin D poisoning are listed below. Vitamin D overdose may cause death as a result of heart, blood vessel, or kidney failure.

If your doctor has prescribed vitamin D to prevent low calcium levels, see him or her regularly to check your progress and reduce the risk of side effects. Tell your doctor if you are taking a calcium supplement and discuss how to best increase the amount of calcium in your diet.

Foods high in vitamin D: some fatty fishes and fish-liver oils, eggs, chicken livers, vitamin D-fortified milk (all are high in cholesterol and/or fat); and bread. Vitamin D is not affected by cooking.

1/2 ounce cod liver oil	1,400 International Units
3 1/2 ounces sardines	1,380 International Units
3 1/2 ounces salmon	300 International Units
1 egg yolk	265 International Units
1 cup vitamin D-fortified milk	100 International Units

Before You Use This Drug
Do not use if you have or have had
❏ high level of calcium in your blood
Tell your doctor if you have or have had
❏ allergies to drugs
❏ hardening of the arteries
❏ kidney problems
❏ heart disease
❏ high blood levels of phosphate
❏ sarcoidosis
Tell your doctor about any other drugs you take, including aspirin, herbs, vitamins, and other non-prescription products.

How To Use This Drug
◆ Take with food to reduce stomach upset.
◆ Liquid form or contents of capsules can be taken alone or can be mixed with juice, cereal, or any other food.

♦ Do not expose to heat, moisture, or strong light. Do not store in the bathroom. Do not let liquid form freeze.

♦ As with all drugs, it is important to take this one regularly. However, because of the length of time required for a vitamin D deficiency to occur, there is no cause for concern if a dose is missed. Take it when you remember. **Do not take double doses.**

Interactions With Other Drugs

The following drugs are listed in *Evaluations of Drug Interactions*, 1991 as causing "highly clinically significant" or "clinically significant" interactions when used together with this drug. There may be other drugs, especially those in the families of drugs listed below, that also will react with this drug to cause severe adverse effects. Make sure to ask your doctor for a complete listing of them and let her or him know if you are taking any of these interacting drugs:

ALTERNAGEL; aluminum hydroxide; AMPHOJEL; DILANTIN; phenytoin.

Adverse Effects
Call your doctor immediately:
❑ **early signs of vitamin D toxicity:** constipation or diarrhea; headache; loss of appetite; metallic taste in mouth; nausea or vomiting; dry mouth and increased thirst; tiredness and weakness
❑ **late signs of vitamin D toxicity:** bone pain; cloudy urine; weight loss; convulsions; high blood pressure; eyes easily irritated by light; irregular heartbeat; itching; mood or mental changes; muscle pain; nausea or vomiting; severe stomach or flank pain; increased urination

Periodic Tests
Ask your doctor which of these tests should be done periodically while you are taking this drug:
For high-dose therapy:
❑ kidney function tests
❑ blood calcium level (weekly, when therapy is started)

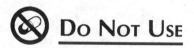 **DO NOT USE**

Alternative treatment: Eat a well-balanced diet with an adequate supply of vitamin E.

Vitamin E

Family: Nutritional Supplements (see p. 553)

Vitamin E is thought to work as an antioxidant, a substance that helps to protect cells from damage. It is found in many foods (see food sources, below), and a well-balanced diet with a variety of healthful foods should supply all the vitamin E that your body needs. The recommended dietary allowance (RDA) of vitamin E is 10 milligrams per day for older men and 8 milligrams per day for older women.

Vitamin E deficiency is rare and has not been known to occur solely from an inadequate diet. It has occurred mainly in people who have certain conditions of their intestines, pancreas, or liver that interfere with their body's ability to absorb the vitamin.

There is no known, proven therapeutic use for vitamin E supplements in older adults. Some have suggested that it may be useful for treating fibrocystic breast disease in women or occasional leg cramps (intermittent claudication), but these uses are unproven. There have been a large number of unsubstantiated claims for vitamin E for a variety of disorders and ailments, from skin problems to schizophrenia, but none of these claims has been validated.

Taking vitamin E in doses that far exceed the RDA can be harmful. Some people who have taken more than 300 milligrams have suffered muscle weakness, fatigue, headaches, nausea, high blood pressure, and increased tendency toward blood clotting.[21] *Foods high in vitamin E:* vegetable oils (corn, cottonseed, soybean, safflower), egg yolk, liver (all of which are high in fat and/or cholesterol); wheat germ and whole-grain cereals. Some vitamin E may be lost in cooking.

1 ounce margarine	15 mgs.
1/2 cup wheat germ	3 mgs.
2 slices whole-wheat bread	2 mgs.

Notes for Nutritional Supplements

1. *The Medical Letter on Drugs and Therapeutics*. New York: The Medical Letter Inc., 1985; 27:66.

2. Schlamowitz P. Treatment of mild to moderate hypertension with dietary fibre. *The Lancet* 1987; 8559:622.

3. Chandra RK. Effect of vitamin and trace-element supplementation on immune responses and infection in elderly subjects. *The Lancet* 1992; 340:1124-7.

4. *The Medical Letter on Drugs and Therapeutics*. New York: The Medical Letter Inc., 1984; 25:73.

5. AMA Department of Drugs. *AMA Drug Evaluations Annual 1992*. Chicago: American Medical Association, 1992:2018-9.

6. Sheikh M. Gastrointestinal absorption of calcium from milk and calcium salts. *New England Journal of Medicine* 1987; 317:532-6.

7. Osteoporosis Part II: Prevention and Treatment. *Public Citizen's Health Research Group Health Letter* 1987; 3(6).

8. Sheikh, op. cit.

9. Osteoporosis Part II, op. cit.

10. AMA Department of Drugs. *AMA Drug Evaluations*. 5th ed. Chicago: American Medical Association, 1983:797.

11. AMA, 1983, op. cit., p. 1144.

12. *The Medical Letter on Drugs and Therapeutics*, 1985, op. cit.

13. Chandra, op. cit.

14. Whelan AM, Price SO, Fowler SF, Hainer BL. The effect of aspirin on niacin-induced cutaneous reactions. *The Journal of Family Practice* 1992; 34:165-8.

15. Hodis HN. Acute hepatic failure associated with the use of low-dose sustained-release niacin. *Journal of the American Medical Association* 1990; 264:181.

16. Henkin Y, Oberman A, Hurst DC, Segrest JP. Niacin revisited: clinical observations on an important but underutilized drug. *American Journal of Medicine* 1991; 91:239-46.

17. *USP DI, Drug Information for the Health Care Professional*. 8th ed. Rockville Md.: The United States Pharmacopeial Convention, Inc., 1988:2077.

18. Colditz GA. Increased green and yellow vegetable intake and lowered cancer deaths in an elderly population. *American Journal of Clinical Nutrition* 1985; 41(32).

19. Gilman AG, Goodman LS, Rall TW, Murad F, eds. *The Pharmacological Basis of Therapeutics*. 7th ed. New York: Macmillan, 1985:1330.

20. Ibid, p. 1570.

21. Roberts H. Perspective on vitamin E as therapy. *Journal of the American Medical Association* 1981; 246:129-30.

Drugs for Eye Diseases

Other Eye Drugs

General Instructions For Application of Eye Drops and Ointment

The normal eye can hold about 10 microliters (10 millionths of a quart) of liquid. A single drop formed by an eye dropper, however, ranges from 25 to 50 microliters. What happens to the excess 15 to 40 microliters when you apply eye drops? Two things occur:

1. Medicine overflows the eyelids and runs down your face, especially if you are upright when applying the drops. This is not a very efficient use of medicine but is relatively harmless.

2. Medicine drains from the eyes into a small opening located at the inside corner of the eye. This small opening is the entrance to a duct (the nasolacrimal duct) through which tears and moisture normally leave the eye and drain into the nose (which is why your nose usually runs when you cry). In the nose, the medicine is absorbed into the blood supply and carried throughout the body, where it can affect the brain, heart, digestive system, lungs and airways, and other areas of the body, causing side effects.

What can be done to maximize drug absorption in the eye and minimize drug absorption through the nasal blood vessels?

1. Do not apply more than one drop of medicine within a 5-minute period, regardless of whether the second drop is the same or a different drug. The eye cannot hold more than one drop at a time, so an extra drop both flushes out the first drop and is diluted by it. It also increases the amount that is absorbed through the nasal blood vessels. Therefore, always wait at least 5 minutes between drops to give adequate time for the drug to be absorbed by the eye.

2. Lie down when applying drops. This helps to prevent "tears" from rolling down your face and through the nasolacrimal duct. As much as 10 times more drug is lost when you are in an upright position than when you are reclining.

3. Using your thumb and middle finger, apply gentle pressure to the inside corner of the eye for 5 minutes after applying each drop, to block the medicine from draining through the nasolacrimal duct.

This technique may be difficult for people who have arthritis, long fingernails, or tremors. An alternative method of decreasing nasolacrimal drainage is to stop "the pump." The nasolacrimal duct relies on the pumping action of the eyelids blinking. If you stop moving your eyelids, you stop the drainage of medicine from the eye. If you squeeze, blink, flutter, etc., the pump is activated. Simple, gentle, relaxed eyelid closure works best to stop the pump.

Either technique, compressing the duct or stopping the pump, if used for 5 minutes, allows enough time for the drug to be absorbed through the eye and decreases side effects.

To avoid contaminating the eye drops, **do not touch the applicator tip to any surface, including the eye.** Store the bottle tightly closed. To ensure sterility, periodically discard used bottles of medicine. Drops can be considered safe for 4 weeks and ointments for 3 months after they have been opened.

To apply drops, first wash your hands. To increase drug absorption, it is best to lie down while applying this medicine. With the middle finger of the hand on the same side as the eye (right eye, right hand, for example), apply pressure to the inside corner of your eye to block the drainage duct. After you have begun to apply pressure with your middle finger, tilt your head back. With the index finger of the same hand, pull the lower eyelid away from the eye to form a pouch. Place a drop of medicine into the pouch, remove the index finger and close your eyes gently, without blinking. Keep your eyes closed and continue to apply pressure for 5 minutes. Do not close your eyes tightly and do not blink.

To apply ointment, first wash your hands. Lie down or tilt your head back. Squeeze about 1/4 to 1/2 inch of ointment inside your lower lid without actually touching the tube to your lid. Close your eye gently and roll your eyeball in all directions while the eye is closed to evenly distribute the medicine. Wait at least 10 minutes before applying other medicines to your eyes. If you need to apply ointment and drops it is best to put in the drops prior to the ointment as the ointment will all but prevent absorption of the drops because of its "Vaseline"-like character.

Glaucoma

Glaucoma is a slowly progressing disorder in which the pressure inside the eye gradually increases. If left untreated, this elevated pressure may lead to nerve damage, decreased vision, and blindness. The higher the pressure inside the eye, the greater the chance of damaging the optic nerve (the nerve to the eye that allows us to see) and losing vision. Most people with glaucoma have no symptoms until extensive, irreversible damage to the optic nerve has occurred, so it is important to have regular eye exams as you grow older. It is also important to take your medicine regularly if you have glaucoma.

To understand what causes glaucoma, it helps to start by discussing how the eye normally works. The eye (shown below as it would appear when cut in half) can be divided into three parts. The vitreous

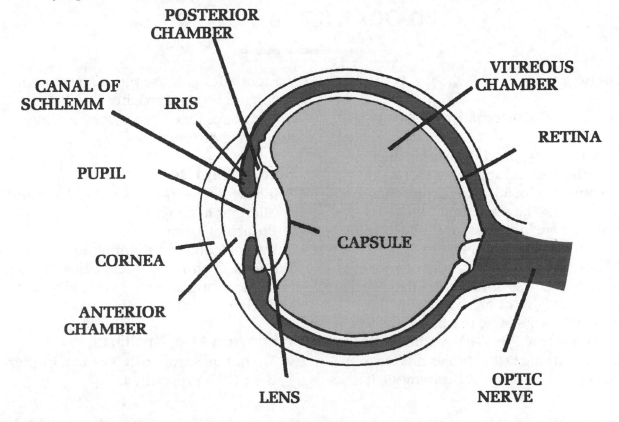

chamber is the large, round area behind the lens. The posterior chamber is the smaller area located behind the iris and in front and to the sides of the lens. The anterior chamber is located in front of the iris. Both the anterior and the posterior chambers are filled with a clear liquid called the aqueous humor. Normally, aqueous humor flows from the posterior chamber through the opening in the iris to the anterior chamber. It leaves the eye through a small opening, called the canal of Schlemm, at the outermost edges of the iris. In glaucoma, less aqueous humor drains from the eye, raising the pressure inside the eye. The disorder is similar to blowing up a balloon: If there is no opening for the air to flow out, the pressure in the balloon steadily increases as the balloon fills with air.

Elevated pressure inside the eye can be treated in two ways:
❏ Increasing the amount of aqueous hu-mor that leaves the eye through the canal of Schlemm or
❏ Decreasing the amount of aqueous humor that is produced.

Drugs such as dipivefrin (Propine), pilocarpine, and physostigmine increase aqueous humor outflow from the anterior chamber, whereas acetazolamide (Diamox) and timolol (Timoptic) decrease aqueous humor production. In either case, the total amount of aqueous humor is reduced and the pressure decreased. Timolol is often used for mild glaucoma, except for older adults who have congestive heart failure, abnormal heart rhythms, asthma, or emphysema. In these patients, pilocarpine is an alternative choice. A combination of drugs may be necessary for more severe forms. Surgery is reserved for those people who continue to have optic nerve destruction and visual loss, in spite of multiple drug therapy.

Pilocarpine
ADSORBOCARPINE, ISOPTO CARPINE (Alcon)
PILOCAR (CooperVision)

Generic: available

Family: Antiglaucoma Drugs (see p. 583)

Pilocarpine (pye loe *kar* peen) is the first-choice drug for treating most forms of glaucoma (see p. 583). Glaucoma is a condition in which the pressure of the fluid inside the eye increases, and pilocarpine lowers the increased pressure.

Pilocarpine makes the pupils of your eyes smaller and affects how quickly they react to light by enlarging or narrowing. Smaller pupils and their slower reaction allow less light to enter the eyes. This can hinder you from performing tasks such as driving at night. Be careful when performing such tasks.

Right after you use pilocarpine, your vision may be blurred, but it will clear. You might notice this more when viewing things at a distance.

Before You Use This Drug
Tell your doctor if you have or have had
❏ allergies to drugs
❏ bronchial asthma
❏ eye infection or inflammation
Tell your doctor about any other drugs you take, including aspirin, herbs, vitamins, and other non-prescription products.

When You Use This Drug
◆ **Do not use more often or in a higher dose than prescribed.**

How To Use This Drug

◆ Directions for applying drops appear on p. 582. If you use an eye system form, follow directions that accompany it. Do not use if system is damaged or if too much medication is being released.

◆ Store gel and eye system forms in refrigerator. Do not store in the bathroom. Do not expose to heat, moisture, or strong light. Do not allow this drug to freeze.

◆ If you miss a dose, apply it as soon as you remember, but skip it if it is almost time for the next dose. **Do not take double doses.**

Interactions With Other Drugs

Some other drugs that you may be taking (either over-the-counter or prescription drugs) can interact with this one, causing adverse effects. Find out from your doctor what these drugs are and let him or her know if you are taking any of them.

Adverse Effects

Call your doctor immediately:
❏ muscle twitches or tremors
❏ nausea, vomiting, or diarrhea
❏ troubled breathing or wheezing
❏ increased sweating
❏ watering of mouth

Call your doctor if these symptoms continue:
❏ blurred vision
❏ eye pain
❏ brow ache
❏ headache
❏ irritation of eyes

Periodic Tests

Ask your doctor which of these tests should be done periodically while you are taking this drug:
❏ eye pressure tests at regular intervals

Cyclopentolate
AK-PENTOLATE (Akorn) CYCLOGYL (Alcon)

Generic: available

Family: Eye Drugs

Cyclopentolate (sye kloe *pen* toe late) is most commonly used to enlarge (dilate) the pupils of the eyes during an eye exam. It is also used to dilate the pupils before or after certain types of eye surgery, and to treat inflammation of the inner eye.

At first, cyclopentolate may cause a stinging sensation, blurred vision, and increased sensitivity to light. Check with your doctor if any of these effects lasts longer than 36 hours after the drug is applied.

Before You Use This Drug

Tell your doctor if you have or have had
❏ allergies to drugs
❏ glaucoma

Tell your doctor about any other drugs you take, including aspirin, herbs, vitamins, and other non-prescription products.

When You Use This Drug

◆ **Do not use more often or in a higher dose than prescribed.**

◆ Do not store in the bathroom. Do not expose to heat, moisture, or strong light. Do not allow to freeze.

◆ If you miss a dose, apply it as soon as you remember, but skip it if it is almost time for the next dose. **Do not take double doses.**

How To Use This Drug

◆ Directions for applying drops appear on p. 582.

Interactions With Other Drugs

Some other drugs that you may be taking

(either over-the-counter or prescription drugs) can interact with this one, causing adverse effects. Find out from your doctor what these drugs are and let him or her know if you are taking any of them.

Adverse Effects
Call your doctor immediately:
❑ clumsiness or unsteadiness
❑ confusion or unusual behavior
❑ flushed or red face
❑ hallucinations

❑ increased thirst, dry mouth
❑ skin rash
❑ slurred speech
❑ fast heartbeat
❑ drowsiness, tiredness, weakness
Call your doctor if these symptoms continue:
❑ blurred vision
❑ increased sensitivity to light
❑ stinging sensation in eyes
❑ headache
❑ irritation of eyes

Levobunolol
BETAGAN (Allergan)

Generic: not available

Family: Antiglaucoma Drugs (see p. 583)
Beta-blockers (see p. 68)

Levobunolol (levo *bewn* o lol) is available as an eye drop, specifically for treating glaucoma. It is well tolerated by most people, especially those who have cataracts or who have problems using another antiglaucoma drug called pilocarpine (see p. 584). Although levobunolol is an eye drop, some of it can be absorbed from the eyes into the bloodstream and the rest of the body, and if this happens you may experience some of the general side effects listed under Adverse Effects. (See p. 582 for directions on how to apply eye drops.)

Levobunolol belongs to the beta-blocker family of drugs and thus is similar in safety and efficacy to timolol (see p. 602).[1,2] Once in the eye, it takes levobunolol about an hour to begin working. If you use levobunolol in only one eye, it may also affect the other eye. Older people are especially sensitive to the harmful effects of levobunolol. Reduced kidney and liver function in the elderly may increase risk of adverse effects.

When used for a long time, the initial improvement sometimes goes away. As with other beta-blockers, long-term use can cause serious heart problems, even in people who did not previously have heart disease. Levobunolol, similarly to timolol, can decrease lung function by 30%, an adverse effect not seen in betaxolol, another beta-blocker.[3] Very rarely, serious harm, even fatalities have occurred, mostly to those with asthma or heart problems.[4] But according to *The Medical Letter*, betaxolol may be less likely than timolol or levobunolol to have adverse side effects on patients with asthma.[5]

At times levobunolol is used along with other medications for glaucoma, such as pilocarpine, dipivefrin, or acetazolamide. Use with epinephrine is controversial.

Before You Use This Drug
Levobunolol can be life-threatening to certain individuals.
Do not use if you have or have had
❑ asthma
❑ congestive heart failure, slow heartbeat or heart block
❑ severe lung disease
Tell your doctor if you have or have had
❑ allergies to drugs

❑ depression
❑ diabetes
❑ emphysema or chronic bronchitis
❑ heart problems
❑ myasthenia gravis
❑ smoked
❑ thyroid problems

Tell your doctor about any other drugs you take, including aspirin, herbs, vitamins, and other non-prescription products.

When You Use This Drug

◆ Restrict your use of caffeine, since it may add to the effect of levobunolol on the heart.[6]

◆ **Caution diabetics:** be aware that levobunolol may mask trembling and pulse rate used to signal low blood sugar.[7]

◆ If you plan to have any surgery, including dental, tell your doctor that you take this drug. Some surgeons prefer to withdraw beta-blockers before surgery.

◆ Be cautious driving until the effect of the drug is complete (about two weeks),[8] and no blurred vision occurs.

◆ **Do not take other drugs without talking to your doctor first — especially non-prescription drugs for appetite control, asthma, colds, coughs, hay fever, or sinus problems.**

Cold Stress Alert

If levobunolol eye drops are absorbed into the body, older people have an increased risk of hypothermia.[9] Early signs are shivering, cold hands and feet, and memory lapse. Stay indoors, especially when it is cold and windy. Keep warm with extra clothes and blankets. If you must go outdoors, dress to protect yourself from the wind and cold. Avoid getting wet. Take along something to eat suitable to your diet such as trail mix.

How To Use This Drug

◆ If you use the compliance cap, whenever you start a new bottle click it until the number corresponding to the day of the week appears.

◆ After opening the cap, do not touch tip of applicator.

◆ Instill only one drop at a time, since the eye sac can only hold that amount (see p. 582 for directions on how to apply eye drops).

◆ Replace the cap. Hold the compliance cap between your thumb and forefinger, then rotate until it clicks.

◆ *If you miss a dose, use the following guidelines:*
  - If you are using levobunolol only once a day, apply the missed dose as soon as you remember, but skip it if you don't remember until the next day.
  - If you are using levobunolol more than once a day, apply the missed dose as soon as you remember, but skip it if it is almost time for the next dose.
  - **Do not apply double doses.**

◆ Flush your eye with water if you accidentally put too many drops in an eye.

◆ Store at room temperature. Avoid high temperatures and freezing. Leave in original container, which protects it from light.

Interactions With Other Drugs

The following drugs are listed in *Evaluations of Drug Interactions,* 1991 as causing "highly clinically significant" or "clinically significant" interactions when used together with this drug. There may be other drugs, especially those in the families of drugs listed below, that also will react with this drug to cause severe adverse effects. Make sure to ask your doctor for a complete listing of them and let her or him know if you are taking any of these interacting drugs:

ADRENALIN (also in bee sting kits); ALDOMET; amiodarone; CALAN; CATAPRES; chlorpromazine; cimetidine; clonidine; cocaine; CORDARONE; DELTASONE; ELIXOPHYLLIN; epinephrine; ESKALITH; FLUOTHANE;

furosemide; HABITROL; halothane; HUMULIN; INDOCIN; indomethacin; insulin ; ISOPTIN; l-thyroxine; LASIX; lidocaine; lithium; LITHOBID; methyldopa; MINIPRESS; NEMBUTAL; nicotine; pentobarbital; prazosin; prednisone; RIFADIN; rifampin; SYNTHROID; TAGAMET; THEO-DUR; theophylline; THORAZINE; thyroid; tobacco (inform your doctor if your smoking habits change while using levobunolol); TUBARINE; tubocurarine; verapamil; XYLOCAINE.

Adverse Effects

Levobunolol can be absorbed into the body through the eye. All adverse effects for oral beta-blockers are possible with levobunolol eyedrops.
Call your doctor immediately:
❑ hives, itching, or skin rash
❑ severe irritation or inflammation of the eye or eyelid
❑ vision change
❑ breathing difficulty, wheezing
❑ chest pain

❑ confusion or mental depression
❑ dizziness, or fainting
❑ headache
❑ slow heartbeat
❑ nausea or vomiting
❑ swelling of ankles, feet or legs
❑ unsteadiness, clumsiness
❑ unusual tiredness or weakness
Call your doctor if these symptoms continue:
❑ burning or stinging of the eye
❑ cold hands and feet
❑ inflammation of eye or eyelids
❑ low blood pressure
Adverse effects to levobunolol can occur even a week after you stop using the drug. *More side effects information appears on p. 68.*

Periodic Tests
Ask your doctor which of these tests should be done periodically while you are taking this drug:
❑ blood pressure and pulse rate
❑ heart function tests, such as electrocardiogram (EKG)
❑ blood glucose levels (for diabetics)
❑ eye pressure exams

Betaxolol (Eye Drops)
BETOPTIC (Alcon)
BETOPTIC S (Alcon)

Generic: not available

Family: Antiglaucoma Drugs (see p. 583)
Beta-blockers (see p. 68)

Betaxolol (bait *ax* o loll) has two dosage forms for different uses: Kerlone tablets for the heart and Betoptic drops for the eyes, specifically for treating glaucoma. This page discusses betaxolol's use as an antiglaucoma drug.

Betaxolol drops are well tolerated by most people, especially those who have cataracts or who have problems using another antiglaucoma drug called pilocarpine (see p. 584). Although betaxolol is an eye drop, some of it can be absorbed from the eyes into the bloodstream and the rest of the body, and if this happens you may experience some of the general side effects listed under Adverse Effects. (See p. 582 for directions on how to apply eye drops.)

When used for a long time, the initial improvement may diminish. As with other beta-blockers, long-term use can cause serious heart problems, even in people who did not previously have heart disease. Two other beta-blockers, levobunolol and timolol, can decrease lung function by 30%, an adverse effect not seen as much in betaxolol.[10] Very rarely, serious harm, even fatalities have occurred, mostly to those with asthma or heart problems.[11] But according to *The Medical Letter*, betaxolol may be less likely than timolol or levobunolol to have adverse side effects on patients with asthma.[12] Older people are especially sensitive to the harmful effects of betaxolol.

At times betaxolol is used along with other eye drugs, such as pilocarpine. As the effect of betaxolol may diminish over time, it is sometimes necessary to supplement its use with other antiglaucoma medication.

Before You Use This Drug

Do not use if you have or have had

❑ congestive heart failure, slow heartbeat or heart block

Tell your doctor if you have or have had

❑ allergies to drugs
❑ asthma
❑ depression
❑ diabetes
❑ emphysema or chronic bronchitis
❑ heart problems
❑ myasthenia gravis
❑ smoked
❑ thyroid problems

Cold Stress Alert

If betaxolol eye drops are absorbed into the body, older people have an increased risk of hypothermia.[16] Early signs are shivering, cold hands and feet, and memory lapse. Stay indoors, especially when it is cold and windy. Keep warm with extra clothes and blankets. If you must go outdoors, dress to protect yourself from the wind and cold. Avoid getting wet. Take along something to eat, suitable to your diet, such as trail mix.

Tell your doctor about any other drugs you take, including aspirin, herbs, vitamins, and other non-prescription products.

When You Use This Drug

◆ Restrict your use of caffeine, since it may add to the effect of betaxolol on the heart.[13]
◆ **Caution diabetics:** be aware that betaxolol may mask trembling and pulse rate used to signal low blood sugar.[14]
◆ If you plan to have any surgery, including dental, tell your doctor that you take this drug.
◆ Be cautious driving until the effect of the drug is complete (about two weeks),[15] and no blurred vision occurs.
◆ **Do not take other drugs without talking to your doctor first — especially non-prescription drugs for appetite control, asthma, colds, coughs, hay fever, or sinus problems.**
◆ Do not expose to heat or direct light.

How To Use This Drug

◆ See general instructions for application of eye drops on page 582.
◆ If you use the suspension form, shake it well first.
◆ Wash your hands.
◆ After opening, avoid touching the tip against your eye or anything else.
◆ *If you miss a dose, use the following guidelines:*
  - If you are using betaxolol only once a day, apply the missed dose as soon as you remember, but skip it if you don't remember until the next day.
  - If you are using betaxolol more than once a day, apply the missed dose as soon as you remember, but skip it if it is almost time for the next dose.
  - **Do not apply double doses.**
◆ Store at room temperature. Protect from freezing.

Interactions With Other Drugs

The following drugs are listed in *Evaluations of Drug Interactions*, 1991 as causing "highly clinically significant" or "clinically significant" interactions when used together with this drug. There may be other drugs, especially those in the families of drugs listed below, that also will react with this drug to cause severe adverse effects. Make sure to ask your doctor for a complete listing of them and let her or him know if you are taking any of these interacting drugs:

ADRENALIN (also in bee sting kits); ALDOMET; CALAN; CATAPRES; chlorpromazine; cimetidine; clonidine; cocaine; DELTASONE; ELIXOPHYLLIN; epinephrine; ESKALITH; FLUOTHANE; furosemide; HABITROL; halothane; HUMULIN; INDOCIN; indomethacin; insulin; ISOPTIN; l-thyroxine; LASIX; lidocaine; lithium; LITHOBID; methyldopa; MINIPRESS; NEMBUTAL; nicotine; pentobarbital; prazosin; prednisone; RIFADIN; rifampin; SYNTHROID; TAGAMET; THEO-DUR; theophylline; THORAZINE; thyroid; tobacco (inform your doctor if your smoking habits change while using betaxolol); TUBARINE; tubocurarine; verapamil; XYLOCAINE.

Adverse Effects

Betaxolol can be absorbed into the body through the eye. All adverse effects for oral beta-blockers are possible with betaxolol eyedrops.

Call your doctor immediately:
❑ difficulty breathing
❑ chills, cold hands or feet
❑ confusion
❑ dizziness
❑ headache
❑ slow heartbeat
❑ hives
❑ eye irritation or visual changes
❑ difficulty swallowing, or painful tongue
❑ unusual tiredness or weakness
Call your doctor if these symptoms continue:
❑ disturbed sleep, nightmares
❑ hallucinations[17]
❑ crusting of eyelashes
❑ depression
❑ diarrhea
❑ eye stinging or irritation when medicine is applied
❑ redness, itching or watering of eye
More side effects information appears on p. 68.

Periodic Tests

Ask your doctor which of these tests should be done periodically while you are taking this drug:
❑ blood pressure and pulse rate
❑ heart function tests, such as electrocardiogram (EKG)
❑ blood glucose levels (for diabetics)
❑ eye pressure exams

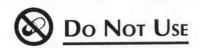 **Do Not Use**

Alternative treatment: An antibiotic alone, if necessary.

Sulfacetamide and Prednisolone (combined)
BLEPHAMIDE (Allergan)
VASOCIDIN (CooperVision)

Family: Antibiotics (see p. 444)
Corticosteroids (see p. 609)

These are eye drops that contain two drugs, sulfacetamide (see p. 600) and prednisolone (see p. 645). The drops are used to treat some eye and eyelid infections caused by bacteria or allergies. **There is no persuasive proof that they are beneficial for this purpose.**

This combination is like several others that contain a drug from the corticosteroid family (in this case prednisolone) and one from the antibiotic family (in this case sulfacetamide). In general, combinations like this are not recommended for treating eye infections externally.[18] Corticosteroids like prednisolone may actually be dangerous because they can hide the signs of an infection or make it spread. Antibiotics such as sulfacetamide may be needed if your eye problem is being caused by a bacterial infection, but otherwise they are unnecessary.

Acetazolamide
DIAMOX (Lederle)

Generic: available

Family: Antiglaucoma Drugs (see p. 583)

Acetazolamide (a set a *zole* a mide) is most commonly used to treat glaucoma (see p. 583). It is also used to treat altitude sickness and to supplement other drugs used for seizure disorders such as epilepsy. In the past, acetazolamide was used as a diuretic (water pill) to treat high blood pressure, but it is outdated for this use because more effective drugs are now available.[19,20]

Acetazolamide beongs to the same family of drugs as methazolamide (Neptazane). These drugs are cousins of sulfa drugs and thiazide diuretics, having the potential for the same adverse effects, but no action against bacteria. This family of drugs may cause kidney stones, gouty arthritis, and depress your bone marrow. Older people with decreased kidney function need to be cautious when taking these drugs. Many individuals cannot tolerate the adverse effects of this family of drugs for a prolonged time.[21]

Do not change brands or manufacturers of acetazolamide. The amount of the drug varies among products, which means that you could receive too much or too little of the drug if you switch brands.

Acetazolamide has caused a few cases of hives, fever, blood cell disorders, and kidney problems.[22] Stop taking the drug and call your doctor if you have any of these reactions.

This drug may also reduce the amount of potassium in your body. To compensate for this loss, eat foods high in potassium (see p. 66).

Before You Use This Drug

Tell your doctor if you have or have had
- ❑ allergies to drugs
- ❑ adrenal gland disease
- ❑ diabetes
- ❑ gout
- ❑ low blood levels of sodium or potassium
- ❑ kidney disease or kidney stones
- ❑ liver disease
- ❑ lung disease

Tell your doctor about any other drugs you take, including aspirin, herbs, vitamins, and other non-prescription products.

When You Use This Drug

- ◆ **Do not use more often or in a higher dose than prescribed. Do not stop taking this drug suddenly. Your doctor must lower your dose gradually.**
- ◆ Until you know how you react to this drug, do not drive or perform other activities requiring alertness. This drug may cause drowsiness, dizziness, lightheadedness, and tiredness.
- ◆ To help prevent kidney stones, drink **at least 6 to 8 glasses (8 ounces each) of fluids each day.**
- ◆ Schedule regular appointments with your doctor to check your progress.
- ◆ **Caution diabetics**: This drug may elevate blood and urine sugar levels.

How To Use This Drug

- ◆ Take with food to decrease stomach upset.
- ◆ Do not store in the bathroom. Do not expose to heat, moisture, or strong light. Do not allow to freeze.
- ◆ If you miss a dose, take it as soon as you remember, but skip it if it is almost time for the next dose. **Do not take double doses.**

Interactions With Other Drugs

The following drugs are listed in *Evaluations of Drug Interactions*, 1991 as causing "highly clinically significant" or "clinically significant" interactions when used together with this drug. There may be other drugs, especially those in the families of drugs listed below, that also will react with this drug to cause severe adverse effects. Make sure to ask your doctor for a complete listing of them and let her or him know if you are taking any of these interacting drugs:

aspirin; cyclosporine; ECOTRIN; ESKALITH; lithium carbonate; LITHOBID; LITHONATE; SANDIMMUNE.

Adverse Effects

Call your doctor immediately:
- ❑ blood in urine, trouble urinating, pain in lower back, pain or burning during urination, or sudden decrease in amount of urine
- ❑ bloody or black, tarry stools
- ❑ clumsiness, unsteadiness
- ❑ convulsions
- ❑ dark urine, pale stools, or yellow eyes and skin
- ❑ dry mouth or increased thirst
- ❑ irregular heartbeat or weak pulse
- ❑ mood or mental changes
- ❑ muscle cramps or pain
- ❑ nausea or vomiting
- ❑ unusual tiredness or weakness
- ❑ fever and sore throat
- ❑ unusual bruising or bleeding
- ❑ fever, hives, itching, or rash
- ❑ mental confusion or depression
- ❑ trouble breathing or shortness of breath
- ❑ ringing or buzzing in ears

Call your doctor if these symptoms continue:
- ❑ diarrhea
- ❑ drowsiness
- ❑ general feeling of discomfort or illness
- ❑ increased frequency of urination
- ❑ loss of appetite, weight loss
- ❑ metallic taste in mouth
- ❑ numbness, tingling, or burning sensation in hands, fingers, feet, toes, mouth, tongue, lips, or rectum

Periodic Tests

Ask your doctor which of these tests should be done periodically while you are taking this drug:
❑ complete blood counts

❑ blood electrolyte (sodium, potassium) tests
❑ tests of kidney function and kidney stone formation

Fluorometholone
FML (Allergan)

Generic: available

Family: Corticosteroids (see p. 609)
Eye Drugs

Fluorometholone (flure oh *meth* oh lone) is a steroid used to treat eye conditions that produce inflammation (swelling and redness), itching, or sensitivity. As with all drugs, you should always use the smallest dose of fluorometholone that works. You should also use it for as short a time as possible. **Check with your doctor if you do not notice improvement after 5 to 7 days of taking the drug, or if your eye condition worsens.**

Corticosteroids (steroids) such as fluorometholone can cause *many* side effects, especially if you use them for a long time so that your entire body absorbs them. Steroids suppress your immune system, lowering your body's defense against disease. Because of this, if you use fluorometholone for a long time, you will be more likely to develop bacterial, fungal, parasitic, and viral infections.

Before You Use This Drug

Do not use if you have or have had
❑ eye infections, such as herpes, tuberculosis, or others caused by a fungus or virus
Tell your doctor if you have or have had
❑ allergies to drugs
❑ glaucoma
❑ cataracts
❑ middle ear infection
❑ other eye or ear infections
Tell your doctor about any other drugs you take, including aspirin, herbs, vitamins, and other non-prescription products.

When You Use This Drug
◆ **Do not use more often or in a higher dose than prescribed.**

How To Use This Drug
◆ If you miss a dose, take it as soon as you remember, but skip it if it is almost time for the next dose. **Do not take double doses.**

Interactions With Other Drugs

Some other drugs that you may be taking (either over-the-counter or prescription drugs) can interact with this one, causing adverse effects. Find out from your doctor what these drugs are and let him or her know if you are taking any of them.

Adverse Effects

Call your doctor immediately:
❑ blurred vision
❑ eye pain
❑ headache
❑ seeing halos around lights
❑ drooping eyelids
❑ unusually large pupils
Call your doctor if these symptoms continue:
❑ burning, stinging, watering of the eyes

Periodic Tests

Ask your doctor which of these tests should be done periodically while you are taking this drug:
❑ eye exams

LIMITED USE

Gentamicin
GARAMYCIN (Schering)
Tobramycin
TOBREX (Alcon)

Generic: available for gentamicin

Family: Antibiotics (see p. 444)
Aminoglycosides

Gentamicin (jen ta *mye* sin) and tobramycin (toe bra *mye* sin) are used in ointment, cream or liquid form to treat eye, ear, and skin infections. **Drugs in this family (aminoglycosides) are also given intravenously in the hospital to treat serious infections, but the information on this page does *not* apply to this use.**

Gentamicin is sometimes used on the skin to treat severe burns that are infected. This is not a recommended use. If you use gentamicin this way, you may develop bacteria that are resistant to the drug, and the injected form of gentamicin might then be ineffective if you ever received it.[23]

Before You Use This Drug
Tell your doctor if you have or have had
❑ allergies to drugs
❑ an unusual reaction to any aminoglycoside (neomycin, for example)
❑ punctured eardrum or other ear problems, *if you are using the ear dosage form*
Tell your doctor about any other drugs you take, including aspirin, herbs, vitamins, and other non-prescription products.

When You Use This Drug
◆ Your eyes may sting or burn just after using. Call your doctor if this problem does not go away in a few days.
◆ Call your doctor if your skin infection does not improve in a week or if it gets worse.

◆ Use all the gentamicin or tobramycin your doctor prescribed, even if you feel better before you finish. If you stop too soon, your symptoms could come back.

How To Use This Drug
◆ *For eye infections:* Follow the instructions on p. 582 for applying eye drops and ointment correctly, so that you won't absorb the drug into your body and possibly suffer serious side effects.
◆ *For skin infections:* Wash affected area with soap and water and dry completely, then apply a small amount of the medication to the skin.
◆ Do not store in the bathroom. Do not expose to heat, moisture, or strong light. Do not let liquid form freeze.
◆ If you miss an application, apply it as soon as you remember, but skip it if it is almost time for the next application. **Do not take double doses.**

Interactions With Other Drugs
The following drugs are listed in *Evaluations of Drug Interactions*, 1991 as causing "highly clinically significant" or "clinically significant" interactions when used together with this drug. There may be other drugs, especially those in the families of drugs listed below, that also will react with this drug to cause severe adverse effects. Make sure to ask your doctor for a complete listing of them and let her or him know if you are taking any of these interacting drugs:
AEROSPORIN; carbenicillin; cephalothin; ether; GEOCILLIN; INDOCIN; indomethacin; KEFLIN; polymyxin B; tubocurarine.

Adverse Effects
Call your doctor immediately:
❑ itching, redness, swelling, or other irritation that has appeared since you started using the drug for a skin infection

---

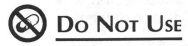 **DO NOT USE**

Alternative treatment: An antibiotic alone, if necessary.

Neomycin, Polymyxin B, and Dexamethasone (combined)
MAXITROL (Burroughs Wellcome)

Family: Antibiotics (see p. 444)
Corticosteroids (see p. 609)

These are eye drops that contain three drugs, neomycin (nee oh *mye* sin), polymyxin (pol i *mix* in) B, and dexamethasone (see p. 620). The drops are used to treat some eye and eyelid infections caused by bacteria and allergies. **There is no persuasive proof that they are beneficial for this purpose.**

One of the drugs in this combination, dexamethasone, belongs to a family called corticosteroids. Drugs in this family are not generally recommended for treating infections because they can hide the signs of an infection or make it spread. The other drugs in this combination, neomycin and polymyxin B, are antibiotics. If your eye problem is caused by a bacterial infection, an antibiotic might be needed. Otherwise, antibiotics are unnecessary and should not be used.[24]

Neomycin commonly causes skin rashes in 8% of the people who use it.[25] Using neomycin can also make it hard for you to use other drugs in its family (aminoglycoside antibiotics, such as gentamicin and tobramycin, see p. 594) that may be needed later in life for serious infections.

Tropicamide
MYDRIACYL (Alcon)

Generic: available

Family: Eye Drugs

Tropicamide (troe *pik* a mide) is most commonly used to enlarge (dilate) the pupils of the eyes during an eye exam. It is also used to dilate the pupils before or after certain types of eye surgery.

At first this drug may

> ***Warning: Special Mental and Physical Adverse Effects***
> Older adults are especially sensitive to the harmful anticholinergic effects of eye drugs such as tropicamide. Drugs in this family should not be used unless absolutely necessary.
> *Mental Effects:* confusion, delirium, short-term memory problems, disorientation, and impaired attention.
> *Physical Effects:* dry mouth, constipation, difficulty urinating (especially for a man with an enlarged prostate), blurred vision, decreased sweating with increased body temperature, sexual dysfunction, and worsening of glaucoma.

cause a stinging sensation, blurred vision, and increased sensitivity to light. Check with your doctor if any of these effects lasts longer than 24 hours after you apply the drug.

Before You Use This Drug
Tell your doctor if you have or have had
- ❑ allergies to drugs
- ❑ glaucoma

Tell your doctor about any other drugs you take, including aspirin, herbs, vitamins, and other non-prescription products.

When You Use This Drug
- ◆ **Do not use more often or in a higher dose than prescribed.**

How To Use This Drug
- ◆ Directions for applying eye drops appear on p. 582.
- ◆ Do not store in the bathroom. Do not expose to heat, moisture, or strong light. Do not allow to freeze.
- ◆ If you miss a dose, apply it as soon as you remember, but skip it if it is almost time for the next dose. **Do not apply double doses.**

Interactions With Other Drugs
Some other drugs that you may be taking (either over-the-counter or prescription drugs) can interact with this one, causing adverse effects. Find out from your doctor what these drugs are and let him or her know if you are taking any of them.

Adverse Effects
Call your doctor immediately:
- ❑ clumsiness or unsteadiness
- ❑ confusion or unusual behavior
- ❑ flushing or redness of face
- ❑ hallucinations
- ❑ increased thirst, dry mouth
- ❑ skin rash
- ❑ slurred speech
- ❑ fast heartbeat
- ❑ drowsiness, tiredness, weakness

Call your doctor if these symptoms continue:
- ❑ blurred vision
- ❑ increased sensitivity to light
- ❑ stinging sensation in eyes
- ❑ headache
- ❑ irritation of eyes

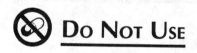 **DO NOT USE**

Alternative treatment: An antibiotic alone, if necessary.

Neomycin and Dexamethasone (combined) NEODECADRON (Merck)

Family: Antibiotics (see p. 444)
Corticosteroids (see p. 609)

These are eye drops that contain two drugs, neomycin (nee oh *mye* sin) and dexamethasone (see p. 620). The drops are used to treat some eye and eyelid infections caused by bacteria and allergies. **There is no persuasive proof that they are beneficial for this purpose.**

One of the drugs in this combination, dexamethasone, belongs to a family called corticosteroids. Drugs in this family are not recommended for treating infections because they can hide the signs of an infection or make it spread. The other drug in this combination, neomycin, is an antibiotic. If your eye problem is being caused by a bacterial infection, an antibiotic may be needed. Otherwise, antibiotics are unnecessary and should not be used.[26]

Neomycin commonly causes skin rashes in 8% of the people who use it.[27] Using neomycin can also make it hard for you to use other drugs in its family (aminoglycoside antibiotics such as gentamicin and tobramycin, see p. 594) that may be needed later in life for serious infections.

Methazolamide
NEPTAZANE (Lederle)

Generic: not available

Family: Antiglaucoma Drugs (see p. 583)

Methazolamide (meth a *zoll* am ide) is an oral drug used to treat glaucoma. It lowers pressure in the eyes, and improves vision. Methazolamide is used long-term for open-angle glaucoma. It may be used temporarily before surgery for angle-closure (narrow angle) glaucoma. Studies of methazolamide to control essential tremor are not yet conclusive.[28]

Methazolamide beongs to the same family of drugs as acetazolamide (Diamox). These drugs are cousins of sulfa drugs and thiazide diuretics, having the potential for the same adverse effects, but no action against bacteria. This family of drugs may cause kidney stones, gouty arthritis, and depress your bone marrow. Older people with decreased kidney function need to be cautious when taking these drugs. Many individuals cannot tolerate the adverse effects of this family of drugs for a prolonged time.[29]

Methazolamide can upset the gastrointestinal tract, and severely deplete your calcium, potassium and other minerals. Unfortunately, stopping methazolamide does not always reverse the damage to bone marrow.[30] Anyone whose liver is impaired risks going into a coma while taking methazolamide.

Before You Use This Drug
Do not use if you have or have had

❑ allergies to acetazolamide, sulfas, or thiazide diuretics
❑ acidosis, hyperchloremic type
❑ adrenal gland failure
❑ kidney or liver disease
❑ very low potassium or sodium levels
Tell your doctor if you have or have had
❑ allergies to drugs
❑ adrenal gland problems (Addison's disease)
❑ breathing or lung problems, including emphysema
❑ diabetes[31]
❑ gout
❑ heart problems
❑ kidney problems, including kidney stones
❑ liver problems, including cirrhosis
❑ mineral imbalance
❑ osteoporosis
Tell your doctor about any other drugs you take, including aspirin, herbs, vitamins, and other non-prescription products.

When You Use This Drug
◆ Until you know how you react to this drug, do not drive or perform other activities requiring alertness. This drug may cause drowsiness, dizziness, lightheadedness, and tiredness.
◆ To help prevent kidney stones, drink **at least 6 to 8 glasses (8 ounces each) of fluids each day.**
◆ Eat foods rich in potassium to compensate for loss of potassium (see p. 66).
◆ Inform your dentist that you take methazolamide.

How To Use This Drug

◆ Swallow tablet whole or break in half. You may take methazolamide with food to decrease stomach upset.

◆ Do not store in the bathroom. Do not expose to heat, moisture, or strong light.

◆ If you miss a dose, take it as soon as you remember but skip it if it is almost time for the next dose. **Do not take double doses.**

Interactions With Other Drugs

The following drugs are listed in *Evaluations of Drug Interactions*, 1991 as causing "highly clinically significant" or "clinically significant" interactions when used together with this drug. There may be other drugs, especially those in the families of drugs listed below, that also will react with this drug to cause severe adverse effects. Make sure to ask your doctor for a complete listing of them and let her or him know if you are taking any of these interacting drugs:

ASA; aspirin, especially in large doses; cyclosporine; ECOTRIN; ESKALITH; lithium; LITHOBID; MEASURIN; SANDIMMUNE.

Additionally, the *United States Pharmacopeia Drug Interactions*, 1992, lists these drugs as having interactions of major significance:

amphetamines; DEXEDRINE; HIPREX; INVERSINE; mecamylamine; methenamine; QUINAGLUTE; QUINIDEX; quinidine; UREX.

Adverse Effects

Call your doctor immediately:

❑ blood in urine, trouble urinating, pain or burning during urination, or sudden decrease in amount of urine

❑ bloody or black, tarry stools
❑ clumsiness, unsteadiness
❑ convulsions
❑ dry mouth or increased thirst
❑ irregular heartbeat
❑ muscle cramps or pain
❑ nausea or vomiting
❑ unusual tiredness or weakness
❑ fever and sore throat
❑ unusual bruising or bleeding
❑ mental confusion or depression
❑ trouble breathing or shortness of breath
❑ ringing or buzzing in ears
❑ hives, itching or skin rash
❑ tremors in hands or feet
❑ vision changes

Call your doctor if these symptoms continue:

❑ constipation or diarrhea
❑ dizziness, lightheadedness
❑ drowsiness
❑ general feeling of discomfort or illness
❑ increased amount or frequency of urination
❑ loss of appetite, weight loss
❑ metallic taste or loss of taste in mouth
❑ numbness or tingling of hands, fingers, feet, toes, mouth, tongue, lips or rectum
❑ hair loss
❑ headache
❑ impotence[32]
❑ irritability, nervousness

Periodic Tests

Ask your doctor which of these tests should be done periodically while you are taking this drug:

❑ complete blood count (CBC)
❑ blood electrolyte (sodium, potassium) tests
❑ platelet count
❑ urological exam

Dipivefrin
PROPINE (Allergan)

Generic: not available

Family: Antiglaucoma Drugs (see p. 583)

Dipivefrin (dye *pi* ve frin) is used to treat the most common form of glaucoma (see p. 583). In glaucoma, the pressure of the fluid inside the eye increases, and dipivefrin controls the pressure by reducing the amount of fluid that is produced and improving its circulation. Pilocarpine (see p. 584) is the first-choice drug for glaucoma, and dipivefrin is usually used as a supplement if pilocarpine alone is not sufficient.

Before You Use This Drug
Tell your doctor if you have or have had
❑ allergies to drugs
❑ the lens in your eye removed
Tell your doctor about any other drugs you take, including aspirin, herbs, vitamins, and other non-prescription products.

When You Use This Drug
◆ Do not use more often or in a higher dose than prescribed.

How To Use This Drug
◆ Do not store in the bathroom. Do not expose to heat, moisture, or strong light. Do not allow to freeze.
◆ If you miss a dose, apply it as soon as you remember, but skip it if it is almost time for the next dose. **Do not take double doses.**

Interactions With Other Drugs
Some other drugs that you may be taking (either over-the-counter or prescription drugs) can interact with this one, causing adverse effects. Find out from your doctor what these drugs are and let him or her know if you are taking any of them.

Adverse Effects
Call your doctor immediately:
❑ rise in blood pressure
❑ fast or irregular heartbeat
Call your doctor if these symptoms continue:
❑ burning, stinging, or irritation of the eyes

Periodic Tests
Ask your doctor which of these tests should be done periodically while you are taking this drug:
❑ eye pressure tests
❑ complete eye exam, including test for visual acuity

Sulfacetamide
SULAMYD (Schering)

Generic: available

Family: Antibiotics (see p. 444)
Sulfonamides

Sulfacetamide (sul fa *see* ta mide) is used to treat some eye infections and is available as a liquid or an ointment. It can cause blurred vision, stinging, or burning after use. It also makes your eyes sensitive to bright light. Wearing sunglasses may help with this problem.

Before You Use This Drug
Tell your doctor if you have or have had
❑ allergies to drugs
❑ an unusual reaction to other sulfa drugs, furosemide, thiazide diuretics (water pills), or diabetes or glaucoma drugs taken by mouth
❑ glucose-6-phosphate dehydrogenase deficiency
Tell your doctor about any other drugs you take, including aspirin, herbs, vitamins, and other non-prescription products.

When You Use This Drug
◆ Call your doctor if your symptoms do not improve in 2 or 3 days.
◆ If the liquid form of sulfacetamide gets dark, throw it away.
◆ **Use all the sulfacetamide your doctor prescribed, even if you feel better before you finish. If you stop too soon, your symptoms could come back.**

◆ Do not give this drug to anyone else. Throw away outdated drugs.

How To Use This Drug
◆ See p. 582 for instructions on applying eye drops and ointment.
◆ Do not let the tip of the applicator touch your eye, your fingers, or anything else. It could become contaminated.
◆ Do not store in the bathroom or expose to heat, moisture, or strong light. Do not allow this drug to freeze.
◆ If you miss a dose, apply it as soon as you remember, but skip it if it is almost time for the next dose. **Do not take double doses.**

Interactions With Other Drugs
Some other drugs that you may be taking (either over-the-counter or prescription drugs) can interact with this one, causing adverse effects. Find out from your doctor what these drugs are and let him or her know if you are taking any of them.

Adverse Effects
Call your doctor immediately:
❑ itching, redness, or swelling not present before using this drug
❑ Because sulfacetamide is absorbed into the body, you may have other side effects like those that occur with the sulfonamides (sulfa drugs). See sulfisoxazole, p. 474, for examples.

Artificial Tears
TEARISOL (CooperVision)
TEARS NATURALE (Alcon)
HYPOTEARS (Iolab)

Generic: available

Family: Eye Drugs

Artificial tears are used to treat people who do not produce tears normally. You can also use them on a temporary basis to moisten dry eyes. Do not use artificial tears for more than 3 days unless your doctor has prescribed them.

Most artificial tears preparations contain either polyvinyl alcohol or a methylcellulose solution for lubrication. Methylcellulose solutions stay in your eye longer, but they tend to form crusts on the eyelids. If you use artificial tears containing polyvinyl alcohol, do not also use an eye solution containing boric acid. The combination may form gummy deposits.[33]

To avoid eye infection, irritation, and other problems, take care to prevent contamination when applying eye drops. Do not allow the applicator tip to touch anything, including your eye. After applying drops, replace the cap tightly on the bottle.

Before You Use This Drug
Tell your doctor if you have or have had
❑ allergies to drugs
Tell your doctor about any other drugs you take, including aspirin, herbs, vitamins, and other non-prescription products.

When You Use This Drug
◆ **Do not use more often or in a higher dose than prescribed.**

How To Use This Drug
◆ Directions for applying eye drops appear on p. 582.
◆ Do not store in the bathroom. Do not expose to heat, moisture, or strong light. Do not allow to freeze.

Interactions With Other Drugs
Some other drugs that you may be taking (either over-the-counter or prescription drugs) can interact with this one, causing adverse effects. Find out from your doctor what these drugs are and let him or her know if you are taking any of them.

Adverse Effects
Call your doctor immediately:
❑ eye irritation that was not present before you started using artificial tears
Call your doctor if these symptoms continue:
❑ blurred vision
❑ matted or sticky eyelids

Timolol (Eye Drops)
TIMOPTIC (Merck)

Generic: available

Family: Antiglaucoma Drugs (see p. 583)
    Beta-blockers (see p. 68)

Timolol (*tim* oh lole) has two forms for different uses: Blocadren tablets for the heart (see p. 80) and Timoptic eye drops for the eyes, specifically for treating glaucoma (see p. 583). This page discusses timolol's use as an antiglaucoma drug.

Timoptic drops are well tolerated by most people, especially those who have cataracts or who have problems using another antiglaucoma drug called pilocarpine (see p. 584). Although Timoptic is an eye drop, some of it can be absorbed from the eyes into the bloodstream and the rest of the body, and if this happens you may experience some of the general side effects listed under Adverse Effects. **(See p. 582 for directions on how to apply eye drops.)**

When used for a long time, the initial improvement sometimes goes away. As with other beta-blockers, long-term use can cause serious heart problems, even in people who did not previously have heart disease. Timolol, similarly to levobunolol, can decrease lung function by 30%, an adverse effect not seen in betaxolol, another beta-blocker.[34] Very rarely, serious harm, even fatalities have occurred, mostly to those with asthma or heart problems.[35] But according to *The Medical Letter*, betaxolol may be less likely than timolol or levobunolol to have adverse side effects on patients with asthma.[36] Timolol taken by mouth has been shown to cause an increased number of adrenal, lung, uterine, and breast cancers in rats. This has not been shown for the eye drops.

Before You Use This Drug
Do not use if you have or have had
❑ congestive heart failure, slow heart beat or heart block
❑ asthma
Tell your doctor if you have or have had
❑ allergies to drugs
❑ emphysema or chronic bronchitis
❑ diabetes
❑ myasthenia gravis
❑ thyroid problems
❑ other heart problems
❑ depression
Tell your doctor about any other drugs you take, including aspirin, herbs, vitamins, and other non-prescription products.

When You Use This Drug
◆ Restrict your use of caffeine, since it may add to the effect of timolol on the heart.[37]
◆ **Caution diabetics:** be aware that timolol may mask trembling and pulse rate used to signal low blood sugar.[38]
◆ If you plan to have any surgery, including dental, tell your doctor that you take this drug.
◆ Be cautious driving until the effect of the drug is complete (about two weeks),[39] and no blurred vision occurs.
◆ **Do not take other drugs without talking to your doctor first — especially**

Cold Stress Alert
If timolol eye drops are absorbed into the body, older people have an increased risk of hypothermia.[40] Early signs are shivering, cold hands and feet, and memory lapse. Stay indoors, especially when it is cold and windy. Keep warm with extra clothes and blankets. If you must go outdoors, dress to protect yourself from the wind and cold. Avoid getting wet. Take along something to eat, such as trail mix suitable to your diet.

**non-prescription drugs for appetite
control, asthma, colds, coughs, hay
fever, or sinus problems.**
◆ Do not expose to heat or direct light.

How To Use This Drug
◆ *If you miss a dose, use the following guidelines:*
  - If you are using Timoptic only once a
    day, apply the missed dose as soon as
    you remember, but skip it if you don't
    remember until the next day.
  - If you are using Timoptic more than
    once a day, apply the missed dose as
    soon as you remember, but skip it if it is
    almost time for the next dose.
  - **Do not apply double doses.**

Interactions With Other Drugs
The following drugs are listed in *Evaluations of Drug Interactions*, 1991 as causing "highly clinically significant" or "clinically significant" interactions when used together with this drug. There may be other drugs, especially those in the families of drugs listed below, that also will react with this drug to cause severe adverse effects. Make sure to ask your doctor for a complete listing of them and let her or him know if you are taking any of these interacting drugs:

ADRENALIN (also in bee sting kits);
BRONKAID; CALAN; CATAPRES;
clonidine; cocaine; DELTASONE;
ELIXOPHYLLIN; EPIFRIN; epinephrine; ESKALITH; FLUOTHANE;
halothane; insulin; lidocaine; lithium;
MINIPRESS; NAPROSYN; naproxen;
prazosin; prednisone; SYNTHROID;
theophylline; thyroid; tubocurarine;
verapamil; XYLOCAINE.

Adverse Effects
Timolol can be absorbed into the body
through the eye. All adverse effects for oral
beta-blockers are possible with timolol
eyedrops.
Call your doctor immediately:
❏ headache
❏ eye irritation or visual changes
❏ itching skin or rash
*Call your doctor if these symptoms
continue:*
❏ anxiety, nervousness
❏ nausea, vomiting, diarrhea
❏ unusual tiredness or weakness
❏ disturbed sleep, nightmares
❏ decreased sexual ability
❏ numbness or tingling of limbs
❏ difficulty breathing
❏ chest pain
❏ hallucinations
❏ cold hands or feet
❏ mental depression
❏ skin rash
❏ swelling of ankles, feet, legs
❏ slow pulse
*More side effects information appears on
p. 68.*

Periodic Tests
*Ask your doctor which of these tests should
be done periodically while you are taking
this drug:*
❏ blood pressure and pulse rate
❏ heart function tests, such as electrocardiogram (EKG)
❏ blood glucose levels (if diabetic)
❏ eye pressure exams

Notes for Drugs for Eye Diseases

1. The Levobunolol Study Group. A four-year study of efficacy and safety in glaucoma treatment. *Ophthalmology* 1989; 96:642-5.

2. Silverstone D, Zimmerman T, Choplin N, Mundorf T, Rose A, Stoecker J, Kelley E, Lue J. Evaluation of once-daily levobunolol 0.25% and timolol 0.25% therapy for increased intraocular pressure. *American Journal of Ophthalmology* 1991; 112:56-60.

3. Dukes MNG, Beeley L. *Side Effects of Drugs Annual* 15, Amsterdam: Elsevier, 1991:510.

4. American Society of Hospital Pharmacists. *American Hospital Formulary Service Drug Information.* Bethesda, MD, 1992:1694-7.

5. *The Medical Letter on Drugs and Therapeutics.* New York: The Medical Letter Inc., 1986; 28:45-6.

6. *USP DI, Drug Information for the Health Care Professional.* 12th ed. Rockville MD: The United States Pharmacopeial Convention, Inc., 1992:1757-61.

7. *USP DI*, 1992, op. cit., p. 656-9.

8. American Society of Hospital Pharmacists, op. cit.

9. *USP DI*, 1992, op cit., p. 1757-61.

10. Dukes, op. cit., p. 510.

11. American Society of Hospital Pharmacists, op. cit.

12. *The Medical Letter on Drugs and Therapeutics,* op. cit.

13. *USP DI*, 1992, op. cit., p. 1757-61.

14. *USP DI*, 1992, op. cit., p. 656-9.

15. American Society of Hospital Pharmacists, op. cit.

16. *USP DI*, 1992, op cit., p. 1751-61.

17. Allen RC, Hertzmark E, Walker AM, Epstein DL. A double-masked comparison of betaxolol vs timolol in the treatment of open-angle glaucoma. *American Journal of Ophthalmology* 1986; 101:535-41.

18. AMA Department of Drugs. *AMA Drug Evaluations.* 1st ed. Chicago: American Medical Association, 1971:526.

19. *USP DI, Drug Information for the Health Care Provider.* 6th ed. Rockville Md.: The United States Pharmacopeial Convention, Inc., 1986:448.

20. AMA Department of Drugs. *AMA Drug Evaluations.* 5th ed. Chicago: American Medical Association, 1983:763-4.

21 AMA Department of Drugs. *AMA Drug Evaluations.* 1992. Chicago: American Medical Association, 1992:1975-7.

22. AMA, 1983, op. cit., p. 763-4.

23. AMA, 1983, op. cit., p. 1686.

24. AMA, 1971, op. cit.

25. Patrick J, Panzer JD. *Archives of Dermatology* 1970; 102:532.

26. AMA, 1971, op. cit.

27. Patrick, op. cit.

28 Koller WC. New drug for treatment of essential tremor? Time will tell. *Mayo Clinic Proceedings* 1991; 66:1085-7.

29. AMA, 1992, op. cit.

30. Moroi-Fetters SE, Metz EN, Chambers RB, Davidorf FH. Aplastic anemia with platelet autoantibodies in a patient after taking methazolamide. *American Journal of Ophthalmology* 1990; 110:570-1.

31. Marmor MF. Hypothesis concerning carbonic anhydrase treatment of cystoid macular edema: example with epiretinal membrane. *Archives of Ophthalmology* 1990; 108:1524-5.

32. Dukes, op. cit, p. 513.

33. *Handbook of Nonprescription Drugs*. 7th ed. Washington, D.C.: American Pharmaceutical Association, 1982:425.

34. Dukes, op. cit., p. 510.

35. American Society of Hospital Pharmacists, op. cit.

36. *The Medical Letter on Drugs and Therapeutics*, op. cit.

37. *USP DI*, 1992, op. cit., p. 1757-61.

38. *USP DI*, 1992, op. cit., p. 656-9.

39. American Society of Hospital Pharmacists, op. cit.

40. *USP DI*, 1992, op. cit., p. 1757-61.

Drugs For Other Conditions

Corticosteroids

Hormones

Muscle Relaxants

Drugs for Urinary Tract Infection

Drugs for Treating Cancer

Skin & Hair Care Drugs

Drugs to Help Stop Smoking

Corticosteroids

Corticosteroids, commonly known as steroids or cortisone, are a class of hormones that regulate vital body functions. They affect carbohydrate, protein, and fat metabolism; maintain the body's water and electrolyte (salt and potassium, for example) balance; support normal heart and blood vessel function; influence mood and sleep patterns; and maintain normal muscle strength. Corticosteroids are produced by the adrenal glands, located just above the kidneys. Prescription corticosteroids are either identical to or a synthetic version of the adrenal hormones. They are given to (1) replace the body's corticosteroids when the adrenal glands are diseased and (2) suppress inflammation in diseases such as arthritis or asthma.

Corticosteroids are taken in many different dosage forms. Nasal dosage, eye dosage, topical, and inhaler forms have been developed to deliver the corticosteroid directly to the affected area, which minimizes side effects. In this section you will find directions common to all corticosteroids, followed by specific information regarding the most common dosage forms.

General Directions
1. Do not allow corticosteroids to freeze.
2. Do not expose corticosteroids to heat or direct light.
3. Do not store in the bathroom. The moisture and heat will alter the structure of the drug, and it will no longer be effective.
4. Do not take more often or in higher doses than your doctor prescribed. **Do not stop taking this drug suddenly. Your doctor must lower your dose gradually to prevent withdrawal symptoms.** When your symptoms improve, ask your doctor about reducing your dosage. Higher doses and/or shorter intervals between doses can stop the body's production of its own corticosteroids. This leads to a lowered defense against disease (a depressed immune system) and can result in a greater likelihood of developing infections and tumors. Do not use the drug to treat problems other than that for which it was prescribed without first checking with your doctor. Corticosteroids should not be used for many bacterial, viral, and fungal infections.

Systemic Dosage Forms
The word *systemic* refers to something which affects the body as a whole. A drug, taken as tablets, capsules, or injections, is distributed throughout the body — to areas that require treatment as well as to those that do not. Because the entire body is exposed to the drug's action, there can be unnecessary adverse side effects.

Side effects from systemic corticosteroids can be minimized by using alternate-day therapy. In this way, the body is only exposed to the drug's full effects every other day. If you will be taking systemic steroids on a long-term basis, ask your doctor about switching to alternate-day therapy.

The body's own corticosteroids are released mostly in the early morning hours between 4:00 a.m. and 8:00 a.m., with very little being released in the evenings. The varying amounts of corticosteroids to which your body is exposed throughout the day help to set your body's clock and to establish sleep and waking cycles. Therefore, a single daily dose or an alternate-day dose should be taken in the morning prior to 8:00 a.m. for the least disruption of your body's natural rhythm.

Prednisone is the drug of choice for systemic steroids, because it is reliable, effective, less expensive, and available in a generic preparation that can be taken by mouth. Oral forms of prednisolone, methylprednisolone, and betamethasone should *not* be used.

Corticotropin (ACTH) has limited use — it should be used only for diagnostic testing of adrenal function. It should not be used for inflammation or disorders which respond to other more preferable corticosteroids.

Nasal Dosage Forms

There are two types of nasal dosage forms: the solution and the aerosol, both of which supply metered-dose sprays of corticosteroid. They are used to treat severe allergies, severe cases of hay fever, and sometimes nasal polyps.

If you have a very runny nose with a lot of secretions or swelling, most of the drug may not reach the nasal mucous membranes and therefore may not be absorbed. Blow your nose before using the spray or take a decongestant first if your nasal passages are blocked. You may require treatment with cortisone tablets or a cream to shrink the nasal blood vessels.

At recommended dosages, absorption of the drug into the body through the lining of the nose is minimal, and side effects are limited primarily to the nose. Nosebleeds, burning, irritation, and sneezing are common.

Eye Dosage Form

While taking this drug you should schedule regular appointments with an eye doctor to check your progress. For both drops and ointments, **call your doctor immediately if symptoms do not improve within 5 to 7 days, if your condition worsens, or if you feel pain, itching or swelling.** Temporary blurring of sight may occur after you apply the medicine. This is normal and will clear shortly. The medicine may also cause sensitivity to bright light. Wearing sunglasses will help. See p. 582 for directions to safely and effectively apply drops and ointments.

Eye pressure should be rechecked approximately 2 weeks after you begin to use corticosteroid drops or ointment on your eye because these drugs can cause or worsen glaucoma.

Topical (Applied to Skin and Mouth) Dosage Form

There are two major categories of corticosteroid preparations that are applied to the skin: those that contain fluorine and those that do not. Neither should be used for prolonged periods on the face or around the eye. Systemic side effects are related to the amount of drug used, and can pose a problem when large areas of skin are treated. Thinning of skin may occur with prolonged use, particularly on the face, armpits and groin, with the exception of weak nonfluorinated creams. If the area which you are treating becomes irritated, stop using the drug and call your doctor.

Fluorinated topical forms

Corticosteroids that contain fluorine are betamethasone (Diprosone, Diprolene, Valisone), desoximetasone (Topicort), dexamethasone (Decadron, Hexadrol), fluocinolone (Synalar, Synemol), fluocinonide (Lidex, Lidex-E), and triamcinolone (Kenalog, Aristocort). Fluorinated topical corticosteroids are generally more effective than those that do not contain fluorine. They are more likely, however, to cause side effects such as skin wasting, loss of pigment, and acne. Because of the potential adverse effects, high strength fluorine-containing steroids should be spread in a very thin layer, covering only the treatment area. Systemic effects are rare if these preparations are used correctly.

Some people find ointments too greasy, especially for hairy areas. In this case, a cream, lotion, or gel may come into better contact with the skin.

Nonfluorinated topical forms

Hydrocortisone (Cortaid) can now be purchased without a prescription in two strengths, 0.25% and 0.50%. The lowest concentration of this drug that is generally considered effective, however, is 0.50%. A soothing emollient, such as a lotion, cream, or ointment, that does not contain hydrocortisone is probably just as effective as the 0.25% hydrocortisone cream.

Inhalation Aerosol for Asthma

Corticosteroid inhalants, used with an inhaler that is placed in the mouth, primarily benefit those people with asthma who require regular, long-term use of corticosteroids to control their symptoms. They are rarely appropriate treatment for nonasthmatic bronchitis or emphysema. The inhalants should not be used when asthma responds to bronchodilators and other nonsteroid drugs, or to systemic (tablets and capsules) steroids used infrequently.

Inhaled aerosol corticosteroids may be used instead of or in addition to systemic corticosteroids. They are preferable to the systemic forms because of the way they deliver the medication to where it is required. Inhaling the medication ensures that more of it is concentrated in the lungs where it is needed and less is available to the rest of the body through general absorption. This is better because it is the drug's actions on the rest of the body that causes most side effects.

Inhaled aerosol corticosteroids can take up to 4 weeks to produce improvement when used alone, and therefore are ineffective if taken on an intermittent basis. People who use corticosterioids infrequently cannot substitute an inhalation aerosol for the medication they use.

Continue to use the inhalant even if you do not notice immediate improvement. It often takes 1 to 4 weeks before seeing full benefit. To receive the most benefit from your inhaler, follow the directions on p. 388.

The inhalant predisposes you to fungal infections of the mouth and throat because some of the drug is absorbed when you inhale the dose. Therefore, *after each dose* you should rinse out your mouth and gargle with water. This flushes out the drug that did not go to your lungs and prevents it from being absorbed.

If you are switching from taking systemic medication to the inhalant, **it is important that you do not suddenly stop taking the tablets or injections.** Your body requires a few weeks or months to adjust to the loss of extra corticosteroids and to start making its own again. In the meantime, your doctor will give you a dosage schedule to slowly taper the amount of systemic steroids that you take each day. Failure to follow this schedule and gradually decrease your dosage can result in serious side effects, including death.

If you have a severe asthma attack, call your doctor immediately. Do *not* inhale an extra dose of the corticosteroid. The inhalant helps to prevent attacks, but it will not control an attack that has already started. You will need to resume taking systemic steroids if the attack occurs while you are changing from tablets or injections to the inhalant. You should carry a card stating that you may need supplementary steroids during periods of stress or illness. If you are only taking corticosteroids via an inhaler, you may still need stronger therapy to treat mucous plugs that may be present.

LIMITED USE

Corticotropin/Adrenocorticotropic Hormone (ACTH)
ACTHAR (Armour) CORTROPHIN-ZINC (Organon)

Generic: available

Family: Corticosteroids (see p. 609)

Corticotropin (kor ti koe *troe* pin) and adrenocorticotropic hormone (ACTH) are two names for the same drug. Both of these drugs act in the same way as natural corticotropin, a hormone which is produced by the pituitary gland in your brain. Natural corticotropin signals your adrenal glands, located just above your kidneys, to produce a type of chemical called corticosteroids (see p. 609).

There are a number of conditions — conditions that produce inflammation, such as arthritis, asthma, and some skin and eye conditions, for example — that can be treated effectively with corticosteroids (also just called steroids). Doctors often prescribe the hormone corticotropin (ACTH) instead of steroids for these conditions, since corticotropin stimulates your body's own production of steroids. However, **you should not take corticotropin for more than 3 consecutive days.** If you need long-term treatment, it is better to take steroids. For treatment lasting 3 days or less, either corticotropin or steroids may be used, but steroids are much less expensive.

If you need steroids and can take them by mouth, prednisone (see p. 622) is the best drug because it is reliable, inexpensive, and available in a generic form.[1]

Corticotropin is also used to test how well the adrenal glands are functioning. For these tests, it is better to use the newer drug Cortrosyn, a synthetic hormone with fewer harmful side effects.

Corticotropin, which is derived from pork products, has caused allergic reactions in some people who have received it.

Before You Use This Drug
Do not use if you have or have had
- ❑ congestive heart failure
- ❑ high blood pressure
- ❑ herpes simplex infection of the eye
- ❑ scleroderma
- ❑ osteoporosis
- ❑ recent surgery
- ❑ an allergy to pork

Tell your doctor if you have or have had
- ❑ allergies to drugs
- ❑ AIDS
- ❑ heart disease
- ❑ high blood pressure
- ❑ liver or kidney disease
- ❑ diabetes
- ❑ inflammation of throat, stomach, or intestines
- ❑ glaucoma
- ❑ fungal infections
- ❑ myasthenia gravis
- ❑ tuberculosis or positive TB test

Tell your doctor about any other drugs you take, including aspirin, herbs, vitamins, and other non-prescription products.

When You Use This Drug
- ◆ Do not drink alcohol. Drinking alcohol while taking this drug increases your chances of developing an ulcer.
- ◆ If you plan to have any surgery, including dental, tell your doctor that you take this drug.
- ◆ Eat a diet low in salt and rich in potassium, protein, and folic acid. Ask your doctor to tell you how you can get more potassium, protein, and folic acid in your diet.

How To Use This Drug
- ◆ **Do not take more than your doctor has prescribed.**

Interactions With Other Drugs

The following drugs are listed in *Evaluations of Drug Interactions*, 1991 as causing "highly clinically significant" or "clinically significant" interactions when used together with this drug. There may be other drugs, especially those in the families of drugs listed below, that also will react with this drug to cause severe adverse effects. Make sure to ask your doctor for a complete listing of them and let her or him know if you are taking any of these interacting drugs:

aspirin; cyclosporine; dicumarol; ECOTRIN; ketoconazole; NIZORAL; SANDIMMUNE; timolol; TIMOPTIC.

Adverse Effects

Call your doctor immediately:
- decreased or blurred vision
- frequent urination
- increased thirst
- numbness, pain, tingling, redness, or swelling at site of injection
- hallucinations
- depression or mood changes
- skin rash or hives

For long-term corticotropin therapy:
- persistent abdominal or stomach pain
- acne or other skin problems
- bloody or black, tarry stools
- rounding out of the face
- hip pain
- increased blood pressure
- swelling of feet or lower legs
- unusual weight gain
- irregular heartbeats
- muscle cramps or pain
- unusual tiredness or weakness
- pain in back, ribs, arms, or legs
- muscle weakness
- nausea or vomiting
- pitting or depression of skin at place of injection
- thin, shiny skin
- unusual bruising
- wounds that will not heal

Call your doctor if these symptoms continue:
- indigestion
- increased appetite
- nervousness or restlessness
- trouble sleeping
- dizziness or lightheadedness
- flushed face
- headache
- increased joint pain
- nosebleeds
- increased body or facial hair

Periodic Tests

Ask your doctor which of these tests should be done periodically while you are taking this drug:
- skin testing for sensitivity to pork products
- blood or urine glucose concentration
- eye exams
- blood levels of potassium, sodium, and calcium
- stool tests for possible blood loss

Triamcinolone
AZMACORT (Rorer) KENALOG (Squibb)

Generic: available

Family: Corticosteroids (see p. 609)

Triamcinolone (trye am *sin* oh lone), like other steroids (corticosteroids), has many uses. It is commonly used to treat inflammation (redness and swelling) and itching caused by certain skin conditions; arthritis and other bone and joint disorders that produce inflammation; and allergies and other breathing problems. In an inhaled form, triamcinolone is used to control asthma that requires regular, long-term use of steroids.

Triamcinolone is available in several forms for different uses. It can be injected into the muscle, joint, lesion, or soft tissue; applied to the skin and mouth (topical form); sprayed into the mouth and inhaled; or taken by mouth as tablets or syrup. You should not use triamcinolone tablets or syrup taken by mouth, because when taken in this form, the drug stays in the body for too long and causes side effects. If you need to take steroids by mouth, prednisone (see p. 622) is the best choice because it is reliable, inexpensive, and available in a generic form.[2]

Steroids suppress your immune system, lowering your defenses against disease and making you more vulnerable to infections. If you use triamcinolone for a long time, you increase your risk of getting bacterial, viral, parasitic, and fungal infections. Older adults using triamcinolone are more likely than younger users to develop the bone-weakening condition called osteoporosis. Older users are also more likely to develop high blood pressure and to retain fluid while taking this drug.

As with all drugs, you should use the smallest dose of triamcinolone that works. You should also use it for the shortest possible time. If you use systemic steroids (ones that are taken by mouth or injected so that your whole body is exposed to them) for a long time, you may suffer many side effects, and you may also suffer withdrawal symptoms if you stop abruptly.

Before You Use This Drug
Do not use if you have or have had
For injections into the joint:
❑ blood clotting disorders
❑ fracture of the joint
❑ infection around the joint
❑ joint surgery
❑ osteoporosis
❑ unstable joint
Tell your doctor if you have or have had
❑ allergies to drugs
❑ AIDS
❑ heart disease
❑ high blood pressure
❑ kidney or liver disease
❑ diabetes
❑ inflammation of throat, stomach, or intestines
❑ glaucoma
❑ fungal infections
❑ myasthenia gravis
❑ osteoporosis
❑ herpes sores
❑ tuberculosis or positive TB skin test
For skin preparations:
❑ infection or ulceration at place where you will be applying the drug
Tell your doctor about any other drugs you take, including aspirin, herbs, vitamins, and other non-prescription products.

When You Use This Drug
For long-term use, if you take the drug by mouth or injection:
◆ **Do not stop taking this drug suddenly.** Your doctor must lower your dose gradually to prevent withdrawal symptoms.

◆ If you plan to have any surgery, including dental, tell your doctor or dentist that you take this drug.

If you are using the inhaled aerosol spray:

◆ Wear a medical identification bracelet or carry a card stating that you may need additional steroids (tablets or injection) in times of unusual stress or sudden, severe asthma attack.

How To Use This Drug

◆ **Use only as prescribed.**

◆ If you miss a dose, take it as soon as you remember, but skip it if it is almost time for the next dose. **Do not take double doses.**

On your skin:

◆ The preparation may sting when applied.

◆ Keep away from eyes.

◆ Apply cream or ointment with cotton applicator. Do not bandage or wrap the area being treated unless your doctor has told you to do so.

◆ If you use the drug correctly, there is no danger that it will be absorbed into your system.

In your mouth:

◆ Apply with cotton applicator by pressing (not rubbing) paste on the sore.

◆ Check with your doctor or dentist if your condition does not improve in 1 week or if it worsens.

◆ See p. 609 for information about the spray.

Interactions With Other Drugs

The following drugs are listed in *Evaluations of Drug Interactions*, 1991 as causing "highly clinically significant" or "clinically significant" interactions when used together with this drug. There may be other drugs, especially those in the families of drugs listed below, that also will react with this drug to cause severe adverse effects. Make sure to ask your doctor for a complete listing of them and let her or him know if you are taking any of these interacting drugs:

aspirin; chlorpropamide; DIABINESE; dicumarol; DILANTIN; ECOTRIN; LUMINAL; phenobarbital; phenytoin; RIFADIN; rifampin; timolol; TIMOPTIC.

Adverse Effects

Call your doctor immediately:

❑ numbness, pain, tingling, redness, or swelling at place of injection
❑ hallucinations
❑ depression or mood changes
❑ skin rash or hives

For long-term use:

❑ persistent abdominal or stomach pain
❑ acne or other skin problems
❑ bloody or black, tarry stools
❑ rounding out of the face
❑ hip pain
❑ increased blood pressure
❑ swelling of feet or lower legs
❑ unusual weight gain
❑ irregular heartbeats
❑ muscle cramps or pain
❑ unusual tiredness or weakness
❑ pain in back, ribs, arms, or legs
❑ muscle weakness
❑ nausea or vomiting
❑ pitting or depression of skin at place of injection
❑ thin, shiny skin
❑ unusual bruising
❑ wounds that will not heal

Call your doctor immediately if these symptoms occur after you stop taking this drug:

❑ abdominal or back pain
❑ dizziness or fainting
❑ low fever
❑ persistent loss of appetite
❑ muscle or joint pain
❑ nausea or vomiting
❑ returning symptoms of the condition for which you were taking the drug
❑ shortness of breath
❑ frequent unexplained headaches
❑ unusual tiredness or weakness
❑ unusual weight loss

Call your doctor if these symptoms continue:

❑ increased appetite
❑ nervousness or restlessness

❑ trouble sleeping
❑ dizziness or lightheadedness
❑ flushed face
❑ headache
❑ increased joint pain
❑ nosebleeds
❑ increase in hair on body or face

Periodic Tests
Ask your doctor which of these tests should be done periodically while you are taking this drug:
❑ blood or urine glucose concentration
❑ eye exams

Hydrocortisone
CORTEF (Upjohn)

Generic: available

Family: Corticosteroids (see p. 609)

Hydrocortisone (hye droe *kor* ti sone), like other steroids (corticosteroids), has many uses. It is commonly used to treat skin conditions, eye infections, and arthritis and other disorders that produce inflammation. It is also used to treat allergies and other breathing problems.

Hydrocortisone has several forms for different uses. It can be taken by mouth (oral form). It can be injected into the muscle, joint, lesion, soft tissue, or blood-stream. It can be applied to the skin (topical form) in one of two strengths available without a prescription, 0.25% and 0.50%. It can be applied to the eye or ear (oph-thalmic-otic form), although it is preferable to see your doctor rather than getting the over-the-counter eye preparation. It is also available as a dental paste and as a rectal suppository or ointment.

You should not use the form of hydrocor-tisone taken by mouth. If you need to take a steroid by mouth, prednisone (see p. 622) is the best choice because it is reliable, inex-pensive, and available in a generic form.[3] You also should not use the weaker (0.25%) form of hydrocortisone applied to the skin, because it is ineffective.

Steroids suppress your immune system, lowering your defenses against disease and making you more vulnerable to infections. If you use hydrocortisone for a long time, you increase your risk of getting bacterial, viral, parasitic, and fungal infections. Older adults using hydrocortisone are more likely than younger users to develop the bone-weakening condition called osteoporosis. Older users are also more likely to develop high blood pressure and to retain fluid while taking this drug.

As with all drugs, you should use the smallest dose of hydrocortisone that works. You should also use it for the shortest possible time. If you use systemic steroids (ones that are taken by mouth or injected so that your whole body is exposed to them) for a long time, you may suffer many side effects, and you may also suffer withdrawal symptoms if you stop abruptly.

Before You Use This Drug
Do not use if you have or have had
For injections into the joint:
❑ blood clotting disorders
❑ fracture of the joint
❑ infection around the joint
❑ joint surgery
❑ osteoporosis
❑ unstable joint
Tell your doctor if you have or have had
❑ allergies to drugs, particularly other hydrocortisone-containing drugs[4]
❑ AIDS
❑ heart disease

❑ high blood pressure
❑ liver or kidney disease
❑ diabetes
❑ inflammation of throat, stomach, or intestines
❑ glaucoma
❑ fungal infections
❑ myasthenia gravis
❑ herpes sores
❑ tuberculosis or positive TB skin test

For topical form:
❑ infection or ulceration at the place where you will be applying the drug

Tell your doctor about any other drugs you take, including aspirin, herbs, vitamins, and other non-prescription products.

When You Use This Drug

◆ If you plan to have any surgery, including dental, tell your doctor that you take this drug.

How To Use This Drug

◆ **Use only as prescribed.**
◆ If you miss a dose, take it as soon as you remember, but skip it if it is almost time for the next dose. **Do not take double doses.**

On your skin:
◆ The preparation may sting when applied.
◆ Keep away from eyes.
◆ Do not bandage or wrap the area you are treating unless your doctor has told you to do so.
◆ If you use the drug correctly, there is no danger that it will be absorbed into your system.

In your mouth:
◆ Apply with cotton applicator by pressing (not rubbing) paste on the sore.
◆ Check with your doctor or dentist if your condition does not improve within 1 week or if it worsens.

Interactions With Other Drugs

The following drugs are listed in *Evaluations of Drug Interactions,* 1991 as causing "highly clinically significant" or "clinically significant" interactions when used together with this drug. There may be other drugs, especially those in the families of drugs listed below, that also will react with this drug to cause severe adverse effects. Make sure to ask your doctor for a complete listing of them and let her or him know if you are taking any of these interacting drugs:

aspirin; chlorpropamide; cyclosporine; DIABINESE; dicumarol; DILANTIN; ECOTRIN; LUMINAL; phenobarbital; phenytoin; SANDIMMUNE; timolol; TIMOPTIC.

Adverse Effects

Call your doctor immediately:
❑ decreased or blurred vision
❑ frequent urination
❑ increased thirst
❑ rectal bleeding, burning, itching
❑ numbness, pain, tingling, redness, or swelling at site of injection
❑ hallucinations
❑ depression or mood changes
❑ skin rash or hives

For long-term use:
❑ persistent abdominal or stomach pain
❑ acne or other skin problems
❑ bloody or black, tarry stools
❑ rounding out of the face
❑ hip pain
❑ increased blood pressure
❑ swelling of feet or lower legs
❑ unusual weight gain
❑ irregular heartbeats
❑ muscle cramps or pain
❑ unusual tiredness or weakness
❑ pain in back, ribs, arms, or legs
❑ muscle weakness
❑ nausea or vomiting
❑ pitting or depression of skin at place of injection
❑ thin, shiny skin
❑ unusual bruising
❑ wounds that will not heal

Call your doctor immediately if these symptoms occur after you stop taking this drug:
❑ abdominal or back pain
❑ dizziness or fainting
❑ low fever

- ❑ persistent loss of appetite
- ❑ muscle or joint pain
- ❑ nausea or vomiting
- ❑ returning symptoms of the condition for which you were taking the drug
- ❑ shortness of breath
- ❑ frequent unexplained headaches
- ❑ unusual tiredness or weakness
- ❑ unusual weight loss

Call your doctor if these symptoms continue:
- ❑ indigestion
- ❑ increased appetite
- ❑ nervousness or restlessness
- ❑ trouble sleeping
- ❑ dizziness or lightheadedness
- ❑ flushed face
- ❑ headache

- ❑ increased joint pain
- ❑ nosebleeds
- ❑ increase in hair on body or face

Periodic Tests
Ask your doctor which of these tests should be done periodically while you are taking this drug:
- ❑ blood or urine glucose concentration
- ❑ eye exams
- ❑ blood levels of potassium, sodium, and calcium
- ❑ stool tests for possible blood loss
- ❑ hypothalamus and pituitary secretion tests

LIMITED USE

Cyclophosphamide
CYTOXAN (Bristol-Meyers) NEOSAR (Adria)

Generic: available

Family: Anticancer Drugs
Antiarthritis Drugs (see p. 261)

Cyclophosphamide (sye kloe *foss* fa mide) is used mainly to treat certain kinds of cancer. It is also used to treat some conditions that produce inflammation (redness, swelling, heat, or pain), such as rheumatoid arthritis (see p. 261) and systemic lupus erythematosus. This page primarily discusses cyclophosphamide's use for conditions causing inflammation.

Cyclophosphamide should be used to treat only the most severe cases of rheumatoid arthritis that have not responded to the progressive use of other drugs for inflammation, such as aspirin, ibuprofen, gold salts (see p. 311), and penicillamine. Cyclophosphamide is the drug of last resort for rheumatoid arthritis because it has serious

side effects, including nausea, vomiting, loss of appetite, blood problems, hair loss, and heart and lung problems. It can also cause other harmful effects such as leukemia and bladder cancer months or years after you stop taking it.

If you are taking cyclophosphamide and a side effect is disturbing you, ask your doctor or other health professional to suggest ways to avoid or decrease the problem. Be aware, however, that some side effects are unavoidable, and that some, in fact, are used to tell whether the drug is working.

Before You Use This Drug
Do not use if you have or have had
- ❑ recent infection or exposure to chicken pox
- ❑ shingles (herpes zoster)

Tell your doctor if you have or have had
- ❑ allergies to drugs

❏ loss of the adrenal glands
❏ bone marrow depression
❏ kidney stones
❏ liver or kidney disease
❏ recent infection

Tell your doctor about any other drugs you take, including aspirin, herbs, vitamins, and other non-prescription products.

When You Use This Drug

◆ **Do not use more or less often or in a higher or lower dose than prescribed.** Check with your doctor before you stop using this drug.

◆ **Check with your doctor to make certain your fluid intake is adequate and appropriate.**

◆ **Because this drug decreases the number of white blood cells, which fight infection, you are more likely to get an infection. Do not get immunizations without your doctor's approval.**

◆ Schedule regular visits with your doctor to check your progress.

◆ If you plan to have any surgery, including dental, tell your doctor that you take this drug.

How To Use This Drug

◆ To reduce stomach upset, your doctor may want you to take smaller doses throughout the day.

◆ Do not store in the bathroom. Do not expose to heat, strong light, or moisture. Do not allow liquid form to freeze.

◆ Call your doctor for instructions if you miss a dose or vomit shortly after taking the drug.

Interactions With Other Drugs

The following drugs are listed in *Evaluations of Drug Interactions,* 1991 as causing "highly clinically significant" or "clinically significant" interactions when used together with this drug. There may be other drugs, especially those in the families of drugs listed below, that also will react with

this drug to cause severe adverse effects. Make sure to ask your doctor for a complete listing of them and let her or him know if you are taking any of these interacting drugs:

chloramphenicol; CHLOROMYCETIN; COUMADIN; digoxin; LANOXIN; succinylchloline; warfarin.

Adverse Effects

Call your doctor immediately:
❏ fever, chills, or sore throat
❏ confusion or agitation
❏ dizziness, tiredness, or weakness
❏ blood in urine
❏ painful urination
❏ cough or shortness of breath
❏ unusually fast heartbeat
❏ flank or stomach pain
❏ swelling of feet or lower legs
❏ joint pain
❏ unusual bleeding or bruising
❏ black, tarry stools
❏ sores in mouth or on lips
❏ unusual thirst
❏ yellow eyes and skin
Call your doctor if these symptoms continue:
❏ hair loss
❏ nausea, vomiting, appetite loss
❏ darkening of skin and fingernails
❏ flushed or red face
❏ headache
❏ rash, hives, or itching
❏ swollen lips
❏ increased sweating

Periodic Tests

Ask your doctor which of these tests should be done periodically while you are taking this drug:
❏ kidney function tests
❏ liver function tests
❏ urine tests
❏ complete blood tests (including hematocrit, platelet count, white blood cell count)

Dexamethasone
DECADRON (Merck) HEXADROL (Organon)

Generic: available

Family: Corticosteroids (see p. 609)

Dexamethasone (dex a *meth* a sone), like other steroids (corticosteroids), has several uses and dosage forms. It can be taken by mouth to treat some types of cancer, to reduce swelling in the brain, and to help doctors diagnose a hormonal condition or depression. It can also be injected into the muscle, joint, lesion, soft tissue, and blood-stream; applied to the skin (topical form), eye (ophthalmic form), or ear (otic form); or sprayed into the nose or mouth. These forms are used to treat conditions that produce inflammation, such as arthritis and other joint and muscle disorders; allergies, hay fever, and other breathing problems; skin infections; and eye infections.

If you need to take a hormone by mouth, prednisone (see p. 622) is the best choice because it is reliable, inexpensive, and available in a generic form.[5]

Steroids suppress your immune system, lowering your defenses against disease and making you more vulnerable to infections. If you use dexamethasone for a long time, you increase your risk of getting bacterial, viral, parasitic, and fungal infections. Older adults using dexamethasone are more likely than younger users to develop the bone-weakening condition called osteoporosis. Older users are also more likely to develop high blood pressure and to retain fluid while taking this drug.

As with all drugs, you should use the smallest dose of dexamethasone that works. You should also use it for the shortest possible time. If you use systemic steroids (ones that are taken by mouth or injected so that your whole body is exposed to them) for a long time, you may suffer many side effects, and you may also suffer withdrawal symptoms if you stop abruptly.

Before You Use This Drug
Do not use if you have or have had
For injections into the joint:
❑ joint surgery
❑ blood clotting disorders
❑ fracture of the joint
❑ osteoporosis
❑ infection around the joint
❑ unstable joint
For eye dosage form:
❑ eye infections such as tuberculosis, herpes simplex, or other fungal or viral diseases
Tell your doctor if you have or have had
❑ allergies to drugs
❑ AIDS
❑ cataracts
❑ diverticulitis
❑ heart disease
❑ high blood pressure
❑ liver or kidney disease
❑ diabetes
❑ inflammation of throat, stomach, or intestines
❑ glaucoma
❑ fungal infections
❑ myasthenia gravis
❑ herpes sores
❑ tuberculosis or positive TB skin test
Tell your doctor about any other drugs you take, including aspirin, herbs, vitamins, and other non-prescription products.

When You Use This Drug
If taken by mouth or injection:
◆ **If you have been taking this drug for a long time, do not stop taking it suddenly.** Your doctor must lower your dose gradually to prevent withdrawal symptoms.
◆ Do not drink alcohol. Drinking alcohol when you are using this drug increases your chances of getting an ulcer.
◆ If you plan to have any surgery,

including dental, tell your doctor that you take this drug.

◆ Avoid becoming constipated.[6] See ways to avoid constipation on p. 356.

◆ If you are taking this drug for a long time, eat a diet low in salt and rich in potassium, protein, and folic acid. Ask your doctor to tell you how you can get more potassium, protein and folic acid in your diet.

If you are using nose or mouth sprays:

◆ Wear a medical identification bracelet or carry a card stating that you may need additional steroids (tablets or injection) in times of unusual stress or sudden, severe asthma attack.

How To Use This Drug

◆ Crush tablet and mix with food or water, or swallow whole with water. Take with food to decrease stomach upset.

◆ **Use only as prescribed.**

◆ If you miss a dose, take it as soon as you remember, but skip it if it is almost time for the next dose. **Do not take double doses.**

◆ See pp. 611 and 610 for information on inhaled mouth and nose sprays.

For eye, ear, skin dosage forms:

◆ Check with your doctor if your condition does not improve in 1 week, or if it worsens.

Interactions With Other Drugs

The following drugs are listed in *Evaluations of Drug Interactions*, 1991 as causing "highly clinically significant" or "clinically significant" interactions when used together with this drug. There may be other drugs, especially those in the families of drugs listed below, that also will react with this drug to cause severe adverse effects. Make sure to ask your doctor for a complete listing of them and let her or him know if you are taking any of these interacting drugs:

aminoglutethimide; aspirin; carbamazepine; chlorpropamide; cyclosporine; CYTADREN; DIABINESE; dicumarol; DILANTIN; ECOTRIN; ketoconazole; LUMINAL; NIZORAL; phenobarbital; phenytoin; PBR/12; RIFADIN; rifampin; SANDIMMUNE; SOLFOTON; TAO; TEGRETOL; timolol; TIMOPTIC; troleandomycin.

Adverse Effects

Call your doctor immediately:

❑ decreased or blurred vision
❑ frequent urination
❑ increased thirst
❑ numbness, pain, tingling, redness, or swelling at site of injection
❑ hallucinations
❑ depression or mood changes
❑ skin rash or hives
❑ muscle weakness

If using eye dosage form:

❑ blurred vision
❑ eye pain
❑ headache
❑ seeing halos around lights
❑ drooping of the eyelids
❑ unusually large pupils

For long-term use:

❑ persistent abdominal or stomach pain
❑ acne or other skin problems
❑ bloody or black, tarry stools
❑ rounding out of the face
❑ hip pain
❑ increased blood pressure
❑ swelling of feet or lower legs
❑ unusual weight gain
❑ irregular heartbeat
❑ muscle cramps or pain
❑ unusual tiredness or weakness
❑ pain in back, ribs, arms, or legs
❑ muscle weakness
❑ nausea or vomiting
❑ pitting or depression of skin at place of injection
❑ thin, shiny skin
❑ unusual bruising
❑ wounds that will not heal

Call your doctor immediately if these symptoms occur after you have stopped taking this drug:

❑ abdominal or back pain
❑ dizziness or fainting
❑ low fever

- ❑ persistent loss of appetite
- ❑ muscle or joint pain
- ❑ nausea or vomiting
- ❑ returning symptoms of the condition for which you were taking the drug
- ❑ shortness of breath
- ❑ frequent unexplained headaches
- ❑ unusual tiredness or weakness
- ❑ unusual weight loss

Call your doctor if these symptoms continue:
- ❑ indigestion
- ❑ increased appetite
- ❑ nervousness or restlessness
- ❑ trouble sleeping

- ❑ dizziness or lightheadedness
- ❑ flushed face

Periodic Tests
Ask your doctor which of these tests should be done periodically while you are taking this drug:
- ❑ blood or urine glucose concentration
- ❑ eye exams
- ❑ blood levels of potassium, sodium, and calcium
- ❑ stool tests for possible blood loss
- ❑ hypothalamus and pituitary secretion tests

Prednisone
DELTASONE (Upjohn) METICORTEN (Schering)
PREDNICEN-M (Central)

Generic: available

Family: Corticosteroids (see p. 609)

Prednisone (*pred* ni sone), like other steroids (corticosteroids), has many uses. It is used to treat asthma, bronchitis, allergies, and other breathing problems; conditions that produce inflammation, such as arthritis and other joint and muscle disorders; skin conditions; and certain kinds of cancer and infections. If you can take a steroid by mouth, prednisone is the drug of choice because it is reliable, inexpensive, and available in a generic form.[7]

Steroids suppress your immune system, lowering your defenses against disease and making you more vulnerable to infections. If you use prednisone for a long time, you increase your risk of getting bacterial, viral, parasitic, and fungal infections. Older adults using prednisone are more likely than younger users to develop the bone-weakening condition called osteoporosis even with short-term use or low doses.[8]

Older users are also more likely to develop high blood pressure and to retain fluid while taking this drug.

As with all drugs, you should use the smallest dose of prednisone that works. You should also use it for the shortest possible time. If you use systemic steroids (ones that are taken by mouth or injected so that your whole body is exposed to them) for a long time, you may suffer many side effects, and you may also suffer withdrawal symptoms if you stop abruptly.

Before You Use This Drug
Tell your doctor if you have or have had
- ❑ allergies to drugs
- ❑ AIDS
- ❑ heart disease
- ❑ high blood pressure
- ❑ liver or kidney disease
- ❑ diabetes
- ❑ inflammation of throat, stomach, or intestines
- ❑ glaucoma
- ❑ fungal infections

- myasthenia gravis
- osteoporosis
- herpes infection of the eye or mouth
- tuberculosis or positive TB skin test

Tell your doctor about any other drugs you take, including aspirin, herbs, vitamins, and other non-prescription products.

When You Use This Drug

- **If you have been using this drug for a long time, do not stop taking it suddenly.** Your doctor must lower your dose gradually, to prevent withdrawal symptoms.
- Do not drink alcohol. Drinking alcohol while taking this drug increases your risk of getting an ulcer.
- If you plan to have any surgery, including dental, tell your doctor that you take this drug.
- Eat a diet low in salt and rich in potassium, protein, and folic acid. Ask your doctor to tell you how you can get more potassium, protein, and folic acid in your diet.

How To Use This Drug

- Crush tablet and mix with food or water, or swallow whole with water. Take with food to decrease stomach upset.
- Do not take more than prescribed.
- If you miss a dose, take it as soon as you remember, but skip it if it is almost time for the next dose. **Do not take double doses.**

Interactions With Other Drugs

The following drugs are listed in *Evaluations of Drug Interactions,* 1991 as causing "highly clinically significant" or "clinically significant" interactions when used together with this drug. There may be other drugs, especially those in the families of drugs listed below, that also will react with this drug to cause severe adverse effects. Make sure to ask your doctor for a complete listing of them and let her or him know if you are taking any of these interacting drugs:

aspirin; chlorpropamide; cyclosporine; DIABINESE; dicumarol; digoxin; DILANTIN; ECOTRIN; ketoconazole; LANOXIN; LUMINAL; NIZORAL; phenobarbital; phenytoin; RIFADIN; rifampin; SANDIMMUNE; timolol; TIMOPTIC; troleandomycin.

Adverse Effects

Call your doctor immediately:
- decreased or blurred vision
- frequent urination
- increased thirst
- hallucinations
- depression or mood changes
- skin rash or hives

For long-term use:
- persistent abdominal or stomach pain
- acne or other skin problems
- bloody or black, tarry stools
- rounding out of the face
- increased blood pressure
- swelling of feet or lower legs
- unusual weight gain
- irregular heartbeat
- muscle cramps or pain
- unusual tiredness or weakness
- pain in back, ribs, arms, or legs
- muscle weakness
- nausea or vomiting
- thin, shiny skin
- unusual bruising
- wounds that will not heal

Call your doctor immediately if these symptoms occur after you stop taking this drug:
- abdominal or back pain
- dizziness or fainting
- low fever
- persistent loss of appetite
- muscle or joint pain
- nausea or vomiting
- returning symptoms of the condition for which you were taking the drug
- shortness of breath
- frequent unexplained headaches
- unusual tiredness or weakness
- unusual weight loss

Call your doctor if these symptoms continue:
- euphoria [9]

❑ depression[10]
❑ indigestion
❑ increased appetite
❑ nervousness or restlessness
❑ trouble sleeping
❑ dizziness or lightheadedness
❑ flushed face
❑ headache
❑ increased joint pain
❑ nosebleeds
❑ increase in hair on body or face

Periodic Tests
Ask your doctor which of these tests should be done periodically while you are taking this drug:
❑ blood or urine glucose concentration
❑ eye exams
❑ blood levels of potassium, sodium, and calcium
❑ stool tests for possible blood loss
❑ hypothalamus and pituitary secretion test

Methylprednisolone
DEPOPRED (Hyrex) MEDROL (Upjohn)

Generic: available

Family: Corticosteroids (see p. 609)

Methylprednisolone (meth ill pred *niss* oh lone), like other steroids (corticosteroids), has many uses. It is used to treat conditions that produce inflammation, such as arthritis and other joint disorders; allergies, asthma (for which it is the drug of last resort) and other breathing problems; and skin infections. It is also used for acute spinal cord injuries.

Methylprednisolone has several forms for different uses. It can be injected into the muscle, joint, lesion, soft tissue or bloodstream, applied to the skin (topical form), or taken by mouth (oral form). The oral form has limited use. If you need to take a steroid by mouth, prednisone (see p. 622) is the best choice because it is reliable, inexpensive, and available in a generic form.[11]

Steroids suppress your immune system, lowering your defenses against disease and making you more vulnerable to infections. If you use methylprednisolone for a long time, you increase your risk of getting bacterial, viral, parasitic, and fungal infections. Older adults using methylprednisolone are more likely than younger users to develop the bone-weakening condition called osteoporosis. Older users are also more likely to develop high blood pressure and to retain fluid while taking this drug.

As with all drugs, you should use the smallest dose of methylprednisolone that works. You should also use it for the shortest possible time. If you use systemic steroids (ones that are taken by mouth or injected so that your whole body is exposed to them) for a long time, you may suffer many side effects, and you may also suffer withdrawal symptoms if you stop abruptly.

Before You Use This Drug
Do not use if you have or have had
For injections into the joint:
❑ blood clotting disorders
❑ fracture of the joint
❑ infection around the joint
❑ joint surgery
❑ osteoporosis
❑ unstable joint
Tell your doctor if you have or have had
❑ allergies to drugs
❑ AIDS
❑ heart disease
❑ high blood pressure
❑ liver or kidney disease
❑ diabetes

❏ inflammation of throat, stomach, or intestines
❏ glaucoma
❏ fungal infections
❏ myasthenia gravis
❏ osteoprorasis
❏ herpes sores
❏ tuberculosis or positive TB skin test

Tell your doctor about any other drugs you take, including aspirin, herbs, vitamins, and other non-prescription products.

When You Use This Drug
If taken by mouth or injected:
◆ **If you have been taking this drug for a long time, do not stop taking it suddenly.** Your doctor must lower your dose gradually to prevent withdrawal symptoms.
◆ Do not drink alcohol. Drinking alcohol while taking this drug increases your risk of getting an ulcer.
◆ If you plan to have any surgery, including dental, tell your doctor that you take this drug.
◆ If you take this drug for a long time, eat a diet low in salt and rich in potassium, protein, and folic acid. Ask your doctor to tell you how you can get more potassium, protein and folic acid in your diet.

How To Use This Drug
◆ Crush tablet and mix with food or water, or swallow whole with water. Take with food to decrease stomach upset.
◆ Use only as prescribed.
◆ If you miss a dose, take it as soon as you remember, but skip it if it is almost time for the next dose. **Do not take double doses.**

Interactions With Other Drugs
The following drugs are listed in *Evaluations of Drug Interactions,* 1991 as causing "highly clinically significant" or "clinically significant" interactions when used together with this drug. There may be other drugs, especially those in the families of drugs listed below, that also will react with this drug to cause severe adverse effects. Make sure to ask your doctor for a complete listing of them and let her or him know if you are taking any of these interacting drugs:

aspirin; cyclosporine; dicumarol; DILANTIN; ECOTRIN; ketoconazole; LUMINAL; NIZORAL; phenobarbital; phenytoin; RIFADIN; rifampin; SANDIMMUNE; TAO; timolol; TIMOPTIC; troleandomycin.

Adverse Effects
Call your doctor immediately:
❏ decreased or blurred vision
❏ frequent urination
❏ increased thirst
❏ numbness, pain, tingling, redness, or swelling at site of injection
❏ hallucinations
❏ depression or mood changes
❏ skin rash or hives
For long-term use:
❏ persistent abdominal or stomach pain
❏ acne or other skin problems
❏ bloody or black, tarry stools
❏ rounding out of the face
❏ hip pain
❏ increased blood pressure
❏ swelling of feet or lower legs
❏ unusual weight gain
❏ irregular heartbeats
❏ muscle cramps or pain
❏ unusual tiredness or weakness
❏ pain in back, ribs, arms, or legs
❏ muscle weakness
❏ nausea or vomiting
❏ pitting or depression of skin at injection site
❏ thin, shiny skin
❏ unusual bruising
❏ wounds that will not heal
Call your doctor immediately if these symptoms occur after you stop taking this drug:
❏ abdominal or back pain
❏ dizziness or fainting
❏ low fever
❏ persistent loss of appetite
❏ muscle or joint pain
❏ nausea or vomiting

❑ returning symptoms of the condition for which you were taking the drug
❑ shortness of breath
❑ frequent unexplained headaches
❑ unusual tiredness or weakness
❑ unusual weight loss
Call your doctor if these symptoms continue:
❑ indigestion
❑ increased appetite
❑ nervousness or restlessness
❑ trouble sleeping
❑ dizziness or lightheadedness
❑ flushed face
❑ headache

❑ increased joint pain
❑ nosebleeds
❑ increase in hair on body or face

Periodic Tests

Ask your doctor which of these tests should be done periodically while you are taking this drug:
❑ blood or urine glucose concentration
❑ eye exams
❑ blood levels of potassium, sodium, and calcium
❑ stool tests for possible blood loss
❑ hypothalamus and pituitary secretion tests

Betamethasone
DIPROLENE, DIPROSONE, VALISONE (Schering)
SELSTOJECT (Mayrand)

Generic: available

Family: Corticosteroids (see p. 609)

Betamethasone (bay ta *meth* a sone), like other steroids (corticosteroids), is used in several different ways. It is commonly used to reduce inflammation (redness and swelling) and relieve itching caused by many kinds of skin conditions or by a type of mouth lesion. It is also used to treat other conditions which produce inflammation, such as arthritis and other joint problems, and allergies, hay fever, and other breathing problems.

Betamethasone has several forms. It can be injected into the muscle, joint, lesion, soft tissue, or bloodstream. It can be applied to the skin (topical form), to the eye (ophthalmic form), or to the ear (otic form). It also has a form that is taken by mouth, but this should not be used. If you need to take a steroid by mouth, prednisone (see p. 622) is the best choice because it is

reliable, inexpensive, and available in a generic form.[12]

Steroids suppress your immune system, lowering your defenses against disease and making you more vulnerable to infections. If you use betamethasone for a long time, you increase your risk of getting bacterial, viral, parasitic, and fungal infections. Older adults using betamethasone are more likely than younger users to develop the bone-weakening condition called osteoporosis. Older users are also more likely to develop high blood pressure and to retain fluid while taking this drug.

As with all drugs, you should use the smallest dose of betamethasone that works. You should also use it for the shortest possible time. If you use systemic steroids (ones that are taken by mouth or injected so that your whole body is exposed to them) for a long time, you may suffer many side effects, and you may also suffer withdrawal symptoms if you stop abruptly.

Before You Use This Drug

Do not use if you have or have had
For injections into the joint:
- [ ] blood clotting disorders
- [ ] fracture of the joint
- [ ] infection around the joint
- [ ] joint surgery
- [ ] osteoporosis
- [ ] unstable joint

Tell your doctor if you have or have had
- [ ] allergies to drugs
- [ ] AIDS
- [ ] heart disease
- [ ] high blood pressure
- [ ] liver or kidney disease
- [ ] diabetes
- [ ] inflammation of throat, stomach, or intestines
- [ ] glaucoma
- [ ] fungal infections
- [ ] myasthenia gravis
- [ ] osteoporosis
- [ ] herpes sores
- [ ] tuberculosis or positive TB skin test

For form applied to skin:
- [ ] infection or ulceration at place where you will be applying the drug

Tell your doctor about any other drugs you take, including aspirin, herbs, vitamins, and other non-prescription products.

When You Use This Drug

- ◆ If you plan to have any surgery, including dental, tell your doctor that you take this drug.

How To Use This Drug

- ◆ **Use only as prescribed.**
- ◆ If you miss a dose, take it as soon as you remember, but skip it if it is almost time for the next dose. **Do not take double doses.**

On your skin:
- ◆ The preparation may sting when applied.
- ◆ Keep away from eyes.
- ◆ Do not bandage or wrap the area being treated unless your doctor has told you to do so.

- ◆ Check with your doctor if your condition does not improve in 1 week, or if it worsens.
- ◆ If you use the drug correctly, there is no danger that it will be absorbed into your system.

Interactions With Other Drugs

The following drugs are listed in *Evaluations of Drug Interactions*, 1991 as causing "highly clinically significant" or "clinically significant" interactions when used together with this drug. There may be other drugs, especially those in the families of drugs listed below, that also will react with this drug to cause severe adverse effects. Make sure to ask your doctor for a complete listing of them and let her or him know if you are taking any of these interacting drugs:

aminoglutethimide; aspirin; chlorpropamide; cyclosporine; CYTADREN; DIABINESE; dicumarol; DILANTIN; ECOTRIN; ketoconazole; LUMINAL; NIZORAL; phenobarbital; phenytoin; RIFADIN; rifampin; SANDIMMUNE; timolol; TIMOPTIC.

Adverse Effects

Call your doctor immediately:
- [ ] decreased or blurred vision
- [ ] frequent urination
- [ ] increased thirst
- [ ] numbness, pain, tingling, redness, or swelling at site of injection
- [ ] hallucinations
- [ ] depression or mood changes
- [ ] skin rash or hives

For long-term use:
- [ ] persistent abdominal or stomach pain
- [ ] acne or other skin problems
- [ ] bloody or black, tarry stools
- [ ] rounding out of the face
- [ ] hip pain
- [ ] increased blood pressure
- [ ] swelling of feet or lower legs
- [ ] unusual weight gain
- [ ] irregular heartbeat
- [ ] muscle cramps or pain

❑ unusual tiredness or weakness
❑ pain in back, ribs, arms, or legs
❑ muscle weakness
❑ nausea or vomiting
❑ pitting or depression of skin at place of injection
❑ thin, shiny skin
❑ unusual bruising
❑ wounds that will not heal

Call your doctor immediately if these symptoms occur after you have stopped taking the drug:
❑ abdominal or back pain
❑ dizziness or fainting
❑ low fever
❑ persistent loss of appetite
❑ muscle or joint pain
❑ nausea or vomiting
❑ returning symptoms of the condition for which you were taking the drug
❑ shortness of breath

❑ frequent unexplained headaches
❑ unusual tiredness or weakness
❑ unusual weight loss

Call your doctor if these symptoms continue:
❑ indigestion
❑ increased appetite
❑ nervousness or restlessness
❑ trouble sleeping
❑ dizziness or lightheadedness
❑ flushed face
❑ headache
❑ increased joint pain
❑ nosebleeds
❑ increase in hair on body or face

Periodic Tests
Ask your doctor which of these tests should be done periodically while you are taking this drug:
❑ blood or urine glucose concentration
❑ eye exams

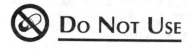 **DO NOT USE**

Alternative treatment: Rest, exercise, physical therapy, and an anti-inflammatory drug such as aspirin.

Orphenadrine
DISIPAL, NORFLEX (Riker)

Family: Muscle Relaxants

Orphenadrine (or *fen a dreen*) is marketed for the relief of severe pain caused by muscle conditions such as sprains and back pain. However, neither the tablet nor the injected form of orphenadrine is effective for these conditions. Instead of taking orphenadrine, you should try rest, exercise, physical therapy, or other treatment recommended by your doctor.

Warning: Special Mental and Physical Adverse Effects
Older adults are especially sensitive to the harmful anticholinergic effects of orphenadrine because of its similarity to the antihistamines. Drugs in this family should not be used unless absolutely necessary.
Mental Effects: confusion, delirium, short-term memory problems, disorientation, and impaired attention.
Physical Effects: dry mouth, constipation, difficulty urinating (especially for a man with an enlarged prostate), blurred vision, decreased sweating with increased body temperature, sexual dysfunction, and worsening of glaucoma.

The level of orphenadrine in this product is not high enough to relax muscles, so this drug will not directly relax tense skeletal muscles. However, the drug is strong enough to have a sedative effect. **Orphenadrine has not been shown to be any more effective than painkillers or anti-inflammatory drugs such as aspirin for relieving the pain of local muscle spasm,[13] yet it has a higher risk of side effects than these painkillers.**

Orphenadrine is similar to a family of drugs called antihistamines, which are used to relieve symptoms of hay fever and other allergies (see p. 382). It may cause some of the same side effects and dangerous drug interactions as antihistamines. Some people taking orphenadrine tablets have experienced blurred vision, dry mouth, mild excitement, temporary dizziness, and lightheadedness as side effects. Many of these effects occur more often in older adults, even at the usual adult dose. Orphenadrine is particularly dangerous for people who have glaucoma, myasthenia gravis, heart problems, or an enlarged prostate.

LIMITED USE

Oxybutynin
DITROPAN (Marion)

Generic: available

Family: Antispasmodics (urinary tract)
Anticholinergics

Oxybutynin (ox i *byoo* ti nin) is used to treat incontinence (loss of bladder control) and frequent urination. The drug decreases spasms in the bladder and increases its ability to hold urine. Oxybutynin has not been proven effective for treating disorders of the stomach and intestines.

This drug has side effects that severely limit its use in older adults. Potential side effects include severe memory impairment, difficulty swallowing, retention of urine, blurred vision, and constipation.[14,15] People over the age of 60 who are taking the usual dose of oxybutynin may experience excitement, restlessness, drowsiness, or confusion.[16]

Before You Use This Drug
Tell your doctor if you have or have had
❑ allergies to drugs
❑ heart disease

❑ reflux esophagitis (a backward flow of stomach contents into the esophagus, which causes heartburn)
❑ abdominal obstruction, disease, or lack of tone

Warning: Special Mental and Physical Adverse Effects

Older adults are especially sensitive to the harmful anticholinergic effects of drugs such as oxybutynin. Drugs in this family should not be used unless absolutely necessary.

Mental Effects: confusion, delirium, short-term memory problems, disorientation, and impaired attention.

Physical Effects: dry mouth, constipation, difficulty urinating (especially for a man with an enlarged prostate), blurred vision, decreased sweating with increased body temperature, sexual dysfunction, and worsening of glaucoma.

❑ glaucoma
❑ liver or kidney impairment
❑ high blood pressure
❑ lung disease
❑ myasthenia gravis
❑ urinary retention
❑ enlarged prostate
❑ enlarged thyroid gland

Tell your doctor about any other drugs you take, including aspirin, herbs, vitamins, and other non-prescription products.

When You Use This Drug
◆ Until you know how you react to this drug, do not drive or perform other activities requiring alertness. Oxybutynin may cause drowsiness, dizziness, and blurred vision.

How To Use This Drug
◆ Take with food or milk to decrease stomach upset.
◆ Use only as prescribed.
◆ Do not expose to heat or direct light. Do not store in the bathroom. Do not let liquid form freeze.
◆ If you miss a dose, take it as soon as you remember, but skip it if it is almost time for the next dose. **Do not take double doses.**

Interactions With Other Drugs
The following drugs are listed in *Evaluations of Drug Interactions,* 1991 as causing "highly clinically significant" or "clinically significant" interactions when used together with this drug. There may be other drugs, especially those in the families of drugs listed below, that also will react with this drug to cause severe adverse effects. Make sure to ask your doctor for a complete listing of them and let her or him know if you are taking this interacting drug:

digoxin; LANOXIN.

Adverse Effects
Call your doctor immediately:
❑ **if you experience signs of overdose:** blurred vision; clumsiness or confusion; convulsions; dizziness; severe drowsiness; severe dry mouth, nose, or throat; fever; hallucinations; shortness of breath; slurred speech; unusual excitement, nervousness, or irritability; unusually fast heartbeat; unusual warmth or dryness of skin
❑ eye pain
❑ skin rash or hives
Call your doctor if these symptoms continue:
❑ constipation
❑ decrease in sweating
❑ dry mouth, nose, throat, or skin
❑ difficulty urinating
❑ difficulty swallowing
❑ drowsiness, headache
❑ nausea or vomiting
❑ trouble sleeping
❑ bloated feeling

Fluorouracil
EFUDEX (Roche) FLUOROPLEX (Herbert)

Generic: available

Family: Anticancer Drug

Fluorouracil (flure oh *yoor* a sill) is used to treat certain kinds of cancer, both inside the hospital in intravenous (IV) form and outside the hospital in a cream and a lotion. **This page only discusses fluorouracil's use outside the hospital in cream or lotion form.**

Fluorouracil cream and lotion are used to treat certain cancers of the skin (basal cell cancers) and certain skin lesions which may lead to cancer. In most cases of cancer, it is better to remove the cancerous cells surgically than to treat them with fluorouracil.

When you apply fluorouracil to a lesion, it causes a sequence of redness, blistering, tenderness, and finally destruction and healing of the abnormal skin. This is a normal reaction. However, treatment may need to be stopped if an extreme reaction occurs in the normal skin around the lesion.

Treatment usually takes 2 to 6 weeks but may take up to 12 weeks. If you are using fluorouracil to treat cancer, or if you are using it to treat a lesion and the lesion comes back after treatment is stopped, you should have a biopsy to make sure that your condition is cured.

When you use fluorouracil on your skin, very little of the drug is absorbed into your system, so side effects such as those caused by intravenous fluorouracil are seldom seen.

Before You Use This Drug
Do not use if you have or have had
❑ recent infection or exposure to chicken pox
❑ shingles (herpes zoster)
Tell your doctor if you have or have had
❑ allergies to drugs

❑ bone marrow depression
❑ liver or kidney disease
❑ recent infection
Tell your doctor about any other drugs you take, including aspirin, herbs, vitamins, and other non-prescription products.

When You Use This Drug
◆ Try to stay out of the sun as much as possible.
◆ Do not use a tight bandage over the area being treated unless your doctor has told you otherwise.
◆ Check with your doctor if the normal skin surrounding the area being treated becomes inflamed.
◆ **Check with your doctor immediately if you notice fever, chills, sore throat, or unusual bleeding or bruising during or after treatment.**
◆ **Because this drug, when absorbed into your body, decreases the number of white blood cells (which fight infection), you may be more likely to get an infection while taking it. Do not get immunizations without your doctor's approval.**
◆ If you plan to have any surgery, including dental, tell your doctor that you take this drug.

Interactions With Other Drugs
Some other drugs that you may be taking (either over-the-counter or prescription drugs) can interact with this one, causing adverse effects. Find out from your doctor what these drugs are and let him or her know if you are taking any of them.

Adverse Effects
Call your doctor if these symptoms continue:
❑ hair loss
❑ nausea, vomiting, appetite loss

❑ rash, hives, or itching
❑ vaginal ulceration, discharge, itching[17]
❑ weakness

Periodic Tests
Ask your doctor which of these tests should

be done periodically while you are taking this drug:
❑ complete blood tests (including hematocrit, platelet count, white blood cell count)

LIMITED USE

Estradiol
ESTRADERM (patch) (Ciba)

Generic: not available

Family: Hormones

> **Warning**
> Estrogen Increases the Risk of Breast and Endometrial (Uterine) Cancer in Postmenopausal Women.

For much more information on estrogens and the risk of breast cancer refer to p. 647.

Estradiol (est ra *dye* all) is an estrogen. In the patch form it is only approved for relief of symptoms of menopause, such as hot flashes, night sweats, and vaginal dryness, itching, or loss of elasticity and for prevention of osteoporosis (see p. 647). The patch form of estradiol may reduce adverse effects on the liver,[18] and be preferred for those who have had side effects from oral contraceptives.

Most women who are using estrogen for symptoms of menopause (such as hot flashes) do not need to take it forever. If you are using estrogen for this reason, you should begin by using it for no more than 6 to 12 months. There is no evidence for increased risk of breast cancer with such short-term use. Then your doctor should slowly take you off the drug, and watch to see if the symptoms return. You should

start taking estrogen again only if the symptoms come back when you stop taking it. If you do keep using it, you should periodically try stopping it, under your doctor's guidance.

Estradiol will not relieve nervousness or depression,[19] nor keep you feeling "young" with soft skin. It is not for minor discomforts of menopause. A drawback for many women is return of monthly vaginal flow

> **Warning**
> Using estrogens increases your risk of endometrial cancer (cancer of the lining of the uterus) by 6 to 8 times. This cancer can be cured by surgery only if it is detected early through a special examination called an endometrial biopsy, and such biopsies are usually done only when a woman is bleeding abnormally. Taking estrogen has also been linked to breast cancer in both men and women. The risk is higher for women who take higher doses or who have used estrogen longer. Experts from the National Cancer Institute and from other countries state that "the prolonged use of estrogens at the time of the menopause may increase the risk of breast cancer by 50% after a 5 to 10 year interval."

after menopause. Adverse effects increase with dose and length of time used.[20,21] Long-term effects whether or not you continue to use the patch are still unknown.[22,23] The lowest dose should be used for the shortest possible time.[24,25,26]

While risks of some diseases fall, other risks rise. Estradiol changes coagulation of blood, and can cause dangerous blood clots or inflame and enlarge veins. At times estrogens increase blood pressure, although the risk is less after menopause.[27]

To reduce the adverse effects of estrogens, a progesterone is often prescribed especially with the oral dosage form but also with the patch.[28] For more information on progesterone, see p. 653.

Menopause is a natural process. As with other changes in the body, disorders may happen. Reassurance should be a valid response from your doctor.

Before You Use This Drug
Do not use if you have or have had
- ❑ history of blood clot formation
- ❑ abnormal or undiagnosed vaginal bleeding
- ❑ breast cancer or a strong family history of breast cancer

Tell your doctor if you have or have had
- ❑ allergies to drugs
- ❑ asthma
- ❑ cancer
- ❑ diabetes
- ❑ endometriosis
- ❑ epilepsy, seizure disorder
- ❑ gallstones or gallbladder disease
- ❑ mental depression
- ❑ migraine headaches
- ❑ kidney disease
- ❑ bone disease
- ❑ breast disease or lumps
- ❑ heart or circulatory disease
- ❑ stroke
- ❑ high levels of calcium in the blood
- ❑ high blood pressure
- ❑ liver disease or jaundice
- ❑ noncancerous growths in uterus

Tell your doctor about any other drugs you take, including aspirin, herbs, vitamins, and other non-prescription products.

When You Use This Drug
- ◆ Take with food to reduce nausea. Estrogen is most likely to cause nausea in the morning.
- ◆ **Do not use more or less often or in a higher or lower dose than prescribed by your doctor.**
- ◆ Do not smoke. Smoking increases your risk of serious side effects such as blood clots, heart attack, or stroke. The risk increases as you get older.
- ◆ Until you know how you react to this drug, do not drive or perform other activities requiring alertness. This drug can cause loss of coordination, blurred vision and drowsiness.
- ◆ If you plan to have any surgery, including dental, tell your doctor that you take this drug.
- ◆ Have your gums cleaned carefully by a dentist at least once a year, as estrogen can cause gum overgrowth.
- ◆ Stay out of the sun as much as possible and do not use sunlamps. Too much sun or sunlamp use while taking estrogen may produce brown, blotchy spots on your skin.

How To Use This Drug
- ◆ If you have been taking an oral estrogen, wait until a week after you stop before applying an estradiol patch.
- ◆ Wash and dry hands.
- ◆ Tear open new patch immediately before use. Do not use scissors to open. The device normally contains bubbles. Discard the liner.
- ◆ Remove old patch.
- ◆ Select an area on the abdomen or buttocks that is clean and dry, and free of hair, oil, breaks or cuts in the skin. Avoid applying to area where the patch is apt to rub loose, such as the waist. Rotate sites so no site is repeated during a week.
- ◆ Never apply patch to a breast.

◆ Press adhesive side of patch firmly on skin, using the palm of your hand and hold for about 10 seconds. Check that contact is good, especially around the edges.

◆ Apply the patch twice a week, the same two days each week, usually three weeks a month. A calendar is enclosed with the patch to aid scheduling.

◆ Reapply the same patch if it loosens or falls off. If necessary put on a new patch. Check patch after bathing, showering, or swimming.

◆ If you forget to change a patch, do so as soon as you remember, then adjust schedule.

◆ Store unopened patches at room temperature. Do not expose to heat. Do not store patches after protective liner has been removed.

Interactions With Other Drugs

The following drugs are listed in *Evaluations of Drug Interactions*, 1991 as causing "highly clinically significant" or "clinically significant" interactions when used together with this drug. There may be other drugs, especially those in the families of drugs listed below, that also will react with this drug to cause severe adverse effects. Make sure to ask your doctor for a complete listing of them and let her or him know if you are taking any of these interacting drugs:

ANECTINE; DELTASONE; LUMINAL; phenobarbital; prednisone; RIFADIN; rifampin; succinylcholine.

Additionally, the *United States Pharmacopeia Drug Information*, 1992 lists these drugs as having interactions of major significance:

bromocriptine; cyclosporine; DANTRIUM; dantrolene; PARLODEL; SANDIMMUME.

Adverse Effects

Call your doctor immediately:
❑ persistent or abnormal vaginal bleeding

❑ drowsiness
❑ dribbling urination
❑ severe headache
❑ sudden loss of coordination
❑ pains in chest, groin, leg, or calf
❑ shortness of breath
❑ slurred speech
❑ vision changes
❑ weakness or numbness in arm or leg
❑ high blood pressure
❑ uncontrolled movements of body
❑ breast lumps or discharge
❑ mental depression
❑ pains in stomach or side
❑ yellowing of eyes or skin
❑ skin rash
❑ thick, white vaginal discharge

Call your doctor if these symptoms continue:
❑ bloating, cramping
❑ nausea, loss of appetite
❑ changes in weight
❑ swelling of ankles and feet
❑ breast swelling and tenderness
❑ changes in sexual desire
❑ changes in hair growth
❑ diarrhea
❑ dizziness, irritability
❑ decreased tolerance to wearing contact lenses

Periodic Tests

Ask your doctor which of these tests should be periodically done while you are taking this drug:
❑ blood pressure
❑ liver function test
❑ pap smear*
❑ yearly mammogram*
❑ physical examination at least every 6 to 12 months, with special attention to the breasts, and including a pelvic exam*
❑ endometrial biopsy

---

* *These should be a part of your normal health care routine.*

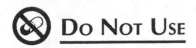 **DO NOT USE**

Alternative treatment: Rest, exercise, physical therapy, and an anti-inflammatory drug such as aspirin.

Cyclobenzaprine
FLEXERIL (Merck)

Family: Muscle Relaxants

Cyclobenzaprine (sye kloe *ben* za preen) tablets are marketed for the relief of severe pain caused by muscle conditions such as sprains and back pain. However, they are not effective for these conditions. Instead of taking cyclobenzaprine, you should try rest, exercise, physical therapy, or other treatment recommended by your doctor.

The level of cyclobenzaprine in the tablets is not high enough to relax muscles, so this drug will not directly relax tense skeletal muscles. However, the drug is strong enough to have a sedative effect. **Cyclobenzaprine has not been shown to be any more effective than painkillers or anti-inflammatory drugs such as aspirin for relieving the pain of local muscle spasm,[29] yet it has a higher risk of side effects than these painkillers.**

Cyclobenzaprine is related to some drugs used to treat depression (tricyclic antidepressants such as amitriptyline, see p. 227, and imipramine, p. 221, and may cause some of the same side effects and dangerous drug interactions. Some people taking cyclobenzaprine have experienced drowsiness, dry mouth, dizziness, nausea, weakness, upset stomach, blurred vision, insomnia, and a fast heartbeat as side effects. If you take cyclobenzaprine for a long time, you can become addicted to it.[30] Cyclobenzaprine is particularly dangerous for people with glaucoma, an enlarged prostate, or heart problems.

LIMITED USE

Nicotine
HABITROL (Basel, Division of Ciba-Geigy)
NICORETTE, NICODERM (Merrell-Dow)
NICOTROL (Warner-Lambert)
PROSTEP (Lederle)

Generic: not available

Family: Aids to Stop Smoking

> **Warning**
> Nicotine has only been shown to be effective when used as an aid to a comprehensive smoking-cessation program. Since the above products contain nicotine, **do not continue to smoke while using them.**

Nicotine (*nick* o teen), whether in a patch or gum, is used to assist quitting smoking. This is the same nicotine found in tobacco, pesticides, and some foods. In patches, gums, and several forms still being developed, nicotine serves as a temporary aid to giving up smoking, by reducing physical withdrawal symptoms. However, unless the nicotine gum or patch is accompanied by a smoking cessation program, the drug works no better than a placebo,[31] because it is treating only the physical, not the psychological addiction.

Withdrawal signs from smoking include fatigue, headache, slowed heart rate, hunger, difficulty concentrating, irritability, and dreams about smoking. These symptoms start about 2 hours after the last cigarette, increase for 24 hours, then decrease over several days or weeks.[32] Signs of withdrawal do not require medical attention. Even people who have severe withdrawal are able to be successful quitting.[33,34]

Simple to use, aids can lull you into unrealistic expectations. To be effective, nicotine patches and gum must be accompanied by changes in behavior. Set a quit date, learn ways to cope with urges to smoke (particularly in the morning, with company, and in response to advertising), and plan ways to cope with relapses.[35] Learn how to deal with anger, anxiety, depression, stress, and tension without smoking. People who smoke are more apt to have a history of being depressed.[36] In addition, those who are anxious or depressed tend to have severe withdrawal.[37,38] Without learning these coping skills, the patch does not work any better than a non-medicated band-aid. While these aids eliminate smoke, they still contain nicotine. **If you continue to smoke while using nicotine replacements, you risk serious heart disease.**[39] Success rates of stopping smoking by using nicotine replacements are low, especially after six months or a year.[40,41,42,43,44,45] However, smokers who try slow withdrawal are apt to smoke less if they resume smoking.[46,47]

Nicotine gum continues to satisfy and reinforce oral habits, and may lessen weight gain.[48] The gum is harder and thicker than regular chewing gums and can loosen dental work. Not everyone masters the chewing technique. Patches are easier to use. The 16-hour patch mimics patterns of smoking, but the 24-hour patches may get you through the strong urge to smoke in the morning. Both types can irritate your skin. Overall, the various patches do not differ in the rate of people who quit smoking.[49]

You must also gradually stop using the gum or patches to prevent addiction to these nicotine products. Quitting smoking reduces your chances of bronchitis, cancers (especially of the lung, mouth, throat, and voicebox), emphysema, heart disease, duodenal ulcers, and dulled sense of smell and taste. People who smoke and take psychotropic drugs often require higher doses of the nicotine and are more apt to have serious adverse effects from the psychotropic drugs, such as akathisia (involuntary restlessness, such as rocking from foot to foot).[50,51] Typically, the amount of weight gain after stopping smoking is a minimal health risk compared to the risks of smoking.[52]

Although most people quit smoking without the aid of organized programs, we recommend such a program especially if you are using these products. Nicotine replacement is not appropriate for light smokers. A number of non-prescription aids to smoking cessation are also available, including plain chewing gum. According to one study, these work just as well as nicotine replacements for light smokers, in the absence of a comprehensive smoking-cessation program.[53] These also are only temporary aids, needing to be augmented by changes in behavior.

Before You Use This Drug
Do not use if you have or have had
❑ myocardial infarction
❑ never smoked
❑ temporomandibular joint (TMJ) disorder, *for gum*
Tell your doctor if you have or have had
❑ allergies to drugs or substances such as adhesives or tapes
❑ angina, chest pain
❑ Buerger's disease
❑ dental work (bridges, crowns, dentures, fillings), *for gum*
❑ depression
❑ diabetes
❑ epilepsy[54]
❑ heart problems

❑ high blood pressure
❑ liver problems[55]
❑ pheochromocytoma
❑ skin problems
❑ throat inflammation or irritation
❑ thyroid problems
❑ ulcers
Tell your doctor about any other drugs you take, including aspirin, herbs, vitamins, and other non-prescription products.

When You Use This Drug
◆ **Stop smoking, or using tobacco in any form. If you continue to smoke and use a nicotine aid, you could get an overdose of nicotine.**
◆ Build social support for your goal to stop smoking, bolstered by counseling and education programs.
◆ Learn skills to avoid giving in to the urge to smoke.
◆ Follow diet recommended by your doctor to avoid weight gain.
◆ Inform your dentist if you are using the gum form.
◆ If you plan to have any surgery, including dental, tell your doctor that you take this drug.

How To Use This Drug
For patches:
◆ Remove patch from outer pouch. A slight discoloration is normal.
◆ Select a site to apply the patch. The site should be clean and dry. The skin should not be broken, irritated, oily, or hairy. Do not use the same site more than once a week. Avoid areas where movement or clothing may dislodge the patch.
◆ Apply sticky side firmly, pressing about 10 seconds, checking that the edges are not loose.
◆ Wash hands after applying the patch.
◆ Leave patch on for the number of hours specified by your doctor.
◆ Replace a patch that falls off, but stay on schedule.
◆ Remove at the same time each day.

◆ Store unopened patches at room temperature. Do not expose to heat. Discard unused opened patches.
◆ Fold used patch with sticky sides together. Place in empty, opened pouch to discard.

For the gum:

◆ Carry the gum with you at all times.
◆ Chew one piece of nicotine gum when you feel the urge to smoke. Chew slowly until you can taste it, or you feel a tingling sensation in your mouth, about 15 chews. When the taste or sensation disappears, resume chewing. Repeat with the same piece of gum for 30 minutes. Avoid swallowing during this time. Do not use carbonated drinks or coffee while chewing nicotine gum.[56]
◆ Do not chew the gum rapidly, or chew more than 30 pieces (60 mg) in one day.
◆ Reduce the number of pieces chewed each day over two to three months. After you are down to one or two pieces of gum a day, stop taking the nicotine gum.
◆ If you accidentally swallow one piece of nicotine gum be alert to gastrointestinal irritation and signs of overdose.
◆ Store gum at room temperature. Protect from light.

Interactions With Other Drugs

The following drugs are listed in *Evaluations of Drug Interactions*, 1991 as causing "highly clinically significant" or "clinically significant" interactions when used together with this drug. There may be other drugs, especially those in the families of drugs listed below, that also will react with this drug to cause severe adverse effects. Make sure to ask your doctor for a complete listing of them and let her or him know if you are taking any of these interacting drugs:

ELIXOPHYLLIN; THEO-DUR; theophylline.

Additionally, the *United States Pharmacopeia Drug Information*, 1992 lists these drugs as having interactions of major significance:

DARVON; HUMULIN; INDERAL; insulin; NOVOLIN; propoxyphene; propranolol.

Adverse Effects

Most adverse effects of nicotine patches and gums are also potential adverse effects from smoking.

Call your doctor or dentist immediately:

❑ damage to dental work or teeth, *for gum*
❑ irregular heartbeat
❑ involuntary movements of arms or legs[57]
❑ **if you experience signs of overdose:** abdominal pain; breathing difficulty; cold sweat; confusion; convulsions; diarrhea; dizziness; fainting; headache; hearing changes; nausea or vomiting; vision changes; severe watering of mouth; severe weakness

Call your doctor if these symptoms continue:

❑ belching, hiccups
❑ body aches
❑ cough
❑ constipation
❑ dry mouth
❑ headache
❑ insomnia, disturbing dreams
❑ irritability
❑ itching, rash, redness of skin,[58] *for patch*
❑ jaw muscle aches, *for gum*
❑ pain in joints or muscles
❑ sore mouth or throat, *for gum*
❑ undesired weight gain

Periodic Tests

Ask your doctor which of these tests should be done periodically while you are taking this drug:

❑ kidney function test
❑ liver function test

Fluocinonide
LIDEX, LIDEX-E (Syntex)

Generic: available

Family: Corticosteroids (see p. 609)

Fluocinonide (floo oh *sin* oh nide) is a steroid that is applied to the skin. It is used to reduce inflammation (redness and swelling) and relieve itching caused by many kinds of skin conditions, such as eczema and psoriasis.

Steroids suppress your immune system, lowering your defenses against disease and making you more vulnerable to infections. If you use fluocinonide for a long time, you increase your risk of getting bacterial, viral, parasitic, and fungal infections

As with all drugs, you should use the lowest possible dose of fluocinonide that works. You should also use it for as short a time as possible and limit the area of your body that you use it on, if possible. A steroid applied to the skin can cause many side effects, especially if you use it for a long time or over a large area so that your whole body absorbs the drug. **If you have used this drug for a long time do not stop suddenly. Your doctor must lower your dose gradually to prevent withdrawal symptoms.**

Before You Use This Drug
Tell your doctor if you have or have had
❑ allergies to drugs
❑ herpes sores
❑ infection or ulceration at place where you will be applying the drug
Tell your doctor about any other drugs you take, including aspirin, herbs, vitamins, and other non-prescription products.

How To Use This Drug
◆ Use only as prescribed.

◆ Spread a very thin layer over the area being treated to minimize absorption of the drug into your body. There is no danger of systemic absorption with correct use.
◆ The preparation may sting when applied.
◆ Do not bandage or wrap the area you are treating unless your doctor has told you to do so.
◆ Do not use around eyes for a long period.
◆ Check with your doctor if your condition does not improve in 1 week or if it worsens.

Interactions With Other Drugs
Some other drugs that you may be taking (either over-the-counter or prescription drugs) can interact with this one, causing adverse effects. Find out from your doctor what these drugs are and let him or her know if you are taking any of them.

Adverse Effects
Call your doctor immediately:
❑ pain, redness, or blisters containing pus
❑ burning, itching, or blistering that was not present before you began using this drug
❑ acne or other skin problems
❑ thinning of skin
❑ bruising
❑ increased hair growth, especially on the face
❑ loss of hair, especially on scalp

Periodic Tests
Ask your doctor which of these tests should be done periodically while you are taking this drug:
❑ blood or urine glucose concentration
❑ eye exams

Flunisolide
NASALIDE (nasal solution spray) (Syntex)
AEROBID (oral aerosol inhaler) (Forest)

Generic: not available

Family: Corticosteroids (see p. 609)

Flunisolide (floo *niss* oh lide) is a steroid (corticosteroid) which is inhaled. It has two forms, a solution that is sprayed into the nose and an inhaler for the mouth. The nose spray is used to treat severe allergies and hay fever and sometimes smooth growths (polyps) in the nose. The inhaler for the mouth mainly benefits people with asthma who need regular, long-term treatment with steroids to control their symptoms. For these people, flunisolide is used after a drug from another family, albuterol or terbutaline (see p. 422) used alone, has not improved the severe chronic symptoms of asthma.[59]

Steroids suppress your immune system, lowering your defenses against disease and making you more vulnerable to infections. If you use flunisolide for a long time, you increase your risk of getting bacterial, viral, parasitic, and fungal infections, especially an infection called oral thrush.

As with all drugs, you should always use flunisolide in the lowest dose that works. You should also take it for the shortest possible time. **If you have used this drug for a long time do not stop suddenly. Your doctor must lower your dose gradually to prevent withdrawal symptoms.**

Before You Use This Drug
Do not use if you have or have had
❑ an allergic reaction to fluorocarbon propellants (the oral inhaler contains fluorocarbons)
Tell your doctor if you have or have had
❑ allergies to drugs
❑ AIDS
❑ heart disease
❑ high blood pressure
❑ liver or kidney disease
❑ diabetes
❑ inflammation of throat, stomach, or intestines
❑ glaucoma
❑ fungal infections
❑ myasthenia gravis
❑ osteoporosis
❑ herpes sores of the eye or mouth
❑ tuberculosis or positive TB skin test
For oral inhaler:
❑ current infection of the mouth
For nose spray:
❑ eye infection
❑ recent nose surgery or injury
❑ ulcers of the nasal septum
Tell your doctor about any other drugs you take, including aspirin, herbs, vitamins, and other non-prescription products.

When You Use This Drug
◆ If you plan to have any surgery, including dental, tell your doctor that you take this drug.
◆ **Do not use this drug to treat a sudden, severe asthma attack. This drug is not strong or fast enough for such an attack.**
◆ Wear a medical identification bracelet or carry a card stating that you may need additional steroids (tablets or injection) in times of unusual stress or sudden, severe asthma attack.

How To Use This Drug
◆ Use only as prescribed.
◆ If you miss a dose, take it as soon as you remember, but skip it if it is almost time for the next dose. **Do not take double doses.**

Oral inhaler:
◆ Clean inhaler every day.
◆ Gargle and rinse your mouth after each time you use the drug, to wash out any of the drug that did not enter your lungs. If your mouth and throat absorb this drug, you may become more susceptible to an infection called thrush.
◆ See p. 388 for information on how to use an inhaler.
◆ See p. 382 for information about drugs taken by nose.

Interactions With Other Drugs

The following drugs are listed in *Evaluations of Drug Interactions*, 1991 as causing "highly clinically significant" or "clinically significant" interactions when used together with this drug. There may be other drugs, especially those in the families of drugs listed below, that also will react with this drug to cause severe adverse effects. Make sure to ask your doctor for a complete listing of them and let her or him know if you are taking any of these interacting drugs:

aspirin; cyclosporine; dicumarol; ECOTRIN; ketoconazole; NIZORAL; SANDIMMUNE; timolol; TIMOPTIC.

Adverse Effects
Call your doctor immediately:
❑ decreased or blurred vision
❑ frequent urination
❑ increased thirst
❑ hallucinations
❑ depression or mood changes
❑ skin rash or hives
❑ muscle weakness
For long-term steroid use:
❑ persistent abdominal or stomach pain
❑ acne or other skin problems
❑ bloody or black, tarry stools
❑ rounding out of the face
❑ hip pain
❑ increased blood pressure
❑ swelling of feet or lower legs
❑ unusual weight gain
❑ irregular heartbeats

❑ muscle cramps or pain
❑ unusual tiredness or weakness
❑ pain in back, ribs, arms, or legs
❑ muscle weakness
❑ nausea or vomiting
❑ unusual bruising
❑ wounds that will not heal
For oral inhaler:
❑ chest pain
❑ chills, cough, fever, sneezing
❑ ear congestion
❑ hoarseness or other voice changes
❑ nose congestion or runny nose
❑ sore throat
❑ white patches inside mouth
❑ difficulty swallowing
❑ eye pain, redness, or tearing
Call your doctor immediately if these symptoms occur after you stop taking this drug:
❑ abdominal or back pain
❑ dizziness or fainting
❑ low fever
❑ persistent loss of appetite
❑ muscle or joint pain
❑ nausea or vomiting
❑ returning symptoms of the condition for which you were taking the drug
❑ shortness of breath
❑ frequent unexplained headaches
❑ unusual tiredness or weakness
❑ unusual weight loss
Call your doctor if these symptoms continue:
❑ indigestion
❑ increased appetite
❑ nervousness or restlessness
❑ trouble sleeping
❑ dizziness or lightheadedness
❑ flushed face
❑ headache
❑ increased joint pain
❑ nosebleeds
❑ increase in hair on body or face
For oral inhaler:
❑ mild abdominal pain, bloated feeling, or gas
❑ constipation or diarrhea
❑ decreased appetite

❑ dry or irritated mouth, nose, tongue, or throat
❑ loss of sense of smell or taste
For nose spray:
❑ bloody mucus or nosebleeds
❑ crusting inside nose
❑ sore throat
❑ trouble breathing
❑ nausea or vomiting
❑ loss of sense of taste or smell

❑ persistent stuffy nose
❑ headache

Periodic Tests
Ask your doctor which of these tests should be done periodically while you are taking this drug:
❑ blood or urine glucose concentration
❑ eye exams

LIMITED USE

ANDROGENS
Methyltestosterone
ORETON METHYL (Schering)
Fluoxymesterone
HALOTESTIN (Upjohn)
ANDROID (Brown)

Generic: available

Family: Hormones

Androgens (*an droe jens*) are male hormones. In older men, they are used to treat impotence (male climacteric), but they are only appropriate in a very limited number of cases. In older women, they are used as a second-choice therapy for advanced breast cancer that is spreading. They are also prescribed for adults with certain rare, hard-to-treat types of anemia.

Most of the prescriptions written for androgens in the United States are for conditions for which they are neither effective nor appropriate. Women have been prescribed androgens to treat a breast condition that most often occurs near or at menopause (fibrocystic disease) and a disorder of the uterine lining (endometriosis), but androgens should not be taken for these conditions. Men suffering

from impotence should take androgens only if their condition is caused by abnormally low androgen levels, which is rare. Most cases of impotence can be more effectively treated by seeking and treating other possible medical causes for the problem, by eliminating medications that can cause impotence, and by counseling. Elderly, bedridden males may react adversely to overstimulation caused by androgens and should not take them.

Long-term, high-dose androgen treatment has been associated with life-threatening liver inflammation and cancer. For older men, taking androgens may increase the risk of developing an enlarged prostate or prostate cancer.

If you are taking androgens, avoid food and drugs containing salt, as they increase the amount of fluid that your body retains. Women who take androgens will notice changes in their body, such as a deeper voice and increased facial hair. Most of these changes are temporary. Women taking androgens for breast cancer should be monitored closely by their doctors because androgen therapy occasionally accelerates the disease.

Before You Use This Drug
Do not use if you have or have had
- ❑ breast cancer
- ❑ prostate cancer

Tell your doctor if you have or have had
- ❑ allergies to drugs
- ❑ diabetes
- ❑ liver or kidney disease
- ❑ heart or blood vessel disease
- ❑ heart attack
- ❑ swelling (edema)
- ❑ high levels of calcium in the blood
- ❑ enlarged prostate gland

Tell your doctor about any other drugs you take, including aspirin, herbs, vitamins, and other non-prescription products.

When You Use This Drug
- ◆ **Do not use more or less often or in a higher or lower dose than prescribed.**
- ◆ **Caution diabetics:** Check urine sugar levels regularly. This drug affects glucose tolerance.

How To Use This Drug
- ◆ *If you use the tablet that is to be swallowed,* take it with or after food to reduce stomach upset.
- ◆ *If you use the buccal tablet,* place it in the space between your cheek and gum and allow it to dissolve slowly. Do not eat, drink, chew, or smoke while the tablet is dissolving. Do not swallow it. After the tablet is dissolved and you can no longer taste it, remove the remaining sugar residue by thoroughly brushing your teeth or rinsing your mouth.
- ◆ Do not store in the bathroom. Do not expose to heat, strong light, or moisture.
- ◆ If you miss a dose, take it as soon as you remember, but skip it if it is almost time for the next dose. **Do not take double doses.**

Interactions With Other Drugs
The following drugs are listed in *Evaluations of Drug Interactions,* 1991 as causing "highly clinically significant" or "clinically significant" interactions when used together with this drug. There may be other drugs, especially those in the families of drugs listed below, that also will react with this drug to cause severe adverse effects. Make sure to ask your doctor for a complete listing of them and let her or him know if you are taking any of these interacting drugs:

carbamazepine; COUMADIN; TEGRETOL; warfarin.

Adverse Effects
Call your doctor immediately:
In women:
- ❑ acne
- ❑ enlarged clitoris
- ❑ deepening of voice, hoarseness
- ❑ changes in hair growth

In men:
- ❑ frequent or continuing erection
- ❑ frequent or difficult urination
- ❑ breast swelling or tenderness
- ❑ unusual increase in sexual desire

In women and men:
- ❑ mental changes
- ❑ shortness of breath
- ❑ changes in skin color
- ❑ dizziness
- ❑ frequent or persistent headache
- ❑ unusual tiredness
- ❑ flushed or red skin
- ❑ nausea, vomiting, loss of appetite
- ❑ skin rash, hives, or itching
- ❑ swelling of feet or lower legs
- ❑ unusual bleeding
- ❑ yellow eyes or skin
- ❑ black, tarry stools
- ❑ vomiting blood
- ❑ pale stools
- ❑ dark urine
- ❑ abdominal pain or swelling
- ❑ sore throat and fever
- ❑ purple-red spots on body, nose, or inside of mouth

Call your doctor if these symptoms continue:
❑ changes in weight
❑ breast swelling and tenderness
❑ changes in sexual desire
❑ changes in hair growth
❑ acne

Periodic Tests
Ask your doctor which of these tests should be done periodically while you are taking this drug:
❑ physical exam, at least every 6 to 12 months
❑ liver function tests
❑ blood levels of calcium and cholesterol
❑ urine levels of calcium
❑ hemoglobin and hematocrit levels

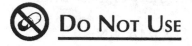 **DO NOT USE**

Alternative treatment: Rest, exercise, physical therapy, and an anti-inflammatory drug such as aspirin.

Chlorzoxazone
PARAFON FORTE DSC (McNeil Pharmaceutical)

Family: Muscle Relaxants

Chlorzoxazone (klor *zox* a zone) tablets are marketed for the relief of severe pain caused by muscle conditions such as sprains and back pain. However, the drug is not effective for these conditions. Instead of using chlorzoxazone, you should try rest, exercise, physical therapy, or other treatment recommended by your doctor.

The level of chlorzoxazone in the tablets is not high enough to relax muscles, so this drug will not directly relax tense skeletal muscles. However, the drug is strong enough to have a sedative effect. **Chlorzoxazone has not been shown to be any more effective than painkillers or anti-inflammatory drugs such as aspirin for relieving the pain of local muscle spasm,[60] yet it has a higher risk of side effects than these painkillers.**

Some people taking chlorzoxazone have experienced drowsiness, headache, upset stomach, nausea, vomiting, heartburn, constipation, diarrhea, and loss of appetite as side effects. If you use this drug for a long time, you can become addicted to it.[61] Some people taking chlorzoxazone have developed liver problems,[62] and the drug is particularly dangerous for people with liver disease.

The brand-name product containing chlorzoxazone was reformulated. The old version, Parafon Forte, contained chlorzoxazone and acetaminophen. The new product, Parafon Forte DSC, contains twice the amount of chlorzoxazone as the old version and no acetaminophen. Both products are equally ineffective.

Prednisolone
PRED FORTE (Allergan) METRETON (Schering)

Generic: available

Family: Corticosteroids (see p. 609)

Prednisolone (pred *niss* oh lone), like other corticosteroids (steroids), has many uses. It is most commonly used to treat eye infections that have produced inflammation. It is also used for other conditions in which there is inflammation, such as arthritis and other joint and muscle disorders; allergies, asthma, hay fever, and other breathing problems; and skin infections.

Prednisolone has several forms for different uses. It can be injected into the muscle, joint, lesion, soft tissue, or bloodstream; applied to the eye (ophthalmic form) or the ear (otic form); or taken by mouth. You should not use the form of prednisolone that is taken by mouth. If you need to take a steroid by mouth, prednisone (see p. 622) is the best choice because it is reliable, inexpensive, and available in a generic form.[63]

Steroids suppress your immune system, lowering your defenses against disease and making you more vulnerable to infections. If you use prednisolone for a long time, you increase your risk of getting bacterial, viral, parasitic, and fungal infections. Older adults using prednisolone are more likely than younger users to develop the bone-weakening condition called osteoporosis. Older users are also more likely to develop high blood pressure and to retain fluid while taking this drug.

As with all drugs, you should use the smallest dose of prednisolone that works. You should also use it for the shortest possible time. If you use systemic steroids (ones that are taken by mouth or injected so that your whole body is exposed to them) for a long time, you may suffer many side effects, and you may also suffer withdrawal symptoms if you stop abruptly.

Before You Use This Drug
Do not use if you have or have had
For injections into the joint:
❑ joint surgery
❑ blood clotting disorders
❑ fracture of the joint
❑ osteoporosis
❑ infection around the joint
❑ unstable joint
For eye dosage form:
❑ eye infections such as herpes, tuberculosis, or others caused by a fungus or virus
Tell your doctor if you have or have had
❑ allergies to drugs
❑ AIDS
❑ cataracts
❑ heart disease
❑ high blood pressure
❑ liver or kidney disease
❑ diabetes
❑ inflammation of throat, stomach, or intestines
❑ glaucoma
❑ fungal infections
❑ myasthenia gravis
❑ osteoporosis
❑ herpes sores
❑ tuberculosis or positive TB skin test
Tell your doctor about any other drugs you take, including aspirin, herbs, vitamins, and other non-prescription products.

When You Use This Drug
If taken by mouth or injected:
◆ **If you have been taking this drug for a long time, do not stop taking it suddenly.** Your doctor must lower your dose gradually, to prevent withdrawal symptoms.
◆ Do not drink alcohol. Drinking alcohol while taking this drug increases your risk of getting an ulcer.
◆ If you plan to have any surgery, including dental, tell your doctor that you take this drug.

◆ If you take this drug for a long time, eat a diet low in salt and rich in potassium, protein, and folic acid. Ask your doctor how you can get more potassium, protein, and folic acid in your diet.

How To Use This Drug
◆ Use only as prescribed.
Eye dosage form:
◆ Follow directions on p. 582 for applying eye drugs.
◆ Check with your doctor if condition does not improve in 1 week, or if it worsens.
◆ If you miss a dose, take it as soon as you remember, but skip it if it is almost time for the next dose. **Do not take double doses.**

Interactions With Other Drugs
The following drugs are listed in *Evaluations of Drug Interactions*, 1991 as causing "highly clinically significant" or "clinically significant" interactions when used together with this drug. There may be other drugs, especially those in the families of drugs listed below, that also will react with this drug to cause severe adverse effects. Make sure to ask your doctor for a complete listing of them and let her or him know if you are taking any of these interacting drugs:

aspirin; chlorpropamide; cyclosporine; DIABINESE; dicumarol; digoxin; DILANTIN; ECOTRIN; ketoconazole; LANOXIN; LUMINAL; NIZORAL; phenobarbital; phenytoin; RIFADIN; rifampin; RIMACTIN; SANDIMMUNE; timolol; TIMOPTIC.

Adverse Effects
Call your doctor immediately:
❑ decreased or blurred vision
❑ frequent urination
❑ increased thirst
❑ numbness, pain, tingling, redness, or swelling at site of injection
❑ hallucinations
❑ depression or mood changes
❑ skin rash or hives

If using eye dosage form:
❑ blurred vision
❑ eye pain
❑ headache
❑ seeing halos around lights
❑ drooping of the eyelids
❑ unusually large pupils
For long-term use:
❑ persistent abdominal or stomach pain
❑ acne or other skin problems
❑ bloody or black, tarry stools
❑ rounding out of the face
❑ hip pain
❑ increased blood pressure
❑ swelling of feet or lower legs
❑ unusual weight gain
❑ irregular heartbeats
❑ muscle cramps or pain
❑ unusual tiredness or weakness
❑ pain in back, ribs, arms, or legs
❑ muscle weakness
❑ nausea or vomiting
❑ pitting or depression of skin at place of injection
❑ thin, shiny skin
❑ unusual bruising
❑ wounds that will not heal
Call your doctor immediately if these symptoms occur after you stop taking this drug:
❑ abdominal or back pain
❑ dizziness or fainting
❑ low fever
❑ persistent loss of appetite
❑ muscle or joint pain
❑ nausea or vomiting
❑ returning symptoms of the condition for which you were taking the drug
❑ shortness of breath
❑ frequent unexplained headaches
❑ unusual tiredness or weakness
❑ unusual weight loss
Call your doctor if these symptoms continue:
❑ indigestion
❑ increased appetite
❑ nervousness or restlessness
❑ trouble sleeping
❑ dizziness or lightheadedness

❏ flushed face
❏ headache
❏ increased joint pain
❏ nosebleeds
❏ increase in hair on body or face
If using eye dosage form:
❏ burning, stinging, or watering of
   the eyes

Periodic Tests
Ask your doctor which of these tests should be done periodically while you are taking this drug:
❏ blood or urine glucose concentration
❏ eye exams
❏ blood levels of potassium, sodium, and calcium
❏ stool tests for possible blood loss
❏ hypothalamus and pituitary secretion tests

LIMITED USE

ESTROGENS
Conjugated Estrogens
PREMARIN (Ayerst)
Estropipate
OGEN (Abbott)
Estradiol
ESTRACE (cream) (Mead Johnson)
Diethylstilbestrol
DES (Lilly)

Generic: available

Family: Hormones

Estrogen (*ess* troe jen) is a hormone normally produced in women's bodies, mainly by the ovaries. When a woman reaches menopause, her body's production of estrogen declines noticeably. Doctors commonly prescribe estrogen for women at menopause to treat symptoms such as hot flashes and vaginal dryness. Doctors also prescribe estrogen to replace normal hormone production in women who have had their ovaries removed (usually as part of a hysterectomy, the removal of the uterus), to prevent a bone disease known as osteoporosis in older women, and to treat certain hormone-sensitive cancers in both men and women. Many women on estrogen pills have been told to take them for the rest of their lives. **Estrogens have several serious risks, and you should therefore take them only if absolutely necessary.**

Estrogens Cause Breast Cancer
The most thorough review of all valid epidemiological studies analyzing the relationship between menopausal estrogens and breast cancer was recently published in the *Journal of the American Medical Association*.[64] The authors, from the Centers for Disease Control (CDC), found that there was a direct linear relationship between the duration of use of menopausal estrogens and the risk of breast cancer such that if a

woman used the pills for 15 years, she had a 30% increased risk of breast cancer. If use were for 25 years, a "goal" toward which many doctors are pointing their patients, there would be a 50% increased risk of breast cancer. The authors divided up the studies according to the quality of the epidemiological research, such as how well the breast cancer cases were matched with the controls who did not have breast cancer to make the comparison more valid.

What is clear is that those studies which failed to show an increase in breast cancer associated with the use of menopausal estrogens were judged by the authors to be of significantly lower quality in terms of the validity of the research than the studies which found an increased risk of breast cancer.

The authors examined the increased risk of breast cancer in the 5 studies which were judged to be of high quality. When just the 5 high quality studies were analyzed, the 15-year risk was an increase of 60% in breast cancer and the 25-year risk would increase 100%, or a doubling in the amount of breast cancer.

Warning

Using estrogens increases your risk of endometrial cancer (cancer of the lining of the uterus) by 6 to 8 times. This cancer can be cured by surgery only if it is detected early through a special examination called an endometrial biopsy, and such biopsies are usually done only when a woman is bleeding abnormally. Taking estrogen has also been linked to breast cancer in both men and women. The risk is higher for women who take higher doses or who have used estrogen longer. Experts from the National Cancer Institute and from other countries state that "the prolonged use of estrogens at the time of the menopause may increase the risk of breast cancer by 50% after a 5 to 10 year interval."[65]

The authors estimate that, based on an increased risk of 30% (the lower estimate, based on high and lower quality studies), the excess number of cases of breast cancer which would be caused by the use of estrogens by 3 million women for 15 years would be 4,708 new cases of breast cancer and 1,468 breast cancer deaths. If the excess risk is 60%, as found in the high quality studies, there would be about 10,000 excess cases of breast cancer and 3,000 deaths. For 25 years of use, these grim statistics would get even worse. National Cancer Institute epidemiologist Dr. Robert Hoover, director of NCI's Environmental Epidemiology Branch, who is a co-author of several of the studies reviewed by the CDC, has told us that:

"The fact that ovarian hormones might relate to increased risk of breast cancer is not on the bizarre fringe of biological reasoning. The biological plausibility was established 100 years ago, so new data which shows that women on replacement therapy have an increased risk is exactly what you would predict."

Because of these risks, any older woman taking estrogen should have a yearly checkup that includes careful breast and pelvic examinations. It may also include an endometrial biopsy and mammography. All women should examine their own breasts monthly (your doctor can teach you how).

Symptoms of Menopause

Most women who are taking estrogen for symptoms of menopause (such as hot flashes) do *not* need to take it forever. If you are taking estrogen for the symptoms of menopause, you should begin by taking it for no more than 6 to 12 months. Then your doctor should slowly take you off the drug and watch to see if the symptoms return. You should start taking estrogen again *only* if the symptoms come back when you stop taking it. If you do keep taking it, you should periodically try stopping it again, under your doctor's guidance.

Some women taking estrogen for symptoms of menopause should not be taking it at all. Estrogen should not be used to treat vague symptoms such as fatigue or sadness. For vaginal dryness, estrogen pills are effective, but there are equally effective alternatives which may be safer. If you need to treat vaginal dryness, you should start by trying lubricant creams without hormones, and if these fail, try a vaginal cream containing estrogen. Although the estrogen in vaginal creams is absorbed into your system, it is not yet clear whether this form has as high a risk as estrogen pills.

Osteoporosis

Estrogen is sometimes prescribed to prevent a bone disease called osteoporosis in older women. In osteoporosis, your bones become frail, placing you at greater risk of hip and other fractures. Many women will never develop this problem. Women who are thin or small-boned, particularly if they are Asian or white, and women who drink more than two alcoholic drinks a day are at higher risk of osteoporosis. Black women, heavy women, and women who get a lot of exercise have a lower risk.

Osteoporosis has no effective treatment, but you can take steps to prevent it. These include getting a lot of calcium in your diet from early adulthood on (see calcium, p. 561) and regularly doing "weight-bearing" exercise such as jogging, walking, tennis, and bicycling. These two steps are enough to prevent osteoporosis in many adults.

Ask your doctor to review your continued need and dose of any drug which causes you to be drowsy or dizzy. Certain diuretics (water pills) may prevent fractures by increasing minerals in the bone,[66] but cause fractures from falls due to dizziness. Paying attention to safety also prevents fractures. Use handrails going up or down stairs, and wear shoes with soles that grip. Use adequate light and vision correction, especially at night. Avoid using throw rugs.

Estrogen therapy, if begun within 6 years after menopause, will slow the weakening of bone in women's bodies. You should only be taking estrogen for this purpose if you are at high risk for osteoporosis. Only for women in the high-risk group may the benefits of estrogen in preventing osteoporosis outweigh the considerable risks of taking the drug. If you are taking estrogen for osteoporosis, you only need a low daily dose of 0.625 milligram.

Preventing Heart Disease?

Researchers are investigating the effect of estrogen therapy on women's risk of heart and blood vessel diseases such as heart attacks, stroke, and blood clots. In general, women are less likely to have heart attacks than men, but their risk increases after menopause. Some researchers have suggested that estrogen protects women from heart and blood vessel diseases and that their risk of these diseases rises after menopause because their bodies are producing less estrogen. This has led to research to see whether taking estrogen after menopause will protect women from heart disease. There is cause for concern, however, because estrogen in birth control pills used by younger women has been shown to increase the risk of heart and blood vessel disease.

A Dutch epidemiologist has seriously questioned the strength of the evidence that estrogens prevent heart disease. He pointed out that in the early 1960s several researchers argued that estrogens were the ultimate protection against all kinds of "senescence" [physical problems of aging] and that estrogens could "delay the 'natural' rise of cardiovascular disease with age." But now the main cardiovascular debate is just beginning "after a lull caused by studies showing an *increased* risk of cardiovascular disease caused by estrogens." Dr. Vandenbroucke, of the Department of Clinical Epidemiology at Leiden University Hospital, referred to studies published in the U.S. in the 1970s raising serious doubts about estrogen's cardioprotective effects.[67]

One set of studies involved the use of higher-dose conjugated estrogens (such as in Premarin) in men with previous proven heart attacks. The Coronary Drug Project, involving men, was randomized so that the drug and placebo groups were the same and the experiment had to be stopped because in the highest estrogen dose group (5 milligrams), men actually had an *increased* incidence of adverse events such as blood clots in the lungs and thrombophlebitis, with an increased incidence of heart attacks. In the lower (2.5 milligrams) dose group, there was also an increased amount of blood clots and thrombophlebitis. Not only did estrogens, at those doses, do more harm than good in men but other estrogens, in the form of the birth control pill (estrogen plus progestagen — a combination of hormones now used by about 1/3 of women taking menopausal estrogens) also caused an increased cardiovascular risk in women. (The current studies on women, with one exception, were not randomized so that the group getting estrogens was not necessarily the same as the control group.)

In one widely-cited study on the beneficial cardiac effects of estrogens in women[68] the authors found a 50% reduction in coronary heart disease in nurses who used estrogen. But, when nurses who had cancer or coronary heart disease at the beginning of the study were excluded for the analysis, the risk reduction for total mortality, which Vandenbroucke correctly points out is more important than just cardiac deaths, was only 10% and was not statistically significant. In other non-randomized studies, after adjusting for factors such as this, there was also a reduction in the apparent benefits of estrogens after the adjustments were made.

It is still entirely possible that a woman who receives a prescription for hormone replacement is, at the start, subtly healthier, or more determined to stay that way, than a woman who forgoes this therapy. A recent study on baseline risk factors in women who were part of a study on hormone replacement therapy found that almost twice as many women who did not take estrogens (28%) were in the top obesity group as women who took estrogens (15.4%) More non-estrogen takers also had diabetes and high blood pressure.[69] Vandenbroucke concludes that the current kind of studies on the benefit of estrogen therapy are unlikely to be useful because they "all have the same defect — i.e., lack of comparability between users and non-users. Perhaps we should demand some colossal well-controlled trials before we let the genie of universal preventive prescription escape from the bottle."

Also of importance, as brought out at a recent Food and Drug Administration hearing on estrogens and heart disease, is the fact that if we would apply what is known about preventing heart disease in women without drugs — increases in exercise, weight loss, eating less cholesterol and harmful fats, stopping smoking and treating high blood pressure — we could reduce heart disease in women by 90%, without significantly increasing the risks of breast and uterine cancer as occurs with the estrogen approach.

To summarize, taking estrogen increases the risk of one serious disease (two kinds of cancer) and protects against another (osteoporosis). Researchers are still trying to define the risks and benefits of estrogen with regard to heart and blood vessel disease in older women. At this time, we do not have enough information to know whether long-term use of estrogen by most older women will, on balance, do more harm or more good.

Internist Dr. Paul Stolley, formerly President of the Society for Epidemiological Research, a Professor at the University of Maryland School of Medicine and an expert on estrogens, has said:

"The famous philosopher Bertrand Russell said that when the experts are not agreed, the non-expert does well to suspend judgement. That could apply to HRT

(hormone replacement therapy). The woman with a predictably high risk of developing osteoporosis might wish to run the known and unknown risks of HRT (with careful monitoring for the fairly certain benefit in the prevention of osteoporosis). However, the woman with no special risk factors of osteoporosis would do well to consider waiting for a few years with the hope that new knowledge will permit a more informed choice."

Doctors frequently prescribe estrogen together with a progestin (see p. 653), a synthetic version of another female hormone normally produced in a woman's body before menopause. It is hoped that a combination of estrogen and progestin will have a lower risk of cancer of the uterine lining than estrogen alone. Progestins carry their own risks of blood clots and breast cancer. It is not yet clear whether adding progestin to estrogen is more protective or more dangerous than taking estrogen alone.

If you are taking estrogen after menopause, you should usually be taking it on a cyclical schedule, such as 3 weeks on and 1 week off. For treatment of menopausal symptoms, estrogen is also available in a skin patch (see p. 632), which releases the drug into your body slowly.

Before You Use This Drug
Do not use if you have or have had
❏ history of blood clot formation
❏ abnormal or undiagnosed vaginal bleeding
❏ breast cancer or a strong family history of breast cancer
Tell your doctor if you have or have had
❏ allergies to drugs
❏ asthma
❏ cancer
❏ diabetes
❏ endometriosis
❏ epilepsy, seizure disorder
❏ gallstones or gallbladder disease
❏ mental depression
❏ migraine headaches

❏ kidney disease
❏ bone disease
❏ breast disease or lumps
❏ heart or circulatory disease
❏ stroke
❏ high levels of calcium in the blood
❏ high blood pressure
❏ liver disease or jaundice
❏ noncancerous growths in uterus
Tell your doctor about any other drugs you take, including aspirin, herbs, vitamins, and other non-prescription products.

When You Use This Drug
◆ **Do not use more or less often or in a higher or lower dose than prescribed by your doctor.**
◆ Do not smoke. Smoking increases your risk of serious side effects such as blood clots, heart attack, or stroke. The risk increases as you get older.
◆ Until you know how you react to this drug, do not drive or perform other activities requiring alertness. This drug can cause loss of coordination, blurred vision and drowsiness.
◆ If you plan to have any surgery, including dental, tell your doctor that you take this drug.
◆ Have your gums cleaned carefully by a dentist at least once a year, as estrogen can cause gum overgrowth.
◆ Stay out of the sun as much as possible and do not use sunlamps. Too much sun or sunlamp use while taking estrogen may produce brown, blotchy spots on your skin.

How To Use This Drug
◆ Take with or right after food to decrease stomach upset. Estrogen is most likely to cause nausea in the morning.
◆ Do not store in the bathroom. Do not expose to heat, strong light, or moisture.
◆ If you miss a dose, take it as soon as you remember, but skip it if it is almost time for the next dose. **Do not take double doses.**
If you are using skin patches see p. 632.

Interactions With Other Drugs

The following drugs are listed in *Evaluations of Drug Interactions*, 1991 as causing "highly clinically significant" or "clinically significant" interactions when used together with this drug. There may be other drugs, especially those in the families of drugs listed below, that also will react with this drug to cause severe adverse effects. Make sure to ask your doctor for a complete listing of them and let her or him know if you are taking any of these interacting drugs:

ANECTINE; DELTASONE: LUMINAL; phenobarbital; prednisone; RIFADIN; rifampin; succinylcholine.

Additionally, the *United States Pharmacopeia Drug Information*, 1992 lists these drugs as having interactions of major significance:

bromocriptine; cyclosporine; DANTRIUM; dantrolene; PARLODEL; SANDIMMUNE.

Adverse Effects

Call your doctor immediately:
- ❏ persistent or abnormal vaginal bleeding
- ❏ drowsiness
- ❏ dribbling urination
- ❏ severe headache
- ❏ sudden loss of coordination
- ❏ pains in chest, groin, leg, or calf
- ❏ shortness of breath
- ❏ slurred speech
- ❏ vision changes
- ❏ weakness or numbness in arm or leg

- ❏ high blood pressure
- ❏ uncontrolled movements of body
- ❏ breast lumps or discharge
- ❏ mental depression
- ❏ pains in stomach or side
- ❏ yellowing of eyes or skin
- ❏ skin rash
- ❏ thick, white vaginal discharge

Call your doctor if these symptoms continue:
- ❏ bloating, cramping
- ❏ nausea, loss of appetite
- ❏ changes in weight
- ❏ swelling of ankles and feet
- ❏ breast swelling and tenderness
- ❏ changes in sexual desire
- ❏ changes in hair growth
- ❏ diarrhea
- ❏ dizziness, irritability
- ❏ decreased tolerance to wearing contact lenses

Periodic Tests

Ask your doctor which of these tests should be done periodically while you are taking this drug:
- ❏ blood pressure
- ❏ liver function test
- ❏ pap smear*
- ❏ yearly mammogram*
- ❏ physical examination at least every 6 to 12 months, with special attention to the breasts, and including a pelvic exam*
- ❏ endometrial biopsy

*These should be a part of your normal health care routine.

LIMITED USE

PROGESTINS
Medroxyprogesterone
PROVERA (Upjohn)
AMEN (Carnrik GW)
Norethindrone Acetate
AYGESTIN (Ayerst)

Generic: available

Family: Hormones

Progesterone is a hormone normally produced in women's bodies. Progestins (proe *jess* tins) are synthetic variations of progesterone. For younger women, doctors prescribe synthetic progesterone to treat irregular menstrual bleeding and endometriosis. Doctors are increasingly prescribing progestins to older women who are taking another hormone, estrogen, to treat symptoms of menopause (such as hot flashes) or to prevent osteoporosis (bone frailty). Progestins are also used in special circumstances to treat uterine, breast, and kidney cancer. If you are taking progestins, you may bleed every month even if you have passed menopause.

Because progestins have potentially significant risks, you should only use them (or progestin and estrogen combinations) to treat serious symptoms, and then for as short a time as possible. It is still unclear whether the benefits of long-term treatment with estrogen and progestins outweigh the risks.

When you take estrogen (for example, to treat symptoms of menopause), the lining of your uterus thickens. Many doctors are prescribing progestins along with estrogen to slow this thickening and to prevent the cancer of the lining of the uterus (endometrial cancer) that estrogen can cause.

Progestin use has been associated with blood clots, strokes, and blindness in women. The drug causes breast and uterine cancers when administered to laboratory mammals, and researchers are investigating whether it causes breast cancer in women by itself or further increases the risk of breast cancer when used with estrogen.

The combination of progestins and estrogen that many doctors are prescribing to older women is similar to that in birth control pills. In birth control pills, this combination has been known to cause serious side effects to the heart and blood vessels, such as heart attack and stroke. These side effects are more common in older women, especially older women who smoke. Using an estrogen-progestin combination later in life for purposes other than birth control may also increase the risk of such side effects.

Before You Use This Drug
Do not use if you have or have had
❑ history of blood clot formation
❑ abnormal or undiagnosed vaginal bleeding
❑ liver disease
Tell your doctor if you have or have had
❑ allergies to drugs
❑ asthma
❑ cancer
❑ diabetes
❑ epilepsy, seizure disorder
❑ mental depression
❑ migraine headaches
❑ kidney disease

❑ breast disease or lumps
❑ heart or circulatory disease
Tell your doctor about any other drugs you take, including aspirin, herbs, vitamins, and other non-prescription products.

When You Use This Drug

◆ **Do not use more or less often or in a higher or lower dose than your doctor has prescribed.**

◆ If you plan to have any surgery, including dental, tell your doctor that you take this drug.

How To Use This Drug

◆ Take with or right after food to decrease stomach upset.

◆ Do not store in the bathroom. Do not expose to heat, strong light, or moisture.

◆ If you miss a dose, take it as soon as you remember, but skip it if it is almost time for the next dose. **Do not take double doses.**

Interactions With Other Drugs

The following drugs are listed in *Evaluations of Drug Interactions*, 1991 as causing "highly clinically significant" or "clinically significant" interactions when used together with this drug. There may be other drugs, especially those in the families of drugs listed below, that also will react with this drug to cause severe adverse effects. Make sure to ask your doctor for a complete listing of them and let her or him know if you are taking this interacting drug:

cyclosporine; SANDIMMUNE.

Adverse Effects

Call your doctor immediately:
❑ persistent or abnormal vaginal bleeding
❑ bulging eyes
❑ double vision, loss of vision
❑ skin rash, itching
❑ severe headache
❑ sudden loss of coordination
❑ pains in chest, groin, leg, calf
❑ sudden shortness of breath
❑ slurred speech
❑ vision changes
❑ weakness or numbness in arm or leg
❑ breast lumps or discharge
❑ mental depression
❑ pains in stomach or side
❑ yellow eyes or skin
Call your doctor if these symptoms continue:
❑ nausea, loss of appetite
❑ changes in weight
❑ swelling of ankles and feet
❑ breast swelling and tenderness
❑ changes in sexual desire
❑ changes in hair growth
❑ acne

Periodic Tests

Ask your doctor which of these tests should be done periodically while you are taking this drug:
❑ physical exam, at least every 6 to 12 months*
❑ breast self-examination, monthly*

---

*These should be a part of your normal health care routine.

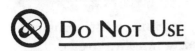 **Do Not Use**

Alternative treatment: Drink plenty of fluids and treat the cause of the pain, such as the urinary tract infection.

Phenazopyridine
PYRIDIUM (Parke-Davis)

Family: Urinary Analgesics (Painkillers)

Phenazopyridine (fen az oh *peer* i deen) is used to treat pain, burning, and other symptoms when the lower part of the urinary tract (bladder) is irritated due to an infection or surgery. **Do not take this drug.** Because older people's bodies eliminate drugs less effectively than younger people's, this drug can stay in your body much longer than it should, and can build up until it reaches dangerously high levels in your bloodstream. This can lead to harmful side effects. Also, this drug can cause cancer, according to the World Health Organization's International Agency for Research on Cancer.[70]

Instead of prescribing this drug to relieve pain and irritation, a physician should find and treat the *cause* of the pain and irritation.

 Do Not Use
(Except for treatment of certain types of skin cancer and severe acne.)

Alternative Treatment: Protection from the sun.

Tretinoin
RETIN-A (Ortho)

Family: Wrinkle Remover

Tretinoin (*tret* in oyn) has been used for a long time to treat certain types of acne. It does not cure acne. Tretinoin cream has been used more recently, despite insufficient information about safety and effectiveness, to reverse skin damage from the sun, which increases with aging. Concern exists that since tretinoin causes increased sensitivity to sunburn, over a long time it could actually increase the risk of skin cancer.[71] Cosmetically, tretinoin may smooth out fine wrinkles, but it is not yet known if wrinkles return. Deep, coarse wrinkles may not improve.[72] Even if tretinoin reduces wrinkles caused by sun damage, it is not known if it works on wrinkles from normal aging, or how older people react to the topical form of tretinoin. At times tretinoin causes a change in pigmentation, which may last months after discontinuing the drug.[73] Some patients cannot tolerate the irritating effect of the drug,[74] and the safety of long-term use on photo-(sun) damaged skin remains to be determined.

To prevent sun damage to the skin, avoid prolonged exposure to the sun, including at work, while driving, and from reflection off water and snow. Wear long sleeves, protective hats, dark sunglasses, and use a sunscreen. Avoid dry air and smoking to reduce premature wrinkling. Alcohol, either regularly taken as a beverage, or applied in cosmetics can aggravate wrinkles. Don't overdo activities that dry the skin, such as frequent bathing or swimming. To abate

dry, wrinkled skin, use a moisturizer, such as products containing lanolin, urea or lactic acid.

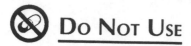 **DO NOT USE**

Alternative treatment: Rest, exercise, physical therapy, and an anti-inflammatory drug such as aspirin.

Methocarbamol
ROBAXIN (Robins)

Family: Muscle Relaxants

Methocarbamol (meth oh *kar* ba mole) is marketed for the relief of severe pain caused by muscle conditions such as sprains and back pain. However, it is not effective for these conditions. Instead of taking methocarbamol, you should try rest, exercise, physical therapy, or other treatment recommended by your doctor.

The level of methocarbamol in this product is not high enough to relax muscles, so this drug will not directly relax tense skeletal muscles. However, the drug is strong enough to have a sedative effect. **Methocarbamol has not been shown to be any more effective than painkillers or anti-inflammatory drugs such as aspirin for relieving the pain of local muscle spasm,[75] yet it has a higher risk of side effects than these painkillers.**

Methocarbamol's side effects include drowsiness, lightheadedness, dizziness, nausea, vomiting, heartburn, abdominal distress, constipation, diarrhea, and loss of appetite. If you use this drug for a long time, you may become addicted to it.

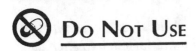 **DO NOT USE**

Alternative treatment: Hair pieces, hair transplants, and accepting baldness as a natural process.

Minoxidil
ROGAINE (Upjohn)

Family: Hair Growth Drugs

Minoxidil (min *ox* id ill) applied to the scalp is used to treat baldness, especially male-pattern baldness. It stimulates hair growth, or at least slows down the rate of hair loss, but does not cure baldness. The same drug in the form of an oral tablet (Loniten) controls high blood pressure. Studies are underway to evaluate the use of topical minoxidil in women and some show effectiveness in women.[76,77,78] It takes four months to a year to promote hair growth, with results varying widely. **Minoxidil works best in men under age 40,** whose hair has been thinning less than 2 years, and when the bald area covers less than 50% of the scalp.

Hair is more apt to regrow on the crown, and less apt on temples and receding hair lines. The first hair growth is usually short and soft, resembling a newborn's. Subsequent growth matches your hair in color (which can be white) and thickness. About 25% of men obtain some regrowth of hair. Less than 1% experience thick regrowth.[79] Complete coverage of a bald area rarely occurs. Expectations often determine satisfaction with the results. At best, one-third rate the results good to excellent.[80] For smokers, a side benefit may be a distaste for smoking cigarettes.[81]

People over age 50 should weigh the risks and benefits carefully,[82] and as indicated above this is a Do Not Use drug for people over the age of 60. Minoxidil is less likely to work the older you are, if baldness has existed more than five years, or is primarily on the sides. Effectiveness in women past menopause has not been studied.

The alcohol in minoxidil solution sometimes irritates the scalp, or eyes if it accidentally gets into the eye. Adverse effects increase with higher strengths of minoxidil. Although absorption of minoxidil is low, when absorbed, all harmful effects of oral minoxidil (Loniten) are possible. Topical minoxidil may cause changes in heart function, such as increased heart rate. Later development of a heart problem or other condition might require discontinuing the drug.

To be effective, treatment must continue. Once minoxidil is stopped, new hair growth disappears over a few months and hair growth returns to the previous pattern. Expenses associated with the use of minoxidil run about $1,000 a year.

Hair regrowth can occur spontaneously when baldness is due to disease, drugs, or radiation once the disease is cured or exposure stopped. Immune diseases, including seasonal allergies, can aggravate hair loss.[83] Options besides minoxidil include hair pieces, hair transplants, and accepting baldness as a natural process.

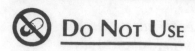 **DO NOT USE**

Alternative treatment: Rest, exercise, physical therapy, and anti-inflammatory drugs such as aspirin.

Carisoprodol
SOMA (Wallace)

Family: Muscle Relaxants

Carisoprodol (kar eye soe *proe* dole) tablets are promoted for the relief of severe pain caused by muscle conditions such as sprains and back pain. However, this drug is not effective for these conditions. Instead of taking carisoprodol, you should try rest, exercise, physical therapy, or other treatment recommended by your doctor.

The level of carisoprodol in the tablets is not high enough to relax muscles, so this drug will not directly relax tense skeletal muscles. However, the drug is strong enough to have a sedative effect. **Carisoprodol has not been shown to be any more effective than painkillers or anti-inflammatory drugs such as aspirin for relieving the pain of local muscle spasm,[84] yet it has a higher risk of side effects than these painkillers.**

Some people taking carisoprodol have experienced drowsiness, lightheadedness, dizziness, nausea, vomiting, heartburn, abdominal distress, constipation, diarrhea, and loss of appetite as side effects. If you take carisoprodol for a long time, you may become addicted to it.[85] Carisoprodol is particularly dangerous for people with acute intermittent porphyria.

Carisoprodol occasionally causes a reaction within the first few minutes or hours after the first dose. Symptoms of a reaction are agitation, confusion, unsteadiness, disorientation, weakness, speech or vision problems, and temporary inability to move arms or legs.

Fluocinolone
SYNALAR, SYNEMOL (Syntex)

Generic: available

Family: Corticosteroids (see p. 609)

Fluocinolone (floo oh *sin* oh lone) is used to reduce inflammation (redness and swelling) and relieve itching caused by many skin conditions, such as eczema and psoriasis.

Steroids suppress your immune system, lowering your defenses against disease and making you more vulnerable to infections. If you use fluocinolone for a long time, you increase your risk of getting bacterial, viral, parasitic, and fungal infections.

As with all drugs, you should use the lowest possible dose of fluocinolone that works. You should also use it for as short a time as possible and limit the area of your body that you use it on, if possible. A steroid applied to the skin can cause many side effects, especially if you use it for a long time or over a large area so that your whole body absorbs the drug. **If you have used this drug for a long time do not stop suddenly. Your doctor must lower your dose gradually to prevent withdrawal symptoms.**

Before You Use This Drug

Tell your doctor if you have or have had

❏ allergies to drugs
❏ herpes sores
❏ infection or ulceration at the place where you will be applying the drug

Tell your doctor about any other drugs you take, including aspirin, herbs, vitamins, and other non-prescription products.

How To Use This Drug

◆ **Use only as prescribed.**
◆ Spread a very thin layer over the area being treated to minimize absorption of the drug into your body. (There is no danger of systemic absorption with correct use.)
◆ The preparation may sting when applied.
◆ Do not bandage or wrap the area you are treating unless your doctor has told you to do so.
◆ Do not use around eyes for a long period.
◆ Check with your doctor if your condition does not improve in 1 week or if it worsens.

Interactions With Other Drugs

Some other drugs that you may be taking (either over-the-counter or prescription drugs) can interact with this one, causing adverse effects. Find out from your doctor what these drugs are and let him or her know if you are taking any of them.

Adverse Effects

Call your doctor immediately:

❏ pain, redness, or blisters containing pus
❏ burning, itching, or blistering that was not present before you began using this drug
❏ acne or other skin problems
❏ thinning of skin
❏ bruising
❏ increased hair growth, especially on the face
❏ loss of hair, especially on scalp

Periodic Tests

Ask your doctor which of these tests should be done periodically while you are taking this drug:

❏ blood or urine glucose concentration
❏ eye exams

THYROID HORMONES
Levothyroxine
SYNTHROID (Flint) NOROXINE (Vortech)
LEVOTHROID (Armour)
Liotrix
EUTHROID (Parke-Davis) THYROLAR (Armour)
Thyroid

Generic: available

Family: Hormones

Thyroid (*thye* roid) hormone pills are prescribed for people whose thyroids do not produce a normal amount of these hormones. Most people, however, are unnecessarily prescribed thyroid hormone even though their own levels are in the normal range. Most people who actually *need* to be on thyroid replacement therapy need to take these hormones for the rest of their lives. **In general, if you are over 60, you need to take only about three-fourths of the usual adult dose.**

Levothyroxine (lee voe thye *rox* een) is the usual first-choice drug for thyroid replacement therapy. Older adults should start at a dose of just 25 micrograms (.025 milligram), with cautious increases every 2 to 4 weeks if necessary. Starting with a low dose will reduce the risk of heart failure or chest pain.[86] Whichever type of thyroid hormone you use, check with your doctor before switching brands. Brands can vary in concentration, so switching brands can cause you to get too much or too little of the hormone.

Natural thyroid extract (thyroid) is an older drug that is now considered obsolete. It can produce hazardous side effects in older people. **You should not take this form of thyroid hormone unless you have already been taking it for years.**[87]

Do not use enteric-coated tablets of thyroid hormone (tablets coated so they will not dissolve in the stomach), as they are not absorbed reliably by your body.

Before You Use This Drug
Tell your doctor if you have or have had
- ❏ allergies to drugs
- ❏ diabetes
- ❏ heart or circulatory disease

Tell your doctor about any other drugs you take, including aspirin, herbs, vitamins, and other non-prescription products.

When You Take This Drug
- ◆ **Do not use more or less often or in a higher or lower dose than prescribed by your doctor.**
- ◆ You may need to take this medicine for the rest of your life. Schedule regular checkups. Do not stop taking this drug without talking to your doctor first.
- ◆ **Talk to your doctor before taking any other prescription or non-prescription drugs. They may interfere with the effects of thyroid hormone.**
- ◆ **Caution diabetics:** see p. 516.
- ◆ If you plan to have any surgery, including dental, tell your doctor that you take this drug.

How To Take This Drug
- ◆ Do not store in the bathroom. Do not expose to heat, strong light, or moisture.
- ◆ If you miss a dose, take it as soon as you remember, but skip it if it is almost time for the next dose. **Do not take double doses.** Check with your doctor if you miss more than 3 doses.

Interactions With Other Drugs

The following drugs are listed in *Evaluations of Drug Interactions*, 1991 as causing "highly clinically significant" or "clinically significant" interactions when used together with this drug. There may be other drugs, especially those in the families of drugs listed below, that also will react with this drug to cause severe adverse effects. Make sure to ask your doctor for a complete listing of them and let her or him know if you are taking any of these interacting drugs:

cholestyramine; COUMADIN; CRYSTODIGIN; digoxin; imipramine; INDERAL; insulin; LANOXICAPS; LANOXIN; propranolol; QUESTRAN; TOFRANIL; warfarin.

Adverse Effects

Call your doctor immediately:
❑ if you experience signs of overdose: changes in appetite; vomiting; weight loss; chest pain; diarrhea; fever; hand tremors; headache; irritability; leg cramps; nervousness; rapid or irregular heartbeat; sensitivity to heat; sweating; shortness of breath; trouble sleeping
❑ skin rash, hives, or itching

Call your doctor if these symptoms continue:
❑ clumsiness
❑ feeling cold
❑ constipation
❑ dry, puffy skin
❑ headache
❑ tiredness
❑ muscle aches
❑ sleepiness
❑ weight gain

Periodic Tests

Ask your doctor which of these tests should be done periodically while you are taking this drug:
❑ thyroid hormone levels
❑ examination for signs of irregular heart rhythm

Desoximetasone
TOPICORT (Hoechst-Roussel)

Generic: available

Family: Corticosteroids (see p. 609)

Desoximetasone (des ox i *met* a sone) is a steroid that is applied to the skin. It is used to reduce inflammation (redness and swelling) and relieve itching of many kinds of skin conditions, such as psoriasis and eczema.

Steroids suppress your immune system, lowering your defenses against disease and making you more vulnerable to infections. If you use desoximetasone for a long time, you increase your risk of getting bacterial, viral, parasitic, and fungal infections.

As with all drugs, you should use the lowest possible dose of desoximetasone that works. You should also use it for as short a time as possible and limit the area of your body that you use it on, if possible. A steroid applied to the skin can cause many side effects, especially if you use it for a long time or over a large area so that your whole body absorbs the drug. **If you have used this drug for a long time do not stop suddenly. Your doctor must lower your dose gradually to prevent withdrawal symptoms.**

Before You Use This Drug

Tell your doctor if you have or have had
❑ allergies to drugs
❑ herpes sores
❑ infection or ulceration at the place where you will be applying the drug

Tell your doctor about any other drugs you take, including aspirin, herbs, vitamins, and other non-prescription products.

How To Use This Drug

♦ Use only as prescribed.
♦ Spread a very thin layer over the area to be treated, to minimize absorption of the drug into your body. (There is no danger of systemic absorption with correct use.)
♦ The preparation may sting when applied.
♦ Do not bandage or wrap the area being treated unless your doctor has told you to do so.
♦ Do not use around eyes for a long period.
♦ Check with your doctor if your condition does not improve in 1 week, or if it worsens.

Interactions With Other Drugs

Some other drugs that you may be taking (either over-the-counter or prescription drugs) can interact with this one, causing adverse effects. Find out from your doctor what these drugs are and let him or her know if you are taking any of them.

Adverse Effects

Call your doctor immediately:
❑ pain, redness, or blisters containing pus
❑ burning, itching, or blistering that was not present before you began using this drug
❑ acne or other skin problems
❑ thinning of skin
❑ bruising
❑ increased hair growth, especially on the face
❑ loss of hair, especially on scalp

Periodic Tests

Ask your doctor which of these tests should be done periodically while you are taking this drug:
❑ blood or urine glucose concentration
❑ eye exams

Bethanechol
URECHOLINE (Merck)

Generic: available

Family: Cholinergics

Bethanechol (be *than* e kole) stimulates the bladder to empty and is used to treat the retention of urine. Although the drug is also used to prevent the backward flow of stomach contents into the esophagus (reflux esophagitis), it is not effective or approved for this purpose.[88]

Before You Use This Drug
Tell your doctor if you have or have had
- [ ] allergies to drugs
- [ ] asthma
- [ ] recent bladder or abdominal surgery
- [ ] slow pulse
- [ ] coronary artery disease
- [ ] epilepsy
- [ ] abdominal obstruction or disease
- [ ] urinary tract obstruction
- [ ] high or low blood pressure
- [ ] enlarged thyroid gland

Tell your doctor about any other drugs you take, including aspirin, herbs, vitamins, and other non-prescription products.

When You Use This Drug
- ◆ You may feel dizzy when rising from a lying or sitting position. When getting out of bed, hang your legs over the side of the bed for a few minutes, then get up slowly. When getting up from a chair, stay by the chair until you are sure that you are not dizzy. (See p. 14.)
- ◆ Until you know how you react to this drug, do not drive or perform other activities requiring alertness. Bethanechol may cause dizziness and blurred vision.

How To Use This Drug
- ◆ Take on an empty stomach to decrease nausea and vomiting.
- ◆ Use only as prescribed.
- ◆ Do not expose to heat or direct light. Do not store in bathroom. Do not let liquid form freeze.
- ◆ If you miss a dose, take it as soon as you remember, but skip it if it is almost time for the next dose. **Do not take double doses.**

Interactions With Other Drugs
Some other drugs that you may be taking (either over-the-counter or prescription drugs) can interact with this one, causing adverse effects. Find out from your doctor what these drugs are and let him or her know if you are taking any of them.

Adverse Effects
Call your doctor immediately:
- [ ] shortness of breath

Call your doctor if these symptoms continue:
- [ ] nausea, vomiting, or diarrhea

Beclomethasone
VANCENASE (nasal aerosol spray) (Schering)
BECLOVENT (Glaxo) VANCERIL (Schering)
(oral aerosol inhalers)

Generic: not available

Family: Corticosteroids (see p. 609)

Beclomethasone (be kloe *meth* a sone) is a steroid (corticosteroid) that is inhaled. It has one form that you spray into your nose and another form that you inhale into your mouth. The nose spray is used to treat severe allergies and hay fever and sometimes smooth growths (polyps) in the nose. The inhaler for the mouth mainly benefits people with asthma who need regular, long-term steroid treatment to control their symptoms. For these people, beclomethasone is used after a drug from another family, albuterol or terbutaline (see p. 422) used alone, has not improved the severe chronic symptoms of asthma.[89]

Steroids suppress your immune system, lowering your defenses against disease and making you more vulnerable to infections. If you use beclomethasone for a long time, you increase your risk of getting bacterial, viral, parasitic, and fungal infections, especially an infection called oral thrush.

As with all drugs, you should always use beclomethasone in the lowest dose that works. You should also take it for the shortest possible time. **If you have used this drug for a long time do not stop suddenly. Your doctor must lower your dose gradually to prevent withdrawal symptoms.**

Before You Use This Drug
Do not use if you have or have had
❑ an allergic reaction to fluorocarbon propellants (found in aerosol sprays)
Tell your doctor if you have or have had
❑ allergies to drugs
❑ AIDS

❑ heart disease
❑ high blood pressure
❑ liver or kidney disease
❑ diabetes
❑ inflammation of throat, stomach, or intestines
❑ glaucoma
❑ fungal infections
❑ myasthenia gravis
❑ osteoporosis
❑ herpes sores of the eyes or mouth
❑ tuberculosis or positive TB skin test
For oral inhaler:
❑ current infection of the mouth, throat, or lungs
For nose spray:
❑ glaucoma
❑ any eye infection
❑ recent nose surgery or injury
❑ ulcers of the nasal septum
Tell your doctor about any other drugs you take, including aspirin, herbs, vitamins, and other non-prescription products.

When You Use This Drug
◆ If you plan to have any surgery, including dental, tell your doctor that you take this drug.
◆ **Do not use to treat a sudden, severe asthma attack. This drug is not strong or fast enough for such an attack.**
◆ Wear a medical identification bracelet or carry a card stating that you may need additional steroids (tablets or injection) in times of unusual stress or sudden, severe asthma attack.

How To Use This Drug
◆ **Use only as prescribed.**
◆ If you miss a dose, take it as soon as you remember, but skip it if it is almost

time for the next dose. **Do not take double doses.**

Oral Inhaler:
◆ Clean inhaler every day.
◆ Gargle and rinse your mouth after each time you use the drug, to wash out any of the drug that did not enter your lungs. If your mouth and throat absorb the drug, you may become more susceptible to an infection called thrush.
◆ See p. 388 for instructions on using an inhaler.

Nose spray:
◆ See p. 382 for information on drugs taken by nose.

Interactions With Other Drugs

The following drugs are listed in *Evaluations of Drug Interactions*, 1991 as causing "highly clinically significant" or "clinically significant" interactions when used together with this drug. There may be other drugs, especially those in the families of drugs listed below, that also will react with this drug to cause severe adverse effects. Make sure to ask your doctor for a complete listing of them and let her or him know if you are taking any of these interacting drugs:

aspirin; cyclosporine; DELTASONE; dicumarol; ECOTRIN; ketoconazole; LUMINAL; NIZORAL; phenobarbital; prednisone; SANDIMMUNE; TAO; troleandomycin.

Adverse Effects

Call your doctor immediately:
❑ decreased or blurred vision
❑ hallucinations
❑ depression or mood changes
❑ skin rash or hives

For long-term use:
❑ persistent abdominal or stomach pain
❑ acne or other skin problems
❑ bloody or black, tarry stools
❑ rounding out of the face
❑ increased blood pressure
❑ swelling of feet or lower legs
❑ unusual weight gain

❑ irregular heartbeats
❑ muscle cramps or pain
❑ unusual tiredness or weakness
❑ pain in back, ribs, arms, or legs
❑ muscle weakness
❑ nausea or vomiting
❑ unusual bruising
❑ wounds that will not heal

If using oral inhaler:
❑ chest pain
❑ chills, cough, fever, sneezing
❑ ear congestion
❑ hoarseness or other voice changes
❑ nose congestion or runny nose
❑ sore throat
❑ white patches inside mouth
❑ difficulty swallowing
❑ eye pain, redness, or tearing

Call your doctor immediately if these symptoms occur after you have stopped taking the drug:
❑ abdominal or back pain
❑ dizziness or fainting
❑ low fever
❑ persistent loss of appetite
❑ muscle or joint pain
❑ nausea or vomiting
❑ returning symptoms of the condition for which you were taking the drug
❑ shortness of breath
❑ frequent unexplained headaches
❑ unusual tiredness or weakness
❑ unusual weight loss

Call your doctor if these symptoms continue:
❑ indigestion
❑ increased appetite
❑ nervousness or restlessness
❑ trouble sleeping
❑ dizziness or lightheadedness
❑ flushed face
❑ headache
❑ increased joint pain
❑ nosebleeds
❑ increase in hair on body or face

If using oral inhaler:
❑ mild abdominal pain or bloated feeling or gas
❑ constipation or diarrhea
❑ decrease in appetite

❑ dry or irritated mouth, nose, tongue, or throat

❑ loss of sense of smell or taste

If using nose spray:

❑ bloody mucus or nosebleeds

❑ crusting inside nose

❑ sore throat

❑ trouble breathing

❑ nausea or vomiting

❑ loss of sense of taste or smell

❑ persistent stuffy nose

❑ headache

Periodic Tests

Ask your doctor which of these tests should be done periodically while you are taking this drug:

❑ blood or urine glucose concentration

❑ eye exams

❑ blood levels of potassium, sodium, and calcium

❑ stool tests for possible blood loss

❑ hypothalamus and pituitary secretion tests

Notes for Drugs for Other Conditions

1. AMA Department of Drugs. *AMA Drug Evaluations.* 5th ed. Chicago: American Medical Association, 1983:893.

2. Ibid.

3. Ibid.

4. Wilkinson SM, Cartwright PH, English JSC. Hydrocortisone: an important cutaneous allergen. *The Lancet* 1991; 337:761-2.

5. AMA, 1983, op. cit.

6. Fadul CE, Lemann W, Thaler HT, Posner JB. Perforation of GI tract in patients receiving steroids for neurologic disease. *Neurology.* 1988; 38:348-52.

7. AMA, 1983, op. cit.

8. Laan RFJM, van Riel PLCM, van Erning LJTO, Lemmens JAM, Ruijs SHJ, van de Putte LBAR. Vertebral osteoporosis in rheumatoid patients. *British Journal of Rheumatology* 1992; 31:91-6.

9. Minden SL, Orav J, Schildkraut JJ. Hypomanic reactions to ACTH and prednisone treatment for multiple sclerosis. *Neurology* 1988; 38:1631-4.

10. Ibid.

11. AMA, 1983, op. cit.

12. Ibid.

13. AMA Department of Drugs. *AMA Drug Evaluations.* 6th ed. Chicago: American Medical Association, 1986:232-3.

14. *USP DI, Drug Information for the Health Care Provider.* 6th ed. Rockville Md.: The United States Pharmacopeial Convention, Inc., 1986:1147.

15. Vestal RE, ed. *Drug Treatment in the Elderly.* Sydney, Australia: ADIS Health Science Press, 1984:250.

16. *USP DI,* 1986, op. cit.

17. Krebs H. Chronic ulcerations following topical therapy. *Obstetrics and Gynecology* 1991; 78:205-8.

18. Boschetti C, Cortellaro M, Nencioni T, Bertolli V, Della Volpe A, Zanussi C. Short- and long-term effects of hormone replacement therapy (transdermal estradiol vs oral conjugated equine estrogens, combined with medroxyprogesterone acetate) on blood coagulation factors in postmenopausal women. *Thrombosis Research* 1991; 62:1-8.

19. Studd J, Watson N, Henderson A. Oestrogen therapy for the menopause. *British Journal of Psychiatry* 1990; 157:931-2.

20. Sillero-Arenas M, Delgado-Rodriguez M, Rodrigues-Canteras R, Bueno-Cavanillas A, Galvez-Vargas R. Menopausal hormone replacement therapy and breast cancer: a meta-analysis. *Obstetrics & Gynecology* 1992; 79:286-94.

21. Steinberg KK, Thacker SB, Smith SJ, Stroup DF, Zack MM, Flanders WD, Berkelman RL. A meta-analysis of the effect of estrogen replacement therapy on the risk of breast cancer. *Journal of the American Medical Association* 1991; 265:1985-90.

22. Hormone replacement therapy in general practice (letters). *British Medical Journal* 1991; 302:1601-2.

23. Miller AB. Risk/benefit considerations of antiestrogen/estrogen therapy in healthy postmenopausal women. *Preventive Medicine* 1991; 20:79-85.

24. L'Hermite M. Sex hormones and cardiovascular risk. *Acta Cardiologica* 1991; 46:357-72.

25. Dukes MNG, Beeley L. *Side Effects of Drugs Annual* 15, Amsterdam: Elsevier, 1991:436.

26. Steinberg, op. cit.

27. L'Hermite, op. cit.

28. Clisham R, Cedars MI, Greendale G, Fu S, Gambone J, Judd HL. Long-term transdermal estradiol therapy on endometrial histology and bleeding patterns. *Obstetrics & Gynecology* 1992; 79:196-201.

29. AMA, 1986, op. cit., p. 232-3.

30. Ibid.

31. Wolfe S. Testimony at Food and Drug Administration advisory committee hearing on nicotine patches, July 14, 1992.

32. Günther V, Gritsch S, Meise U. Smoking cessation—gradual or sudden stopping? *Drug and Alcohol Dependence* 1992; 29:231-6.

33. West R. The focus and conduct of clinical trials. *British Journal of Addiction* 1991; 86:663-6.

34. West R. The 'nicotine replacement paradox' in smoking cessation: how does nicotine gum really work? *British Journal of Addiction* 1992; 87:165-7.

35. Morgan GD, Villagra VG. The nicotine transdermal patch: a cautionary note. *Annals of Internal Medicine* 1992; 116:424.

36. Benowitz NL. Cigarette smoking and nicotine addiction. *Medical Clinics of North America* 1992; 76:415-37.

37. Breslau N, Kilbey MM, Andreski P. Nicotine withdrawal symptoms and psychiatric disorders: findings from an epidemiologic study of young adults (abstract). *American Journal of Psychiatry* 1992; 149:464-9.

38. West, 1991, op. cit.

39. Wolfe, op. cit.

40. American Society of Hospital Pharmacists. *American Hospital Formulary Service Drug Information*. Bethesda, MD, 1992:754-9.

41. *The Medical Letter on Drugs and Therapeutics.* New York: The Medical Letter Inc., 1992; 34:37-8.

42. Russell MAH, Jarvis MJ. Skin patches to prevent lung cancer. *European Journal of Cancer* 1991; 27:223-4.

43. Säwe U. From smoking behaviour to nicotine addiction:the history of research (letter). *Journal of the Royal Society of Medicine* 1992; 85:184.

44. Tonnesen P, Norregaard J, Simonsen K, Säwe U. A double-blind trial of a 16-hour transdermal nicotine patch in smoking cessation. *The New England Journal of Medicine* 1991; 325:311-5.

45. Transdermal Nicotine Study Group. Transdermal nicotine for smoking cessation: six-month results from two multicenter controlled clinical trials. *Journal of the American Medical Association* 1991; 266:3133-8.

46. Günther, op. cit.

47. Transdermal Nicotine Study Group, op. cit.

48. Perkins KA. Metabolic effects of cigarette smoking. *Journal of Applied Psychology* 1992; 72:401-9.

49. Transdermal nicotine patch for smoking cessation (letters). *The New England Journal of Medicine* 1992; 326:344-5.

50. Kirch DG. Where there's smoke...nicotine and psychiatric disorders. *Biological Psychiatry* 1991; 30:107-8.

51. Menza MA, Grossman N, Van Horn M, Cody R, Forman N. Smoking and movement disorders in psychiatric patients. *Biological Psychiatry* 1991; 30:109-15.

52. Perkins, op. cit.

53. Jensen EJ, Schmidt E, Pederson B, Dahl R. Effect on smoking cessation of silver acetate, nicotine and ordinary chewing gum. *Psychopharmacology* 1991; 104:470-4.

54. Yokota T, Kagamihara Y, Hayashi H, Tsukagoshi H, Tanabe H. Nicotine-sensitive paresis. *Neurology* 1992; 42:382-8.

55. Kyerematen G, Vesell E. Metabolism of nicotine. *Drug Metabolism Reviews* 1991; 23:3-41.

56. Gilman AG, Rall TW, Nies AS, Taylor P, eds. *The Pharmacological Basis of Therapeutics.* 8th ed. New York: Pergamon Press, 1990:545-9.

57. Yokota, op. cit.

58. Bircher AJ, Howald H, Rufli T. Adverse skin reactions to nicotine in a transdermal therapeutic system. *Contact Dermatitis* 1991; 25:230-6.

59. AMA, 1986, op. cit., p. 399.

60. AMA, 1986, op. cit., p. 232-3.

61. Ibid.

62. Ibid.

63. AMA, 1983, op. cit.

64. Steinberg, op. cit.

65. *International Journal of Cancer,* 1986; 37:173-7.

66. Forbes AP. Fuller Albright: his concept of postmenopausal osteoporosis and what came of it. *Osteoporosis* 1991; 269:128-40.

67. Vandenbroucke JP. Postmenopausal oestrogen and cardioprotection. *The Lancet* 1991; 337:833-4.

68. Stampfer MJ, Willett WC, Colditz GA, Rosner B, Speizer FE, Hennekens CH. *New England Journal of Medicine* 1985; 313:1044-9.

69. Wolf PH, Madans JH, Finucane FF, Higgins M, Kleinman JC. Reduction of cardiovascular disease—related mortality among postmenopausal women who use hormones: evidence from a national cohort. *American Journal of Obstetrics and Gynecology* 1991; 161:489-94.

70. *International Agency for Research on Cancer Monographs on the Evaluation of the Carcinogenic Risk of Chemicals to Humans, Vol. 24: Some Pharmaceutical Drugs*. Lyon, France: International Agency for Research on Cancer, 1980:163.

71. Randall T. FDA scrutinizes 'off-label' promotions. *Journal of the American Medical Association* 1991; 266:11.

72. American Society of Hospital Pharmacists, op. cit., p. 2158-9.

73. *USP DI, Drug Information for the Health Care Professional*. 12th ed. Rockville MD: The United States Pharmacopeial Convention, Inc., 1992:2695-7.

74. *The Medical Letter on Drugs and Therapeutics*, 1992, op. cit., p. 28-9.

75. AMA, 1986, op. cit., p. 232-3.

76. Olsen EA. Topical minoxidil in the treatment of androgenetic alopecia in women. *CUTIS* 1991; 48:243-8.

77. Saxena U, Ramesh V, Misra RS. Topical minoxidil in monilethrix. *Dermatologica* 1991; 182:252-3.

78. Wilson C, Walkden V, Powell S, Shaw, S, Wilkinson J, Dawber R. Contact dermatitis in reaction to 2% topical minoxidil solution. *Journal of the American Academy of Dermatology* 1991; 24:661-2.

79. Gilman, op. cit., p. 1587.

80. AMA Department of Drugs. *AMA Drug Evaluations Annual* 1992. Chicago: American Medical Association, 1992:1123.

81. Trattner A, Ingber A. Topical treatment with minoxidil 2% and smoking intolerance. *The Annals of Pharmacotherapy* 1992; 26:198-9.

82. American Society of Hospital Pharmacists, op. cit., p. 2180-5.

83. Fiedler V. Alopecia areata: current therapy. *Journal of Investigative Dermatology* 1991: 96:69S-70S.

84. AMA, 1986, op. cit., p. 232-3.

85. Ibid.

86. *Drugs for the Elderly*. Denmark: World Health Organization, 1985, 92-9.

87. AMA, 1986, op. cit., p. 802.

88. *The Medical Letter on Drugs and Therapeutics*. New York: The Medical Letter Inc., 1980; 22:27.

89. AMA, 1986, op. cit., p. 399.

CHAPTER 4

Action To Stop the Drug-induced Disease Epidemic in Older Adults: Helping Your Doctor Toward Safer Drug Prescribing

When you read about problems with prescription drugs for older adults, most suggestions for patients are aimed at getting patients to better "comply" with doctors' prescriptions and other strategies also put the main "blame" on the patient. If you read about this same problem from the perspective of the doctor or pharmacist, materials again stress the need to educate the patient to "behave" better. Occasionally, some also put the "blame" on the doctor for misprescribing and overprescribing, and, more rarely, on the drug industry for overselling drugs for older people. Even when the doctor is portrayed as the partial culprit, however, the proposed solution is a ritual of faith, hoping the system of medical education will do a better job of teaching and that doctors will do a better job of learning about the proper use of drugs by older people. In reality, the problem of adverse drug reactions in older adults is due to a complex brew of overselling, misprescribing, poor communication between doctors and patients and some patient misuse of drugs.

While separate patient-modifying or doctor-modifying behavioral changes are important, they are not enough, and they are not likely to occur without another, more primary change.

Activating Yourself and Your Doctor: 10 Rules for Safer Drug Use

What is needed is a process of activating older patients, their families, and friends to approach the doctor, with the help of their pharmacist, and to begin working with the doctor to reduce the number of drugs and the dosage of drugs being used. In most cases, this will result in not only fewer adverse reactions, including life-threatening ones, but also in fewer drugs being used. Equally important, this process will improve patients' ability to properly take the drugs that are actually needed. Studies show that more drugs lead to poorer patient compliance with instructions, while fewer drugs lead to better compliance.[1]

This chapter assumes that most doctors who take care of older patients have not had adequate training in the special problems of drug prescribing and use in people of this age group. Therefore, they usually use the same decisionmaking process (when to treat and what drug and dose to use) for older adults as for younger people. This too often results in their prescribing too many drugs at doses which are too high. In addition, many older people see multiple doctors — an internist, a gynecologist, and a heart specialist, for example. Communications among physicians about what drugs are prescribed is often deficient. We also assume that *most doctors are quite willing to learn to prescribe fewer and safer drugs, but this is most likely to occur if you begin the activation process we outline in this chapter.* Shyness is not only inappropriate but may be dangerous to your health. If there are any of the sections on the drug worksheet or any of the 10 Rules which you do not understand — ask. Remember — the doctor is working *for* you, *with* you.

Rule 1: Have "Brown Bag Sessions" With Your Primary Doctor. Fill Out Drug Worksheet.

It is impossible to overemphasize the importance of this first and most crucial step in the process of patient and doctor activation: **Whenever you go to a doctor you have not previously seen or to one with whom you have never had a brown bag session, put all prescription and over-the-counter drugs you are using, have used in the last month, or are likely to use in a bag, and bring them to the doctor so a list can be made and you can start to fill out your drug worksheet.** (See p. 674 for a sample of this worksheet which you can use.)

Doctors should never prescribe a drug or renew a prescription on an old drug, nor should you or your parents be willing to get a new prescription, without full up-to-date knowledge of all drugs already being taken or likely to be taken.

Before your brown bag session with the doctor, your neighborhood pharmacist may help you to fill out some of the blanks on your **drug worksheet**.

Once you have brought all drugs in, ask your doctor to help you fill out the **drug worksheet**. You will probably be able to fill out more of the information concerning over-the-counter drugs yourself, since doctors often do not know that you are taking them or for what purpose. The doctor will be able to help you to fill out most of the information concerning prescription drugs, at least the ones that he or she has prescribed for you.

Explanation of items on drug worksheet

a. *Name of drug, of doctor who wrote prescription, and date drug started or changed*: Drugs should be listed by both brand and generic names since both are commonly used. All drugs prescribed by all doctors should be listed. Over-the-counter drugs and the amount of alcohol, tobacco, and caffeine used should also be indicated. There are many dangerous interactions between drugs and between drugs and alcohol, so this information is extremely important in avoiding adverse drug interactions.

b. *Purpose for the drug*: Identify the reason for which each drug is being taken. Often, because physicians are frustrated at not being able to do anything else for the patient, or sometimes because the doctor believes that the patient will not be satisfied unless a pill is recommended, prescriptions are written without a valid medical reason. In one recent study, patients reported that one out of every four times (25.4%) they received a prescription, they were not told the purpose of the drug being prescribed.[2]

c. *Dose, freqency of use, and duration of use*: It is important to know what the dose is, how often it is supposed to be taken, at what hours, and for how long.

d. *When the drug should be stopped or the need for its use reevaluated*: For any drug, new or old, the assumption should be that it should be used for as short a time as possible unless there is evidence that its continued use is necessary. Evaluation at least every 3 to 6 months for each drug being used will reduce the number of drugs being taken. For some drugs, such as tranquilizers, sleeping pills, antidepressants, and others, much more frequent reevalution is necessary.

e. *Important possible adverse effects of the drug*: Because many of the most serious perceptible adverse effects of drugs are often wrongly attributed to "growing old," it is important for patients to know about the adverse effects of the drugs they take so they can recognize them and report them to the doctor. A recent study found that 37% of adverse drug reactions had not previously been recognized by the patient and reported to the doctor, and that the majority of these patients had not been informed about possible adverse drug reactions.[3]

f. *Important possible drug and food interactions, especially with over-the-counter drugs and diet recommendations*: Ask your doctor which foods and other drugs taken along with your drug can interact and cause side effects and ask for dietary recommendations.

g. *How you are actually taking the drug:* Always be straightforward with your doctor about whether or not you are taking your medicine and how often. Do this even if you had no defined reason for stopping. This is important because not giving your doctor this information can lead to mistaken conclusions about dosage or what works.

h. *New problems or complaints noticed by the patient, friends, or family since any of the drugs listed on the worksheet have been started:* As mentioned above, patients themselves often do not notice a change, especially older adults who are inclined to blame many of their problems on aging. Friends and relatives are often the first to notice adverse drug reactions, especially ones which affect thinking or mood. An additional difficulty is that patients are often reluctant to tell their doctors that something the doctor did to try to make them better actually made them worse. **The safest assumption is that any worsening of a patient's condition or any new symptoms that develops after a drug is started is an adverse drug reaction, until proven otherwise.**

i. *In the judgment of you, your family and your doctor, is the drug working?* Have the purposes for which the drug is being prescribed (as in b) been achieved?

"Do Not Use" drugs

If a drug already being used or being considered for use is one of the 119 drugs that we list as "Do Not Use" (see **Drug Index,** p. xviii) ask your doctor about alternative therapy which could be either nondrug therapy or a safer drug. If the drug you are using is listed in this book as "Limited Use," it may also be a good idea to discuss the drug with your doctor to see if a better alternative might be found.

How to use the drug worksheet
The story of Beatrice

Beatrice is a 68-year-old woman who went to see her family practitioner, Dr. Jackson. Dr. Jackson checked her blood pressure at several visits and found it too high each time.

February 2, 1992: Dr. Jackson started Beatrice on hydrochlorothiazide, a diuretic, to lower her pressure. Beatrice asked Dr. Jackson to fill out her drug worksheet at this first visit when the medicine was prescribed. She had, of course, remembered to bring the worksheet with her! Dr. Jackson wrote down that the medicine was for her blood pressure, which was 180/100 that day, under the "reason why prescribed." She wrote down under "dose" that Beatrice should take 12.5 milligrams, or half a hydrochlorothiazide pill. Under "times per day" Dr. Jackson wrote once, and under "what time of day," she wrote that it should be taken in the morning. She also noted that Beatrice should take the medicine at least until her next visit in 1 month.

She explained to Beatrice that this drug can cause the body to lose potassium, resulting in weakness and muscle cramps in some people. She also explained that she might urinate more frequently. These things were written down under "problems to watch out for." Because of the effects of the drug, she recommended that Beatrice eat foods high in potassium, and listed some of these under "diet recommendations." To help lower her blood pressure, she also suggested that Beatrice avoid salt, and wrote this down under "diet recommendations." Although Beatrice does not have diabetes, Dr. Jackson warned her that if she were to develop diabetes, hydrochlorothiazide may lessen the effectiveness of diabetes drugs taken by mouth, and that should the problem arise, she should use other diabetes treatments. This was written under "interactions with other drugs and foods," in the same column with "diet recommendations." Beatrice did not take any other prescription or nonprescription drugs, so her worksheet has only one drug on it.

Beatrice filled her prescription at the pharmacy, where the pharmacist explained to her how much less expensive it was to buy the generic hydrochlorothiazide instead of HydroDIURIL — a brand name. He also showed her how to break the pills. After going home she started taking her pills, but occasionally forgot on weekends when she would go for long walks in the morning. She didn't notice any side effects except going to the bathroom slightly more often. She wrote down on her worksheet that she was taking the medicine 5 to 6 times a week and feeling fine, under "how are you actually taking the drug" and "new problems since drug started."

March 8, 1992: Beatrice returned to see Dr. Jackson, who found that her blood pressure was still high at 165/100. She therefore increased the dose to 25 milligrams daily (one whole pill) in the morning, and wrote the changes down on Beatrice's worksheet. She recommended that she stay on this dose until her next visit in 2 months. Beatrice started taking the medicine, but after 2 weeks (3/22/92) she began to feel very tired and weak. She also didn't like the high potassium foods. She was able to avoid salt in her diet. On April 1 she stopped taking her pills. She wrote down how she was feeling and how she was taking her medicines, as well as the dates, on her worksheet under " how are you actually taking the drug" and "new problems or complaints." She called for a new appointment with Dr. Jackson.

April 15, 1992: Dr. Jackson found that Beatrice's blood pressure was slightly better, 165/95, even though she was off her medicine. She explained that this was probably because Beatrice was eating less salt. Since her pressure was now lower, and she had had no problems with the lower dose of medicine, Dr. Jackson restarted Beatrice on 12.5 milligrams of hydrochlorothiazide once a day, and wrote down the date and the new blood pressure and dosages of medicine. Beatrice crossed out the earlier dosage with a single line, so as not to confuse past dosages with her current one, but still to be able to read it. Beatrice started taking the medicine, and on this lower dosage she was not bothered by any side effects. She also learned to remember to take her pills by having them with breakfast. When she returned to see Dr. Jackson 2 months later, her blood pressure was 160/89. (Not noted on drug worksheet, since no changes were made.)

October 10, 1992: In October, Beatrice moved to Texas to be nearer her daughter, and she found a new doctor there, Dr. Lewis. Dr. Lewis was not used to using this low dose of hydrochlorothiazide, but when he saw Beatrice's worksheet, he realized that she was doing well on this dose of medicine and a low salt diet, and that she had not tolerated the higher dose well. Her blood pressure was 155/87. He decided to leave what was working well alone.

Rule 2: Find Out If You Are Having Any Adverse Drug Reactions.

Even before you have a brown bag session with your doctor, if you develop any of the following reactions after beginning to use any of the drugs on the appropriate lists, contact your doctor. Ask if you really need a drug in the first place and, if you do, whether a safer drug can be substituted or whether a lower dose could be used to reduce or eliminate the adverse effect. For each of the adverse effects listed below, look in Chapter 2, *Adverse Drug Reactions*, p. 9, for the lists of widely used drugs that can cause each of these problems:

❑ *Mental adverse drug reactions*: depression, hallucinations, confusion, delirium, memory loss, impaired thinking and insomnia

❑ *Nervous system adverse drug reactions*: parkinsonism, involuntary movements of the face, arms, and legs (tardive dyskinesia), dizziness on standing, falls which can sometimes result in hip fractures, injurious automobile accidents, and sexual dysfunction

❑ *Gastrointestinal adverse drug reactions*: loss of appetite, nausea, vomiting,

Sample Page of Drug Worksheet for Patients, Family, Doctor and Pharmacist

Name Beatrice Jones

Primary Doctor's Name Dr. Jackson

Page 1

Doctor's Telephone 555-1212

	a.	b.	c.		d.	e.	f.	g.	h.	i.
Generic Name of Drug / Brand Name of Drug	Doctor, date started & changes	Reason why prescribed or changed?	Dose? (Each time)	Times per day?	What time of day?	How long should you take drug? days / weeks / months	Problems to watch out for which this drug can cause	Interactions of this drug with other drugs or food; diet recommendations	How are you actually taking the drug?	New problems or complaints since drug started (Date it began)	Is drug working?
Example: hydrochlorothiazide HydroDIURIL [This is an example only.]	Dr. Jackson 2/10/92	high blood pressure 180/100	12.5 mg 1/2 pill	once	morn-ing	at least till next visit in 1 month	muscle weakness; cramps from low potassium; frequent urination common	1) Eat raisins, bananas wheat germ & drink or-ange juice for potassium	most days 5-6/wk	No	No
	3/8/92	pressure still high 165/100	25 mg 1 pill	once	morn-ing	fill next visit, 2 months		2) Avoid salt	stopped 4/1 — felt too weak	feeling tired 3/22/92	No
	4/15/92	pressure 165/95	12.5 mg 1/2 pill	once	morn-ing	fill next visit, 2 months		3) may lower effectiveness of diabetes drugs	every day	NONE	No
	Dr. Lewis 10/10/92	pressure 155/87	same	same	same	fill next visit, 6 months			every day	NONE	Yes

Instructions:
1. Include all over-the-counter drugs you take as well as prescription drugs.
2. When you change doses draw a single line through the old dose.
3. Bring this with you every time you go to a doctor or pharmacist.
4. Be straightforward with your doctor and yourself about how often you take medicine and why.

abdominal pain, bleeding, constipation, and diarrhea

❏ *Urinary adverse drug reactions*: difficulty urinating and loss of bladder control (incontinence)

If you or a relative or friend has any of the above problems and is taking any of the drugs listed under each problem in Chapter 2, notify your doctor or tell your friend or relative to notify theirs.

Another way of identifying possible adverse drug reactions you may be having is to look in the Index, p. xviii, for the name of the drug you are using. Then find the page with the details on adverse reactions caused by the drug.

Next, we will discuss other rules or principles of safer drug use (or nonuse) that doctors and patients who are involved in drug therapy should know. These rules are compiled from a number of lists, but particularly from the World Health Organization's *General Prescribing Principles for the Elderly*.[4,5,6,7]

Rule 3: Assume That Any New Symptom You Develop After Starting a New Drug Might Be Caused By the Drug. Call Your Doctor to Report This.

See the individual drug pages in Chapter 3 beginning on p. 55, for adverse drug reactions to specific drugs, or look at the lists of adverse drug reactions in Chapter 2 on p. 17, to see which drugs may be causing specific side effects you are having.

Rule 4: Make Sure Drug Therapy Is Really Needed for the Patient's Problem.

Often, drugs are prescribed for older (or younger) people to treat situational problems such as loneliness, isolation, and confusion. Whenever possible, try to use nondrug approaches to these problems. These include hobbies, socializing with others, and getting out of the house. When a person is suffering from an understandable depression after losing a loved one, support from friends, relatives, or a psychotherapist is preferable to drugs such as antidepressants. (See discussion

on depression for proper use of antidepressant drugs, p. 215.)

Nondrug therapy such as weight loss is preferable to drugs for such problems as mild high blood pressure and adult-onset diabetes. (See discussions of these two problems on pp. 62 and 516.) Increasing fiber and liquid in the diet is preferable to using laxatives (see p. 356). For swollen legs due to "bad" veins in the legs (not due to heart disease), wearing support hose is less expensive, safer, and probably more effective than taking heart pills or water pills.

Anxiety or difficulty sleeping are two situations for which drugs should rarely if ever be prescribed in older adults. See discussions of these problems and nondrug solutions on p. 204 and 205.

A last category of "disease" for which drug therapy is rarely if ever appropriate is drug-induced disease or adverse drug reactions. The proper treatment for drug-induced parkinsonism is not a second drug to treat the problem caused by the first drug, but stopping the first drug.

For any condition, always consider and discuss with the doctor whether the drug that is being selected may cause problems (side effects) worse than the disease being treated. A very common example of this is the extraordinary overtreatment of older people with slightly high blood pressure but without any symptoms of high blood pressure. In most cases, the person will feel worse because of the treatment, without any evidence of benefit. *Always consider the seriousness of the condition which your doctor is considering treating, and try to make sure that the treatment is not worse than the disease.*

The guiding principle is to use as few drugs as possible, in order to reduce adverse reactions and increase the odds of properly taking the ones that are really necessary.

Rule 5: If Drug Therapy Is Indicated, In Most Cases It Is Safer To Start With a Dose That Is Lower Than the Usual Adult Dose.

"Start low, go slow." The lowest effective dose in any patient is always the best because a lower dose will cause fewer adverse effects, which are almost always related to dose in older adults. Some experts suggest starting with one-third to one-half of the usual adult dose for most drugs and watching for side effects, increasing the dose slowly only if necessary to get the desired effect.

Rule 6: When Adding a New Drug, See If It Is Possible to Discontinue Another Drug.

Considering the addition of a new drug should always be used as an opportunity to reevaluate existing drugs and eliminate those which are not absolutely essential. The possibility of an adverse drug interaction between the new drug and one of the old ones may force dropping or changing a drug.

Rule 7: Stopping a Drug Is As Important As Starting It.

Regularly review with your doctor, at least every 3 to 6 months, the need to continue each drug being taken. For many mind-affecting drugs, such as sleeping pills, tranquilizers, and antidepressants, and for antibiotics this reevaluation should be more frequent and sooner. *The prevailing principle for doctors and patients should be to discontinue any drug unless it is essential.* Many adverse drug reactions are caused by drugs which were continued long after any rational duration of use ended. Many drugs such as sleeping pills, tranquilizers, digoxin, antiarrhythmia drugs and others that are started for an acute problem are not needed beyond a short period, and cause risks without providing benefits. Slow and careful weaning off these drugs may significantly improve the user's health. In addition to considering whether to stop the drug, you and your doctor should discuss the possibility of lowering the dose.

Although there are not enough doctors with training in geriatric medicine, a blunt restatement of this rule is **"one of the functions of geriatricians is to take patients off drugs prescribed by other doctors."**[8]

Rule 8: Make Sure Your Drug-using Instructions Are As Clear As Possible To You and At Least One Other Person.

Regardless of how old someone is, the chance of adverse reactions is high enough that at least one other person — a spouse, child or friend — should know about these possibilities. In the presence of such adverse reactions as confusion and memory loss, this is especially critical. For older adults, the complexities of drug use may be greater, especially for people taking more than one drug or people with physical or mental disabilities. In these cases, it is even more important to inform another person about possible adverse drug reactions.

Ask your doctor to make sure that the label on the drug states, if at all possible, the purpose for which the drug is being used. This is especially important when you are using multiple drugs, but is always important as a way of increasing your and your family's or friend's participation. All information concerning the proper use of the drug should also be on the label. In addition to the label, you should get and have explained to you, a separate instruction sheet.

Rule 9: Discard All Old Drugs Carefully.

Many people are tempted to keep and reuse drugs obtained in the past, even though reasons for their use have changed. Additional drugs used may make the earlier drugs much more dangerous. In addition, you may be tempted to give drugs to a friend or relative whom you believe may benefit from them. Resist these temptations and avoid further problems caused by using outdated drugs, by throwing them away when you are done with your course of therapy.

Rule 10: Ask Your Primary Doctor to Coordinate Your Care and Drugs.

If you see a specialist and he or she wants to start you on new medicines in addition to the ones you are on, check with your primary doctor first — usually an internist or general or family practitioner. It is equally important to use one pharmacist, if possible.

In summary, perhaps the best way of ending this chapter is to quote from a pamphlet called *Observations on Geriatric Medicine*, published 14 years ago by the then Department of Health, Education, and Welfare: **"Generally, stopping a drug is more beneficial than starting one."** Especially in older adults, but in many other people who are overmedicated, this statement, in the context of the above 10 rules, may be the best guide to better health.

Special Problems in Nursing Homes

All of the problems of dangerous misprescribing of drugs for people living in the community are even worse in many nursing homes, where, for example, one study found that almost 40% of nursing home residents were being given antipsychotic drugs even though only a small fraction of them actually were psychotic. Another study found that one-third of people in nursing homes were getting seven or more prescription drugs. (See Chapter 1, *Are Older Adults Prescribed Too Many Drugs?*, p. 1, for more information on the extent of prescription drug use in nursing homes.) Most of the above rules apply in the nursing home situation, but there are some differences. The main one is that the brown bag session and filling out the **drug worksheet** should be done by the nursing home staff, including the nurse, doctor, and pharmacist.

As the child, other relative, or friend of a nursing home resident, with his or her permission, you have the right to demand and receive a completed drug worksheet for that person and an explanation of the reasons for each drug being used. The process of obtaining this information, with the help of your own pharmacist and, possibly your own doctor, will very likely lead to a reduced number of drugs being given and, where appropriate, reduced doses of those still judged to be necessary. In doing this, you will have made a major contribution to the health and well-being of your loved one(s) in nursing homes.

Notes for Chapter 4

1. Hulka BS, Kupper LL, Cassel JC, Efrid RL, Birdette JA. Medication use and misuse: physician and patients discrepancies. *Journal of Chronic Diseases* 1975; 28:7-21.

2. German PS, Klein LE. Adverse drug experience among the elderly. In *Pharmaceuticals for the Elderly*. Pharmaceutical Manufacturers Association, November 1986.

3. Ibid.

4. *Drugs for the Elderly*. Denmark: World Health Organization: 1985.

5. Vestal RE, ed. *Drug Treatment in the Elderly*. Sydney, Australia: ADIS Health Science Press, 1984:24-6.

6. Carruthers SG. Clinical pharmacology of aging. In *Fundamentals of Geriatric Medicine*. New York: Raven Press, 1983.

7. Avorn JL, Lamy PP, Vestal RE. Prescribing for the elderly—safely. *Patient Care* June 1982:14-62.

8. Gryfe CI, Gryfe BM. Drug therapy of the aged. *Journal of the American Gerontology Society* 1984; 32:301-7.

CHAPTER 5

Saving Money By Buying Generic Drugs

According to current estimates, one-third of all elderly Americans spent over $650 in 1992 on drugs, while 20% spent over $1,000.[1] Many other older adults spend thousands of dollars they can often ill-afford each year filling the prescriptions for drugs their doctors write for them. Is this necessary?

Take the example of Lucy, a 62-year-old woman with rheumatoid arthritis. She was diagnosed as having this disease last year and was started on Feldene, an arthritis drug which, because it causes an increased risk of ulcers and bleeding, we recommend that you "Do Not Use" (see p. 285). Within a month after starting to take one pill a day, at a projected annual cost of $1,008 a year, Lucy began having an upset stomach and some abdominal pain which her doctor attributed to the Feldene. Although the drug had relieved many of her symptoms, the doctor thought it was too dangerous and switched her to Motrin, one of the brand name versions of ibuprofen. When Lucy went to the drugstore to have the prescription filled, her pharmacist told her that the drug was available in a generic version which was just as safe and effective, but much less expensive. It turned out that the brand name Motrin would have cost $360 a year but the generic version, ibuprofen, cost $128 a year. Lucy has had no adverse effects from ibuprofen and has gotten just as much relief as she did from Feldene, and is further relieved to be saving almost $880 a year in comparison with what Feldene would have cost, and to be saving $232 a year by purchasing generic ibuprofen instead of Motrin.

But Lucy is only one of 42 million people 60 and older, most of whom get multiple prescriptions filled in a year. In Chapter 1,

Are Older Adults Prescribed Too Many Drugs (p. 1), we discussed the 650 million prescriptions a year that are filled by people 60 and over. Although about one out of every five prescriptions is now filled with a generic drug, at the very least **another two out of five prescriptions which could be filled by a generic drug are being filled with the much more expensive brand name version.**

Using the figure cited by former Food and Drug Administration Commissioner Dr. Jere Goyan at a congressional hearing, projected to reflect drug price increases by 1992, **we conclude that the average saving per prescription by purchasing the generic version of a drug instead of the brand name version is $11.11.**[2] If another two-fifths of the 650 million prescriptions a year filled by older adults would be filled by generic instead of brand name drugs, this would amount to an additional 260 million generic prescriptions a year with an average cost saving of $11.11, **for a total additional saving of $2.9 billion dollars a year for older adults.**

Of the 245 drugs in this book which are *not* "Do Not Use" drugs, 168 of them or 69% are available in a generic form. This is indicated at the beginning of the discussion on the drug. Always ask your pharmacist, as more drugs may now have a generic version available.

FDA Repels Attacks on Generics

If you worry about the health hazards of prescription drugs, should you be more worried about brand name or about the less-expensive copies of those brand name drugs which are no longer on patent, the ones called generic drugs? **In reviewing the major prescription drug disasters of the** last decade, in every case in which there were deaths or serious injuries, the cause was a brand name drug, never a generic one.

Examples of such disasters, which collectively have killed hundreds of Americans and injured thousands more, include the arthritis drugs or painkillers **Oraflex**, **Suprol**, and **Zomax**, the antidepressant **Merital** and the high blood pressure drug **Selacryn**. Because of the serious dangers of these five drugs, all were taken off the market.

In fact, all of these tragedies involved brand name drugs which had only recently come onto the market, making it impossible for there to even be a generic version because the patent had not yet expired. In other words, once a drug has been on the market long enough for the patent to have expired and for there to be a generic equivalent, there is very little chance that some previously undetected danger will come to light. This is much more likely to happen with drugs on the market for only a short time.

But what about those drugs which have been on the market for a long enough time for the patents to have expired and which are available in both brand name and generic versions? Which is safer or more effective? It has always been our position that there is no difference between generic and brand name drugs on the odds that there will be something found wrong with the amount of active ingredient or the purity. Over the years, there have been recalls because of these kinds of problems with both generic and brand name drugs. Fortunately, even in these instances, there has never been any evidence that there was any harm to the public.

In the past several years, however, there has been some concern by doctors, pharmacists and patients because of illegal activities by officials of several generic drug companies and FDA officials following the passage of legislation which speeded up the time for generic copies of brand name drugs to get approved and marketed once the brand name patent had expired. Some generic companies, overly eager to get drugs on the market as quickly as possible, stooped to criminal activity such as bribing Food and Drug Administration (FDA) officials to push their drug more quickly. There has been successful prosecution of both the FDA and drug company officials for these actions and, as a result, the process of looking at data upon which to base a decision to approve a generic drug is probably tighter and more patient-protective than ever. Again, fortunately, even though these procedural irregularities occurred, there is no evidence that any patients were harmed as a result of taking the generic drugs made by these companies.

A new study, by Food and Drug Administration laboratories from all over the country, has found that those classes of prescription drugs which theoretically could be most likely to pose safety or effectiveness problems if they were not manufactured properly, met the applicable standards in virtually all cases. The classes of drugs tested included contraceptives, antibiotics, and ones prescribed for asthma, epilepsy, high blood pressure, and abnormal heart rhythms. Of the 424 samples of 24 different drugs which were tested, including both brand name and generic drugs, there were no samples tested which posed a health hazard to patients when examined for potency and, where applicable, dissolution rate and content uniformity.

The reason that these 24 different drugs were chosen is that they all have a narrow therapeutic range. This means that, unlike most kinds of drugs, for which there is a relatively large range of dosages which are both effective and relatively safe, for these drugs the amount which gets into the body must be more tightly controlled. If it is not, the drug may too easily lose its effectiveness (if the dose is too low) or become toxic (if the dose is too high).

The drugs which were tested included seven asthma drugs, five for treating epilepsy, four high blood pressure drugs, four drugs for treating heart arrhythmias, a birth control pill, one antibiotic, a drug for treating depression and a so-called blood-thinning drug. Only in the case of the birth control pill, where all of the major brand names were tested, was no generic version tested. For the other six categories of drugs, both brand name and generic versions were tested.

For 23 of the 24 different drugs, there was no difference between the brand name and the generic versions in passing the tests for purity or quality done by the FDA laborato-ries. Only for **aminophylline**, an asthma drug which we do not recommend as a first line treatment, did five batches from two manufactures fail to meet the FDA standards. Although none of these five batches posed a health hazard, all were recalled.

We list below the names, both brand and generic, by therapeutic class, of all the drugs studied except for the birth control pill (because no generic version was studied) and aminophylline (see p. 392).

Asthma Drugs

Brand Name	Generic Name	Manufacturers of brand name or generic drugs
Lufyllin	dyphylline	Altana Inc., Lemmon Company, Wallace Laboratories
	isoetharine mesylate	Reedco, Inc.
Medihaler, Isuprel	isoproterenol inhaler	Abbott Laboratories, Barre-National Inc., Sterling Drug Inc.
Alupent, Metaprel	methaproterenol inhaler	American Thepapeuits, Inc., Boehringer Ingelheim Pharmacy, Pharmaceutical Basics Inc., Sandoz Pharmaceuticals
Choledyl	oxtriphylline	Bolar Pharmaceutical Co. Inc., Warner Lambert Company
Quibron-T-Sr, Slo-Phyllin	theophylline	Banner Gelatin Products, Bristol-Myers USPNG, Central Pharmaceuticals, Cord Laboratories, Graham, DM Laboratories I, Inwood Labs, KV Pharmaceutical Co., Paco PR, Inc., Riker Labs/3M Pharmaceuticals, Rorer Pharmaceutical Corp., Schering-Plough Products, Searle & Co., Inc.

Epilepsy Drugs

Tegretol	carbamazepine	Geigy Pharmaceuticals, Inwood Labs, Pharmaceutical Basics Inc., Purepac, Sidmark Laboratories, Teva Pharmaceuticals, Warner Chilcot
Dilantin	phenytoin	Bolar Pharmaceutical Co., Inc., Lannett Company, Inc., Mason Distributors, Inc., Warner Lambert, Inc., Zenith Labs Inc.

Brand Name	Generic Name	Manufacturers of brand name or generic drugs
Mysoline	primidone	Bolar Pharmaceutical Co., Inc., Danbury Pharmacal., Inc., Lannett Company Inc., Wyeth-Ayerst Labs
Depakote	valproate sodium	Abbott Laboratories, Pharmaceutical Basics Inc.
Depakene	valproic acid	Abbott Laboratories, Chase Chemical Co., Pharmaceutical Basics Inc., Scherer, R.P. , North America

High Blood Pressure Drugs

Catapres	clonidine	American Thepapeuits Inc., Barr Labs Inc., Boehringer Ingelheim Pharm., Bolar Pharmaceutical Co. Inc., Cord Laboratories, Danbury Pharmacal. Inc., Duramed Pharmaceuticals, Interpharm Inc., Kalipharma Inc., Lederle Laboratories, Par Pharmaceutical, Warner Lambert
Esimil, Ismelin	guanethidine	Bolar Pharmaceutical Co. Inc., Ciba Geigy Corp.
Loniten	minoxidil	Danbury Pharmacal Inc., Par Pharmaceutical, Quantum Pharmics Ltd., Upjohn Company
Minipress	prazosin	Danbury Pharmacal Inc., Kalipharma Inc., Mylan Pharmaceuticals, Inc., Pfizer Inc., Zenith Labs Inc.

Antiarrythmic Drugs

Norpace	disopyramide	Barr Labs Inc., Bocraft Labs Inc., Cord Laboratories, Danbury Pharmacal Inc., Interpharm Inc., KV Pharmaceutical Co., Searle & Co., Inc., Zenith Labs Inc.
Pronestyl	procainamide	Bolar Pharm Co. Inc., Chelsea Labs Copley Pharmaceutical Inc., Cord Laboratories, Danbury Pharmacal Inc., Sidmak Laboratories, Squibb Corp., Warner Lambert, Zenith Labs Inc.

Brand Name	Generic Name	Manufacturers of brand name or generic drugs
Quinaglute	quinidine gluconate	Berlex Labs, Bolar Pharmaceutical Co. Inc., Cord Laboratories, Halsey Drug Co. Inc.,
Quinide	quinidine sulfate	American Cyanamid Co., Barr Labs Inc., Chelsea Labs, Cord Laboratories, Danbury Pharmacal., Inc., Halsey Drug Co. Inc., Kalipharma Inc., Lannett Company Inc., Lilly, Eli & Co., Mutual Pharmaceutical Co., Private Formulations Inc., Reid-Rowell Inc., Richlyn Labs Inc., Robins, A.H. Company, Inc., Roxane Laboratories Inc., Vitarine Pharmaceuticals, Warner Lambert

Antibiotic

Cleocin	clindamycin	Upjohn Company, Vitarine Pharmaceuticals

Antidepressant

Eskalith	lithium carbonate	Bolar Pharmaceutical Co. Inc., Pfizer Inc., Reid-Rowell Inc., Roxane Laboratories Inc., Smith Kline & French

Blood-Thinner

Coumadin	warfarin	Abbott Laboratories, Bolar Pharmaceutical Co. Inc., DuPont Pharmaceuticals, Pharmaceutical Basics Inc.

Costs to Pharmacists of Brand Name vs Generic Drugs[3]				
Brand Name Drug	Price	Generic Drug	Price	Duration of Treatment
Calan	$37.73	verapamil	$19.74	(1 month)
Bactrim	21.78	trimethoprim sulfamethoxazide	4.44	(10 days)
Keflex	46.90	cephalexin	17.80	(10 days)
Tofranil	79.08	imipramine	6.79	(1 month)
Motrin	23.78	ibuprofen	12.94	(1 month)

In an article reprinted in the World Health Organization's *Essential Drugs Monitor* in 1988, the FDA rebuts what it calls "ten charges or myths currently being raised, under the guise of independent dialogue, aimed at discouraging health professionals from prescribing or dispensing generic drugs":

Myth 1: The 1984 action by Congress has eliminated safety and effectiveness testing requirements for generic drugs and has thus reduced the confidence that physicians and patients can have in the safety and effectiveness of generic drugs.

Fact 1: What the new law in fact does is eliminate the unnecessary requirement for duplicative testing to redemonstrate the safety and effectiveness of active drug ingredients that have already been shown to be safe and effective by adequate and well-controlled studies and that have been widely used and accepted by the medical community for many years.

Myth 2: FDA requires pioneer drug manufacturers to study their drugs in thousands of patients, but it requires generic firms to test their drug products in 20 or 30 healthy volunteers.

Fact 2: This statement is misleading. Testing in a large number of patients is required for the pioneer drug in order to establish the safety and effectiveness of the new active drug ingredient. Once this has been established, FDA need ensure only that others wanting to market a copy of the innovator's product make their product correctly. Because of reformulations, most marketed brand name products have the same status as their generic counterparts in their relationship to the formulations that were originally tested for safety and effectiveness.

Myth 3: Plasma level studies do not show how a drug acts at the site of action and therefore are not indicative of how well a drug will perform.

Fact 3: Once the active ingredient is shown to enter the bloodstream at the same rate and extent as that same active ingredient from another drug product, there is no currently recognized scientific basis to allege that the therapeutic effects of the two drugs will differ.

Myth 4: Bioequivalence studies are performed in healthy volunteers, who are usually in their twenties, while many of the drugs are used primarily in elderly patients. These elderly patients can be expected to absorb and metabolize the drug differently than do the healthy volunteers. Therefore bioequivalence testing is not an indicator of how the drug will perform in patients.

Fact 4: The testing in healthy volunteers, which shows an equivalent blood level between the generic and the brand name product, is a strong indicator that the two tested dosage forms will behave the same under the same conditions. No one has demonstrated that two products found by conventional tests to be bioequivalent perform inequivalently in different patients. It is also preferable to subject healthy people, rather than already weakened or disabled patients, to the blood sampling and other discomforts of bioequivalence testing.

Myth 5: FDA applies lower standards for generic approval compared to those required for the brand name products.

Fact 5: The lesser standard that is usually implied in such a statement relates to the safety and efficacy testing mentioned earlier. FDA in fact requires that the manufacturers in both instances follow good manufacturing practice, that they show that their drug is stable, that it is bioequivalent, and that it meets the same standards of identity, strength, quality and purity.

Myth 6: FDA has no written rules or criteria for how it determines bioequivalence.

Fact 6: FDA has required generic drugs to be bioequivalent to innovator products since the mid-1970s, and it published final regulations on bioequivalence in January 1977.

Myth 7: Because FDA allows a variation of ± 20 or 30% in the blood levels between the brand name and the generic products, generics may differ by as much as 60% from each other.

Fact 7: The test that FDA employs and the standard that is applied is a statistical one. It is virtually impossible for a generic product to pass if it in fact differs in its average plasma level by 20% from the standard product. Deviations of more than 10% between generic and brand name products are rare; usually the differences are much less than 10%.

Myth 8: Brand-name drugs are made in modern facilities, while generics are often made in sub-standard facilities. Thus generics are of generally inferior quality.

Fact 8: No one has been able to demonstrate that the quality of generic drugs differs from that of the brand name counterparts. The rates of defects found by FDA in both brand name and generic products are extremely low and speak well of the pharmaceutical industry's care in producing prescription drugs. In fact, the innova-

tor drug firms themselves account for an estimated 70-80% of the generic drug market. Thus, to believe generics are inferior, one would have to accept the premise that the research-oriented drug firms can't adequately manufacture products other than the ones they pioneered. It is also true that many innovator drug firms distribute products made by smaller generic firms. It is unlikely they would continue such arrangements if they really doubted the ability of generic firms to manufacture quality products.

Myth 9: In calling drugs bioequivalent, FDA overlooks documented cases of bioinequivalence.

Fact 9: While there have been a few well-known, documented cases of bioinequivalence, they are either examples from many years ago that have long since been corrected or problems resulting from drugs which have never gone through FDA's approval system. FDA is not aware of a single documented bioinequivalence involving any generic drug product that has been approved by FDA as bioequivalent.

Myth 10: Patients using generic products are more likely to suffer adverse reactions than those taking the brand name drug.

Fact 10: There is no evidence of a different rate of adverse drug reactions (ADRs) between brand name products and their generic equivalents. There have been some efforts recently by several brand name firms to stimulate reporting to FDA's voluntary ADR system of adverse reactions to the products of their generic competitors. FDA has vigorously opposed any such attempts.

The FDA has a public obligation to investigate thoroughly all allegations of drug product defects or failures. The agency has not found any of the allegations raised thus far in the brand name versus generic drug controversy to be valid. FDA also has an obligation to make known to health care professionals and to the public its conclusions that false or misleading reports are being generated.

Should You Use Generic Drugs?

Do not use any new drug for at least five years after it was first marketed unless it is one of the rare examples of a real breakthrough drug (only one out of 10 new drugs approved by the FDA are important advances over existing therapy). This will go a long way toward protecting you from previously undiscovered dangers of drugs which usually come to light within the first five years of marketing.

The new FDA study makes it clear that generic drugs are as good as brand name drugs. Unless you want to waste a large amount of money — often hundreds of dollars a year — by using brand name instead of generic drugs, you should, especially if starting on a drug for the first time, ask for the generic version. (See chart, p. 683)

Notes for Chapter 5

1. Statement of Representative Fortney H. Stark. Introduction of the Medicare Prescription Drug Act of 1991.

2. Committee on the Judiciary, Subcommittee on Antitrust and Business Rights. Hearing on Generic Drugs, October 21, 1987.

3. *1992 Drug Topics Red Book* and supplements. Medical Economics, Inc.: Montvale, NJ, 1992.

Glossary

ACE inhibitor: Angiotensin-converting enzyme inhibitor. Drugs such as captopril, mainly used to treat high blood pressure or heart failure.

Akathisia: Restless leg syndrome. Can be drug-induced, involving an inability to remain in a sitting position, promoting restlessness and a feeling of muscular jitters.

Akinesia: Weakness and muscular fatigue. Can be drug-induced, involving nerve problems which make patient appear listless, disinterested and depressed. Additional problems can include infrequent blinking, slower swallowing of saliva with drooling, and a lack of facial expression.

Allergy: Hypersensitivity (overreaction) to substances such as drugs, food, and pollen.

Analgesic: A drug used to relieve pain.

Anemia: Decrease in red blood cells or in hemoglobin of the blood.

Antacid: A drug used to neutralize excess acid in the stomach.

Antiarrhythmic: A drug used to treat abnormal heart rhythms.

Antibiotic: A drug derived from molds or bacteria which is used to treat bacterial infections.

Anticholinergic: A drug that blocks the effects of acetylcholine, a substance produced by the body which is responsible for certain nervous system activities (parasympathetic). Drugs with anticholinergic effects (including antidepressants, antihistamines, antipsychotics, drugs for intestinal problems, antiparkinsonians) inhibit the secretion of acid in the stomach; slow the passage of food through the digestive system; inhibit the production of saliva, sweat, and bronchial secretions; and increase the heart rate and blood pressure. Adverse effects of these drugs include dry mouth, constipation, difficulty urinating, confusion, worsening of glaucoma, blurred vision, and short-term memory problems.

Anticoagulant: A drug that inhibits or slows down blood clotting.

Anticonvulsant: A drug that prevents or treats seizures (convulsions or fits).

Antidepressant: A drug used to treat mental depression.

Antiflatulent: A drug used to relieve "excess gas" in the stomach or intestines.

Antifungal: A drug used to treat infections caused by a fungus (such as ringworm, thrush, or athlete's foot).

Antihistamine: A drug used to prevent or relieve the symptoms of allergy (such as hay fever).

Antihypertensive: A drug used to lower high blood pressure.

Antiparkinsonian: A drug used to control the symptoms of Parkinson's disease.

Antiprotozoal: A drug used to treat infections caused by protozoa (tiny, one-celled animals).

Antipsychotic: A drug used to treat certain serious mental conditions such as schizophrenia.

Antispasmodic: A drug used to reduce smooth muscle spasms (for example, stomach, intestinal, or urinary tract spasms).

Antitubercular: A drug used to treat tuberculosis (TB).

Aortic stenosis: Narrowing of one of the valves (aortic valve) in the heart or of the aorta itself (one of the major blood vessels in the body).

Arthritis: A chronic disease marked by painful, stiff, swollen, and sometimes red joints.

Asthma: A chronic disorder characterized by wheezing, coughing, difficulty in breathing, and a suffocating feeling. Can be caused by allergies or infections.

Barbiturate: A drug used to produce drowsiness and/or a hypnotic state. It can become addictive if taken for a long period of time.

Benzodiazepines: A family of drugs that are prescribed for nervousness and sleeping problems and to relax muscles and control seizures. They can be addictive if taken for an extended period of time. Adverse effects include confusion, drowsiness, hallucinations, mental depression, and incoordination that can result in falls and hip fractures.

Beta-blockers: Drugs used to treat high blood pressure, angina, and irregular heart rhythms and to prevent migraine headaches. They work to dilate (open) the blood vessels and to decrease the number of heartbeats per minute thereby lowering blood pressure.

Bone marrow depression: The body produces new red and white blood cells by making blood cells in the bone marrow, the core of the bones. Certain types of drugs reduce the ability of the marrow to produce new blood cells, leaving fewer blood cells to circulate in the body to carry oxygen or fight infection.

Bronchodilator: A drug used to open the bronchial tubes (air passages) of the lungs to increase the flow of air through them, in patients who have asthma, chronic bronchitis, or emphysema.

Bronchospasm: Temporary narrowing of the air passages in the lungs decreasing the flow of air to the lungs. This occurs in patients who have asthma, chronic bronchitis, or emphysema.

Calcium channel blocker: A drug used to control high blood pressure (hypertension) and heart rate and to improve blood flow to the heart. It works by lowering the calcium concentrations in certain smooth muscles in the blood vessels, causing blood vessels to dilate (open) and heart rate to decrease thereby lowering blood pressure.

Cardiovascular system: The system which allows circulation of oxygen and blood. It consists of the heart and blood vessels.

Carotid sinus: A special receptor in the carotid artery, a major blood vessel in the body, which is sensitive to changes in blood pressure.

Cephalosporins: A family of antibiotics which have antibacterial activity similar to the penicillins, but which can work against a wider range of infections than the penicillins and kill some bacteria resistant to penicillins.

Cholesterol: A fat-like substance found in blood and most tissues. Too much cholesterol is associated with such health risks as hardening of the arteries and heart attacks.

Cholesterol-lowering Drug: Drugs which work — by various mechanisms including blocking cholesterol synthesis or increasing cholesterol breakdown — to lower blood cholesterol levels.

Colitis: Inflammation of the colon (large bowel).

Complete Blood Count (CBC): An examination of the blood to detect red cell and white cell counts.

Congestive heart failure: A medical condition in which the heart does not pump adequately and fluid accumulates in the lungs and in the legs. Body tissues also do not receive an adequate blood supply.

Corticosteroids: A family of drugs similar to the chemical cortisone, produced by the adrenal gland, which are used as anti-inflammatory agents and to control the body's salt/water balance, if it is not working properly.

Dementia: Deterioration or loss of intellectual faculties, reasoning power, will, and memory due to organic brain disease; characterized by confusion, disorientation, and stupor of varying degrees.

Diabetes mellitus: Also known as sugar diabetes. A disorder in which the body cannot process sugars to produce energy, due to lack of a hormone called insulin. This leads to too much sugar in the blood (hyperglycemia), and an increased risk of coronary artery disease, kidney disease, and other problems.

Diuretic: Also known as a water pill. A drug that increases the amount of urine produced, by helping the kidneys get rid of water and salt.

Diverticulitis: Inflammation of an outpouching (abnormal sac) protruding from the lining of the intestine.

Eczema: Inflammation of the skin marked by itching, redness, swelling, blistering, watery discharge, and scales.

Edema: Swelling in the body, most notably feet and legs, caused by accumulation of fluid. This may be due to diseases in the veins of the legs or heart problems.

Electrolytes: Important chemicals such as sodium, potassium, calcium, magnesium, chloride, and bicarbonate, found in the body tissues and fluids.

Emphysema: Condition of the lungs characterized by swelling of the alveoli (small air cells of the lungs) which causes breathlessness and difficulty breathing.

Endogenous depression: Serious depression not precipitated by outside factors, such as death of spouse, job loss, etc.

Endometriosis: Condition in which material similar to the lining of the womb (uterus) is present at other sites outside of the womb (including the pelvic cavity, intestines, and lung). This condition may cause pain and bleeding.

Enzyme: A chemical which acts on other substances to speed up a chemical reaction. Enzymes in the intestines help to break down food.

Expectorant: A drug used to thin mucus in the airways, so that the mucus may be coughed up more easily. None of these drugs are effective.

Fecal impaction: A collection of stool in the rectum or colon which is difficult to pass.

Fixed-ratio combination drug: A combination of two or more ingredients, each ingredient in a set amount. This means that you cannot take more of less or one ingredient without also changing the amount of the other ingredient.

G6PD (glucose-6-phosphate dehydrogenase) deficiency: An inherited medical condition marked by a lack of or reduced amounts of an enzyme (glucose-6-phosphate dehydrogenase) that breaks down certain sugar compounds in the body.

Glaucoma: A condition in which partial or complete loss of vision occurs because of abnormally high pressure in the eye.

Gout: A form of arthritis caused by too much uric acid buildup in the blood which then becomes deposited around the joints.

Heart block: Failure of the electrical conduction tissue of the heart to conduct impulses normally from one part of the heart to another, causing altered rhythm of the heartbeat. There are varying degrees of severity. Slow heartbeat with fainting, seizure, or even death can result from this abnormality.

Heart failure: **see congestive heart failure**

Herpes simplex: Also known as cold sores. Inflammation of the skin, caused by a virus, resulting in groups of small, painful blisters. They may occur either around the mouth or, in the case of genital herpes, around the genitals (sex organs).

Histamine: A chemical made by the body especially during an allergic reaction.

It produces dilation of small blood vessels causing redness, localized swelling, and often itching; lowers the blood pressure; and increases secretions from the stomach, the salivary glands, and other organs.

Hormone: Substance produced in one part of the body (usually a gland) which then passes into the bloodstream and is carried to other organs or tissues, where it helps them to function.

Hypersensitivity: An exaggerated response to a foreign stimulus.

Hypertension: High blood pressure.

Hypoglycemia: A low blood sugar level.

Hypothermia: A condition resulting from overexposure to cold temperatures. The symptoms include shivering, cold hands and feet, and memory lapse.

Infection: Disease resulting from presence of certain microorganisms or matter in the body.
 Viral: flu or cold, for example; cannot be treated with drugs except for herpes, flu, or AIDS.
 Bacterial: often treated with antibiotics.

Laxative: A drug used to encourage bowel movements.

Myasthenia gravis: A chronic disease marked by abnormal weakness, and sometimes paralysis of certain muscles.

Narcotic: A drug used to relieve pain but which also may produce insensibility or stupor.

Nervous system: The brain, spinal cord, and nerves throughout the body.

Nonsteroidal anti-inflammatory drug (NSAID): A drug (such as aspirin or ibuprofen) used to treat pain, fever, and swelling. It does not contain corticosteroids.

Osteomalacia: Softening of the bones due to lack of vitamin D.

Osteoporosis: Loss of bone tissue which occurs most often in older women (thin, small-boned, white women in particu-

lar), resulting in bones that are brittle and easily broken.

Parkinson's disease: Disorder of the nervous system marked by tremor (shaking), muscular rigidity, slow movements, stooped posture, salivation, and an immobile facial expression.

Peptic ulcer: A localized loss of tissue, involving mainly the lining of areas of the digestive tract exposed to acid produced by the stomach. Usually involves the lower esophagus, the stomach, or the beginning of the small intestine (duodenum).

Pneumonia: Disease of the lungs in which the tissue becomes inflamed, hardened, and watery. Causes include bacteria, viruses, chemical inhalation, and trauma.

Polyps: Swollen or tumerous tissues which may or may not be cancerous. They may be found in various parts of the body such as the lining of the digestive tract, bladder, nose, or throat.

Porphyria: Rare, inherited blood disease.

Prostate: A walnut-sized gland found only in males located deep inside the abdomen just below the bladder. The prostate gland surrounds the urethra, the canal which carries urine from the bladder. The prostate gland is responsible for producing semen, the liquid which carries sperm. It enlarges with age and can cause difficulty with starting and stopping urination.

Psoriasis: Chronic skin condition marked by itchy, scaly, dry, red skin patches.

Psychosis: Severe mental illness marked by loss of contact with reality, often involving delusions, hallucinations, and disordered thinking.

Raynaud's phenomenon: Condition marked by paleness, numbness, redness, and discomfort in the toes and fingers when they are exposed to cold. It rarely occurs in males.

Salicylates: Drugs used to treat rheumatism and relieve pain.

Sarcoidosis: A chronic disorder in which the lymph nodes in many parts of the body are enlarged, and small fleshy swellings develop in the lungs, liver, and spleen.

Schizophrenia: Serious mental illness (the most common type of psychosis) marked by a breakdown of the thinking process, of contact with reality, and of normal emotional responses. People with schizophrenia often have hallucinations.

Scleroderma: Persistent hardening and shrinking of the body's connective tissue.

Sick sinus syndrome: Abnormality in the wiring system of the heart marked by periods of rapid and/or extremely slow heartbeats which may cause fainting, chest pain, or palpitations.

Sjogren's syndrome: Condition marked by swollen glands, dryness of the mouth and often the eyes, and arthritis.

Spasm: A sudden contraction of a muscle which can cause pain and restrict movement.

Stool: Bowel movement.

Sulfonamide: An antibiotic drug derived from sulfa compounds.

Sympathomimetics: Drugs that increase blood pressure and heartbeat. They are related to the chemical produced naturally in the body, adrenaline. These drugs also relieve nasal congestion by causing constriction of blood vessels.

Systemic lupus erythematosus: Also known as lupus or SLE. A chronic disease affecting the skin, blood vessels, and various internal organs, often accompanied by arthritis.

Tardive dyskinesia: Slow, involuntary movements of the tongue, lips, arms, and other body parts often brought on by certain drugs, especially antipsychotic drugs.

Thalassemia: An inherited blood disorder which causes anemia that is most often seen in persons of Mediterranean descent.

Thyroid: A large gland in front and on either side of the trachea which secretes thyroxine, a hormone regulating the growth of the body. Malfunctioning of the gland (hyperthyroidism, hypothyroidism) can cause medical problems.

Toxic: Poisonous; potentially deadly.

Tuberculosis: Also known as TB. An infectious disease, usually of the lungs, marked by fever, night sweats, weight loss, and coughing up blood.

Ulcer: Localized loss of surface tissue of the skin or mucous membrane.

Uric acid: One of the products made when protein is broken down in the body. It is normally eliminated from the body by the kidneys. Too high levels of uric acid in the body cause gout.

Urinalysis: An examination of the urine to detect abnormalities such as sugar, protein, bacteria, or crystals, and to check the pH.

Ventricular fibrillation: A life-threatening rapid, irregular contraction of the heart.

Vertigo: Dizziness. A sensation of irregular or whirling motion, either of oneself or of external objects. Elderly people often experience "postural vertigo" when rising from a lying or sitting position.

Vitamin: A substance found in foods which does not provide energy, but is needed by the body in small amounts for normal functioning.

Wolff-Parkinson-White syndrome: Also known as WPW syndrome. An abnormality of the heart marked by periods when the heart rate is very fast and must be controlled with medication or electrical shock to the heart (defibrillation).

Fed up with business as usual?

Public Citizen has the prescription for change!

Read on and learn how you can make a difference:

1   Become a Public Citizen member today.

2   Receive the Public Citizen *Health Letter.*

3   Join the Public Citizen Action Network.

4   Order Public Citizen's other important books on health, safety and citizen involvement.

Join Public Citizen Today!

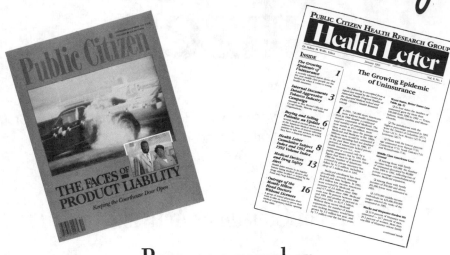

Become a member...

HELP lead the fight for consumer justice and open and clean government...

HELP take on the big-money interests and their lobbyists...

HELP fight for health care reform, campaign finance reform, a national energy policy, and consumer health and safety...

HELP provide sound and important information for consumers through publications like *Worst Pills, Best Pills II.*

Join with thousands of Public Citizen members to help us speak out strongly and effectively in Washington. Your contribution is vital—we accept no corporate or government funds. Join today!

Benefits of membership:

1 **For a membership contribution of $20,** our award-winning bimonthly magazine *Public Citizen*, filled with provocative, hard-hitting articles that give you the "inside story" and help you to be a better-informed consumer. Plus a FREE health awareness poster with easy-to-use tips on drug safety and nutrition.

2 **For a membership contribution of $35 or more,** you will also receive a full year's subscription to Dr. Sidney Wolfe's monthly *Health Letter.* This respected newsletter brings you critical information about health issues such as long-term care insurance, questionable doctors and hospitals, the outrageous costs of obtaining quality care, and updates on prescription drug dangers.

Look for the membership order form at the back of the book.

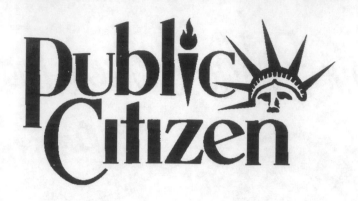

Public Citizen

Buyers Up • Congress Watch • Critical Mass • Health Research Group • Litigation Group
Ralph Nader, Founder

22 Years of Consumer Activism

Dear Friend:

Public Citizen is a nonprofit membership organization based in Washington, D.C., representing consumer interests through lobbying, litigation, research and publications. Since its founding by Ralph Nader in 1971, Public Citizen has fought for consumer rights in the marketplace, for safe and secure health care, for clean and renewable energy sources, and for corporate and government responsibility.

With five divisions and a staff of 75, Public Citizen is active in every public policy forum: Congress, the courts, government agencies and the media.

In the past year alone, Public Citizen finally persuaded the Food and Drug Administration to restrict the sale of silicone gel-filled breast implants, prevented the White House from destroying valuable electronic mail messages, organized grassroots support for sweeping changes in political campaign financing, and bared the deadly design flaws in General Motors' "firebomb" pickup trucks.

To retain its independence, Public Citizen does not accept government or corporate grants. Support funding comes from contributions from our 140,000 members, plus foundation grants and publication sales. Please join us.

Sincerely,

Joan Claybrook
President

2000 P Street NW • Suite 600 • Washington, D.C. 20036 • (202) 833-3000

Five Divisions — One Mission

CONGRESS WATCH champions consumer-related legislation on Capitol Hill, exposes campaign financing abuses, demands fair U.S. trade and banking policies and lobbies to strengthen U.S. health and safety regulations. Most of all it seeks to bring the democratic process back to the people, by trying to diminish the influence of moneyed interests who make meaningful change impossible.

THE HEALTH RESEARCH GROUP fights for safe foods, drugs and medical devices; for greater consumer control over personal health decisions; and for universal access to quality health care. As the country's leading consumer watchdog group on health issues, HRG has exposed the tobacco industry's pervasive influence on Capitol Hill, the failure of state medical boards to discipline incompetent doctors, and the unnecessarily high rate of caesarean section deliveries.

THE LITIGATION GROUP is the nation's preeminent public interest law firm. Its attorneys bring precedent-setting lawsuits on behalf of citizens in order to protect the health, safety and rights of consumers. Litigation Group attorneys have won two-thirds of the more than 30 cases they have argued before the U.S. Supreme Court, helping forge new public policy and laws that ensure public access to government documents, challenge the actions and inactions of federal regulators, and challenge unconstitutional government actions.

THE CRITICAL MASS ENERGY PROJECT is a powerful voice in the movement to decrease reliance on nuclear and fossil fuels and to promote safe, economical and environmentally sound energy use through conservation and renewable sources. Critical Mass prepares and disseminates reports, lobbies Congress, and acts as a watchdog of key federal and state energy regulatory agencies.

BUYERS UP is a home heating-oil cooperative group buying program that acts as an information resource on home energy and environmental issues. Its reports have yielded important data on the over-promotion of high-octane gasoline by the oil companies, and the failure of many states to ensure the quality of gasoline sold to consumers.

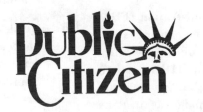

Public Citizen's Greatest Hits

Some important milestones of our first twenty-two years

1971: Public Citizen is founded by Ralph Nader. • The Health Research Group and the Aviation Consumer Action Project are created. • The Citizen Action Group, the organizing arm of Public Citizen, organizes Student Public Interest Research Groups.

1972: The Litigation Group and the Tax Reform Research Group are founded.

1973: The Litigation group wins a court decision that Nixon's firing of Special Watergate Prosecutor Archibald Cox was illegal. • Congress Watch, the legislative lobbying arm of Public Citizen, is formed.

1974: Critical Mass Energy Project founded to mobilize opposition to nuclear power. • Congress Watch convinces Congress to pass major improvements to the Freedom of Information Act, overriding President Ford's veto.

1975: Congress Watch successfully lobbies for major new energy conservation legislation, including fuel economy requirements for cars, and price control legislation for oil and gas. • HRG, suing with several unions, obtains a court order requiring the Labor Department to reconsider its inadequate rules to protect workers from 14 carcinogenic chemicals.

1976: The Food and Drug Administration (FDA) bans the use of the cancer-causing agent chloroform in cough medicines and toothpastes, in response to an HRG petition. • The FDA bans Red Dye No. 2, four years after HRG began its campaign against the carcinogenic food dye. • Consumers win the right to obtain meaningful price information about prescription drugs as a result of a Litigation Group victory in the Supreme Court.

1977: Congress Watch is instrumental in passing the Toxic Substances Control Act and antitrust reform legislation giving state attorneys general the right to sue price fixers. • Critical Mass mobilizes citizens and persuades President Carter to stop construction of the Clinch River Breeder Reactor.

1978: Cyclamates, a popular artificial sweetener, are banned in response to concerns raised by HRG. • Congress passes the National Consumer Cooperative Bank bill, drafted by Congress Watch, providing $300 million "seed money" for consumer cooperatives.

1979: In response to a 1977 HRG petition, EPA bans DBCP, a pesticide that causes sterility in human males and cancer in laboratory animals.

1980: HRG publishes *Pills That Don't Work*, which quickly climbs onto the best seller lists. • Congress Watch plays a critical role in passage of the Superfund law to require cleanup of toxic waste dumps.

1981: Congress Watch helps thwart Reagan's attempt to bury the Consumer Product Safety Commission in the Commerce Department.

1982: Oraflex, an arthritis drug that caused dozens of deaths and hundreds of injuries, is withdrawn from the market after HRG's campaign • Congress Watch stops passage of President Reagan's Regulatory Reform bill, which would have given OMB Director David Stockman extraordinary powers over government agency decisions. • Congress

Watch convinces Congress not to exempt doctors, lawyers and other professionals from Federal Trade Commission (FTC) oversight. • Publication of bi-monthly *Public Citizen* magazine begins.

1983: The Litigation Group wins a landmark separation-of-powers case in the Supreme Court, stopping Congress from vetoing governmental regulations. • HRG publishes *Over the Counter Pills That Don't Work.* • Public Citizen and Ralph Nader found Buyers Up, a cooperative consumer buying group. • Critical Mass finally gets Congress to stop funding the Clinch River Breeder Reactor revived by President Reagan. • Litigation Group publishes *Representing Yourself.* • Supreme Court overrules Reagan revocation of air bag standard.

1984: Public Citizen publishes *Retreat from Safety.*

1985: After a four-year battle by HRG, the FDA requires aspirin labels to warn of the risk of Reye's Syndrome. • HRG begins publishing the *Health Letter.*

1986: Litigation Group lawsuit strikes down the Gramm-Rudman-Hollings deficit reduction law as unconstitutional. • Congress passes a law requiring health warnings on the labels of snuff and chewing tobacco, capping HRG's two-year campaign.

1987: Public Citizen plays an instrumental role in the defeat of Judge Robert Bork's Supreme Court nomination. • Congress Watch helps pass a strong "check hold" bill that restricts the time banks can hold checks. • Litigation Group suit forces the chemical companies who produced Agent Orange to make all relevant documents and materials public.

1988: HRG publishes *Worst Pills, Best Pills*, a guide to dangerous drugs for the elderly. By 1991, almost one million copies are sold. • Proposition 103 wins in the California polls and rolls back auto insurance rates.

1989: A law requiring air bags or passive seat belts in all cars goes into effect after a 20-year battle. • Ralph Nader and Public Citizen successfully oppose a $40,000 Congressional pay raise and focus the nation's attention on the need for campaign finance and Congressional ethics reform. • Critical Mass wins a great victory when Californians vote to shut down the Rancho Seco nuclear power plant.

1990: HRG publishes *6,892 Questionable Doctors,* a nationwide listing of doctors sanctioned by state medical boards and federal agencies. • Public Citizen wins court victory requiring Nuclear Regulatory Commission to issue mandatory training requirements for nuclear plant personnel. • Litigation Group establishes Supreme Court Project to assist lawyers with public interest cases in the Supreme Court. • Congress Watch publishes an account of the savings and loan scandal, entitled *Who Robbed America?* • Lobbying and educational program to clean up Congress focuses attention on public financing of House and Senate elections.

1991: Public Citizen celebrates its 20th anniversary. • Litigation Group wins all three cases it argues in the Supreme Court, bringing its record to 19–9. • HRG publishes *Women's Health Alert,* a handbook on women's health issues. • Congress Watch publishes *They Love to Fly and It Shows,* a study of lobbyist-funded House travel during 1989–90. • Public Citizen initiates its Trade Watch Campaign • Public Citizen gets major auto safety legislation enacted to save 11,000 lives a year.

1992: Twenty-eight victims of corporate negligence help Public Citizen to defeat a bill, sponsored by the insurance industry and manufacturers, that would restrict the use of the courts by consumers injured by defective products. • Congress Watch exposes the threat to government health and safety standards posed by Vice President Dan Quayle's secretive Council on Competitiveness. • Public Citizen helps pass ground-breaking legislation that, if not vetoed by President Bush, would have resulted in sweeping campaign finance reform. • Litigation Group wins a landmark case limiting abuses of the congressional free-mailing privilege. • Health Research Group, after a four-year campaign, wins nearly complete ban on the use of silicone gel breast implants. • Buyers Up releases a report criticizing big oil companies for exaggerating the benefits of high-octane gasolines in their advertising. • Critical Mass Energy Project presses successfully to strike down provisions in the Energy Policy Act that would have allowed the disposal of radioactive waste in landfills, sewers and incinerators.

"Thank you for calling. No one's here to take your call right now, but if you leave your name and message at the sound of the tone. . ."

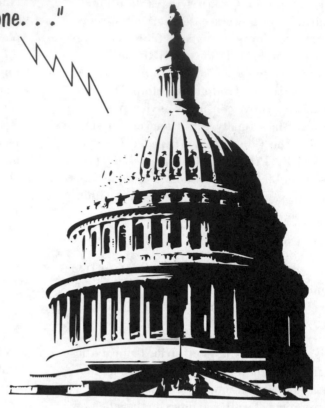

Can't get through to Washington?

3 Join the Public Citizen Action Network

Stop the special interests and their high-paid lobbyists.

Help win health care coverage for all Americans.

Protect the environment and the safety of consumers.

Let Public Citizen Show You How!

You saw the nation's economy and health care in crisis, and demanded change. But will Congress and the new Administration deliver? Only if you take part, and join with those who have the experience and expertise to get your message heard in Washington.

The Public Citizen Action Network is thousands of citizens working to shake up the status quo. To loosen the pharmaceutical and insurance lobbyists' stranglehold on the health care debate. To end a campaign finance system that turns our lawmakers into fundraisers. To stop banking policies that could cause another S&L crisis.

Others Talk—We Act!

By joining the Action Network, you learn how to become *involved*, using the techniques that make politicians sit up and take notice. We alert you when to take action, help you understand the issues, and recommend who you should contact to make your views known.

Strengthening your efforts are activists with over 20 years of experience fighting for citizens' rights in Washington. Public Citizen has been there, on the inside: beating back the Congressional pay raise, getting dangerous drugs and medical devices taken off the market, blowing the whistle on wasteful government spending.

Get Ready, Get Set—Get Involved

For a one year membership of only $14, we'll send you:

- The Action Kit—written by Washington insiders, with details on how to communicate effectively with lawmakers, the press and other opinion-makers.
- Regular Action Alerts—asking for your support, and suggesting ways for you to get involved. Organize a petition. Write a letter or postcard to your member of Congress. Set up a meeting with a lawmaker or reporter. Write a letter to the editor. Action Alerts let *you* decide how to become active.
- Action Updates—progress reports on the issues you care about.

Public Citizen Action Network—People CAN!

Special interests will continue to put our democracy on hold—unless we work together!

Join with us and get heard. Join now and tell the politicians: People CAN make a difference!

(Complete the order form at the back of this book and mail it with your check in the envelope provided.)

4 Give a copy to your friends...

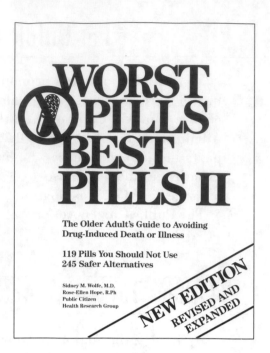

...since it's easy to get additional copies of WORST PILLS, BEST PILLS II. *Just use the form on the last page of this book.*

An older adult's guide to avoiding drug-induced death or illness. This is a revised and expanded edition of the landmark guide to commonly prescribed drugs that can cause harm or even death. It includes an update on 287 drugs reviewed in the first edition and information on 60 new drugs. Safer alternatives are also described. Sidney Wolfe, M.D., *et al.*, 1993, 720 pages, $15 (paperback).

Also from Public Citizen:

MEDICAL RECORDS: GETTING YOURS

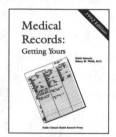

If you needed them for an insurance policy or to check their accuracy, would you know how to obtain your medical records? Do you know if your state allows full access? This useful guide for consumers and professionals includes:

- Definitions of medical records
- Step-by-step guide to getting your medical records
- Glossary of terms to help you understand your own records
- State-by-state access guide

Also, how to deal with medical records held in federal facilities and your right to access under the Privacy Act. 1992, 69 pages, $10 individuals/non-profits, $20 businesses (saddle stitched).

CRIMINALIZING THE SERIOUSLY MENTALLY ILL: THE ABUSE OF JAILS AS MENTAL HOSPITALS

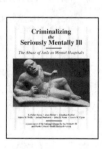

Twenty-nine percent of jails surveyed hold seriously mentally ill individuals without any criminal charges against them. Civil rights are violated when jails are used as a substitute for appropriate mental health care. Public Citizen and National Alliance for the Mentally Ill, 1992, 158 pages, $10 (paperback).

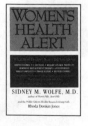

WOMEN'S HEALTH ALERT

What most doctors won't tell you. This book gives the straight facts and unbiased, expert opinion on health practices, operations, drugs, and products that adversely affect 85% of women of all ages in this country. Sidney Wolfe, M.D., *et al.*, 1991, 324 pages, $7.95 (paperback).

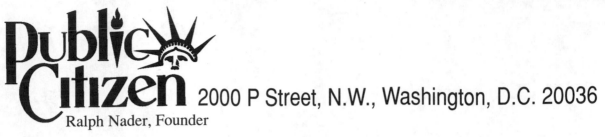

Public Citizen

Ralph Nader, Founder

2000 P Street, N.W., Washington, D.C. 20036

Order Form

Join Public Citizen

1
2

Item	Reference #	Amount	Quantity	Total
Basic membership*	01054040	$20.00		
Membership with Health Letter	01054040	$35.00		

*Basic membership includes our bimonthly magazine and a **free** health awareness poster.

Join the Network

3

Public Citizen Action Network package	01054040	$14.00		

Books from Public Citizen

4

Worst Pills, Best Pills II	01804070	$15.00		
Medical Records: Getting Yours	06154070	$10.00		
Criminalizing the Seriously Mentally Ill	06154070	$10.00		
Women's Health Alert	06154070	$ 7.95		

Overseas/Canada please add $6 shipping for book orders.   **TOTAL**

Allow 6-8 weeks for book deliveries.

NAME (MR. / MS. / MRS. / MISS) _____

STREET _____

CITY _____ STATE _____ ZIP _____

☐ CHECK ENCLOSED / PAYABLE TO PUBLIC CITIZEN

Use the pre-addressed envelope in this book or send this form to: **Public Citizen, Worst Pills Best Pills II,** 2000 P Street, N.W., Suite 600, Washington, D.C. 20036

WPII 4/93

Let the Clintons know that the only viable solution to the national health care crisis is a Canadian style single-payer system.

First Lady Hillary Rodham Clinton is charged with develping a health care system for the nation. The American people want a health care system which controls costs and provides universal coverage for all Americans. The only way to control costs sufficiently to expand coverage to all Americans is to eliminate the over $100 billion currently wasted on insurance overhead and allow the government to control physicians fees and drug prices.

That's where you come in: in order to convince our First Lady and President that the single payer solution is the right one, we are joining with dozens of other national and local organizations to launch a postcard campaign. As this book goes to press, we have collected half a million postcards and are about to present them to the First Lady. Until we have enacted national health care legislation, we want to keep the postcards flowing in to let the President know how strongly the American people feel about this issue.

You can help by:
1. Getting postcards signed by colleagues, friends and relatives.
2. Sending them to us so we can present them to Mrs. Clinton.
3. Publicizing the postcard campaign through meetings and the media.

To participate, paste or copy this postcard-sized notice to a postcard and send to us at: Public Citizen, Postcards to Hillary, 215 Pennsylvania Ave., SE, Washington, D.C. 20003.

Dear Hillary Rodham Clinton,

Congratulations on your work to provide all Americans with universal, affordable health care. When you write your bill, please base it on the Canadian model. Only by replacing the 1,500 private insurers with a single payer of health care costs can we use the over $100 billion wasted on paper pushing now to provide health care to the people who need it.

Please work for a plan which is universal, controls costs, provides comprehensive benefits, emphasizes prevention, is accessible, publicly accountable, portable and assures quality care, including long term care.

You have my support for a bill that meets these goals and lets the American people—not the insurance companies—run our health care system.

NAME _____

STREET _____

CITY _____ STATE _____ ZIP _____

Public Citizen
Postcards to Hillary
215 Pennsylvania Ave., SE
Washington, D.C. 20003